SIXTH EDITION

LANGE Q&A™

PHYSICIAN ASSISTANT

Anthony A. Miller, MEd, PA-C
Professor & Director
Division of Physician Assistant Studies
Shenandoah University
Winchester, Virginia

Albert F. Simon, DHSc, PA-C
Vice Dean and Associate Professor
School of Osteopathic Medicine in Arizona and
Associate Professor
Department of Physician Assistant Studies
A.T. Still University of Health Sciences
Mesa, Arizona

Rachel A. Carlson, MSBS, PA-C
Associate Professor & Associate Director
Division of Physician Assistant Studies
Shenandoah University
Winchester, Virginia

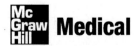 **Medical**

New York   Chicago   San Francisco   Lisbon   London   Madrid   Mexico City
Milan   New Delhi   San Juan   Seoul   Singapore   Sydney   Toronto

Lange Q&A™: Physician Assistant, Sixth Edition

3 4 5 6 7 8 9 0   QDB/QDB   14 13 12

Set ISBN 978-0-07-162828-0; MHID 0-07-162828-2
Book ISBN 978-0-07-162826-6; MHID 0-07-162826-6
CD ISBN 978-0-07-162827-3; MHID 0-07-162827-4

Notice

Medicine is an ever-changing science. As new research and clinical experience broaden our knowledge, changes in treatment and drug therapy are required. The authors and the publisher of this work have checked with sources believed to be reliable in their efforts to provide information that is complete and generally in accord with the standards accepted at the time of publication. However, in view of the possibility of human error or changes in medical sciences, neither the authors nor the publisher nor any other party who has been involved in the preparation or publication of this work warrants that the information contained herein is in every respect accurate or complete, and they disclaim all responsibility for any errors or omissions or for the results obtained from use of the information contained in this work. Readers are encouraged to confirm the information contained herein with other sources. For example and in particular, readers are advised to check the product information sheet included in the package of each drug they plan to administer to be certain that the information contained in this work is accurate and that changes have not been made in the recommended dose or in the contraindications for administration. This recommendation is of particular importance in connection with new or infrequently used drugs.

This book was set in Palatino by Aptara, Inc.
The editors were Catherine A. Johnson and Cindy Yoo.
The production supervisor was Catherine Saggese.
Project management was provided by Samir Roy at Aptara, Inc.
The cover designer was The Gazillion Group.
Quad/Graphics Dubuque was printer and binder.

This book is printed on acid-free paper.

Library of Congress Cataloging-in-Publication Data

Lange Q & A. Physician assistant / [edited by] Anthony A. Miller, Albert F. Simon, Rachel Carlson.—6th ed.
    p. ; cm.
  Other title: Lange Q and A
  Other title: Physician assistant
  Includes bibliographical references and index.
  ISBN-13: 978-0-07-162828-0 (pbk. : alk. paper)
  ISBN-10: 0-07-162828-2 (pbk. : alk. paper)
  1. Physicians' assistants—Examinations, questions, etc.   I. Miller, Anthony A.   II. Simon, Albert F.
III. Carlson, Rachel.   IV. Title: Lange Q and A.   V. Title: Physician assistant.
  [DNLM: 1. Physician Assistants—Examination Questions.   W 18.2 L2737 2010]
  R697.P45A67 2010
  610.76—dc22

                                            2010012156

McGraw-Hill books are available at special quantity discounts to use as premiums and sales promotions, or for use in corporate training programs. To contact a representative, please e-mail us at bulksales@mcgraw-hill.com

Contents

SECTION VII: HEALTH PROMOTION & DISEASE PREVENTION

Contributors

Frank A. Acevedo, MS, PA-C, DFAAPA
Academic Coordinator/Associate Director
Department of Physician Assistant Studies
New York Institute of Technology
Old Westbury, New York
Thoracic Cardiovascular Physician Assistant
Division of Surgical Critical Care
Winthrop University Hospital
Mineola, New York

Mark E. Archambault, DHSc, PA-C
Assistant Professor and Academic Coordinator
Department of Physician Assistant Studies
Wake Forest University Health Sciences
Winston-Salem, North Carolina

Rachel A. Carlson, MSBS, PA-C
Associate Professor & Associate Director
Division of Physician Assistant Studies
Shenandoah University
Premier Health Resources, Inc.
Winchester, Virginia

James F. Cawley, MPH, PA-C
Professor and Vice Chair
Department of Prevention and Community Health
School of Public Health and Health Services
Professor of Health Care Sciences
The George Washington University
Washington, D.C.

Michelle DiBaise, MPAS, PA-C
Adjunct Associate Professor
Department of Physician Assistant Studies
AT Still University
Mesa, Arizona

Raymond Eifel, MS, PA-C
City Urgent Care
Martinsburg, West Virginia

Cynthia D. Ferguson, MHS, PA-C
Clinical Faculty, Department of Dermatology
Eastern Virginia Medical School
Norfolk, Virginia

Michelle Heinan, EdD, DFAAPA, PA-C
Associate Professor and Director
Department of Physician Assistant Studies
Lincoln Memorial University-DeBusk College of
    Osteopathic Medicine
Harrogate, Tennessee

Rex L. Hobbs, MPAS, PA-C
Assistant Professor, Director of Didactic Education
Physician Assistant Program
Lincoln Memorial University-DeBusk College of
    Osteopathic Medicine
Harrogate, Tennessee

Jennie A. Hocking, MPAS, PA-C
Assistant Professor & Academic Coordinator
Department of Physician Assistant Studies
UT Southwestern Medical Center
Dallas, Texas

Robert W. Jarski, PhD, PA
Professor, School of Health Sciences and
    The OU William Beaumont School of Medicine
Director, Complementary Medicine and Wellness
    Program
Oakland University
Rochester, Michigan

Matthew A. McQuillan, MS, PA-C
Associate Professor & Assistant Director
Physician Assistant Program
University of Medicine and Dentistry of New Jersey
Piscataway, New Jersey

Anthony A. Miller, MEd, PA-C
Professor & Director
Division of Physician Assistant Studies
Shenandoah University
Winchester, Virginia

Carla J. Moschella, PA-C, MS, RD
Saugus, Massachusetts

Sue M. Nyberg, MHS, PA-C
Associate Professor & Chair
Department of Physician Assistant
College of Health Professionals
Wichita State University
Wichita, Kansas

Raymond J. Pavlick, Jr., PhD
Assistant Dean for Curriculum & Professor
    of Physiology
School of Osteopathic Medicine in Arizona
AT Still University
Mesa, Arizona

Paula B. Phelps, MHE, PA-C
Associate Professor & Clinical Coordinator
Idaho State University Physician Assistant Program
Pocatello, Idaho
Bingham Memorial Women's Center
Blackfoot, Idaho

Maura Polansky, MS, PA-C
Director, PA Education Programs
Physician Assistant, Gastrointestinal Medical Oncology
University of Texas MD Anderson Cancer Center
Houston, Texas

Brenda L. Quincy, MPH, PA-C
Associate Professor
Division of Physician Assistant Studies
Shenandoah University
Winchester, Virginia

Jill Reichman, MPH, PA-C
Associate Professor & Associate Director
Physician Assistant Program
University of Medicine and Dentistry of New Jersey
Piscataway, New Jersey

Christina M. Robohm, MS, PA-C
Associate Professor and Associate Director —
    Admissions and Student Life
Department of Pediatrics, Child Health
    Associate/Physician Assistant Program
University of Colorado Denver
Aurora, Colorado

Rebecca Lovell Scott, PhD, PA-C
Associate Clinical Professor & Academic Coordinator
Physician Assistant Program
Northeastern University
Boston, Massachusetts

Michel Statler, MLA, PA-C
Associate Professor & Associate Director
Department of Physician Assistant Studies
UT Southwestern Medical Center
Dallas, Texas

Gary R. Uremovich, DMin, MPAS, PA-C, DFAAPA
Distinguished Fellow, American Academy of
    Physician Assistants
Assistant Professor and Director, Physician
    Assistant Program
Wingate University
Wingate, North Carolina

Mary L. Warner, MMSc, PA-C
Associate Dean and Program Director
Assistant Professor, Internal Medicine
Physician Associate Program
Yale University School of Medicine
New Haven, Connecticut

Thomas A. Woods, DHSc, MEd, PA-C
Associate Professor
Department of Physician Assistant Sciences
Saint Francis University
Loretto, Pennsylvania

Donna L. Yeisley, MEd, PA-C
Associate Professor & Chair/MPAS
Program Director School of Health Sciences
Department of Physician Assistant Sciences
Saint Francis University
Loretto, Pennsylvania

Reviewers

The editors wish to thank the physician assistant students at Shenandoah University who reviewed manuscripts and provided helpful feedback to the authors. Specifically we wish to thank the following individuals:

Josh Adili
Erin Abernethy
Michael Beliew
Alix Gilbert
Richard Gilbert
Korrine Klieman
Nicole Kane
Megan Leach
Adam Lunnie
Kristin Matushevski
Candice Moreland
Taylor Murphy

Susie Parrish
Marina Shvarts
Caitlin Woodruff
Jennifer Writsel

In addition, we wish to thank the following faculty at Shenandoah University for their invaluable feedback:

Jessica Trompeter, PharmD
Amanda Welbourne, MSPAS, PA-C

Preface

In this sixth edition of *Lange Q&A™: Physician Assistant*, we have responded to the changing aspects of health care by including many of the new treatments and diagnostic tests from modern medical practice in extensively updated questions, while maintaining the basic format and quality our readers have grown to expect. With this edition, overall 25% of the questions are new or substantially revised, a new chapter on basic science concepts has been added, and we have expanded the total number of questions in the book. An exciting change in this edition is the CD practice test, so you can experience an electronic testing format similar to the one found on the certifying examination. Furthermore, revisions have been made to respond to changes in the format and blueprint of the NCCPA certification examination. For example, all matching type questions have been removed or revised to conform to the NCCPA format of examination questions.

We believe that you will find this review book a helpful and useful resource as you prepare for your initial or recertification examination. Your comments and constructive criticisms are welcome and will be considered in future editions.

We would like to thank our families, friends, and coworkers for their support, encouragement, and patience during the long hours spent working on this project. We also wish to thank Catherine Johnson and Cindy Yoo from McGraw-Hill for their editorial assistance and our contributors for their hard work and dedication. Finally, we thank you, the readers, for choosing this book as one of your resources. We wish you success on the examination.

Your comments and constructive criticisms are welcome and will be considered in future editions. Please send your comments to *PA@mcgraw-hill.com.* Note the title of the book in the subject line.

Anthony A. Miller, MEd, PA-C
Albert F. Simon, DHSc, PA-C
Rachel A. Carlson, MSBS, PA-C

Introduction

This book has been designed as a study aid to review for the Physician Assistant National Certification and Recertification Examination. Here, in one package, is a comprehensive review resource with 1,300 questions presented in the format seen in the national examinations. Each question is answered with a referenced, paragraph-length answer. The entire book has been organized by specialty area to help evaluate your areas of relative strength and weakness and to further direct your study effort with the available references.

ORGANIZATION

This book is divided into seven major sections preceded by an Introduction and a chapter on test-taking tips and techniques. Chapter 1 provides helpful hints on how to prepare for and take certification examinations. Section I, Chapters 2 through 12, reviews the major areas of internal medicine using the question-and-answer format. Sections II through V cover the major subspecialty areas and pharmacology. Section VI, Surgery, is subdivided into five chapters (13 through 17) covering its subspecialties, and Section VII includes preventive medicine and basic science concepts, which is new in this edition.

This introduction provides information on question types, methods for using this book, and specific information on the national certifying and recertifying examinations. The reader is also urged to consult the National Commission on Certification of Physician Assistants' Web site for up-to-date information on the examination procedures and content. The Web site is *www.nccpa.net.*

QUESTIONS

The National Certifying Examination is made up of "one best answer–single item" questions. In addition, some questions have illustrative materials (graphs, x-rays, and tables) that require understanding and interpretation on your part. Finally, some of the items are stated in the negative. In such instances, we have highlighted in bold or italics the negative word (eg, "All of the following are correct EXCEPT"; "Which of the following choices is NOT correct"; and "Which of the following is LEAST correct"). These items are discouraged, and now there are very few. Many examinees will not encounter a negative question when they take the certifying exams.

One Best Answer–Single Item Question

This type of question presents a problem or asks a question and is followed by four to five choices, only one of which is entirely correct. The directions preceding this type of question will generally appear as below:

DIRECTIONS: Each of the numbered items or incomplete statements in this section is followed by answers or by completion of the statement. Select the ONE-lettered answer or completion that is BEST in each case.

An example for this item type follows:

1. An obese 21-year-old woman complains of increased growth of coarse hair on her lip, chin, chest, and abdomen. She also notes menstrual irregularity with periods of amenorrhea. Which of the following is the most likely cause?

(A) polycystic ovary disease
(B) an ovarian tumor
(C) an adrenal tumor
(D) Cushing disease
(E) familial hirsutism

In this type of question, choices other than the correct answer may be partially correct, but there can be only one best answer. In the question above, the key word is "most." Although ovarian tumors, adrenal tumors, and Cushing disease are causes of hirsutism (described in the stem of the question), polycystic ovary disease is a much more common cause. Familial hirsutism is not associated with the menstrual irregularities mentioned. Thus, the most likely cause of the manifestations described can only be "(A) polycystic ovary disease."

Answers, Explanations, and References

In each of the sections of this book, the question sections are followed by a section containing the answers, explanations, and references for the questions. This section (1) tells you the answer to each question; (2) gives you an explanation, reviews the reason the answer is correct, and supplies background information on the subject matter (and in most cases, the reason the other answers are incorrect); and (3) tells you where you can find more indepth information on the subject matter in other books and journals. We encourage you to use this section as a basis for further study and understanding.

If you choose the correct answer to a question, you can read the explanation for reinforcement and to add to your knowledge of the subject matter. If you choose the wrong answer to a question, you can read the explanation for an instructional review of the material in the question. Furthermore, you can note the reference cited, look up the complete source in the references at the end of the chapter (eg, McPhee SJ, Papadakis MA. *Current Medical Diagnosis and Treatment, 2009*, 48th ed. New York: McGraw-Hill; 2009), and refer to the pages cited for a more in-depth discussion. With this edition, we have provided more detailed citations that include the chapter author in edited books in order to make it easier to find the references.

Practice Test

On the basis of user feedback, we no longer provide a chapter with a typewritten practice test. Instead, a CD has been included to allow the reader to practice their test skills in a format similar to that encountered with the national (re)certification examination. Questions from throughout the book are delivered in random order.

HOW TO USE THIS BOOK

There are two logical ways to get the most value from this book. We will call them Plan A and Plan B.

In Plan A, you go straight to the Practice Test on the CD and complete it according to the instructions provided. This will be a good indicator of your initial knowledge of the subject and will help to identify specific areas for preparation and review. You can then use the earlier chapters of the book to help you improve your relative weak points.

In Plan B, you go through each section checking off your answers and then comparing your choices with the answers and discussions in the book. Once you have completed this process, you can take the Practice Test and see how well prepared you are. If you still have a major weakness, it should be apparent in time for you to take remedial action. In Plan A, by taking the Practice Test first, you get quick feedback regarding your initial areas of strength and weakness. You may find that you have a good command of the material, indicating that perhaps only a cursory review of each section is necessary. This, of course, would be good to know early in your exam preparation. On the other hand, you may find that you have many areas of weakness. In this case, you could then focus on these areas in your review—not just with this book but also with appropriate textbooks. (It is, however, unlikely that you will not study before taking the National Boards, especially because you have this book.) Therefore, it may be more realistic to take the Practice Test after you have reviewed the seven sections (as in Plan B). This is likely to provide you with a more realistic type of testing situation, as very few of us merely sit down to a test without studying. In this case, you will have done some reviewing (from superficial to in-depth) and your Practice Test will reflect this study time. If, after reviewing the first seven sections and taking the Practice Test, you still have some weaknesses, you can then go back to the first of these sections and supplement your review with the reference texts.

We hope that through careful use of this book, whether through Plan A or Plan B, you find this text a useful and beneficial study guide.

SPECIFIC INFORMATION ON THE EXAMINATIONS

The official source for all information on the certification or recertification process is the National Commission on Certification of Physician Assistants, Inc. (NCCPA), Suite 100, 12000 Findley Road, Johns Creek, Georgia 30097. This organization comprises representatives from the major organizations of medicine, including the American Academy of Physician Assistants and the Physician Assistant Education Association. Their function is to formulate and administer the annual certification examination and to provide the means for recertification.

Eligibility requires completion of a Physician Assistant program that is accredited by the Accreditation Review Commission on Education for the Physician Assistant (ARC-PA). Details regarding registration are available from the NCCPA.

The entry-level examination (PANCE) consists of 360-questions addressing all aspects of physician assistant education, including basic science concepts, history taking, physical examination, laboratory and radiographic interpretation, as well as treatment modalities. Tips for improving your score on the exam are provided in Chapter 1. Currently, the recertification (PANRE) examination consists of 300 questions constructed in a similar format as the entry-level examination. Recently, the NCCPA has implemented a process whereby recertification candidates may choose alternate forms for the PANRE. Sixty percent of the examination will be a generalist focus. Examination candidates may select primary care, adult medicine, or surgery for the remaining 40%. An alternative pathway (Pathway II) for recertification was discontinued by NCCPA in 2010. More details on this option are found through the NCCPA Web site www.nccpa.net.

CHAPTER 1

Test-Taking Skills: Tips and Techniques

Anthony A. Miller, MEd, PA-C

Robert W. Jarski, PhD, PA

To become certified and maintain their recertification status, physician assistants are required to successfully respond to multiple-choice questions that appear on Board exams. Passing these exams requires not only medical knowledge but also test-taking skills. By providing examples, helpful explanations, and opportunities for experience and practice, this chapter and the subsequent chapters will help the physician assistant student, or graduate, prepare for the Board exams and use effective test-taking strategies for answering the types of questions found on these standardized tests.

For initial certification, new graduates are required to complete and pass the Physician Assistant National Certifying Examination (PANCE). This 360-item multiple-choice exam covers primary care medical knowledge. For recertification, graduates are required to complete, in addition to a prescribed number of continuing medical education credits, one of the recertification exams, the Physician Assistant National Recertifying Examination (PANRE), which contains 300 multiple-choice questions. Recently, the NCCPA has adopted a practice-focused approach to the PANRE. Sixty percent of the content will be generalist in nature, and the candidate can select remaining 40% to be focused in adult medicine, surgery or primary care.

These exams are designed by the National Commission on Certification of Physician Assistants (NCCPA). The PANCE and PANRE are timed, multiple-choice tests that are presented and answered on a computer screen in local commercial testing centers. Information about exam development and scoring is available at the NCCPA Web site (http://www.nccpa.net). Examination candidates are encouraged to review the content blueprint to better understand the types of practices, tasks, and diseases covered by the Board examinations.

Three conditions are generally necessary for successfully passing multiple-choice examinations: (1) knowing about or recognizing the medical information contained in the questions; (2) using appropriate test-taking skills and strategies; and (3) avoiding situations that are likely to cause mistakes or impede performance. Test anxiety is an example; any standardized exam can produce anxiety that leads to error. However, remembering that most test questions were created by clinicians like yourself who aim to be fair can help you keep the exam's purpose in perspective. Multiple-choice questions are limited in what they can evaluate; they generally assess only fundamental cognitive knowledge (*Ballantyne, 2002; Burton and Miller, 1999*) and test-wise individuals use strategies that enable them to respond correctly to these types of questions.

The fact is, written tests—even at their psychometric "best"—are crude evaluation devices (*Ballantyne, 2002; Burton and Miller, 1999*). Multiple-choice questions cannot reflect a clinician's total fund of clinical skills. For example, patient rapport and the mechanics of examining patients are not accurately measured through multiple-choice questions. These questions can, however, successfully measure certain cognitive or knowledge skills. Computer-administered and scored exams have limited assessment capabilities. Test taking is a discrete skill that is different from clinical skills, and expert clinicians are not necessarily expert test takers.

Clinicians who must pass standardized tests should master the skill of test taking the same way they have mastered clinical skills. This may be accomplished by practicing the methods suggested in this chapter—answering the questions in the chapters and on the CD provided with this book. Reading and answering questions directly on a computer screen may be unfamiliar to some physician assistants, and learning to become accustomed and at ease with this format are skills well worth mastering prior to test time.

This chapter is organized into four sections: (1) what to do when preparing for the exam; (2) what to do during the exam; (3) illustrative questions; and (4) "dos" and "don'ts" that bring together the strategies explained in the previous three sections.

Objectives

In this chapter, the student or graduate physician assistant will:

1. Identify proven techniques from the psychology of learning and educational measurement that will enhance test performance
2. Identify information from testing theory that will help avoid "careless" errors
3. Practice using clues to help identify correct and incorrect responses to exam questions

WHAT TO DO WHEN PREPARING FOR THE EXAM

Getting into Practice

To develop test-taking skills, you must *actively* practice what you will be doing on the test, that is, answering multiple-choice questions. Reading and reviewing without active practice are rarely sufficient. To become proficient in suturing wounds, you need to not only *read* about suturing but also *practice* suturing. Some physician assistants have not taken a written exam in weeks, months, or years. Do not attempt to sit for Board exams without practicing answering multiple-choice questions any sooner than you would suture a facial laceration without having sutured skin in weeks, months, or years. You will have the opportunity to practice responding to questions presented on a computer screen by using the enclosed practice examination CD

Areas to Emphasize

Although you may enjoy studying the areas related directly to your own practice specialty, the task at hand is to pass the Boards. This is best accomplished by achieving a fundamental knowledge of all the medical disciplines represented on the exam. Therefore, it is suggested that you direct your studying to the primary care areas with which you are *least* familiar.

The certification and recertification exams are divided into two general dimensions: (1) organ systems, and the disorders and assessments physician assistants encounter; and (2) the knowledge and skills physician assistants should exhibit (*NCCPA, 2010*). Up-to-date knowledge and skill content areas by percentages, additional testing categories, and a sampling of the diseases and disorders that are included in the content blueprint are available on the NCCPA Web site (www.nccpa.net).

As you prepare, you are strongly encouraged to write several of your own test questions. Those who do so frequently comment that their questions were surprisingly similar to those on the Boards. This occurs because only a limited amount of knowledge is amenable to the written exam format. In addition to identifying clinical information that is likely to be tested, you will gain valuable insight into the logic of test-item construction, which, in turn, helps you to select the intended correct answers from among the foils.

Scheduling Preparation Time

Using a planner, schedule specific periods for test preparation, setting aside specific times for actively reviewing and answering multiple-choice questions. Regular preparation over several months is preferred to cramming; studying just before the exam is usually nonproductive.

For the recertification exam, the amount of preparation needed depends largely on your practice. If your knowledge in primary care family medicine is current, you will need less preparation time than a physician assistant practicing a subspecialty. Primary care knowledge will enhance test performance because in designing the Boards it is assumed that all physician assistants should have fundamental and broad knowledge in primary care medicine regardless of specialty.

The usual learning aids, such as the use of mnemonics, are highly recommended. The reader is referred to appropriate references for general information about study skills (*Academic Skills Center, 2010; Kelman and Straker, 2000; Study Skills Self-help Information, 2010*). The remainder of this chapter addresses specific information about the Board examinations.

WHAT TO DO DURING THE EXAM

Meeting Your Physical Needs

Your anticipated physical and environmental needs during the testing period should be considered when sitting for the PANCE or PANRE. Arriving early may allow you to select a computer terminal in an optimal location. If permitted, choose one that has few or no distractions, avoiding places near doorways and thoroughfares. Repeated interference can hinder your test performance.

Observe the lighting conditions. Extremely bright fore- and overhead lights or glare on computer screens have been reported. Examine the conditions when you arrive and, if possible, request a terminal that meets your needs.

Temperature extremes may be possible. Therefore, dress in layers that will allow you to be comfortable if the temperature is too low or too high. The room situation and your own thermoregulatory mechanisms may change over the course of the day, so be prepared and avoid conditions that may prevent your best performance. In addition, you may wish to consider bringing ear plugs if you are easily distracted by environmental noises.

The exam is divided into several blocks of questions, approximately 60 questions per block for the PANRE and 90 questions per block for the PANCE. Even though the time frame within each block is conveniently provided on the computer screen, you are responsible for the amount of time taken between blocks and completing all blocks within the designated time frame. (See "Time Allowance.") Therefore, you should take a watch (non-digital) in case a clock is not easily visible. However, a timer is generally embedded in the examination and can be accessed via a keystroke.

You are entitled to a comfortable and quiet environment. However, be alert for potential distractions and make reasonable requests that may be honored by the testing center.

Consider Your Nutritional Needs

Consider nutritional and other personal needs. It is recommended that a heavy meal not be eaten within 2 hours prior to the exam, but a complex carbohydrate snack approximately 30 minutes before test time and between blocks of questions may be beneficial. You may also wish to bring with you packaged drinks and other supplies, such as tissues and cough drops. Although these items are not allowed in the testing room, keep snacks, food for lunch, and drinks handy for breaks taken between blocks of questions.

Get Proper Rest

Your exam performance should reflect your knowledge fund rather than mental and physical endurance. You are encouraged to experience the energy required for answering hundreds of multiple-choice questions by using the online testing provided on the CD included with this book.

Research has demonstrated that lack of sleep may result in deterioration of normal cognitive and psychomotor functioning similar to that seen with alcohol intoxication (*Williamson and Feyer, 2000*). No one could be expected to perform optimally on an exam while intoxicated! Lacking even 1 hour of sleep can be expected to impede your test performance. Try to get adequate sleep and rest before the exam by practicing the same sleep hygiene advice given to patients.

Time Allowance

You are allowed a specified number of hours to complete the test on exam day. The amount of time you spend on breaks for rest, bathroom breaks, and meals between blocks of questions is up to you, but you must complete the entire exam within the designated time frame. You may check the number of questions per block and the number of blocks for the entire exam on the NCCPA Web site.

Before beginning each block of questions, calculate the average amount of time you can spend on each question. Typically, you have approximately 1 minute per question. Never go over the calculated time limit on your first attempt at each question. If you do not know an answer, you can mark it by clicking on the appropriate icon and return to it at the end of the block. Always allow for a few extra minutes at the end for returning to marked items and checking your answers. Your subconscious processes items you have previously encountered while you work on other questions. Also, clues often appear in other items. (See "Test Mechanics.") Candidates with learning disabilities who require extended time for examinations should contact the NCCPA significantly before the anticipated test date to schedule accommodations and provide necessary documentation.

Maintain a Positive Attitude

Set yourself up for success by maintaining a positive, confident attitude. Remind yourself that you prepared as best you could. Practice other self-coaching suggestions presented here and use others that have been successful for you in the past.

Do not become discouraged by questions you cannot answer. Test questions with a predetermined discrimination level are retained for use in future exams. If too many test takers answer a particular test item correctly, it is not used again. Therefore, many of the items you will be answering are those that other test takers have failed to answer. So keep in mind that there will be a number of questions you are not expected to answer correctly.

Also, be aware that some experimental questions appear on standardized exams. Experimental questions are those being field-tested, and they are not counted in your score. Because you do not know which items these are, assume that any absurd or very difficult question is experimental. Try not to become irate or unnecessarily concerned about any question.

Self-coaching and imaging or visualization techniques are helpful for all test takers (*Davis et al., 2000; Rossman, 2000*). Stress management methods may be especially useful for anxious test takers (*Davis et al., 2000*). Resources are also available to assess your own level of test anxiety (*Kelman and Straker, 2000*). Most professional athletes and stage performers master and routinely use these techniques to manage their stress and avoid situations likely to interfere with optimal performance.

Techniques should be learned and practiced several weeks before the exam and used the day of the exam. These techniques will not bring to mind medical information you have never studied, but they help you retrieve learned information and avoid exam errors due to extreme stress. Effectively managing stress generally results in improved concentration and the ability to reason logically. The suggested techniques may be learned through special courses and by consulting appropriate references (*Davis et al., 2000; Rossman, 2000*). Certain brief imaging procedures and breathing techniques described by Davis et al. (2000) and Paul et al. (2007) may be used for relaxing and improving concentration during the exam.

Keeping Your Concentration

During the exam, think of nothing except the questions in front of you. When working in the operating room, you concentrate on the operative field. Similarly, give the exam your full, serious, and undivided attention. Problems at work or home should be left at the exam room doorstep knowing you will later have the opportunity to return to them. Your one and only task during the exam period is to answer questions to the best of your ability.

Test Mechanics

The mechanics of navigating through the computer-administered Board exams may be unfamiliar to most. However, the instructions are explained in detail and practice opportunities are provided on the NCCPA Web site. To conserve your mental focus and energy on the exam day, and to maximize the time allotted for rest between blocks, it is helpful to thoroughly master the test instructions well before exam day on a computer without any time constraints. Never find yourself confused because you arrived at the testing center uninformed. In addition, always read the instructions as you begin each section of the exam.

Once you are into the exam, if you do not know the answer to a question, mark it on the computer screen. You will be able to return to it at the end of the block. Unanswered questions are counted incorrect, so it is beneficial to answer the questions you plan to return to, just in case you run out of time at the end. Continue answering the questions you know. Frequently, you will find clues in other questions. In addition, your subconscious will have processed the questions you marked. It has been found that a great deal of information is successfully stored in your memory, but information *retrieval* is often the problem during exam time. Retrieval is enhanced by getting proper rest before the exam, using well-practiced stress management skills, and varying mental tasks during the exam to help keep your mind fresh and alert.

Should You Change Your Answer?

Contrary to some popular misconceptions, if you doubt an answer selection and want to change it, it is suggested that you do so. In numerous studies across disciplines examining thousands of changed responses, answers were changed approximately twice as often from incorrect responses to correct ones (*Welch and Leichner, 1988*; *Fischer et al., 2005*). It might not seem this way because we tend to remember mistakes when we have changed answers from right to wrong, but pay no attention to the times we changed answers correctly. On the other hand, if you really have no idea which response is correct and you find yourself purely guessing, perhaps your first instinct will have been accurate. However, if you do have a reason to change your answer, you will probably change from an *incorrect* to a *correct* response.

Answering by Elimination

Answering multiple-choice questions resembles the process of elimination used when arriving at a diagnosis from a differential diagnosis list. Selecting an answer on the exam by the process of elimination increases the probability of choosing the correct response. Using the stem of the question, form a sentence with each choice provided. After reading the stem, it may be helpful to think out the answer before examining the foils. However, be cautioned against selecting the first answer you think is correct; consider *all* possibilities before making a final selection.

Most test questions have in common the following anatomic features: (1) one choice is easily recognized as an outlier and incorrect; (2) two choices appear plausible as either slightly off the topic or the opposite of the correct answer (eg, artery vs arteriole, left vs right hemithorax); and (3) two choices are correct, but one is better than the other.

The test taker's job is to first (1) eliminate the outlier; next (2), identify the two plausible choices and reject them after weighing them against the two that are more likely to be correct; and finally (3) select the better answer of the remaining two. As with a differential diagnosis, this job is most effectively accomplished through the process of elimination.

By using the process of elimination, almost anyone can eliminate the outlier. By doing so, the probability of selecting the wrong answer by guessing alone is now decreased by 20%. If the two plausible but incorrect choices are identified, you now have two remaining items, and the more correct choice should be selected. At this point, even a pure guess will have a 50–50 chance of being correct. When in doubt, play the odds to your advantage.

Always Triage First

Some exam questions involve dangerous, invasive, expensive, or potentially harmful choices. On the exam, as in real life, you must be alert for such errors. Screen each and every question for potentially harmful or invasive choices. Just as patients are triaged, you should similarly triage each test item encountered. There are three question categories that should be identified.

The first is the "friendly" question—the one that assesses your medical knowledge simply by asking for information. The second category includes those questions designed to trap. Unlike the "friendly" question, the item designed to trap has a preconceived attractor or distracter that may catch the test taker off guard. The third type of question is the one containing a potentially harmful choice. It may refer to a treatment, procedure, finding, or diagnosis.

The third category might not be necessarily tricky, but the test-item writer had in mind a possible pitfall that must *not* be selected. Examples of each question type are presented and discussed in the section "Illustrative Questions."

Some General Hints

Certain "hints" of test taking apply to most multiple-choice questions. These hints are not, however, as likely to work on standardized exams as on other tests, because standardized examinations are subject to many reviews and statistical analyses; but they may be useful as a last resort instead of guessing randomly.

The choices "all of the above" or "none of the above" have an increased probability of being correct. If a single-answer multiple-choice question contains two alternatives that mean exactly the same thing, they probably are both incorrect.

Finally, if you must make a pure guess, (C) is most likely the correct choice. The next most likely choice is (B). Board exam test writers try to guard against these probabilities, but the odds might prove useful to you if all else fails.

ILLUSTRATIVE QUESTIONS

You may encounter the following types of questions on Board exams. Each example presented illustrates a strategy to help identify correct choices. As always, first triage each question and identify its category as (1) friendly, (2) designed to identify a harmful choice, or (3) designed to trap.

The Oversimplification

Some questions appear tricky because you think, "No question could be this simple!" If you really know the answer to a question, answer it without belaboring or looking for booby traps that are not there. The following is an example.

A 22-year-old woman presents with abdominal pain and fever of 2 days' duration. During the digital pelvic exam, she experiences exquisite pain when the cervix is moved. This suggests a diagnosis of

(A) uterine fibroids
(B) vaginitis
(C) peritonitis
(D) cystitis
(E) cervical carcinoma

The item least likely to cause pain, (E), is eliminated. Any of the remaining four are possibilities, but peritonitis of any etiology is usually a safe diagnostic consideration. Do not get bogged down considering the unlikely diagnostic possibilities when an obvious choice is present. The oversimplification in this case is the correct answer, (C).

The Oversimplification that is Dangerous by Omission

As always, triage questions for traps. In the following question, the correct choice is an oversimplification that is dangerous by omission.

A painless testicular mass is found in an otherwise normal 29-year-old. Which of the following diagnoses should be pursued?

(A) varicocele
(B) carcinoma
(C) furuncle
(D) torsion
(E) strangulation

Choices (C), (D), and (E) are ruled out because they usually are painful. (A) and (B), however, usually are painless. Because of its prognosis if left untreated, a testicular mass should be considered cancer until proven otherwise. Not to do so would be considered a life-threatening omission. The correct choice is (B).

Always screen questions for dangerous or critical choices whether harmful by omission or commission. A potentially harmful choice may present itself as an oversimplification.

Clues from Logic

Sometimes a logical (and correct) answer is contained in the stem, as shown in the following example.

The diagnosis of congenital hip dislocation is made

(A) in utero
(B) at birth
(C) at 6 weeks of age
(D) at 6 months of age
(E) fluoroscopically

The term *congenital* means "present at birth." This is when the diagnosis of congenital hip dislocation is made. The correct choice is (B).

Clues from Related Areas

Similar to clues from logic, knowledge about related disciplines can provide additional hints.

An obese 45-year-old woman presents with acute genital pain. Upon examination, you find a 2- to 3-cm soft mass in the right labia majora. This is most likely

(A) marked lymphadenopathy
(B) an inguinal hernia
(C) a femoral hernia
(D) a femoral aneurysm
(E) neurofibroma

If the mass were located in the scrotum of an obese man, you would probably not miss the common diagnosis of inguinal hernia. Remembering from developmental anatomy that the labia majora and scrotum are corresponding tissues, (B) would be selected as the correct response, even if the test taker had minimal knowledge about surgical emergencies.

The "Odd" Choice

This test-taking clue is demonstrated by way of two examples. The first example comes from psychiatry.

Which of the following is **NOT** a sign of trans-sexualism?

(A) rejecting one's anatomic sex
(B) sex identity problems during childhood
(C) dressing in clothing of the opposite sex
(D) aversion toward one's own genitalia
(E) sex identity problems during adolescence

Transsexualism is considered pathological because the patient considers a serious and invasive procedure preferable to living as his/her designated gender. Each choice except (C) implies pathology—rejecting one's own anatomy, sex identity problems, and aversion. The odd choice, (C), has, however, no associated pathology and is the correct response.

The second example follows.

A 65-year-old man complains of burning pain in the distal extremities especially upon exposure to heat. Upon examination, the hands and feet are warm and erythematous. The findings are most consistent with

(A) diabetes mellitus
(B) arteriosclerosis
(C) Raynaud phenomenon
(D) thromboembolism
(E) erythromelalgia

With the limited amount of information provided in the stem, it is unlikely that you can differentiate precisely among the choices provided. Your only clue is the odd choice. Even if you are unfamiliar with the infrequently seen problem of erythromelalgia, notice that choices (A) through (D) are associated with problems causing impaired circulation and cold extremities. "Erythro" or "red" implies *increased* circulation and warmth. (E), the odd choice among the options provided, is the correct answer.

Qualifying Words

Test-item stems containing qualifying words, such as *most, more, usually, often, less, seldom*, and *few*, will sometimes lead you to the correct answer.

You see in the outpatient clinic a 32-year-old man who you suspect is suffering from alcohol withdrawal. The most likely finding would be

(A) visual hallucinations
(B) auditory hallucinations
(C) fine motor tremors
(D) major motor seizures
(E) autonomic hyperactivity

Any of the above may be seen with alcohol withdrawal. However, fine motor tremors are the most common by far. The stem contains a qualifying word suggesting (C) as the correct choice.

If a qualifying word appears among the choices presented, it deserves special attention. Words such as *best, entirely, completely, always*, and *all* imply that something is always true; words such as *worst, never, no*, and *none* imply that something is never true. In clinical practice, *always* and *never* are rarely correct.

The Overqualified Choice

To make an answer acceptable, test-item writers sometimes must qualify a choice to the point at which the savvy test taker recognizes the ploy. The following example illustrates an overqualified choice.

In a 66-year-old emphysematous man with a 100-pack-per-year smoking history, clubbing is most appropriately described as

(A) discoloration
(B) a flattened angle between the dorsal surface of the distal phalanx and the proximal nail
(C) an abnormal inwardly curved nail
(D) a measurably increased eponychium

The overqualified (lengthy) choice, (B), is likely to be correct, as in this example.

However, remember the "odd choice" described earlier! Sometimes the very short "odd choice" is correct. You will recognize this variation because it will be attractively precise and succinct. Having at least some knowledge about the item, you will identify it as accurate.

Strange Terms

Choices containing completely unfamiliar words are likely to be distracters. Do not assume that you somehow missed an important chapter of Harrison's or that there is a gap in your education. If the choice appears completely bizarre, the test-item writer was probably scraping the barrel for a distracter.

On a routine peripheral blood smear from a 13-year-old boy, you see a nucleated cell that is filled with bright red granules and is approximately three times the diameter of a typical red blood cell. This should be recognized as a (an)

(A) Franz-Kulig cell

(B) myelocyte

(C) eosinophil

(D) Olson cell

(E) Kupffer cell

Choices (A), (D), and (E) are completely fictitious. The test-item writer obviously did not lack imagination. (B) is familiar—remember basic anatomy or hematology? However, identifying a myelocyte on the peripheral smear is not basic primary care that the Board exam covers. Physician assistants should recognize the morphology and significance of an eosinophil; thus, the correct response is (C).

"Apple Pie" Choices

There are some responses to which no one would object. Consider the following test question.

When evaluating a 23-year-old woman with vaginal bleeding, the most important clinical information is gained from the

(A) prothrombin time

(B) partial thromboplastin time

(C) CBC and iron studies

(D) physical exam

(E) detailed history

A patient's history provides a clinician's best information and is almost never incorrect. (E) is an "apple pie" choice.

The "apple pie" choice, however, can also be used by test-item writers to set traps.

The most important physical exam component(s) in the emergency evaluation of an unconscious patient is (are)

(A) body symmetry

(B) a carefully performed and prompt neurological exam

(C) the cardiopulmonary exam

(D) vital signs

(E) blood gases

The initial triage of this question would identify it as a "trap" question because of the critical nature of the scenario combined with an incorrect "apple pie" choice. Blood gases are promptly dismissed because they are not physical exam components, for which the stem asks. (B) appears attractive because of its "apple pie" component. Nevertheless, remember your ABCs of emergency care! The correct response is (D).

Hints from Inconsistencies in Terminology

Grammar inconsistencies between the stem and a choice (eg, tense, number, gender) are usually recognized by expert educational evaluators who screen Board exam test questions. You will, therefore, seldom encounter this type of "hint" on Board exams, although it will be found more frequently in classroom situations. Hints due to inconsistencies in terminology are more frequent than other types and you may benefit from being alert for this inconsistency.

A 19-year-old unconscious motorcycle accident victim with suspected multiple trauma is brought to the emergency department. The most significant physical findings usually will result from

(A) undressing the patient

(B) a prompt neurological exam

(C) interviewing the family

(D) interviewing a witness to the accident

(E) all the above

Choices (C) and (D) can be excluded because they refer to historical, not physical, findings. This also excludes foil (E). Although indicated, at this point of presentation, the neurological exam is too focused. A more general, overall assessment provides the best clinical information. Therefore, critical, life-saving information across organ systems may be gained from observing the patient. Choice (A) is correct. Similarly, choice (E), blood gases, in the previous example was eliminated because it was inconsistent with the information asked for in the stem.

Rank Orders

When given a list of numbers or other rank orders, the correct response most often occurs somewhere between the extremes, as shown in these examples.

A 17-year-old woman presents with a history of pelvic discomfort during menses. Through questioning, you determine that the amount of blood lost during each cycle is normal. The amount of her blood loss would be approximately

(A) 25 mL
(B) 35 mL
(C) 70 mL
(D) 100 mL
(E) 125 mL

Here is the second example.

In reviewing the chart of a 45-year-old man, you notice a past diagnosis of chronic schizophrenia. To be termed *chronic*, this disorder should have been present for at least

(A) 3 months
(B) 1 year
(C) 2 years
(D) 3 years
(E) 4 years

Most test-item writers try to bury the correct answer somewhere in the middle. (C) is the correct answer in each example.

As with hints from inconsistencies in terminology, this clue does not work as often on Board exams as it does on classroom tests. Educational evaluators try to randomize the position of correct responses as much as possible. However, when in doubt, it is better to avoid the extremes when presented with rank-ordered options.

DOS AND DON'TS

The following dos and don'ts summarize some of the important points made earlier in this chapter.

DO practice what you will be doing during the exam, that is, answering multiple-choice questions on a computer. Answering these questions is a skill different from knowing clinical information. Get into practice for answering Board questions by actually answering similar questions. This is imperative for the clinician who has not taken a written or computer-based exam recently.

DO direct your studying to the primary care areas with which you are *least* familiar. Passing the Boards is best accomplished by achieving a fundamental knowledge level in each medical discipline assessed on the exam. This is especially important for PANRE candidates who have worked in a narrow subspecialty.

DO write your own multiple-choice questions. Not only will you gain insights into the mechanics of test-item writing and correctly answering questions, but also it is likely that many of your items will resemble actual Board exam questions.

DO get adequate sleep and rest before the exam. Some individuals elect to stay at a hotel located near the testing center in order to help get a good night's sleep and to avoid being late due to traffic conditions.

DO dress comfortably in layers that prepare you for temperature extremes, hot or cold. Coats or jackets may not be allowed.

DO arrive alert, calm, and well-rested.

DO bring beverages, food for lunch, and between-question block snacks. They are not allowed in the exam room but may be checked outside and accessed during breaks.

DO reread instructions provided by the testing agency the night before to ensure you arrive on time, at the right place, and with the right supplies. Recheck directions to the test center.

DO review in detail the information on the PANCE or PANRE content, instructions, and format found at www.nccpa.net

DO remember to bring admissions materials (such as your permit and government-issued identification).

DO examine the computer station you are assigned. Be alert for glare or other lighting problems, and potential traffic flow as others arrive and leave throughout the day.

DO consider that the proctor is there to support you. Ask for any reasonable support or change of computer location that will help you do your best.

DO pace yourself, allowing a calculated amount of time per question. In your time allocation, allow for some extra minutes at the end for returning to items you have marked as unsure.

DO avoid situations that might put you in an unfavorable mindset before the exam. For example, if you anticipate heavy highway traffic, arrive at the exam site a day early. If disturbances bother you during an exam, come early and request a computer in a far corner of the testing room. Let nothing interfere with your best possible performance on the day of the exam.

DO relate test questions to your own practice and experience. Test-item writers are people who have derived many of the test questions from their own clinical experience. What would *you* expect a primary care physician assistant to know? Use this mindset to understand the goal of a question and to keep a positive attitude throughout the exam.

DO practice effective stress management techniques daily several weeks before the exam. During the exam, slow breathing always induces a parasympathetic response that will calm the mind and increase your concentration and focus. If you have any tendency for test anxiety, participate in programs designed to help you do your best.

DO change your answer if you have a good reason to do so. You are twice as likely to change from an incorrect response to a correct one. However, if you are only playing a hunch with no information about the topic at all, your first "gut" reaction might be correct.

DO triage each and every question before selecting your answer. Evaluate it as a question designed: (1) to test knowledge in a "friendly" way; (2) to trap by including common pitfalls; or (3) to evaluate your knowledge about potentially dangerous choices. In the first case, the apparent oversimplification is probably the correct choice. In questions designed to trap, beware of the "apple pie" choice—by omission or commission.

DO use the process of elimination. Your job is to find the single-best answer. As with a patient's differential diagnosis, this usually is done by *elimination*. Avoid choosing an answer until after you have considered all of the choices.

DO read the question stem and combine it with each foil to form a sentence. After doing this, use the process of elimination to arrive at the final answer.

DO mark items if you are not sure of the answer. Return to these items when you finish the question block.

DO make *educated* guesses, if you must guess. Use the information provided in this chapter to help in your decision. By also using your medical knowledge and judgment, your chances will be much improved.

DO be alert for qualifying words such as *most*, *more*, *usually*, *often*, *less*, *seldom*, and *few*, which will sometimes lead you to the correct answer.

DO eliminate choices containing completely unfamiliar words as distracters. If the choice appears completely unfamiliar, it is probably incorrect.

DO consider "apple pie" choices as probably correct. However, beware that they may also be used to trap.

DO consider choices that are different from the others—the "odd choice." This may involve the choice having the "odd" meaning or the "odd" length—long or short. The overqualified choice often is correct.

DO select item (C) when purely guessing. It is most frequently the correct response on many one-choice-only multiple-choice questions. If you eliminate (C) as a possibility, (B) is the next most likely choice. This is a "last-ditch" strategy that works more often on classroom tests than on Board exams.

DO select "all the above" or "none of the above" as a last-ditch strategy. When appearing as choices, they are more likely to be correct.

DO consider taking the exam as a positive experience. Keep your motivation high through self-coaching and imaging techniques. Use recommended stress management methods, especially if you are anxious when taking tests.

DO plan to reward yourself for a good performance after the exam. This facilitates a positive attitude.

DON'T cram at the last minute. This kind of preparation will not be adequate for an exam that covers mostly primary care breadth rather than depth.

DON'T eat a large meal within 2 hours of the beginning of the exam. Be well nourished, but not full.

DON'T leave any item blank at the end of the exam. Unanswered items will be counted wrong.

DON'T discuss the exam during the administration, during breaks, or after the exam; this adds to anxiety and may result in disqualification or revocation of your certification.

DON'T become irate over seemingly absurd or difficult questions. Answer them to the best of your ability, realizing that they probably are experimental questions that will not affect your score. Other test takers probably will also consider them absurd.

DON'T guess randomly. Even if you are completely unsure of the answer to a question, use the hints suggested in this chapter to increase the probability of guessing the correct response. Make educated, not random, guesses.

DON'T think of anything except the exam in front of you. Think of it as your "operative field." Concentrate on giving your best possible performance.

DON'T engage in any behavior that could be interpreted by the proctor as cheating or unprofessional conduct. All examination administration irregularities are reported to the NCCPA and could result in severe sanctions.

REFERENCES

Academic Skills Center. Study Skills Library. California Polytechnic State University, 2010. http://www.sas.calpoly.edu/asc/ssl.html. Accessed January 31, 2010.

Ballantyne C. *Multiple Choice Tests*. Perth, Western Australia: The Teaching and Learning Centre of Murdoch University; 2002.

Burton RF, Miller DJ. Statistical modelling of multiple-choice and true/false tests. Assessment & Evaluation in Higher Education. 1999;24:399-411.

Davis M, Eshelman ER, McKay M. The Relaxation and Stress Reduction Workbook. Oakland, CA: New Harbinger Publications; 2000.

Fischer MR, Herrmann S, Kopp V. Answering multiple-choice questions in high-stakes medical examinations. *Med Educ*. 2005;39:890-894.

Kelman EG, Straker KC. *Study Without Stress*. Thousand Oaks, CA: Sage Publications; 2000.

NCCPA Connect. National Commission on Certification of Physician Assistants. 2010. http://www.nccpa.net. Accessed May 18, 2010.

Paul G, Elam B, Verhulst SJ. A longitudinal study of students' perceptions of using deep breathing meditation to reduce testing stresses. *Teac Learn Med*. 2007;19:287-292.

Rossman ML. *Guided Imagery for Self-Healing*. Tiburon, CA: H.J. Kramer, Inc; 2000.

Study Skills Self-help Information. Online Study Skills Workshops, Virginia Polytechnic Institute and State University. http://www.ucc.vt.edu/stdyhlp.html. Accessed January 28, 2010.

Welch J, Leichner P. Analysis of changing answers on multiple-choice examination for nationwide sample of Canadian psychiatry residents. *J Med Educ*. 1988; 63(6): 133-135.

Williamson AM, Feyer AM. Moderate sleep deprivation produces impairments in cognitive and motor performance equivalent to legally prescribed levels of alcohol intoxication. *Occup Environ Med*. 2000; 57:649-655.

SECTION I
Internal Medicine Topics

CHAPTER 2

Cardiology

Mary L. Warner, MMSc, PA-C

DIRECTIONS: Each of the numbered items or incomplete statements in this section is followed by answers or by completion of the statement. Select the ONE-lettered answer or completion that is BEST in each case.

1. A patient with a long history of innocent palpitations comes to the clinic complaining now of presyncopal symptoms. She is admitted for evaluation and definitive therapy. Which condition is a likely indication for implantation of a permanent cardiac pacemaker in this patient?

    (A) first-degree atrioventricular (AV) block
    (B) Mobitz type I heart block with a heart rate of 72 bpm
    (C) third-degree heart block
    (D) fascicular block without AV block

2. Your patient's wife calls asking for advice. Her husband was admitted this morning with acute coronary syndrome and the doctors are recommending he have coronary artery bypass graft (CABG). What are the indications for bypass versus percutaneous coronary intervention?

    (A) 2 lesions both with 80% occlusion
    (B) 1 lesion with 95% occlusion and diabetes
    (C) an ostial left main lesion
    (D) lesions both with greater than 95% occlusion

3. The use of a bioprosthetic valve replacement versus a mechanical valve is based on several key factors. One of the important factors to consider relates to the patient's age. In which age range would a surgeon most likely consider using a mechanical valve for valvular replacement?

    (A) 55 to 65 years
    (B) 66 to 75 years
    (C) 76 to 82 years
    (D) older than 83 years

4. A 62-year-old woman comes into the office complaining of substernal chest pain and diaphoresis. Her electrocardiograph (ECG) indicates ST elevation in leads II, III, and aVF. What is the next step of care for this patient?

    (A) obtain a stat chest radiograph
    (B) start a verapamil drip
    (C) have the patient chew an aspirin
    (D) repeat the ECG

5. An 81-year-old woman is admitted to the hospital with new-onset atrial fibrillation. When considering whether to heparinize her, which of the following is an absolute contraindication for the use of thrombolytic therapy?

    (A) blood pressure of 170/102 mm Hg on admission
    (B) age greater than 72
    (C) active peptic ulcer disease
    (D) suspicion of aortic dissection

6. Anticoagulation therapy for a mechanical valve should target what international normalized ratio (INR) range?

(A) 1.0 to 2.0
(B) 2.1 to 3.0
(C) 2.5 to 3.5
(D) 3.5 to 4.5

7. Indications for abdominal aortic aneurysm repair include

(A) asymptomatic aneurysm greater than 5.5 cm
(B) 5-cm aneurysm in a patient with coronary artery disease
(C) asymptomatic aneurysm of 3.4 cm in diameter
(D) 4-cm aneurysm in a patient with a recent cerebrovascular accident

8. Which of the following risk factors is *not* associated with increased perioperative mortality in a patient undergoing CABG?

(A) underlying congestive heart failure
(B) presence of diabetes mellitus
(C) advanced age greater than 80
(D) history of sustained ventricular tachycardia

9. Early thrombolytic therapy reduces mortality and limits myocardial infarction size. Four thrombolytic agents have been evaluated extensively in acute infarction. Which antithrombolytic agent should be avoided if the patient previously received it within the past 2 years?

(A) streptokinase
(B) reteplase (r-PA)
(C) alteplase (t-PA)
(D) tenecteplase (TNK)

10. The definitive treatment of aortic dissection that involves the ascending aorta (type A) should include

(A) conservative therapy, admit to the step-down unit
(B) emergent operative intervention

(C) admit to the intensive care unit and manage the hypertension with intravenous (IV) labetalol
(D) serial computed tomography scans to follow changes

11. A 57-year-old man comes to your office for a routine checkup. He has a long history of hypertension that is not well controlled. He has been experiencing more fatigue over the last 2 months. He has smoked two packs of cigarettes daily for the past 25 years. The physical examination findings are 4+/4 carotid pulse, S_3, and 5-cm jugular venous pressure (JVP) at sternal angle with the head of bed at 30 degrees. Which of the following additional findings would be most likely found on this examination?

(A) varicose veins of the lower extremities
(B) more rapid capillary refill time
(C) enlarged and sustained apical impulse
(D) murmur of mitral stenosis

12. A 62-year-old woman with pulmonary hypertension called 911 complaining of sweating and difficulty in breathing. Upon arrival to her home the paramedics found her to have pallor, diaphoresis, tachypnea, hypotension, and tachycardia. Her pulse oxymetry was 89%, so they gave her oxygen via nonrebreather mask and transported her to the emergency department (ED). She was not complaining of angina. The ED physician assistant noted her to be in acute distress with elevated jugular venous pressure, a medial heave, a tender palpable liver, a systolic murmur of tricuspid regurgitation, and an S_4 gallop. ECG demonstrated right axis deviation and right ventricular hypertrophy with no ST-T changes. Her arterial blood gas (ABG) demonstrated a low PaO_2 and a low $PaCO_2$. What is her likely diagnosis?

(A) acute coronary syndrome
(B) cor pulmonale
(C) heart failure
(D) pulmonary embolus

13. A 33-year-old healthy woman during a routine physical examination 3 months ago was found to be hypertensive with a blood pressure of

150/98 mm Hg. She has no family history of hypertension but her provider was concerned, so she was started on an angiotensin-converting enzyme (ACE) inhibitor. Her blood pressure improved slightly but on a routine blood draw her creatinine was noted to be 2.3. She is asymptomatic but is noted to have an abdominal bruit. Based on her history and laboratory evaluation, which of the following is her most likely diagnosis?

(A) essential hypertension

(B) isolated systolic hypertension

(C) secondary hypertension

(D) pheochromocytoma

14. A 73-year-old man with a history of rheumatic fever and coronary atherosclerosis presents to the emergency department with dyspnea on exertion and orthopnea. He called 911 because he could not catch his breath. On examination, he was found to have jugular venous distention (JVD), hepatic congestion, and peripheral edema. A blowing holosystolic murmur along the left sternal border that is intensified during a Valsalva maneuver and inspiration is noted. Atrial fibrillation is noted on his ECG. What is his most likely diagnosis?

(A) aortic stenosis

(B) mitral regurgitation

(C) mitral stenosis

(D) tricuspid regurgitation

15. A retired operating room nurse comes to the clinic complaining of a dull ache in her legs after prolonged standing. She notes her legs feel heavy and she has mild ankle edema when she spends the day shopping. The aching pain and the edema resolve spontaneously if the patient elevates her legs. She denies calf tenderness or dyspnea. Physical examination reveals +1 ankle edema bilaterally. What is her most likely diagnosis?

(A) deep venous thrombosis

(B) lymphedema

(C) varicose veins

(D) intermittent claudication

16. What is the most common primary tumor that metastasizes to the heart?

(A) leukemia

(B) lymphoma

(C) prostate

(D) malignant melanoma

17. A 55-year-old man presents to the ED with chest pain that started 30 minutes ago, diaphoresis, and nausea. An ECG shows ST elevation in I, aVL, and V_2 through V_6. What is the diagnosis?

(A) inferior infarction

(B) lateral infarction

(C) anterior infarction

(D) posterior infarction

18. A 71-year-old woman with a history of hypertension presents to the office with an ulcer on the anterior aspect of the right leg. She presents to the office because she shopped all day yesterday and has developed significant edema. The skin in the pretibial region appears thin and has excessive brown pigment. What is the most likely diagnosis?

(A) venous insufficiency

(B) arterial insufficiency

(C) expected complication of diabetes mellitus

(D) peripheral neuropathy

19. A 35-year-old Asian man presents to your office with burning pain and numbness in his right hand. The patient admits the pain intensifies when working with his hands and may continue for several minutes upon resting. This process began about 1 month ago and now he has developed a persistent ulcer on the nail margin of his right thumb. He has a 20-pack-year history of smoking. He denies using any medications or any illegal drug or alcohol abuse. What is the most likely diagnosis?

(A) venous insufficiency

(B) thromboangiitis obliterans

(C) Raynaud phenomenon

(D) acute arterial thrombosis

20. A 34-year-old woman with a history of tobacco use comes to the emergency department complaining of severe substernal anginal symptoms. She has never had these symptoms before. She states that she had been watching TV this afternoon and the pain was not related to physical exertion. ECG demonstrates ST elevation. What is this patient's most likely diagnosis?

    (A) acute coronary syndrome
    (B) stable angina
    (C) unstable angina
    (D) Prinzmetal angina

21. What is the most common primary tumor of the heart?

    (A) atrial myxoma
    (B) rhabdomyoma
    (C) fibrous histiocytoma
    (D) hemangioma

22. Patients with systemic lupus erythematosus have a predilection to which cardiovascular abnormality?

    (A) congestive heart failure
    (B) acute myocardial infarction
    (C) abdominal aortic dissection
    (D) pericarditis

23. A 68-year-old man comes to the hospital complaining of fatigue and generalized weakness that has been getting worse over the past month or so. He denies angina and palpitations but complains of a 3-day history of dyspnea. He denies any changes in his weight. He has weak pulses and distant heart sounds. His ECG demonstrates sinus bradycardia and prolongation of his QT interval. His chest x-ray demonstrates a water-bottle appearance of the cardiac silhouette with pleural effusions. What is his most likely underlying diagnosis?

    (A) diabetes mellitus
    (B) hypothyroidism
    (C) hyperthyroidism
    (D) pheochromocytoma

24. What ECG change may be noted when a patient has a potassium level of 6.0 mEq/L?

    (A) prolongation of the ST segment
    (B) peaked T waves
    (C) loss of P waves
    (D) prominent U waves

25. An 82-year-old woman with a history of hypertension and coronary artery disease presents to the ED with orthopnea and dyspnea on exertion. She denies angina. Over the past several days, she has noted a worsening of her dyspnea and now sleeps using four pillows. She now complains of dyspnea when she climbs the stairs to her bedroom. On physical examination, you note she is comfortably resting in the sitting position, her vitals are within normal limits, she has 3 cm of JVD, and 4+ pitting edema. She is not using accessory muscles to breathe and her pulse oximetry is 92% on room air. She has normal heart sounds other than an S_4. Rales are heard at the bases of her lung fields bilaterally; there is dullness to percussion over the lung bases as well. What is the laboratory test that you should order to confirm her diagnosis?

    (A) arterial blood gas
    (B) B-type natriuretic peptide
    (C) dobutamine stress test
    (D) CBC (complete blood cell count) and troponin levels

26. The differential diagnosis of a patient with an ECG demonstrating prominent U waves includes

    (A) potassium depletion
    (B) calcium depletion
    (C) digitalis toxicity
    (D) hypothermia

27. A 45-year-old patient with a history of hypertension, diabetes mellitus, and cocaine abuse presents to the emergency department with acute 10/10, nonradiating, substernal chest pain. She denies recent cocaine use but appears very anxious. ECG reveals sinus tachycardia with no other significant changes. Which test(s) should be ordered to determine this patient's disease?

(A) arterial blood gases

(B) CPK enzymes

(C) troponin levels

(D) AST and ALT

28. A patient in the ED who is suspected as having cardiac ischemia has an initial troponin level of 0.08 ng/dL. What can be concluded from this finding?

(A) The patient is having a myocardial infarction.

(B) This is a normal laboratory result, so the patient may be discharged.

(C) This is a normal finding but a repeat level must be obtained.

(D) This level confirms the patient is suffering from angina.

29. A 48-year-old patient with a history of ionizing radiation to the chest wall presents to the ED with dyspnea and fatigue. Physical examination reveals tachycardia, 4-cm JVD, and slight peripheral edema of the extremities. ECG shows low-voltage QRS complexes and CXR demonstrates normal lung fields and cardiac silhouette. What test should be ordered next in this patient?

(A) Holter monitor

(B) echocardiogram

(C) cardiac catheterization

(D) stress test

30. A febrile patient with petechiae and a new-onset murmur of aortic regurgitation should have which of the following diagnostic tests to determine if surgical intervention is required?

(A) Holter monitor

(B) transthoracic echocardiogram

(C) cardiac catheterization

(D) transesophageal echocardiogram

31. Radiographic findings associated with aortic dissection include

(A) widened mediastinum

(B) elevation of the left hemidiaphragm

(C) consolidation in the right lower lobe

(D) pleural effusion on the right side

32. Which of the following ECG findings is associated with tetralogy of Fallot?

(A) right ventricular hypertrophy

(B) right axis deviation with an rSr' pattern

(C) left ventricular hypertrophy

(D) atrial fibrillation

33. The most common cause of myocarditis is

(A) Coxsackie virus

(B) *Staphylococcus aureus*

(C) human immunodeficiency virus (HIV)

(D) Lyme disease

34. A late systolic murmur that may be preceded by a systolic click describes this valvular abnormality

(A) aortic stenosis

(B) mitral valve prolapse

(C) aortic regurgitation

(D) mitral valve stenosis

35. A murmur detected in both systole and diastole is most likely associated with

(A) atrial myxoma

(B) patent ductus arteriosus

(C) mitral regurgitation

(D) aortic regurgitation

36. A 21-year-old woman who is otherwise healthy comes to the ED very anxious, complaining of a severe headache and diaphoresis. She has no history of tobacco use or family history of atherosclerosis. She was found to be hypertensive with a blood pressure of 170/109 mm Hg while her heart rate was noted to be 122 bpm. Based on this presentation, what is the most likely diagnosis?

(A) pheochromocytoma

(B) acute coronary syndrome

(C) aortic dissection

(D) atrial fibrillation

37. A 23-year-old woman with a history of congenital heart disease who has been asymptomatic for the past several years comes to the clinic for counseling about pregnancy. Which congenital heart malformation confers the least risk of complications in pregnancy?

(A) pulmonary hypertension
(B) aortic coarctation
(C) patent foramen ovale
(D) cyanotic heart disease

38. Which of the following radiographic findings is associated with tetralogy of Fallot?

(A) boot-shaped heart
(B) dilated left subclavian artery
(C) right atrial enlargement
(D) normal heart size

39. Which patient population is most predisposed to developing varicose veins?

(A) men
(B) women
(C) those with a history of deep venous thrombosis
(D) those with a history of lymphedema

40. A patient found to have a split of the second heart sound that persists unchanged with expiration may have which of the following conditions?

(A) pulmonary embolus
(B) increased pulmonary vascular resistance
(C) pulmonary valve stenosis
(D) atrial septal defect

41. A 53-year-old man who is of relatively good health except his history of tobacco use is brought to the emergency department complaining of severe substernal chest pain that radiates to his back. The pain began with an acute onset of "a ripping sensation." He called 911 immediately. After arriving in the ED, he was placed on the monitor. His blood pressure was recorded at 190/128 mm Hg. Based

on this history, what is his most likely diagnosis?

(A) acute coronary syndrome
(B) mitral valve stenosis
(C) cardiogenic shock
(D) aortic dissection

42. An 81-year-old woman with a 10-year history of well-controlled atrial fibrillation complains of a 3-day history of fatigue, dyspnea, and a 10-lb weight gain. She denies angina or diaphoresis. Based on this history what would the most likely diagnosis be?

(A) acute coronary syndrome
(B) congestive heart failure
(C) sinus tachycardia
(D) cardiac tamponade

43. A 66-year-old woman with an 11-year history of hypertension takes hydrochlorothiazide for her disease. Recently, she complained of self-limiting presyncopal episodes associated with a "few minutes" of palpitations. She went to her primary care provider and he sent her for Holter monitoring. Which cardiac arrhythmia was the practitioner looking for?

(A) atrial fibrillation
(B) sinus bradycardia
(C) sick sinus syndrome
(D) ventricular tachycardia

44. A 35-year-old woman with no medical history complains of an occasional fluttering sensation in her chest. She denies any associated anginal or presyncopal symptoms. What is the most likely diagnosis?

(A) atrial fibrillation
(B) atrial extrasystoles
(C) sinus bradycardia
(D) ventricular tachycardia

45. A 55-year-old diabetic patient who has a history of tobacco use complains of a sudden onset of severe pain and paresthesias in his right leg. He denies any history of trauma and states he has not had these symptoms before. What is the most likely diagnosis?

(A) arterial insufficiency

(B) venous stasis disease

(C) Raynaud syndrome

(D) arterial occlusion

46. Which of the following descriptions are characteristic of venous stasis ulcers?

(A) painful, erythematous

(B) painful, purulent

(C) painless, erythematous

(D) painless, pallorous

47. Which of the following is the most likely cause of paradoxical splitting of S_2?
(A) pulmonic stenosis
(B) left bundle branch block
(C) atrial septal defect
(D) right ventricular failure

48. Orthostatic hypotension is defined as a drop in systolic blood pressure of at least ___ or a drop of diastolic blood pressure of at least ___ within 3 minutes of standing from the sitting position.

(A) 5 mm Hg; 10 mm Hg

(B) 10 mm Hg; 20 mm Hg

(C) 10 mm Hg; 5 mm Hg

(D) 20 mm Hg; 10 mm Hg

49. A 65-year-old man with a 15-year history of HIV presents to the emergency department in florid congestive heart failure. Which class of medication should be given to this patient immediately?

(A) vasopressors

(B) beta-blockers

(C) calcium channel blockers

(D) diuretics

50. A 55-year-old hypertensive man comes to the office for a routine check after his myocardial infarction. His blood pressure is 145/98 mm Hg and his blood urea nitrogen (BUN) is 22 mg/dL and his creatinine is 1.5 ng/dL. Three years ago, you had placed him on hydrochlorothiazide for

his essential hypertension. Which medication class might you add first to improve his symptoms and decrease his blood pressure?

(A) beta-blockers

(B) calcium channel blockers

(C) ACE inhibitors

(D) spironolactone

51. A 50-year-old stockbroker called 911 when he developed severe substernal chest pain. In the ambulance, he is given three sublingual nitroglycerin tablets, which improved his pain but did not alleviate it completely. His blood pressure is stable and he is noted to have ST-T elevations on his ECG. When he presents to the ED, which medication will you begin while you are evaluating this patient?

(A) oral angiotensin II blocking agents

(B) IV calcium channel blockers

(C) nitroprusside drip

(D) nitroglycerin drip

52. Which medication should be used to control the ventricular rate during rapid atrial fibrillation?

(A) beta-blocker

(B) digoxin

(C) warfarin

(D) nitroglycerin

53. Amiodarone (Cordarone) may cause all of the side effects listed below *except*

(A) thyroid abnormalities

(B) photodermatitis

(C) liver abnormalities

(D) kidney failure

54. Which of the following antiarrhythmic drugs most potently blocks sodium channel current in the myocardium?

(A) lidocaine

(B) procainamide

(C) amiodarone

(D) flecainide

55. The Adult Treatment Panel III guidelines recommend screening initially for hyperlipidemia at what age?

(A) 20 years
(B) 35 years
(C) 50 years
(D) 65 years

56. According to the American Diabetes Association, risk reduction for cardiovascular events in patients with diabetes can be achieved by the use of

(A) antioxidant vitamins
(B) statins
(C) cholesterol absorption inhibitors
(D) aldosterone

57. Patients who are known to be diabetic are at an increased risk of developing diabetic dyslipidemia and cardiovascular disease. Which of the following would *least* likely be recommended to your female patient with diabetes who is 60 years old?

(A) strict control of blood glucose levels
(B) utilize HMG-CoA reductase inhibitor therapy
(C) begin estrogen/progestin combination therapy
(D) utilize ACE inhibitors to control her hypertension

58. When counseling a patient with a history of severe congestive heart failure about how to avoid the precipitating causes of this disease, what would you tell her about her sodium intake?

(A) Ask her to maintain a 1-g sodium diet.
(B) Ask her to maintain a 2-g sodium diet.
(C) Ask her to maintain a 4-g sodium diet.
(D) She does not need to worry about her sodium intake.

59. Secondary prevention of an ST-elevation myocardial infarction should include all *except* which of the following measures?

(A) beta-blockade
(B) ACE inhibition
(C) calcium channel blockers
(D) aspirin

60. A patient presents to the ED with ST elevation in leads II, III, and aVF. The patient is hemodynamically stable. What measure should you use to limit the size of infarction in this patient?

(A) nonsteroidal anti-inflammatory medication
(B) glucocorticoids
(C) calcium channel blockers
(D) fibrinolytic agents

61. An increase in which factor is most likely to increase the preload?

(A) arterial vascular tone
(B) stroke volume
(C) heart rate
(D) intravascular volume

62. During the first half of pregnancy the cardiac output increases. Which of the following factors is responsible for this change?

(A) hormonal changes and arteriovenous (AV) shunt effect of uteroplacental circulation
(B) increases in mean arterial pressure
(C) increased blood viscosity
(D) decrease in heart rate

63. Cardiac tamponade is potentially life-threatening. What is the mechanism by which the effusion impedes stroke volume?

(A) direct compression increases end-diastolic volume
(B) increased pressure in pericardium decreases coronary blood flow
(C) increased pressure decreases sinus rhythm
(D) compression of inferior vena cava decreases preload

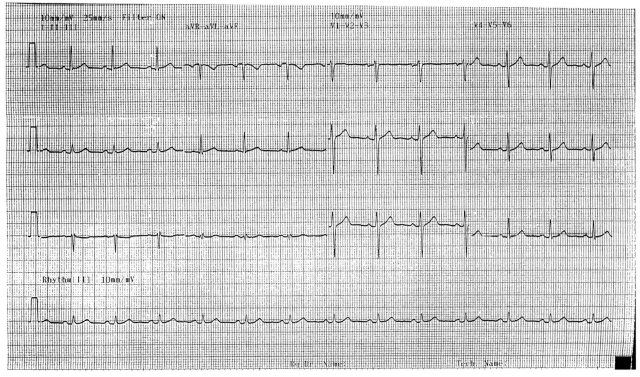

Figure 2-1. ECG A.

64. Diastolic dysfunction is characterized by

    (A) increased systemic vascular resistance
    (B) decreased ventricular compliance
    (C) decreased stroke volume
    (D) decreased afterload

65. The fall in right atrial pressure during inspiration is associated with

    (A) an increase in right atrial and ventricular preloads
    (B) a decrease in right atrial and ventricular preloads
    (C) no change in the right atrial and ventricular preloads
    (D) an initial decrease in the pressures with a rebound

66. Arterial baroreceptors are found in all of the following locations *except*

    (A) right and left atria
    (B) aortic arch
    (C) pulmonary veins
    (D) external jugular vein

67. A 44-year-old woman with a history of diabetes presents to the emergency department complaining of "indigestion." She has an ECG in the triage area. What is your diagnosis? (Refer to Figure 2-1.)

    (A) normal sinus rhythm
    (B) atrial fibrillation
    (C) tachycardia
    (D) nodal rhythm

68. A 35-year-old man comes to the ED complaining of palpitations. What is the abnormality noted in this ECG? (Refer to Figure 2-2.)

    (A) bradycardia
    (B) premature ventricular contractions
    (C) bundle branch block
    (D) atrial fibrillation

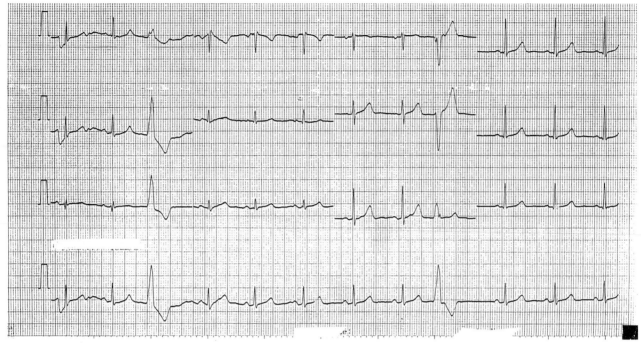

Figure 2-2. ECG C.

69. The treatment recommended for malignant hypertension without encephalopathy includes

(A) oral labetolol
(B) IV nitroprusside
(C) oral phentolamine
(D) IV esmolol

70. You have started your patient who has giant cell arteritis on her glucocorticoid therapy. Which test should you use to monitor her response to this therapy?

(A) urine sodium
(B) serum creatinine kinase
(C) sedimentation rate
(D) complete blood cell count

71. A 72-year-old woman comes to the office complaining of a recent history of substernal chest pain. Her symptoms occur most notably when she brings her laundry up the two flights of stairs from her basement and when she is out shopping for a long period of time. The pain is relieved with rest. She is not complaining of pain now. Her physical examination and ECG are normal. What is the next test you would order?

(A) troponin levels
(B) technitium 99 sesta-mibi
(C) treadmill exercise test
(D) echocardiogram

72. A 70-year-old diabetic patient comes to the clinic for a routine examination and his physical examination reveals an irregular heartbeat. His blood pressure is 130/80 mm Hg and his pulse is 84 bpm. ECG reveals atrial fibrillation, whereas his ECG from 2 years ago revealed sinus rhythm. Upon further questioning, you learn he has felt his heart "flutter" every once in a while for the past 6 months but he did not think to call the office. What is the first drug this patient should receive?

(A) digoxin
(B) amiodarone
(C) metoprolol
(D) heparin

73. The treatment of an asymptomatic patient with first-degree atrioventricular (AV) block with a heart rate of 80 bpm is

(A) pacemaker
(B) atropine

(C) isoproterenol

(D) no treatment

74. Which of the following is *not* an etiology of atrioventricular block?

(A) hypokalemia

(B) Lyme disease

(C) acute myocardial infarction

(D) lithium ingestion

75. A 24-year-old woman with premature atrial contractions (PACs) is quite symptomatic with her irregular heartbeat. Her heart rate is causing her to be very anxious about her health as well. What is the first-line therapy for this woman?

(A) Class Ic antiarrhythmics

(B) digoxin

(C) metoprolol

(D) radiofrequency ablation

76. What ECG finding can be seen in patients taking ibutilide for their atrial fibrillation?

(A) sinus bradycardia

(B) AV block

(C) atrial fibrillation

(D) torsades de pointes

77. A 69-year-old woman comes to the ED with dull chest pain and hypotension. You are trying to distinguish cardiac tamponade from right ventricular infarction. Which of the following clinical features is absent in tamponade but present in right ventricular infarction?

(A) elevated jugular pressures

(B) Kussmaul sign

(C) hypotension

(D) absent y descent in jugular venous pulse

78. What is the recommended treatment of a patient who has been diagnosed with the first episode of cardiac tamponade?

(A) observe to watch for an increase in the effusion

(B) echocardiograph-guided pericardiocentesis

(C) conservative therapy with aspirin and analgesics

(D) pericardial window

79. The etiology of Chagas disease is

(A) *Mycobacterium tuberculosis*

(B) *Trypanosoma cruzi*

(C) Coxsackie B virus

(D) thiamine deficiency

80. Which of the following is *not* considered a key feature of tetralogy of Fallot?

(A) obstruction to right ventricular outflow

(B) malaligned ventricular septal defects

(C) aortic override of ventricular septal defect

(D) constriction of the aortic lumen

81. A 75-year-old patient with a 5-year history of mild angina comes to the clinic complaining of a 1-week history of fatigue and dyspnea when climbing a flight of stairs. Her symptoms resolve if she rests for 10 minutes halfway up the stairs. She denies pain at rest. What is the functional classification of this patient's heart failure, based on the New York Heart Association classification?

(A) Class I

(B) Class II

(C) Class III

(D) Class IV

82. Activation of neurohormonal systems in heart failure involves multiple physiologic pathways. The first step in the cascade is

(A) release of antidiuretic hormone (ADH)

(B) stimulation of baroreceptors in aortic and carotid sinus

(C) retention of sodium and water

(D) sympathetic stimulation of the kidneys

83. Preventing additional episodes of ventricular tachycardia in patients with structural abnormalities of the heart remains an important strategy to decrease the prevalence of hemodynamic compromise. What is the first-line medication you would prescribe for a patient with a history of heart disease who has just survived a bout of polymorphic ventricular tachycardia?

    (A) lidocaine
    (B) quinidine
    (C) procainamide
    (D) sotalol

84. What is the most common proarrhythmic manifestation of amiodarone?

    (A) sinus bradycardia
    (B) torsades de pointes
    (C) atrial fibrillation
    (D) accelerated junctional rhythm

85. A 61-year-old healthy man presents to the ED with a presyncopal episode and a 1-month history of palpitations. He is anxious but is not in respiratory distress. Physical examination reveals vital signs that are stable except tachycardia with an irregularly irregular rhythm. The remainder of his examination is normal. A 12-lead ECG reveals an irregular rhythm with no P waves noted. He is admitted for anticoagulation therapy and cardioversion is planned for a later date. What is the minimum target INR recommended before proceeding with electrocardioversion?

    (A) 1.5
    (B) 1.8
    (C) 2.5
    (D) 2.8

86. A 71-year-old man with a history of third-degree AV block and subsequent pacemaker insertion complains of a 2-week history of increasing fatigue, dyspnea on exertion, a slight nonproductive cough, and a funny sensation in his neck. He has no change in his weight and denies angina. His pulse is irregular. Respiratory rate is 14, nonlabored and his lungs are clear

bilaterally. JVP is 3.5 cm. What test would you order first in this patient?

    (A) chest x-ray
    (B) CBC and chemistries
    (C) 12-lead ECG
    (D) ABG

87. What ECG finding is suggestive of Wenckebach heart block?

    (A) PR interval greater than 0.2 seconds
    (B) progressive lengthening of the PR interval with a dropped beat
    (C) fixed PR intervals with an occasional dropped beat
    (D) dissociation between P waves and QRS complexes

88. A 78-year-old woman with a history of coronary disease and mild LV dysfunction is admitted to the hospital when she is found to have a heart rate of 46 bpm. She is in sinus rhythm and is noted to be taking a beta-blocker. About 36 hours after presentation, the nurse calls you because the patient's heart rate is 130 bpm and her monitor tracing lacks P waves. The nurse states the patient is asymptomatic and her vitals are stable. Given this patient's history, what is her likely diagnosis?

    (A) acute coronary syndrome
    (B) sinoatrial (SA) node dysfunction
    (C) premature atrial contractions
    (D) AV node re-entrant tachycardia.

89. A 55-year-old otherwise healthy man comes to the office for his annual evaluation. He denies any history of fatigue, dyspnea, or exercise intolerance. He is noted to have a grade II midsystolic murmur. What is the next step in his work-up?

    (A) echocardiogram
    (B) electrocardiogram
    (C) coronary arteriogram
    (D) dobutamine stress test

90. A patient in the ICU who has just had a minimally invasive CABG is noted to have a decrease in his cardiac output. Hemodynamic monitoring suggests his intravascular fluid status is appropriate. What is the most efficient way to improve his cardiac output?

    (A) increase his heart rate
    (B) increase his systemic vascular resistance
    (C) decrease his preload
    (D) decrease his myocardial contractility

91. Metabolic syndrome which increases a patient's risk of atherosclerotic heart disease has several key clinical features. Which of the following is *not* a risk factor for metabolic syndrome?

    (A) triglyceride level greater than 150 mg/dL
    (B) blood pressure greater than 130/85 mm Hg
    (C) fasting blood sugar greater than 110 mg/dL
    (D) male abdominal girth greater than 35 inches

92. The goal of treatment for pulmonary arterial hypertension (PAH) is to decrease pulmonary artery pressures in an effort to unload the right ventricle. Which drug should be tried in a patient who had a marked reduction in pulmonary artery (PA) pressures with vasodilators during the cardiac catheterization?

    (A) nifedipine
    (B) bosentan
    (C) sildenafil
    (D) iloprost

93. A 68-year-old woman is admitted to the hospital for further evaluation of her syncopal episodes after a Holter monitor reveals three runs of sustained ventricular tachycardia that lasted between 20 and 30 seconds. While in the hospital, her monitor tracings reveal multifocal premature ventricular contractions. She has no symptoms or 12-lead ECG evidence of ST-segment elevation or depression. What study would you recommend to evaluate her ventricular excitability?

    (A) repeat the ECG
    (B) electrophysiology study
    (C) stress echocardiogram
    (D) transesophageal echocardiogram

94. Pharmacologic management of peripheral arterial disease (PAD) includes

    (A) papaverine
    (B) calcium channel blockers
    (C) cilostazol
    (D) pentoxifylline

Answers and Explanations

1. **(C)** The American College of Cardiology recommendations for permanent pacing include symptomatic third-degree heart block. First-degree AV block is not an indication for a pacemaker unless the PR interval is longer than 300 ms. Mobitz type I heart block generally does not progress to complete heart block, so it is unlikely to require permanent pacing. Asymptomatic fascicular block without AV block is considered a rare indication for pacemaker insertion. *(Tomaselli, 2008, p. 1424)*

2. **(C)** Indications for PCI have changed over the past several years. Drug-eluting stents have decreased restenosis rates to less than 5% for most patients. Still, ostial left main lesions should be treated with coronary artery bypass grafting. *(Baim, 2008, p. 1544)*

3. **(A)** Patients who are younger than 65 years are generally good candidates for a mechanical valve replacement. Bioprostheses deteriorate over time so that while anticoagulation is not required with this type of prosthesis, the revision of these prostheses is very high over time. Nearly half of all replacements will need to be revised within 15 years. Patients who are older than 65 years should be screened to determine what their life span may be, and whether the inherent risk of anticoagulation is worth the benefit of a longer prosthetic reliability. While the durability of new bioprostheses has increased their use in patients younger than 65 years, they remain the mainstay of therapy for patients older than 65 years. *(O'Gara and Braunwald, 2008, p. 1480)*

4. **(C)** Evidence suggests that aspirin in a patient with acute ischemia is beneficial. There is no need to get further tests to confirm this patient's condition until the patient gets to the hospital. Time delay should be minimized. Verapamil in acute ischemia is contraindicated. *(Cannon and Braunwald, 2008, p. 1530)*

5. **(D)** Suspicion of aortic dissection precludes the use of thrombolytic medications because of the risks associated with hemorrhagic shock. Patients with severe sustained hypertension (systolic of greater than 180 mm Hg or diastolic of greater than 110 mm Hg) should not be given thrombolytic medications. Patients who are elderly may be at a higher risk for hemorrhagic complications, but, to date, the evidence suggests that the benefits for thrombolysis generally outweigh the risks. Patients who have active peptic ulcer disease are at a relative risk for complications with this class of medications but the risk–benefit ratio must be discussed. *(Antman and Braunwald, 2008, pp. 1537-1538)*

6. **(C)** The INR range recommended for patients with a mechanical valve replacement is 2.5 to 3.5. Prophylaxis of thrombotic events may require an INR of less than 2.0. Generally, patients who require anticoagulation for other reasons are monitored to maintain an INR of 2.0 to 3.0. Patients with an INR greater than 3.5 are at a high risk of developing warfarin-associated bleeding. *(Weitz, 2008, pp. 744-745)*

7. **(A)** An aneurysm that is 5.5 cm in size requires surgical intervention. Patients who have an aneurysm between 4 and 5 cm require surgical

intervention but only if their co-morbidities are low. *(Creager and Loscalzo, 2008a, p. 1565)*

8. **(D)** A patient with a history of sustained ventricular tachycardia has an improved survival with coronary revascularization. The mortality rates of CABG are less than 1% overall. Factors that increase the morbidity and mortality of the procedure include those listed above as well as a surgeon's lack of operative experience. *(Antman, 2008, p. 1525)*

9. **(A)** Streptokinase should not be given to patients who have received it before because they may acquire streptococcal antibody levels sufficient to neutralize its activity. The other medications listed are not associated with this outcome. *(Antman and Braunwald, 2008, p. 1538)*

10. **(B)** Ascending aortic dissections are associated with an extremely high mortality rate. Emergent surgical correction is required. Even with surgical intervention in the hospital, mortality rate is up to 25%. Patients with descending aortic dissections (type B) and hemodynamically stable may be treated with conservative therapy and should be followed every 6 months with serial CT scans. In addition, both patients with type A and type B dissections benefit from intravenous beta blockade as well as intravenous nitroprusside. *(Merrick, 2006, pp. 413-415)*

11. **(C)** The findings in this case are associated with heart failure and left ventricular hypertrophy likely related to long history of poorly controlled hypertension. The patient may also have other cardiovascular findings but they are not associated with the history presented. If anything, the capillary refill would be decreased and not increased secondary to the myocardial dysfunction. *(LeBlond et al., 2009, p. 360)*

12. **(B)** Patients with all of these conditions may be diaphoretic and complaining of dyspnea. Marked hypotension in acute coronary syndrome occurs when the right coronary artery is affected. Acute coronary syndromes do not usually present with systolic murmurs, but patients will complain of angina and the ECG changes will include ST-segment changes.

Patients who have severe heart failure will have similar symptoms but also have pulsus alternans and pulmonary rales. Finally, patients with pulmonary embolus may have hemodynamic changes but usually have a low PaO_2 and a normal $PaCO_2$. ECG may show right-axis deviation in a pulmonary embolus as well. *(Cannon, 2008, p. 1527; Goldhaber, 2008, p. 1652; Mann, 2008, pp. 1450-1455)*

13. **(C)** This patient likely has renovascular disease, which is responsible for her secondary hypertension. Patients with renovascular stenosis have decreased blood flow to one kidney. This ischemic state initiates renin release, which increases the vascular tone in the remaining normal renal artery. Essential hypertension usually responds to medication and is more likely to be diagnosed in a patient who is older. Secondary hypertension is also associated with pheochromocytoma, but these patients generally have headaches, palpitations, anxiety attacks, and hyperglycemia as well. Pheochromocytomas are not associated with an abdominal bruit. Isolated systolic hypertension is defined as a systolic blood pressure of greater than 140 mm Hg but a diastolic blood pressure of less than 90 mm Hg. *(Kotchen, 2008, pp. 1554-1556)*

14. **(D)** Tricuspid regurgitation is associated with a holosystolic soft murmur heard best at the left sternal border and the intensity may increase with inspiration. Aortic stenosis is associated with a paradoxical split of S_2, a murmur that is loudest mid systole and is heard best at the base of the heart. Severe disease also is associated with a murmur, which can be heard near the carotid arteries. The murmur of mitral regurgitation is heard best at the apex and radiates to the axilla. The Valsalva maneuver reduces it. Mitral stenosis is associated with an opening snap, which is followed by a low-pitched rumbling murmur in diastole. *(O'Gara and Braunwald, 2008, pp. 1467, 1470, 1473-1474, 1479)*

15. **(C)** Varicose veins develop when individuals spend a prolonged amount of time on their feet. Lymphedema is a condition also associated with calf heaviness and edema but the

symptoms do not resolve spontaneously. Deep venous thrombosis edema is usually unilateral, may be associated with calf tenderness or a palpable cord, and does not resolve on its own. Intermittent claudication is not associated with peripheral edema generally and while the pain is resolved with rest, walking exacerbates the pain. (*Creager and Loscalzo, 2008b, pp. 1569-1575*)

16. **(D)** Malignant melanoma is the most common tumor responsible for metastasis to the heart. Lymphomas, prostate cancer, and leukemias also metastasize to the heart but less frequently than melanoma. Patients present with dyspnea, pericarditis, and tamponade symptoms and/or tachyarrhythmias. (*Awtry and Colucci, 2008b, p. 1497*)

17. **(C)** Anterior infarctions are characterized by ST elevation in I, aVL, and chest leads. Inferior wall myocardial infarction is consistent with elevations in II, III, and aVF. Lateral wall and posterior infarctions have a loss of depolarization, which may be noted simply by increases in the R-wave amplitude in V_1 and V_2. (*Goldberger, 2008, pp. 1393-1394*)

18. **(A)** Patients with chronic venous insufficiency note occasional pain with prolonged standing, edema, hyperpigmentation, dermatitis, and erythema. Patients with arterial insufficiency complain of claudication and they are found to have decreased pulses, distal hair loss, thick nails, and pallor. Patients with diabetes that is well controlled may have no symptoms in the lower extremities. Peripheral neuropathies are not associated with pigmentation changes or edema, although ulcers may develop if the patients have lost their proprioception. (*Creager and Loscalzo, 2008b, pp. 1569-1575*)

19. **(B)** Thromboangiitis obliterans or Buerger disease is an inflammatory disease affecting the small and medium arteries of the distal extremities. It is seen most commonly in Asian men younger than 40 years. Little is known about the etiology, although one of the risk factors appears to be smoking. Venous insufficiency is most commonly seen in the lower extremities and while associated with ulcers, there are

other examination findings noted. Raynaud phenomenon is most commonly seen in women between the age of 20 and 40, who complain of severe pain in one or two digits, usually of the hand. Acute arterial thrombosis is not a chronic condition, and so the presentation will be different for acute arterial occlusion. (*Creager and Loscalzo, 2008b, pp. 1569-1575*)

20. **(D)** Prinzmetal angina occurs in younger patients at rest, with no preceding angina. It is associated with ECG changes and is thought to be related to transient coronary vasospasm rather than atherosclerosis. A squeezing chest pressure that is crescendo–decrescendo in nature, which lasts from 2 to 5 minutes, characterizes stable angina. It is often exacerbated by exertion. Unstable angina is noted in an individual with coronary artery disease who notes severe, new-onset pain at rest lasting greater than 10 minutes that is crescendo in character. It may be associated with ECG changes as well. Acute coronary syndrome is usually seen in older patients who have a history of anginal symptoms. (*Antman, 2008, p. 1521; Cannon, 2008, pp. 1527, 1531; Goldberger, 2008, p. 1393*)

21. **(A)** Atrial myxoma is the most common primary cardiac tumor overall. Rhabdomyomas and fibromas are the most common tumors in infants and children. Hemangiomas are small intracardiac tumors that generally affect the AV conduction and may cause sudden death. (*Awtry and Colucci, 2008b, p. 1497*)

22. **(D)** Pericarditis occurs in about two-thirds of patients with lupus. It generally follows a benign course. Patients with lupus may also develop valvular endocardial lesions. It is less common for patients to develop acute coronary syndrome, dissection, or congestive heart failure although these complications are seen in patients with antiphospholipid syndromes. (*Libby, 2008, p. 1501*)

23. **(B)** Patients with hypothyroidism will complain of fatigue, dyspnea when pleural effusions are present, and deny changes in their weight. The bradycardia and prolonged QT interval also should help distinguish this condition from

others. Diabetic patients may have ST changes and evidence of silent ischemia on their ECG. Sinus bradycardia does not usually occur in these patients. Both pheochromocytoma and hyperthyroidism are associated with tachycardia. *(Awtry and Colucci, 2008, p. 1500; Jameson, 2008, p. 2231)*

24. **(B)** Peaked T waves are the first electrocardiographic changes seen in hyperkalemia. Late changes associated with higher morbidities and mortalities and potassium levels higher than 7.0 mEg/L include prolonged PR interval and QRS duration, atrioventricular conduction delays, and loss of the P wave. Prominent U waves are associated with hypokalemia and antiarrhythmic medication toxicity. *(Goldberger, 2008, pp. 1395-1396; Singer and Brenner, pp. 281-284)*

25. **(B)** The diagnosis of mild to moderate congestive heart failure is made using the clinical signs and symptoms and an echocardiogram to determine the underlying etiology of the heart failure. In heart failure associated with both normal and depressed LV function, B-type natriuretic peptide level is elevated. An arterial blood gas in this patient may show a slight decrease in her PaO$_2$; however, because she is not in acute distress and her pulse oximetry on room air is 92%, this test is not critically important at this time. Dobutamine stress tests are used to assess the myocardial perfusion and function. CBC and troponin levels may help elucidate the related causes of congestive heart failure but an echocardiogram is needed to document the severity of the systolic or diastolic dysfunction. *(Mann, 2008, p. 1447)*

26. **(A)** Prominent U waves are noted on ECG when there are ventricular repolarization abnormalities, which are associated with hypokalemia or antiarrhythmic medications. Very prominent U waves are related to the development of torsades de pointes. Hypocalcemia prolongs the QT interval. Buildup of procainamide metabolite *N*-acetylprocainamide (NAPA) is associated with QT-interval prolongation. Hypothermia is associated with J-point elevation. *(Goldberger, 2008, pp.1391, 1395)*

27. **(C)** We must determine whether there is a life-threatening etiology of her chest pain. Troponin levels are useful in the diagnosis of acute coronary syndrome because this amino acid does not exist in skeletal muscle. Troponins have a high sensitivity and specificity for acute coronary syndromes. The enzyme levels rise after 6 hours and peak at 12 hours. Abnormalities in arterial blood gases exist for many reasons but are not sensitive or specific to acute coronary syndromes. CPK enzymes vary in their specificity because of the distribution of these enzymes in other parts of the body. CPK release can occur from the myocardium as well as skeletal muscle. AST and ALT levels may be elevated but these are not specific markers for acute coronary syndrome. *(Cannon and Braunwald, 2008, p. 1528)*

28. **(C)** This troponin level is considered normal. If one suspects that the individual is suffering from acute coronary syndrome, serial samples must be obtained to confirm the diagnosis. Additional testing of a normal level is required to evaluate the potential serum markers of ischemia longitudinally. A normal troponin level does not aid in making the diagnosis of angina. *(Cannon and Braunwald, 2008, p. 1528)*

29. **(B)** This patient is suffering from pericarditis. Pericarditis is diagnosed using the Doppler echocardiography. Holter monitor should be used to aid in the diagnosis of arrhythmias and to work up syncope. Cardiac catheterization is generally used to evaluate individual coronary arteries and cardiac function. Electrocardiographic stress tests are used to screen for coronary artery disease in an ambulatory patient who is complaining of chest discomfort. *(Braunwald, 2008, pp. 1489, 1491)*

30. **(D)** The most likely diagnosis in this patient is infective endocarditis. Evaluation of the blood flow and the functional status of the myocardium can be evaluated with either transthoracic or transesophageal echocardiogram. However, vegetations can be detected with more sensitivity and specificity using the transesophageal echocardiogram. Holter monitors and cardiac catheterization do not detect valvular lesions or vegetations. *(Karchmer, 2008, pp. 789-792)*

31. **(A)** Widened mediastinum is associated with aortic dissection. Pneumothorax and consolidation are not seen with this condition. Pleural effusion may occur with a dissection but it is usually an effusion on the left side. *(Creager and Loscalzo, 2008a, p. 1566)*

32. **(A)** Right ventricular hypertrophy is associated with tetralogy of Fallot. This condition is characterized by a malaligned ventricular septal defect and obstruction of the right ventricle outflow tract. Right axis deviation with an rSr' pattern is associated with an ostium secundum defect. Left ventricular hypertrophy is associated with coarctation of the aorta. Atrial fibrillation is associated with Epstein anomaly and atrial septal defects. *(Child, 2008, p. 1463)*

33. **(A)** The most common cause of myocarditis is the Coxsackie B virus. The most common bacterial agent related to myocarditis is diphtheria, not *Staphylococcus aureus*. Diphtheria is a very rare cause of myocarditis. Both HIV and Borrelia infection can cause myocarditis but these infections are less common than the one caused by the Coxsackie virus. *(Wynne and Braunwald, 2008, p. 1486)*

34. **(B)** Mitral valve prolapse is characterized by a midsystolic click and a late systolic murmur. The murmur associated with aortic stenosis is a midsystolic murmur, also known as a systolic ejection murmur. Aortic regurgitation is characterized by a high-pitched decrescendo murmur in early diastole. Mitral valve stenosis is associated with a low-pitched, mid-diastolic murmur. *(O'Gara and Braunwald, 2008, pp. 1468-1474)*

35. **(B)** Patent ductus arteriosus is the known cause of a continuous murmur, unless the patient has pulmonary hypertension. Patients with atrial myxoma may have a mid-diastolic or presystolic murmur. Mitral and aortic regurgitation are associated with systolic or diastolic murmurs, respectively. *(O'Rourke and Braunwald, 2008, pp. 1386-1388)*

36. **(A)** Pheochromocytoma is associated with a sudden onset of hypertension, tachycardia, and other findings consistent with catecholamine stimulation. Sick sinus syndrome and/or atrial

fibrillation may be associated with tachycardia but is not associated with hypertension. This patient is not complaining of chest pain, and so it is unlikely that the patient has either acute coronary syndrome (ACS) or aortic dissection. *(Neumann, 2008, p. 2271)*

37. **(C)** The foramen ovale usually closes soon after birth. Patients whose foramen remains open most commonly have normal pulmonary pressures with small left-to-right shunts. Patients with Marfans and coarctation of the aorta risk aortic dissection during pregnancy. Patients with pulmonary hypertension are also at risk of death during pregnancy. *(Child, 2008, pp. 1458-1459)*

38. **(A)** A boot-shaped heart is noted in patients with tetralogy of Fallot. A dilated left subclavian is associated with coarctation of the aorta. Right atrial enlargement is seen in atrial septal defects, whereas a normal heart silhouette is associated with pulmonary stenosis. *(Child, 2008, pp. 1460-1463)*

39. **(B)** Women are two to three times more likely than men to develop varicosities of their lower extremities. Patients who develop secondary varicosities may have a history of deep venous insufficiency. Patients with lymphedema generally have a different physical presentation, which is inconsistent with varicose veins. Lymphedema does not increase one's risk of developing varicosities. *(Creager and Loscalzo, 2008b, p. 1574)*

40. **(D)** Physiologic splitting of the second heart sounds occur in inspiration as the aortic and pulmonic valves close at different times. Fixed splitting of the S_2 heart sound is heard in patients with atrial septal defects. Patients with pulmonary embolus and pulmonary valve stenosis have a split that is prolonged and is noted in expiration. Patients with increased pulmonary vascular resistance have a narrowing of the second heart sound split. *(O'Rourke and Braunwald, 2008, p. 1385)*

41. **(D)** The differential diagnosis includes acute coronary syndrome. However, if the patient is hypertensive, a tobacco user, and complains of

a severe pain that radiates to the back, the patient most likely is experiencing an aortic dissection. Mild mitral stenosis may be asymptomatic but moderate stenosis is associated with dyspnea on exertion and cough. Cardiogenic shock is characterized by hypotension and chest pain. *(Lee, 2008, pp. 87-91)*

42. **(B)** Congestive heart failure is associated with fatigue, dyspnea, and sudden weight gain. Myocardial infarction may be a precipitating case for the patient's congestive heart failure but would generally present with chest pain. Sinus tachycardia is unlikely because this patient has had long-standing atrial fibrillation. Cardiac tamponade is a possibility; however, generally while there is fatigue and dyspnea, patients with this condition do not experience such a sudden change in their weight. *(Lee, 2008, pp. 87-89; Mann, 2008, pp. 1446-1447)*

43. **(D)** Ventricular tachycardia is associated with bursts of tachycardia and presyncope. Patients who are taking diuretics that are not potassium sparing may develop hypokalemia as a result of the medication. This deficit predisposes patients to ventricular arrhythmias. Atrial fibrillation is generally characterized by a sustained irregular rhythm. Sinus bradycardia is a slow regular rhythm and is associated with abrupt syncopal episodes rather than presyncope. Sick sinus syndrome is associated with heart rates that are slow, normal, and fast and are associated with sinus pauses. *(Carlson, 2008, pp. 139-141)*

44. **(B)** This patient is experiencing palpitations as a result of premature atrial contractions. She does not have atrial fibrillation or sinus bradycardia because her symptoms are transient. Atrial fibrillation is characterized by sustained irregular rhythm. Sinus bradycardia is characterized by a slow, often regular rhythm, whereas ventricular tachycardia is characterized by sustained bursts of rapid heart rate. Ventricular tachycardia usually presents with presyncopal symptoms. *(Loscalzo, 2008b, p. 236)*

45. **(D)** The pain associated with arterial occlusion occurs as a sudden onset of severe pain and associated paresthesias. Arterial insufficiency is characterized by intermittent claudication, pain at rest, and it generally has a gradual onset. Venous insufficiency presents with edema that is relieved with leg elevation. Venous stasis ulcers are large, painless ulcerations. Patients with Raynaud syndrome complain of pallor, rubor, limb coldness, and paresthesias and pain. The cycles of vasoconstrictions responsible for these symptoms are often triggered by exposure to stress or cold environments. *(Creager and Loscalzo, 2008b, pp. 1568-1575)*

46. **(C)** Ulcerations associated with venous stasis disease are painless, whereas ulcerations associated with peripheral arterial insufficiency are painful. With severe arterial disease, thickened nails, hair loss, pallor with elevation of the extremity, and dependent rubor are common findings. The skin changes with venous disease may include erythema and hyperpigmentation. *(Rapp, 2006, p. 805; Wakefield, 2006, pp. 858-860)*

47. **(B)** Paradoxical splitting of S_2 occurs on expiration and disappears on inspiration: the opposite of physiologic splitting. The most common cause is left bundle branch block. Atrial septal defect and right ventricular failure are associated with fixed splitting. Pulmonic stenosis is associated with a wide split. *(Bickley and Szilagyi, 2009, p. 380)*

48. **(D)** Orthostatic hypotension, which may occur for many reasons, is related to autonomic nervous system abnormalities or intravascular volume deficits. Orthostasis is defined as a drop of greater than 20 mm Hg in the systolic pressure or a drop of greater than 10 mm Hg in the diastolic pressure within 3 minutes of posture change. When the drop in pressure is related to neurogenic causes, the compensatory change in the pulse rate is not seen. *(Low and Engstrom, 2008, p. 2578)*

49. **(D)** The treatment of congestive heart failure includes preventive measures, control of excess fluid, and enhancement of myocardial contractility. Diuretics should be used to decrease the fluid overload. ACE inhibitors, beta-blockers, and sympathomimetic agents are important adjuncts to emergent treatment. Calcium

channel blockers have no role in the treatment of congestive heart failure. (*Mann, 2008, pp. 1448-1453*)

50. **(A)** Drug therapy is recommended for patients with a blood pressure of greater than or equal to 140/90 mm Hg. For a patient who has underlying cardiac disease, beta-blockers have been shown to decrease morbidity and mortality if the patient has hypertension. If the patient's hypertension remains recalcitrant, ACE inhibitors may help if the patient has left ventricular dysfunction but should be used cautiously in patients with renal insufficiency. Calcium channel blockers have not been shown to improve the survival of patients who are hypertensive and have known cardiac disease. Spironolactone should be used in patients with heart failure. (*Kotchen, 2008, p. 1559*)

51. **(D)** Nitroglycerin is indicated in this patient. It will improve the myocardial oxygen availability because of its vasodilatory effects. Medications by mouth are not indicated at this time. Nitroprusside will decrease the systemic vascular resistance and decrease the blood pressure. It is not indicated in this acute stage because of its potent hypotensive effects. Calcium channel blockers do not have a role in the therapy of an acute myocardial infarction. (*Antman, 2008, p. 1535*)

52. **(A)** Beta-blockers should be used to control the ventricular rate in rapid atrial fibrillation. While digoxin will slow the ventricular rate, it is no longer the drug of choice. Warfarin is used for anticoagulation and the prevention of clot formation that is a risk with the occurrence of atrial fibrillation. There is not a clear need for nitroglycerin at the time because the patient is not complaining of angina. (*Marchlinski, 2008, p. 1428*)

53. **(D)** Major side effects of amiodarone are photosensitivity, thyroid, central nervous system, and liver abnormalities. (*Hume, 2007, p. 228*)

54. **(D)** Flecainide is a Class Ic antiarrhythmic whose mechanism of action blocks sodium channels. Class Ic medications are indicated

for life-threatening ventricular tachycardia or fibrillation. They may also be used in refractory supraventricular tachycardia. (*Tomaselli, 2008, p.1414*)

55. **(A)** The Expert Panel on Detection, Evaluation, and Treatment of High Blood Cholesterol recommends initial screening of all patients older than 20 years. (*Libby, 2008, p. 1505*)

56. **(B)** Statins are recommended if the total cholesterol is greater than 135 mg/dL. ACE inhibitors have also been shown to be effective in this patient group. (*Libby, 2008, p. 1507*)

57. **(C)** Microvascular complications of diabetes can be reduced by strict glucose controls. The VA HDL Intervention Trial demonstrated a decrease in strokes and cardiovascular events when gemfibrozil was given to patients. The Women's Health Initiative study concludes that there was no reduction in coronary events with the use of estrogen/progestin tablets. ACE inhibition has been shown to decrease coronary events in diabetic patients. (*Libby, 2008, pp. 1506-1507*)

58. **(A)** For patients with a history of heart failure, sodium excess can have an adverse effect on the patient's fluid homeostasis. Patients should restrict their sodium intake to 1 g if they have severe disease. (*Mann, 2008, p. 1448*)

59. **(C)** Calcium channel blockers have been shown to increase mortality in patients who have had a previous myocardial infarction. However, beta-blockers, ACE inhibitors, and aspirin have been shown to improve the morbidity and mortality rates in patients who have had a myocardial infarction. (*Antman, 2008, pp. 1539-1540*)

60. **(D)** Fibrinolytic agents should be initiated within 30 minutes of presentation if there are no contraindications. NSAIDs and glucocorticoids have not been helpful to reduce the size of infarction and are known to impair infarct healing. Calcium channel blockers are not indicated in the treatment of myocardial infarction. (*Antman, 2008, pp. 1538-1540*)

61. (D) Preload is defined as the ventricular end-diastolic volume. Factors that increase the ventricular end-diastolic volume include an increase in the intravascular volume. Arterial vascular tone increases the blood pressure, which may decrease the venous return to the heart. Increases in the stroke volume occur when the ventricle is more efficient, thus increasing the cardiac output; increases in the stroke volume have little to no effect on the end-diastolic volume. The heart rate does not increase the ventricular end-diastolic volume. In fact, if the heart rate increases, it provides less time for ventricular filling so that it may decrease the ventricular end-diastolic volume. *(Loscalzo, 2008a, p. 1373)*

62. (A) The cardiac output increases by about 40% as a result of hormonal changes and effects of uteroplacental circulation, with the highest levels achieved between weeks 20 and 24. Heart rate generally increases during pregnancy, which also impacts the cardiac output. Women have up to a 50% increase in their blood volume during pregnancy and a decrease in blood viscosity. Systemic pressure in pregnant women generally decreases earlier in pregnancy and then returns to prepregnancy levels. *(Kahn and Koos, 2007, pp. 149-151)*

63. (D) Compression caused by cardiac tamponade decreases the preload, which is an important component of stroke volume. Direct compression prevents inflow of blood to the heart muscle, which will decrease the end-diastolic volume. While tamponade does increase the pressure in the heart muscle itself, stroke volume is the amount of blood that is ejected with each contraction. The increased intracardiac pressure associated with tamponade affects the patient's cardiac output. Tamponade has no intrinsic effect on the heart rate. *(Braunwald, 2008, pp. 1490-1491; Ganong, 2006, p. 325)*

64. (B) Diastolic dysfunction affects stroke volume by decreasing it. This is true of systolic dysfunction as well. The distinction between the two is that the increase in intrapericardial pressure and the increased stiffness of the ventricle decreases the end-diastolic volumes in diastolic dysfunction. *(Kusumoto, 2006, pp. 273-275)*

65. (A) Inspiration makes the negative pressure in the intrathoracic cavity more negative. This increases the thoracic blood volume and increases venous return to the heart. Valsalva maneuvers, positive pressure ventilation, and excessive coughing increase the intrathoracic pressure that decreases venous return. *(O'Rourke and Braunwald, 2008, p. 1387)*

66. (D) Baroreceptors are stretch receptors found in the walls of the heart and blood vessels. They are also noted in the carotid sinus, the atria, and the pulmonary veins. *(Kotchen, 2008, p. 1550)*

67. (A) This patient has normal sinus rhythm. Atrial fibrillation is characterized by the absence of P waves. Tachycardia exists when the heart rate is greater than 100 bpm. Nodal rhythm is characterized by heart rates in the 40s and the lack of P waves. *(Goldberger, 2006, pp. 157-161)*

68. (B) Premature ventricular contractions are generally isolated widened QRS beats followed by a compensatory pause seen here. The patient's heart rate is greater than 60 bpm, so he does not have bradycardia. Bundle branch block is characterized by a wide QRS complex, well visualized throughout most of the precordial leads. *(Goldberger, 2006, pp. 161, 189, 209-211)*

69. (A) The treatment goal of malignant hypertension without encephalopathy is to decrease the blood pressure slowly with short-acting oral agents. IV nitroprusside and IV esmolol should be reserved for hypertensive emergencies because their impact on blood pressure is dramatic and sudden. Phentolamine is used to treat pheochromocytoma. *(Kotchen, 2008, p. 1562)*

70. (C) Patients with giant cell arteritis present with elevated erythrocyte sedimentation rates (ESRs), which are useful for monitoring therapy because they decrease with steroid intervention. Patients with giant cell arteritis do initially present with anemia but this condition does not respond to steroids. Serum creatinine kinase level is not generally elevated in this disease, and so it would not be a good test to follow the response to treatment. *(Langford and Fauci, 2008, pp. 2126-2127)*

71. **(C)** In this patient, her exercise intolerance needs to be evaluated more formally. She may have stable exertional angina. Troponin levels should be ordered if the patient either has ECG changes consistent with ischemia or if the pain is acute. Technetium 99 should be ordered if the baseline ECG shows pre-excitation, left bundle branch block, or ST-segment changes. Echocardiogram should be performed if the patient has a positive exercise stress test result. *(Antman et al., 2008, pp. 1516-1519)*

72. **(D)** This patient has stable atrial fibrillation (AF) that likely began in the past 6 months. He is hemodynamically stable and is not tachycardic. His age and diabetes predispose him to emboli formation; therefore, he would benefit from anticoagulation. Digoxin can be used to control the rate of atrial fibrillation if tachycardia is present but is not used alone in acute atrial fibrillation. Amiodarone is used to prevent AF recurrence but does not work well to convert patients with a 6-month history of an irregular heartbeat. Beta-blockade is used to control the heart rate in cases of tachycardia. *(Marchlinski, 2008, pp. 1428-1429)*

73. **(D)** First-degree AV block does not require treatment unless the patient is profoundly bradycardic and has left ventricular dysfunction. Pacemakers are used for those who are bradycardic or have an irreversible second- or third-degree AV block. Atropine and isoproterenol can increase conduction through the AV node. These medications can be used for diagnostic purposes. *(Tomaselli, 2008, pp. 1421, 1423)*

74. **(A)** AV block can be precipitated by hyperkalemia, Lyme disease, myocardial infarction, and lithium. *(Tomaselli, 2008, p. 1419)*

75. **(C)** Most patients with PACs do not require intervention unless the patient is profoundly symptomatic. If a patient requires intervention, beta-blockade should be initiated as a first-line therapy. Class Ic antiarrhythmics can be tried if there is no structural disease. Digoxin is used to control heart rate in atrial flutter and fibrillation. *(Marchlinski, 2008, pp. 1427, 1429)*

76. **(D)** Ibutilide is a Class III antiarrhythmic agent used to cardiovert patients with atrial fibrillation and atrial flutter to sinus rhythm. Torsades de pointes and QT prolongation are side effects of ibutilide therapy. Sinus bradycardia and AV block can be noted in patients taking amiodarone. Atrial fibrillation is rhythm associated with adenosine administration. *(Marchlinksi, 2008, p. 1430)*

77. **(B)** Kussmaul sign (JVP rise with inspiration) is absent in tamponade and present in right ventricular infarction. Cardiac tamponade and right ventricular infarctions share many clinical features such as hypotension, elevated jugular venous pressure, absent y descent in JVP, and occasionally, pulsus paradoxicus. *(Braunwald, 2008b, p. 1491)*

78. **(B)** Cardiac tamponade should be treated with pericardiocentesis urgently because of the hemodynamic compromise. Patients with acute pericarditis should be monitored for changes in effusion size. Aspirin (acetylsalicylic acid [ASA]) and analgesics can be used to treat idiopathic acute pericarditis. Pericardial window should be used for recurrent tamponade episodes and cases of chronic constructive pericarditis. *(Braunwald, 2008b, pp. 1492, 1494)*

79. **(B)** Chagas disease is caused by the protozoan parasite *Trypanosoma cruzi*, which is found most commonly in patients from Central and South America and may present with manifestations of cardiac abnormalities. Tuberculosis is associated with chronic pericardial effusion, whereas the Coxsackie virus is associated with acute myocarditis. Thiamine deficiency causes high output cardiac failure and is associated with cardiomyopathy. *(Braunwald, 2008b, pp. 1495; Wynne and Braunwald, 2008, pp. 1487-1488)*

80. **(D)** Constriction of the aortic lumen is noted with coarctation of the aorta not tetralogy of Fallot. Tetralogy of Fallot is characterized by maligned ventricular septal defect (VSD), obstruction to right ventricular (RV) outflow, aortic override of VSD, and RV hypertrophy. *(Child, 2008, pp. 1462-1463)*

81. **(B)** This patient has Class II symptoms characterized by angina with exertion but no pain at rest. Class I symptoms are noted in patients with cardiac disease but without limits of physical activity and no anginal (or equivalent) symptoms. Class III symptoms are noted in patients who have marked limitations because less than ordinary activity causes angina or equivalent symptoms. Class IV symptoms are noted in patients who cannot carry on any physical activity without discomfort. These patients have pain at rest as well. *(Mann, 2008, p. 1448)*

82. **(B)** Baroreceptors detect less circulating blood volume because of a decrease in left ventricular function. They signal the brain to release ADH in an effort to increase peripheral vasoconstriction. Free water is reabsorbed by the kidneys, by stimulation of the renin-angiotensin cascade and subsequent retention of salt and water, which increases the afterload. *(Mann, 2008, p. 1445)*

83. **(D)** Sotalol and amiodarone are indicated to prevent recurrent ventricular tachycardia (VT) in a patient with cardiac disease. Lidocaine can be used during the ventricular tachycardia episode to convert the rhythm and is used acutely because of its intravenous form. Quinidine and procainamide should not be used in patients with a history of VT and structural heart abnormalities because of its proarrhythmic effect unless an implantable cardioverter defibrillator (ICD) has been placed. *(Marchlinksi, 2008, p. 1437)*

84. **(A)** Amiodarone causes sinus bradycardia, AV block, and an increase in the defibrillation threshold. Torsades de pointes is rarely associated with amiodarone use. Atrial fibrillation can be associated with adenosine toxicity, and junctional rhythms may occur commonly in patients treated with digoxin. *(Marchlinksi, 2008, p. 1430)*

85. **(B)** An INR of 1.8 for 3 weeks is recommended before cardioversion. INRs between 2.0 and 3.0 are recommended for patients with long-standing atrial fibrillation in which cardioversion has failed. *(Marchlinksi, 2008, pp. 1428-1429)*

86. **(C)** This patient has symptoms of pacemaker syndrome. This entity is cause by atrial and ventricular pacing that is asynchronous. The treatment for this condition is pacemaker exchange. The best initial test to diagnose this condition is the ECG. Chest x-ray and other laboratory data will not help you to diagnose this condition. *(Tomaselli, 2008, p. 1423)*

87. **(B)** Wenckebach (type I second-degree AV block) is characterized by a progressive lengthening of the PR interval. First-degree heart block is characterized by a PR interval that is longer than 0.2 seconds. Type II second-degree block has a fixed PR interval with occasional dropped beats, while dissociation between the electrical activity of the atrium and the ventricle is noted in third-degree AV block. *(Tomaselli, 2008, pp. 1420-1421)*

88. **(B)** This patient has a short history of both profound bradycardia and tachycardia consistent with SA node dysfunction (also called tachy–brady syndrome). The patient is asymptomatic so it is unlikely that she has acute coronary syndrome. Premature atrial contractions have P waves before the QRS complex and AV node re-entrant tachycardia usually generates a faster rhythm. *(Tomaselli, 2008, pp. 1418, 1426; Marchlinksi, 2008, p. 1433).*

89. **(B)** Patients who have a grade I or grade II systolic murmur with no symptoms can be followed conservatively with a chest x-ray and a 12-lead ECG. Echocardiogram should be performed in patients with diastolic or continuous murmurs and in patients with a systolic murmur that is greater than grade II. Also, patients with grade I or II murmurs that have other cardiac symptoms should be evaluated using an echocardiogram. Coronary arteriogram and dobutamine stress tests are used to evaluate patients with anginal symptoms. *(Braunwald, 2008a, p. 1381)*

90. **(A)** Cardiac output is impacted by the heart rate and the stroke volume. Stroke volume is

impacted by volume status (preload), myocardial contractility, and systemic vascular resistance (afterload). While impacting the preload, afterload, and the myocardial contractility will improve cardiac output, the contribution of each factor is far less than that of the heart rate. *(Loscalzo, 2008a, p. 1373)*

91. **(D)** The abdominal girth associated with metabolic syndrome for women is greater than 35 inches whereas the girth for men is greater than 40 inches. All other criteria are suggestive of metabolic syndrome. *(Libby, 2008, p. 1507)*

92. **(A)** The calcium channel blocker nifedipine is recommended in this patient as the vasodilator challenge demonstrated PA responsiveness. Bosentan (an endothelial receptor antagonist), sildenafil (a phosphodiesterase-5 inhibitor), and iloprost (a prostacyclin analog) all are indicated when the PAH is not responsive to the vasodilator challenge. *(Rich, 2008, pp. 1577-1578)*

93. **(B)** Electrophysiology studies are used to evaluate the excitability of the myocardium and to reproduce the ventricular tachycardia.

Repeating the ECG in the face of documented ventricular tachycardia on Holter monitor and evidence of multifocal PVCs is unnecessary. Dobutamine stress tests are used to access the myocardial perfusion and function. Transesophageal echocardiography is used most commonly to evaluate the aorta for evidence of dissection, to elucidate evidence of atrial clots, and to assess for evidence of valvular vegetations. *(Nishimura et al., 2008, pp. 1397, 1399)*

94. **(C)** Cilostazol (a phosphodiesterase inhibitor with a mechanism of action that is unknown) increases claudication distance by 40% to 60% in patients with PAD. Pentoxifylline has been shown to improve the exercise tolerance in patients with PVD, by decreasing blood viscosity and increasing the red blood cell flexibility, but this finding has not been confirmed in all trials. Papaverine, calcium channel blockers, and alpha-adrenergic blockers, while known for the vasodilatory effects, have been shown to be ineffective in improving tissue oxygenation in patients with PVD. *(Creager and Loscalzo, 2008b, p. 1569)*

REFERENCES

Antman EM, Braunwald E. ST-Segment elevation myocardial infarction. In: Fauci AS, et al., eds. *Harrison's Principles of Internal Medicine*. New York, NY: McGraw-Hill; 2008.

Antman EM, et al. Ischemic heart disease. In: Fauci AS, et al., eds. *Harrison's Principles of Internal Medicine*. New York, NY: McGraw-Hill; 2008.

Awtry E, Colucci WS. Cardiac manifestations of systemic disease. In: Fauci AS, et al., eds. *Harrison's Principles of Internal Medicine*. New York, NY: McGraw-Hill; 2008a.

Awtry E, Colucci WS. Tumors and trauma of the heart. In: Fauci AS, et al., eds. *Harrison's Principles of Internal Medicine*. New York, NY: McGraw-Hill; 2008b.

Baim DS. Percutaneous coronary intervention. In: Fauci AS, et al., eds. *Harrison's Principles of Internal Medicine*. New York, NY: McGraw-Hill; 2008.

Bickley LS, Szilagyi PG. *Bates' Guide to Physical Examination and History Taking*. Philadelphia, PA: Lippincott Williams & Wilkins; 2009.

Braunwald E. Approach to the patient with possible cardiovascular disease. In: Fauci AS, et al., eds. *Harrison's Principles of Internal Medicine*. New York, NY: McGraw-Hill; 2008a.

Braunwald E. Pericardial disease. In: Fauci AS, et al., eds. *Harrison's Principles of Internal Medicine*. New York, NY: McGraw-Hill; 2008b.

Cannon CP, Braunwald E. Unstable angina and non-ST-elevation myocardial infarction. In: Fauci AS, et al., eds. *Harrison's Principles of Internal Medicine*. New York, NY: McGraw-Hill; 2008.

Carlson MD. Syncope. In: Fauci AS, et al., eds. *Harrison's Principles of Internal Medicine*. New York, NY: McGraw-Hill; 2008.

Child JS. Congenital heart disease in the adult. In: Fauci AS, et al., eds. *Harrison's Principles of Internal Medicine*. New York, NY: McGraw-Hill; 2008.

Creager MA. Loscalzo J. Diseases of the aorta. In: Fauci AS, et al., eds. *Harrison's Principles of Internal Medicine*. New York, NY: McGraw-Hill; 2008a.

Creager MA, Loscalzo J. Vascular diseases of the extremities. In: Fauci AS, et al., eds. *Harrison's Principles of Internal Medicine.* New York, NY: McGraw-Hill; 2008b.

Ganong WF. Cardiovascular disorders: vascular disease. In: McPhee SJ, et al., eds. *Pathophysiology of Disease.* New York, NY: Lange Books/McGraw-Hill; 2006.

Goldberger AL. *Clinical Electrocardiography.* Philadephia, PA: Mosby-Elsevier; 2006.

Goldberger AL. Electrocardiography. In: Fauci AS, et al., eds. *Harrison's Principles of Internal Medicine.* New York, NY: McGraw-Hill; 2008.

Goldhaber SZ. Deep venous thrombosis and pulmonary thromboembolism. In: Fauci AS, et al., eds. *Harrison's Principles of Internal Medicine.* New York, NY: McGraw-Hill; 2008.

Hume JR. Agents used in cardiac arrhythmias. In: Katzung BG, et al., eds. *Basic and Clinical Pharmacology.* New York, NY: McGraw-Hill; 2007.

Jameson JL, Weetman AP. Disorders of the thyroid gland. In: Fauci AS, et al., eds. *Harrison's Principles of Internal Medicine.* New York, NY: McGraw-Hill; 2008.

Kahn DH, Koos BJ. Maternal physiology during pregnancy. In: DeCherney AH, et al., eds. *Current Diagnosis & Treatment: Obstetrics & Gynecology.* 10th ed. New York, NY: McGraw-Hill; 2007.

Karchmer AW. Infective endocarditis. In: Fauci AS, et al., eds. *Harrison's Principles of Internal Medicine.* New York, NY: McGraw-Hill; 2008.

Kotchen TA. Hypertensive vascular disease. In: Fauci AS, et al., eds. *Harrison's Principles of Internal Medicine.* New York, NY: McGraw-Hill; 2008.

Kusumoto FM. Cardiovascular disorders: heart disease. In: McPhee SJ, et al., eds. *Pathophysiology of Disease.* New York, NY: Lange Books/McGraw-Hill; 2006.

Langford CA, Fauci AS. The vasculitis syndromes. In: Fauci AS, et al., eds. *Harrison's Principles of Internal Medicine.* New York, NY: McGraw-Hill; 2008.

LeBlond RF, Brown DD, DeGowin RL. *DeGowin's Diagnostic Examination.* 9th ed. New York, NY: McGraw-Hill: 2009.

Lee TH. Chest discomfort. In: Fauci AS, et al., eds. *Harrison's Principles of Internal Medicine.* New York, NY: McGraw-Hill; 2008.

Libby P. The pathogenesis, prevention and treatment of atherosclerosis. In: Fauci AS, et al., eds. *Harrison's Principles of Internal Medicine.* New York, NY: McGraw-Hill; 2008.

Loscalzo J. Basic biology of the cardiovascular system. In: Fauci AS, et al., eds. *Harrison's Principles of Internal Medicine.* New York, NY: McGraw-Hill; 2008a.

Loscalzo J. Palpitations. In: Fauci AS, et al., eds. *Harrison's Principles of Internal Medicine.* New York, NY: McGraw-Hill; 2008b.

Low PA, Engstrom JW. Disorders of the autonomic nervous system. In: Fauci AS, et al., eds. *Harrison's Principles of Internal Medicine.* New York, NY: McGraw-Hill; 2008.

Mann DL. Heart failure and cor pulmonale. In: Fauci et al., eds. *Harrison's Principles of Internal Medicine.* New York, NY: McGraw-Hill; 2008.

Marchlinski F. The tachyarrhythmias. In: Fauci AS, et al., eds. *Harrison's Principles of Internal Medicine.* New York, NY: McGraw-Hill; 2008.

Merrick SH. The heart: 1. Acquired diseases. In: Doherty GM, et al., eds. *Current Surgical Diagnosis and Treatment.* New York, NY: Lange Medical Books/McGraw-Hill; 2006.

Neumann HPH. Pheochromocytoma. In: Fauci AS, et al., eds. *Harrison's Principles of Internal Medicine.* New York, NY: McGraw-Hill; 2008.

Nishimura RA, et al. Noninvasive cardiac imaging: echocardiography, nuclear cardiology, and MRI/CT imaging. In: Fauci AS, et al., eds. *Harrison's Principles of Internal Medicine.* New York, NY: McGraw-Hill; 2008.

O'Gara P, Braunwald E. Valvular heart disease. In: Fauci AS, et al., eds. *Harrison's Principles of Internal Medicine.* New York, NY: McGraw-Hill; 2008.

O'Rourke RA, Braunwald E. Physical examination of the cardiovascular system. In: Fauci AS, et al., eds. *Harrison's Principles of Internal Medicine.* New York, NY: McGraw-Hill; 2008.

Rapp JH, et al. Arteries. In: Doherty GM, et al., eds. *Current Surgical Diagnosis and Treatment.* New York, NY: Lange Medical Books/McGraw-Hill; 2006.

Rich S. Pulmonary hypertension. In: Fauci AS, et al., eds. *Harrison's Principles of Internal Medicine.* New York, NY: McGraw-Hill; 2008.

Singer GG, Brenner, BM. Fluid and Electrolyte Disturbances. In: Fauci et al., eds. Harrison's Principles of Internal Medicine. New York, NY: McGraw-Hill; 2008.

Tomaselli GF. The bradyarrhythmias. In: Fauci AS, et al., eds. *Harrison's Principles of Internal Medicine.* New York, NY: McGraw-Hill; 2008.

Wakefield TW. Veins and lymphatics. In: Doherty GM, et al., eds. *Current Surgical Diagnosis and Treatment.* New York, NY: Lange Medical Books/McGraw-Hill; 2006.

Weitz JI. Antiplatelet, anticoagulant and fibrinolytic drugs. In: Fauci AS, et al., eds. *Harrison's Principles of Internal Medicine.* New York, NY: McGraw-Hill; 2008.

Wynne J, Braunwald E. Cardiomyopathy and myocarditis. In: Fauci AS, et al., eds. *Harrison's Principles of Internal Medicine.* New York, NY: McGraw-Hill; 2008.

CHAPTER 3

Dermatology

Michelle DiBaise, MPAS, PA-C

DIRECTIONS: Each of the numbered items or incomplete statements in this section is followed by answers or by completion of the statement. Select the ONE-lettered answer or completion that is BEST in each case.

1. Erythema with yellowish scale-forming plaques on the eyebrows, nasolabial folds, glabella, and presternal area best describes (see Figure 3-1)

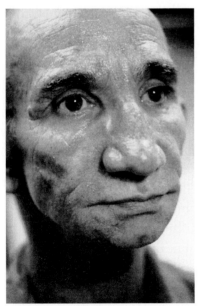

Figure 3-1
(Courtesy of Jack Cohen, DO)

   (A) bacterial folliculitis
   (B) allergic contact dermatitis
   (C) rosacea
   (D) seborrheic dermatitis

2. A 36-year-old patient reporting sudden hair loss is found to have a round, well-circumscribed, 3-cm area of alopecia on the parietal scalp area with exclamation point hair. The most likely diagnosis is

   (A) anagen effluvium
   (B) androgenetic alopecia
   (C) alopecia areata
   (D) tinea capitis

3. A Tzanck smear demonstrating multinucleated giant cells indicates which of the following conditions? (Figure 3-2)

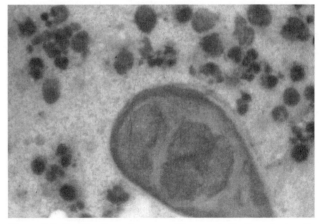

Figure 3-2. Positive Tzanck smear with arrow indicating giant mult-inucleated cell. (*Courtesy of William H. Fenn. From Rodney M (ed). Primary Care for Physician Assistants, 2nd ed. McGraw-Hill, Inc, 2001, with permission.*)

   (A) scabies
   (B) tinea versicolor
   (C) impetigo
   (D) herpes simplex

4. An acute eruption of violaceous, pruritic, polygonal, shiny, flat-topped papules involving the flexor surfaces is suggestive of which of the following?

   (A) lichen planus
   (B) pityriasis rosea
   (C) psoriasis
   (D) seborrheic dermatitis

5. Bites that typically reveal a central blue color of impending necrosis with a surrounding white area of vasospasm and a peripheral red halo of inflammation are associated with

   (A) scabies
   (B) black widow spiders
   (C) brown recluse spiders
   (D) deer ticks

6. Linear, pruritic, vesicles with underlying erythema on the hands, arms, and legs best describes

   (A) impetigo
   (B) varicella zoster virus
   (C) toxicodendron dermatitis
   (D) herpes simplex virus

7. Velvety, hyperpigmented, papillomatous lesions of the neck, axillae, and groin would warrant what further testing?

   (A) KOH (potassium hydroxide) test of skin scrapings
   (B) fasting blood sugar
   (C) mineral oil skin scraping
   (D) chest x-ray

8. A patient known to have allergic rhinitis and asthma presents with chronic pruritic inflammatory lesions of the flexor surfaces, wrists, and dorsal areas of the feet. The lesions are excoriated and lichenified with crusted patches and plaques. The most likely diagnosis is

   (A) nummular eczema
   (B) psoriasis

   (C) seborrheic dermatitis
   (D) atopic dermatitis

9. Which of the following diseases can affect the skin, nails, and joints?

   (A) erythema nodosum
   (B) psoriasis
   (C) pityriasis rosea
   (D) lichen planus

10. Using the "rule of nines" to calculate body surface area, what would the percentage of burned area be in an adult patient with second-degree burns involving the entire right arm, the anterior chest and abdomen, and the entire right leg?

    (A) 27
    (B) 36
    (C) 45
    (D) 52

11. A 65-year-old patient presents with a 4-week history of dark red pruritic urticarial plaques on the flexor surfaces. The plaques begin developing tense bullae on the surface. This clinical presentation is most suggestive of

    (A) bullous pemphigoid
    (B) bullous impetigo
    (C) pemphigus vulgaris
    (D) dermatitis herpetiformis

12. Mupirocin (Bactroban) ointment is indicated for the treatment of mild to moderate

    (A) impetigo
    (B) ecthyma gangrenosum
    (C) tinea pedis
    (D) cellulitis

13. Organ transplant recipients have a significantly increased risk for developing (see Figure 3-3)

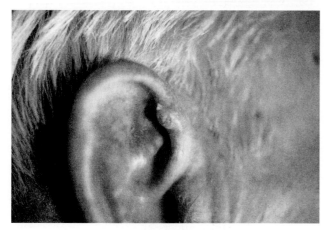

Figure 3-3
(*Courtesy of Jack Cohen, DO*)

(A) squamous cell carcinoma
(B) erythema multiforme
(C) bullous pemphigoid
(D) pseudomonas folliculitis

14. A predisposing condition for recurrent cellulitis of the lower extremity is

(A) onychomycosis
(B) tinea pedis
(C) verruca vulgaris
(D) erythema nodosum

15. A patient presents with complaints of the development of a slate-gray hyperpigmentation on the lower extremities. Which of the following agents is most likely responsible?

(A) minocycline (Minocin)
(B) erythromycin (E-Mycin)
(C) trimethoprim-sulfamethoxazole (Septra DS)
(D) Naproxen (Aleve)

16. A 12-year-old girl presents with complaints of pruritis of the scalp for 2 weeks that started at the occiput and postauricular areas but has now spread. Based on Figure 3-4, the most likely diagnosis is

(A) psoriasis
(B) seborrheic dermatitis
(C) pediculosis capitis
(D) tinea capitis

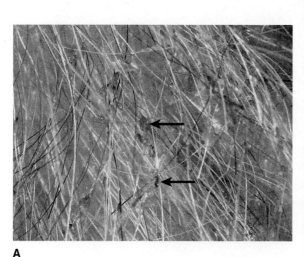
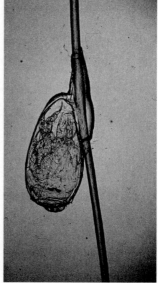

A   B

Figure 3-4
(*Reproduced with permission from Fitzpatrick, Johnson, Wolff, et al. Dermatology in General Medicine, 4th ed. New York: McGraw-Hill, 1993.*)

17. A 22-year-old patient presents with multiple, flat, round, light brown lesions measuring 1 to 5 mm in diameter as noted in Figure 3-5.

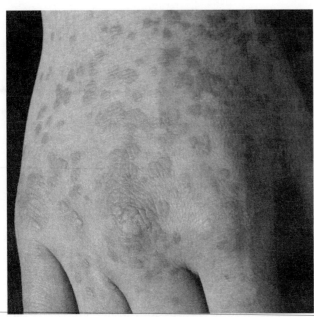

Figure 3-5
(*Reproduced, with permission, from Wolff K, Johnson RA, Suurmond D. Fitzpatrick's Color Atlas & Synopsis of Clinical Dermatology. 5th ed. New York: McGraw-Hill, 2005:781.*)

Several are noted to form a linear pattern. The most likely diagnosis is

(A) lichen planus
(B) verruca plana
(C) seborrheic keratoses
(D) syringomas

18. A nursing home patient with a history of diabetes develops an indurated, painful, crusted ulcer with surrounding erythema on the anterior shin as seen in Figure 3-6. The most likely diagnosis is

(A) ecthyma
(B) porphyria cutanea tarda
(C) decubitus ulcer
(D) bullous pemphigoid

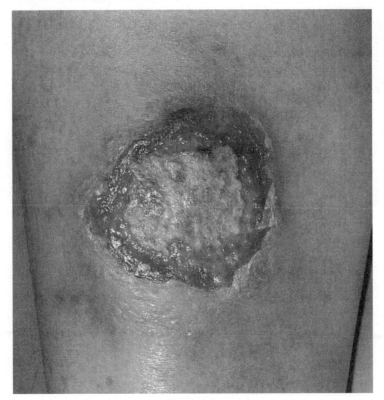

Figure 3-6
(*Reproduced, with permission, from Wolff K, Johnson RA, Suurmond D. Fitzpatrick's Color Atlas & Synopsis of Clinical Dermatology. 5th ed. New York: McGraw-Hill, 2005:594.*)

19. Perifollicular purpura, corkscrew hair, and gingival bleeding are most likely due to what deficiency?

   (A) vitamin A
   (B) vitamin B$_{12}$
   (C) vitamin C
   (D) vitamin K

20. A 19-year-old presents with the minimally pruritic rash seen in Figure 3-7. The lesion on the right chest was the first to appear, followed a week later by the remaining lesions. He states he had cold-like symptoms about a week before the eruption, but feels fine now. The most likely diagnosis is

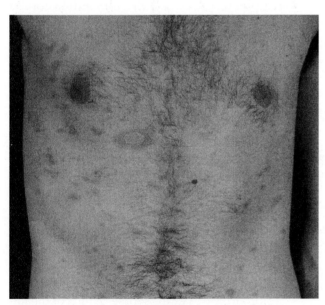

Figure 3-7
(Reproduced, with permission, from Wolff K, Johnson RA, Suurmond D. Fitzpatrick's Color Atlas & Synopsis of Clinical Dermatology. 5th ed. New York: McGraw-Hill, 2005:119.)

   (A) tinea corporis
   (B) scabies
   (C) guttate psoriasis
   (D) pityriasis rosea

21. A 17-year-old white female presents to a family practice office to clear up a rash that has come and gone for a number of years, but now wants to wear a strapless dress to prom. The lesions are discrete, hyperpigmented, and velvety on the chest, shoulders, and upper back. Which of the following is the best treatment option?

   (A) topical glucocorticoid
   (B) selenium sulfide shampoo
   (C) topical 4% hydroquinone
   (D) cryotherapy

22. A 45-year-old African American woman presents with an indurated, reddish orange lesion on her cheek and indurated painful nodules on the shins bilaterally. The most important diagnostic test to order is

   (A) an erythrocyte sedimentation rate
   (B) a complete blood cell count
   (C) an electrocardiogram
   (D) a chest x-ray

23. The best management for a 4-mm macular lesion that is asymmetrical, black and red, located on the left forearm, and has progressed rapidly over the past 6 months, would be to

   (A) have the patient document changes to the lesion in a journal for 4 months
   (B) schedule visits with a provider every 6 months to photograph changes
   (C) remove the lesion with a vascular laser
   (D) completely excise the lesion as soon as possible

24. A patient with recurrent erythema multiforme minor lesions approximately every month should be treated prophylactically with

   (A) oral steroids
   (B) acyclovir
   (C) dapsone
   (D) oral terbinafine

25. Painful, erythematous, indurated nodules on the lower extremities of a woman on an oral contraceptive pill is most likely

   (A) erythema nodosum
   (B) erythema multiforme
   (C) erythema annulare centrifugum
   (D) erythema chronica migrans

26. Thickening of the epidermis secondary to scratching best describes

    (A) lichen striatus
    (B) lichen planus
    (C) lichen simplex chronicus
    (D) lichen nitidus

27. Onycholysis with oil spots is pathognomonic for

    (A) liver disease
    (B) tinea unguium
    (C) eczema
    (D) psoriasis

28. The presence of 1- to 2-mm, dome-shaped, umbilicated, waxy papules is due to what etiology?

    (A) varicella zoster virus
    (B) pox virus
    (C) chronic sun damage
    (D) *Staphylococcus aureus*

29. Folliculitis under occlusion of a bathing suit is most likely secondary to

    (A) *Staphylococcus aureus*
    (B) *Candida albicans*
    (C) group A β-hemolytic streptococcus
    (D) *Pseudomonas aeruginosa*

30. Pink lesions on the distal extremities and face that rapidly depigment best describes

    (A) vitiligo
    (B) pityriasis alba
    (C) guttate psoriasis
    (D) contact dermatitis

31. Which of the following is the best treatment option for a 2-cm plaque of Bowen's disease (squamous cell carcinoma in situ) on the lower leg of a young woman with concerns about her cosmetic outcome?

    (A) topical imiquimod
    (B) topical clobetasol
    (C) intralesional glucocorticoid
    (D) surgical excision

32. A 1-cm pearly papule with central ulceration and telangiectasias on the left temple of a 67-year-old man is most likely

    (A) rosacea
    (B) basal cell carcinoma
    (C) ecthyma
    (D) sebaceous gland hyperplasia

33. Comedonal acne is best treated with

    (A) benzoyl peroxide
    (B) topical antibiotics
    (C) oral antibiotics
    (D) topical retinoids

34. A 64-year-old man with a history of Hodgkin lymphoma presents with a 6-month history of a fish-like scale most prominent on the lower extremities that is getting progressively worse. He has no history of atopy and is currently on no medications. Which of the following is the most likely diagnosis?

    (A) ichthyosis vulgaris
    (B) eczema craquelé
    (C) acquired ichthyosis
    (D) lichen simplex chronicus

35. A 53-year-old white woman presents with flushing that she notes is worse when she has her morning coffee and when she is stressed at work. She is starting to get broken blood vessels on her face. She notes an increase in acne lesions that are getting worse. Which of the following is the most likely diagnosis?

    (A) impetigo
    (B) folliculitis
    (C) acne vulgaris
    (D) rosacea

36. The causative organism of erythema chronica migrans is

    (A) *Treponema pallidum*
    (B) *Borrelia burgdorferi*
    (C) *Bartonella henselae*
    (D) *Rickettsia rickettsii*

37. A 16-year-old female patient with type 1 diabetes mellitus presents with a lesion on the finger pad of the fourth digit of the left hand. She states it came up rapidly and bleeds easily if she bumps it. On physical examination, you note a vascular, sessile, dome-shaped lesion. What is the most likely diagnosis?

    (A) pyoderma gangrenosum
    (B) nodular melanoma
    (C) pyogenic granuloma
    (D) cherry angioma

38. A 47-year-old man presents to clinic with complaints of blisters that form on sun-exposed areas of skin, leaving behind scars. He admits to being an alcoholic but has been sober for the past 6 months. On physical examination you note atrophic scars and milia on the dorsum of the hands. He has a tense bulla noted on his fifth digit of the right hand. He is also noted to have hypertrichosis of the face. Which of the following disorders would you test for?

    (A) human immunodeficiency virus
    (B) hepatitis C virus
    (C) herpes simplex virus
    (D) Coxsackie virus

39. A 32-year-old patient presents with grouped vesicles that are intensely pruritic noted on the elbows, knees, sacral area, and buttocks. The patient has also noted a chronic diarrhea. Immunofluorescence of a skin biopsy shows IgA deposits. The most effective course of treatment for this patient's skin rash would be which of the following?

    (A) acyclovir
    (B) a gluten-free diet
    (C) topical glucocorticoids
    (D) dapsone

40. Which of the following forms of alopecia occur because of sensitivity to dihydrotestosterone (DHT)?

    (A) alopecia areata
    (B) androgenetic alopecia
    (C) telogen effluvium
    (D) anagen effluvium

Answers and Explanations

1. **(D)** This is a classic distribution pattern for seborrheic dermatitis, a common, chronic inflammatory dermatitis associated with *Pityrosporum ovale* as well as genetic and environmental factors. Bacterial folliculitis presents as dome-shaped pustules with small erythematous halos arising in the center of hair follicles. Allergic contact dermatitis is characterized by vesicles, edema, erythema, and pruritus. Rosacea presents as eruptions of erythema, telangiectasias, pustules, and papules localized to the face. *(Schwartz et al., 2007, p. 807)*

2. **(C)** Alopecia areata is an autoimmune process presenting as localized, well-circumscribed loss of hair in oval or round patterns without visible evidence of inflammation, most commonly on the scalp with exclamation point hair at the periphery of alopecia. Anagen effluvium is diffuse hair loss involving the entire scalp and is commonly caused by drugs or chemotherapy. Androgenetic alopecia is progressive balding secondary to genetic predisposition and the influence of androgen and typically spares the parietal region. Tinea capitis is uncommon in adults. It has "black dots" in the area of alopecia from broken-off hair, also with scale and possibly inflammation. There also may be adenopathy. *(Eickhorst and Levit, 2010, pp. 776-780; Kelso and Raimer, 2010, pp. 836-837)*

3. **(D)** The Tzanck smear is a microscopic examination of cells obtained from the base of vesicles and bullae for multinucleated giant cells seen in herpes simplex, herpes zoster, and varicella. Scabies is diagnosed with a scabies prep, a microscopic examination for mites, scybala (fecal pellets), or eggs. Tinea versicolor is a dermatophyte infection diagnosed with a potassium hydroxide (KOH) test looking for hyphae and spores in a classic spaghetti-and-meatballs pattern. Impetigo is caused by streptococci and/or staphylococci typically diagnosed by the clinical presentation, but culture and sensitivity tests can isolate the causative organism(s). *(Kelso and Raimer, 2010, pp. 836-837; Losi-Sasaki and Moore, 2010, pp. 828-830; Nichols, 2008, pp. 824-827)*

4. **(A)** Lichen planus is an inflammatory reaction pattern of unknown etiology, with characteristic "five P" clinical features: pruritic, planar (flat), polyangular/polygonal, purple (violaceous) papules. Pityriasis rosea is typically confined to the trunk, beginning with a single red oval plaque that is followed by a number of similar smaller plaques with spontaneous resolution in 4 to 8 weeks. Psoriasis is a papulosquamous disease commonly presenting as scaly plaques involving the elbows, knees, and scalp. Seborrheic dermatitis is a common, chronic inflammatory disease commonly seen on the scalp and scalp margins, eyebrows, nasolabial folds, and presternal areas. *(Moses, 2010, pp. 31-35)*

5. **(C)** Brown recluse (*Loxoscelidae recluses*) spider bites in fatty areas such as thighs and buttocks can become necrotic within 4 hours; with a rapidly expanding blue-gray halo around the puncture site surrounded by a white area of vasospasm and a peripheral red halo of inflammation. Scabies (*Sarcoptes scabiei*) lesions are pleomorphic and often vesicular, pustular, or excoriated with linear, curved, or S-shaped burrows. Black widow (*Latrodectus mactans*) bites result in slight swelling with small red fang

marks. Deer tick (*Ixodes dammini*) lesions can present as a small papule with a slowly enlarging ring (erythema migrans), a bluish red nodule (Borrelia lymphocytoma), or an atrophic plaque (acrodermatitis chronica atrophicans). *(Haroz and Roberts, 2010, p. 1136; Katsambas and Nicolaidou, 2010, pp. 834-835; Weinstein and Wani, 2010, pp. 138-141)*

6. **(C)** Allergic phytocontact dermatitis due to the toxicodendrons occurs most commonly on areas at risk of contact (hands, arms, and legs) with the plants of poison ivy, poison sumac, or poison oak. They form linear pruritic vesicles caused by the resin of the plant being dragged by scratching. Impetigo may or may not be pruritic but occurs mainly on the face (nose and mouth). Varicella is pruritic, unilateral (in zoster form), and predominantly noted on the trunk. Herpes simplex virus, generally more painful than pruritic, occurs either around the lips and nose or on the genitalia. *(Anderson and Marks Jr., 2007, pp. 1277-1279; Losi-Sasaki and Moore, 2010, pp. 828-830; Nichols, 2008, pp. 824-827)*

7. **(B)** Acanthosis nigricans is commonly associated with obesity, insulin resistance, and diabetes mellitus. A fasting blood sugar is a first step in screening patients for insulin resistance. Potassium hydroxide (KOH) of skin scrapings is used to look for hyphae and spores indicating a fungal infection or tinea versicolor. While tinea versicolor is velvety and can be hyperpigmented, it is not papillomatous. Mineral oil skin scrapings are used to look for the mites of scabies. Scabies can occur in the axillae but appear as erythematous papules or nodules. A chest x-ray would be used to look for pulmonary changes associated with cutaneous findings, such as sarcoidosis. Acanthosis nigricans is not associated with pulmonary changes. *(Katsambas and Nicolaidou, 2008, pp. 834-835; Kong et al, 2007; Raimer, 2010, pp. 836-837; Sharma and Mohan, 2010, pp. 271-272)*

8. **(D)** Atopic dermatitis often occurs in association with a family or personal history of atopy, to include allergic rhinitis, asthma, and eczema. It is characterized as the "itch that rashes" and is associated with dry skin, ichthyosis vulgaris, keratosis pilaris, sensitivity to wool, and hyper-

linear palmar creases. Psoriasis is a papulosquamous disease commonly presenting as scaly plaques involving the elbows, knees, and scalp. Nummular eczema presents as chronic, coin-shaped plaques with small papules and vesicles on an erythematous base, typically seen on the lower legs of older men in winter months. Seborrheic dermatitis presents as erythema with yellowish scale-forming plaques on the eyebrows, nasolabial folds, glabella, and presternal area of the chest. *(Chamlin, 2010, pp. 848-850; Lee and Koo, 2010, pp. 789-792; Moses, 2010, pp. 31-35; Schwartz et al., 2007, p. 807, Morelli, 2007c)*

9. **(B)** In addition to erythematous scaly papules and plaques, psoriasis may present with oil spots, nail pitting, and onycholysis. Psoriatic arthritis occurs in 5% to 8% of those affected with psoriasis. Erythema nodosum is an inflammatory nodular pattern of panniculitis typically involving only the lower extremities. Pityriasis rosea is an epidermal papulosquamous disorder typically confined to the trunk, with no nail or joint involvement. Lichen planus is characterized as an inflammatory reaction pattern with mucous membrane, nail, scalp, and cutaneous lesions but no associated joint involvement. *(Lee and Koo, 2010, pp. 789-792; Moses, 2010, pp. 31-35; Schwartz and Nervi, 2007, pp. 695-700)*

10. **(C)** The anterior chest and abdomen are 18%, the entire right leg is 18%, and the entire right arm is 9%, for a total of 45% body surface area. *(Latenser, 2010, p. 1121)*

11. **(A)** Bullous pemphigoid is a subepidermal blistering disease presenting on the flexor surfaces of elderly patients. A hallmark is the presence of tense bullae overlying erythematous plaques. Direct immunofluorescence is positive for IgG and C3 deposition at the dermal—epidermal junction. Bullous impetigo is a superficial skin infection caused by streptococci and/or staphylococci, with flaccid vesicles typically distributed on the face and distal extremities in children and adolescents. Pemphigus vulgaris presents as multiple flaccid (suprabasilar intraepidermal) blisters from one to several centimeters in diameter, often

involving the oral mucosa and skin from the neck to the knees. Direct immunofluorescence is positive for epidermal intercellular IgG deposition. Dermatitis herpetiformis is a gluten-sensitive enteropathy presenting with severe pruritus and clustered herpetiform grouped vesicles on the elbows, knees, sacrum, nuchal area, shoulders, and buttocks. Direct immunofluorescence is positive for granular deposition of IgA in the dermal papillary tips. *(Dick and Werth, 2008, pp. 854-858)*

12. **(A)** Mupirocin is the first topical antibiotic approved for the treatment of impetigo. Ecthyma gangrenosum is typically treated with oral or parenteral antibiotics. Tinea pedis is a dermatophyte infection treated with antifungals. Cellulitis typically requires treatment with oral or parenteral antibiotics. *(Nichols, 2008, pp. 824-827)*

13. **(A)** Immunosuppressive agents required following organ transplant greatly increase the risk (65- to 250-fold) for developing squamous cell carcinoma. Erythema multiforme, a reaction pattern of idiopathic, drug, and infectious origin, is unrelated to organ transplant immunosuppression, as is bullous pemphigoid, an autoimmune subepidermal blistering disease. Pseudomonas folliculitis is an acute skin infection that follows exposure to contaminated water and is also known as "hot tub folliculitis." *(Ajithkumar, 2007; pp. 921-932; Dick and Werth, 2008, pp. 854-858; Nichols, 2008, pp. 824-827)*

14. **(B)** Fungal infection of the interdigital spaces can result in breaks in the dermal barrier, permitting bacterial entry through the skin, and requires careful examination of the feet in lower extremity cellulitis. Onychomycosis typically involves the nail plate and not the surrounding soft tissue. Common warts (verruca vulgaris) are not likely to lead to breaks in the dermis because they arise from the epidermis. Erythema nodosum, a hypersensitivity reaction to a variety of antigenic stimuli, typically presents as erythematous nodules over the anterior shin area and is not associated with the development of cellulitis. *(Housman and Williford, 2010, pp. 811-816, 840; Nichols, 2008, pp. 824-827;*

Piraccini and Lorizzo, 2010, pp. 804-808; Schwartz and Nervi, 2007, pp. 695-700)

15. **(A)** Slate-gray hyperpigmentation is an adverse effect of minocycline. Cutaneous side effects of erythromycin typically include urticaria, maculopapular rash, erythema, and acute generalized exanthematous pustulosis (AGEP). Adverse cutaneous effects to trimethoprim-sulfamethoxazole include Stevens–Johnson syndrome, toxic epidermal necrolysis (TEN), erythema multiforme, exfoliative dermatitis, angioedema, Henoch-Schönlein purpura (leukocytoclastic vasculitis), serum sickness-like syndrome, maculopapular rash, erythema nodosum, conjunctival and scleral injection, lupus-like symptoms, periarteritis nodosa, photosensitivity, and urticaria. Adverse cutaneous effects to naproxen include pruritus, ecchymoses, urticaria, alopecia, pseudoporphyria, epidermolysis bullosa, and photosensitive dermatitis. *(Physicians' Desk Reference, 2009)*

16. **(C)** *Pediculosis capitis* (head lice) begins most commonly at the occiput and postauricular area where grayish white, oval-shaped nits are seen adhered to the hair shaft. Psoriasis presents with well-demarcated, erythematous plaques with silvery white scale. Seborrheic dermatitis presents with diffuse erythema with a greasy yellow scale throughout the scalp. Tinea capitis appears as an area of alopecia with scale and broken off hair or "black dots". *(Katsambas and Nicolaidou, 2010, pp. 834-835; Lee and Koo 2010, pp. 789-792; Moses, 2010, pp. 31-35; Raimer, 2008, pp. 836-837; Schwartz et al., 2007, p. 807)*

17. **(B)** Flat warts or verruca plana are light brown- or flesh-colored papules ranging from 1 to 5 mm in diameter. Because the virus spreads with scratching or shaving, a linear pattern forms. Lichen planus lesions are pruritic, planar (flat), polyangular/polygonal, purple papules, generally seen on the volar aspects of the wrist and forearm as opposed to the dorsum. Seborrheic keratoses range from 2 mm to 3 cm, can be tan, brown, or black in color, can appear on the dorsum of the hands, but do not form a linear pattern secondary to trauma. Syringomas are small firm yellowish white

papules that occur on the lower eyelids, forehead, chest, and abdomen. *(Duvic, 2010, pp. 2957-2959; Housman and Williford, 2008, pp. 811-816, 840; Morelli, 2007b, p. 2766; Moses, 2010, pp. 31-35)*

18. **(A)** Ecthyma is caused by group A β-hemolytic streptococcus and seen most commonly in diabetic patients, the elderly, alcoholic patients, and patients with poor hygiene. It is usually found on the lower extremities. Porphyria cutanea tarda is caused by a combination of genetic predisposition and alcohol abuse or hepatitis C infection and presents with vesicles, scarring, and milia on sun-exposed surfaces, most commonly the dorsum of the hands. Decubitus ulcers occur from pressure over bony prominences (ie, the sacrum, ischial tuberosities, iliac crest, heels, elbows, knees, malleoli, and scapula) in bedridden patients. Bullous pemphigoid is an autoimmune disease that presents with multiple tense bullae that can rupture or ulcerate most commonly on the lower abdomen, groin, and flexural areas on the arms and legs. *(Dick and Werth, 2008, pp. 854-858; Morelli, 2007a, p. 2740; Thomas, 2010, pp. 846-848)*

19. **(C)** Scurvy (vitamin C deficiency) presents with petechiae around the hair follicles, corkscrew hair, and gingival bleeding. Vitamin A deficiency presents with phrynoderma or "toad-skin," which is perifollicular hyperkeratosis, in addition to keratomalacia. Vitamin B_{12} deficiency, or pernicious anemia, is associated with vitiligo, alopecia areata, and premature graying of the hair. Vitamin K deficiency leads to clotting abnormalities and the presence of purpura but will not have corkscrew hair present. *(Mason, 2008, pp. 1626-1639)*

20. **(D)** Pityriasis rosea starts with the herald patch and then 7 to 10 days later smaller ovoid lesions with inverse collarette of scale erupt following the skin lines in a Christmas tree pattern. It is usually preceded by symptoms of an upper respiratory infection before the eruption begins. The lesions do not follow the skin lines. A KOH will help confirm a diagnosis of tinea. Scabies presents with burrows at the edge of vesicles or papules and excoriations in the interdigital web spaces, axillae, groin, breasts,

buttocks, wrist, and waist-band area. Guttate psoriasis presents as a sudden eruption of small 2- to 10-mm scattered, discrete, salmon-pink plaques that may still retain the silvery white scale of psoriasis. Up to two-thirds of patients have a preceding streptococcal pharyngitis. *(Katsambas and Nicolaidou, 2010, pp. 834-835; Lee and Koo, 2010, pp. 789-792; Raimer, 2008, pp. 836-837; Nahary et al., 2008, pp. 441-449)*

21. **(B)** Tinea versicolor comes and goes but tends to flare in hot and humid weather. Treatment options include selenium sulfide shampoo daily in the warm months and 2 to 3 times per week in the cooler months. Alternatively, patients can be treated with ketoconazole 400 mg po once followed by vigorous exercise (to induce sweating) or with topical ketoconazole shampoo. Topical glucocorticoids will exacerbate the condition. Topical hydroquinone (4%) is a bleaching agent that could even out skin pigment but will not affect the tinea versicolor. Cryotherapy is not indicated as a therapy option and could leave permanent hypopigmentation of the skin. *(Raimer, 2008, pp. 836-837)*

22. **(D)** Sarcoidosis is commonly seen in middle-aged, African American women. The lesions are reddish orange to purple indurated nodules and plaques with a predilection for the central face. It is associated with erythema nodosum and elevated angiotensin-converting enzyme levels in up to 60% of all patients with sarcoidosis. Sarcoidosis affects many organs but most commonly the lungs and eyes; therefore, a chest x-ray looking for pulmonary infiltrates and an ophthalmology examination are necessary diagnostic steps. *(Sharma and Mohan, 2010, pp. 271-272)*

23. **(D)** Based on the ABCDE criteria, this lesion falls into four categories: asymmetrical, irregular borders, two colors particularly black and red, which are ominous, and rapid enlargement or elevation. It is less than 6 mm in diameter. However, this lesion is highly suspicious for a melanoma and should be excised as soon as possible for diagnosis. *(Haluska, 2010, pp. 891-892)*

24. **(B)** Recurrent erythema multiforme is most commonly due to recurrent herpes simplex virus outbreaks. Prophylactic treatment with acyclovir or related compound should suppress future herpes simplex virus outbreaks, and therefore, future erythema multiforme recurrences. *(Losi-Sasaki and Moore, 2010, pp. 828-830)*

25. **(A)** Erythema nodosum presents with painful nodules generally on the lower extremities. The most common causes are oral contraceptive use, sarcoidosis, and Behçets. Erythema multiforme is usually due to herpes simplex virus infection or a drug reaction, but the lesions are targetoid in appearance. Erythema annulare centrifugum presents as one or more urticarial-type papules that enlarge to form indurated ringed lesions that may herald a systemic lupus, Lyme disease, or internal malignancy. Erythema chronica migrans is the classic rash associated with Lyme disease and is usually a solitary ringed lesion at the site of the tick bite. *(Requena and Yus, 2008, pp. 425-438; Tonneson, 2010, pp. 850-851; Weinstein and Wani, 2010, pp. 138-141; Ziemer et al., 2009, pp. 119-126)*

26. **(C)** Lichen simplex chronicus is the name for lichenification that occurs secondary to scratching. Lichen striatus presents as tiny 1- to 2-mm, flat-topped, scaly erythematous papules, in a linear configuration along Blaschko lines, most commonly occurring on the limbs, and less frequently on the trunk, face, neck, or buttocks. Lichen planus presents as purple, polygonal, planar papules. Lichen nitidus is multiple, discrete smooth, flat papules that are flesh-colored and can appear throughout the body. *(Morelli, 2007b, pp. 2706-2707; Moses, 2010, pp. 31-35)*

27. **(D)** Nail disease in psoriasis presents with onycholysis and a yellowish brown discoloration under the nail plate resembling oil spots. Nail pitting can also be seen, but nail pits are also noted in eczema. Liver disease can present with Terry nails where the nail bed is white with a normal distal band (cirrhosis) or in the case of Wilson disease, azure (blue) lunulae. Tinea unguium presents as thickened, yellow, crumbly nails. *(Piraccini and Lorizzo, 2010, pp. 804-808)*

28. **(B)** Molluscum contagiosum is described as 1- to 2-mm, dome-shaped, umbilicated waxy papules. Varicella starts as erythematous papules that progress to vesicles, then pustules that umbilicate and crust in crops. Basal cell carcinoma can have central ulceration but are not waxy lesions and generally are larger than 1 to 2 mm. In addition, they usually have telangiectasias on the lesion that are not seen in molluscum. Impetigo begins as vesicles or bulla that umbilicate and then rapidly becomes a honey-colored crust. *(Losi-Sasaki and Moore, 2010, pp. 828-830; Morelli, 2007a and d , p. 2766; Nichols, 2008, pp. 824-827)*

29. **(D)** Hot tub folliculitis occurs under areas of occlusion of the bathing suit and is usually due to improperly cleaned hot tubs caused by *Pseudomonas aeruginosa*. *Staphylococcus aureus* tends to occur in areas of trauma, such as shaving with a predilection of the beard area in men and the legs in women. Group A β-hemolytic streptococcus does not generally cause a folliculitis. It tends to cause impetiginization of open skin areas. *Candida albicans* folliculitis is seen in febrile bedridden patients generally on the back due to occlusion. *(Nichols, 2008, pp. 824-827; Raimer, 2008, pp. 836-837)*

30. **(A)** Vitiligo presents as pink lesions that depigment on the acral extremities and central face (periorbital and perioral areas). Pityriasis alba is hypopigmentation secondary to an inflammatory rash of eczema. Guttate psoriasis are pink–red teardrop lesions of psoriasis but do not depigment. Contact dermatitis presents as erythematous areas that on resolution can leave postinflammatory hypopigmentation but not depigmentation. *(Chamlin, 2010, pp. 848-850; Lee and Koo, 2010, 789-792; Nahary et al., 2008, pp. 441-449; Szepietowski and Reich, 2010, pp. 866-867)*

31. **(A)** Intralesional steroids are of no benefit in the treatment of squamous cell carcinoma in situ. Topical clobetasol, a glucocorticoid, will also have no effect on squamous cell carcinoma. Of the other two modalities, imiquimod topically and surgical excision will both lead to resolution of Bowen disease or squamous cell carcinoma in situ. However, because the plaque is 2 cm in size, the use of imiquimod will lead to resolution

without scarring, so it is the better choice in this scenario. *(Jacobs and Orengo, 2010, pp. 781-784)*

32. **(B)** Basal cell carcinoma is most commonly found on the sun-exposed areas of the face (temples, nose, cheeks), behind the ears in men, and upper back/shoulders. They generally appear in the fifth and sixth decades of life and are noted to have central ulceration and telangiectasias. Rosacea is adult acne characterized by papules, pustules, a notable absence of comedones, and flushing that can lead to permanent telangiectasia formation on the central face. Ecthyma is caused by group A β-hemolytic streptococcus and seen most commonly in diabetic patients, the elderly, and alcoholic patients and is usually found on the lower extremities. Sebaceous gland hyperplasia are enlarged oil glands, approximately 2 to 4 mm, yellowish white, with telangiectasias and generally more than one are noted on the forehead, nose, and cheeks, but rarely, if ever, get as large as 1 cm. *(Duvic, 2008, pp. 2957-2959; Feldman and Fleischer, 2010, pp. 773-774; Jacobs and Orengo, 2010, pp. 781-784; Morelli, 2007, p. 2740)*

33. **(D)** The four treatment areas for acne are decrease sebum production, normalize abnormal desquamation of follicular epithelium, inhibit *Propionibacterium acnes* proliferation and colonization, and reduce the inflammatory response. Topical retinoids normalize follicular desquamation, which is the key factor in comedonal production. They also reduce the inflammatory response preventing the development of papules and pustules. Benzoyl peroxide and topical and oral antibiotics have a weak effect on comedones and follicular desquamation, but rather all three work to inhibit *P. acnes* proliferation and colonization as well as reduce the inflammatory response. *(Feldman and Fleischer, 2010, pp. 773-774)*

34. **(C)** HIV infection, lymphoma, sarcoidosis, and thyroid disease are all associated with the development of acquired ichthyosis, a sudden appearance of fish-like scales, usually on the lower extremities, but possibly throughout the entire body. Ichthyosis vulgaris is a heritable form of ichthyosis that presents with the triad of atopic dermatitis, keratosis pilaris, and ichthyosis generally on the lower extremities. Eczema craquelé is also referred to as asteatotic eczema or winter itch and occurs in high temperature/low humidity environments (heated homes and desert climates). It is more common in older patients and presents as dry, cracked skin with pruritis. Lichen simplex chronicus is the name for lichenification that occurs secondary to scratching. *(Chamlin, 2010, pp. 848-850; Moore and Devere, 2008, pp. 17-29; Morelli, 2007c, pp. 2708-2714; Moses, 2010, pp. 31-35; Roberts, 2006, pp. 271-280)*

35. **(D)** Impetigo presents with vesicles that rapidly become honey-colored crusts around the nose and mouth predominantly. Folliculitis and acne vulgaris both have pustules that arise from hair follicles. Neither will have associated flushing and telangiectasia. Rosacea presents with erythematous papules and pustules, a noted absence of comedones, and flushing that is exacerbated by caffeine, alcohol, stress, extremes of temperature, and certain foods. *(Feldman and Fleischer, 2010, pp. 773-774; Nichols, 2008, pp. 824-827)*

36. **(B)** *Borrelia burgdorferi* is the causative organism of Lyme disease of which erythema chronica migrans is the distinctive rash. *Treponema pallidum* is the causative organism of syphilis. *Bartonella henselae* is the causative organism of cat scratch disease, bacillary angiomatosis, and bacillary peliosis hepatitis. *Rickettsia rickettsii* is the causative organism of Rocky Mountain spotted fever. *(Anderson and Sexton, 2010, pp. 175-176; Shah, 2010, pp. 744-745; Smith, 2010, pp. 167-169; Weinstein and Wani, 2010, pp. 138-141)*

37. **(C)** Pyogenic granulomas occur frequently after trauma and can occur anywhere on the body. They arise rapidly and are sessile and friable. Nodular melanoma should be kept in the differential and a biopsy considered. However, based on the history and the fact that nodular melanomas in this age group are quite rare, it is less likely to be the diagnosis. Cherry angiomas are generally not sessile, but rather small, red papules that predominantly occur on the trunk. They are hereditary and do not arise from trauma. Pyoderma gangrenosum lesions begin as a pustule that enlarges into a

violaceous plaque, which eventually ulcerates. It is associated most commonly with inflammatory bowel disease and rheumatoid arthritis. *(Baran and Richert, 2006, pp. 297–311; Duvic, 2008, pp. 2957-2959; Gedalia, 2007, p. 1033; Haluska, 2010, pp. 891-892; Jacobs and Orengo, 2010, pp. 781-784)*

38. **(B)** The patient has symptoms that would indicate a diagnosis of porphyria cutanea tarda (PCT). This can be an acquired or inherited defect in hepatic uroporphyrinogen decarboxylase. PCT can manifest in the presence of iron overload, ethanol abuse, hepatitis C, and estrogen use, although most patients in the United States have concomitant hepatitis C. Therefore, all patients with PCT should be screened for hepatitis C. The other diseases do not impact the formation or course of PCT. *(Bonkovsky and Thapar, 2010, p. 473)*

39. **(D)** Dermatitis herpetiformis (DH) is an IgA-mediated presentation of celiac sprue with intense pruritus, grouped papules and vesicles on the extensor surfaces of the elbows, knees, buttocks, and back. Dapsone is the first-line therapy for DH. Other medications that can be used include sulfapyridine, tetracycline, niacinamide, heparin, colchicine, azathioprine, prednisone, and cholestyramine. A gluten-free diet is important for the long-term management of celiac sprue, but it may not clear the skin lesions without the use of dapsone. *(Dick and Werth, 2010, pp. 854-858)*

40. **(B)** In androgenetic alopecia in men, 5-α reductase activity and DHT are increased as opposed to nonbalding scalp skin. Therefore, finasteride (Propecia), a 5-α reductase inhibitor, can halt or slow further hair loss in men. Alopecia areata is due to an autoimmune disorder in which antibodies to the hair follicles are produced leading to alopecia. Telogen effluvium occurs after trauma and physical and emotional stressors, which leads to an increase in diffuse shedding. Anagen effluvium occurs generally after chemotherapy or radiation therapy. *(Eickhorst and Levit, 2010, p. 779)*

REFERENCES

Ajithkumar TV. Management of solid tumours in organ transplant recipients. *Lancet Oncol.* 2007;8(10):921-932.

Anderson DJ, Sexton DJ. Rickettsial and ehrlichial infections. In: Rakel RE, Bope ET, eds. *Conn's Current Therapy.* Philadelphia, PA: Saunders, Elsevier, Inc; 2010.

Anderson BE, Marks JG Jr. Plant-induced dermatitis: In: Auerbach PS, ed. 5th ed. *Wilderness Medicine.* Philadelphia, PA : MOSBY ELSEVIER, 2007:127.

Baran R, Richert B. Common nail tumors. *Dermatol Clin.* 2006;24(3):297-311.

Bonkovsky HL, Thapar M. Porphyria. In: Rakel RE, Bope ET, eds. *Conn's Current Therapy.* Philadelphia, PA: Saunders, Elsevier, Inc; 2010.

Chamlin SL. Atopic dermatitis. In: Rakel RE, Bope ET, eds. *Conn's Current Therapy.* Philadelphia, PA: Saunders, Elsevier, Inc; 2010.

Dick SE, Werth V. Bullous diseases. In: Rakel RE, Bope ET, eds. *Conn's Current Therapy.* Philadelphia, PA: Saunders, Elsevier, Inc; 2010.

Duvic M. Urticaria, drug hypersensitivity rashes, nodules and tumors, and atrophic diseases. In: Goldman L, Ausiello D, eds. *Cecil Medicine.* 23rd ed. Philadelphia, PA: Saunders, Elsevier, Inc; 2008.

Eickhorst KM, Levit E. Diseases of the hair. In: Rakel RE, Bope ET, eds. *Conn's Current Therapy.* Philadelphia, PA: Saunders, Elsevier, Inc; 2010.

Feldman SR, Fleischer AB. Acne vulgaris and rosacea. In: Rakel RE, Bope ET, eds. *Conn's Current Therapy.* Philadelphia, PA: Saunders, Elsevier, Inc; 2010.

Gedalia A. Hereditary periodic fever syndromes. In: Kliegman RM, Behrman RE, Jenson HB, Stanton BF, eds. *Nelson Textbook of Pediatrics.* Philadelphia, PA: Saunders, Elsevier, Inc; 2007.

Haluska FD. Melanoma. In: Rakel RE, Bope ET, eds. *Conn's Current Therapy.* Philadelphia, PA: Saunders, Elsevier, Inc; 2010.

Haroz R, Roberts JR. Spider bites and scorpion stings. In: Rakel RE, Bope ET, eds. *Conn's Current Therapy.* Philadelphia, PA: Saunders, Elsevier, Inc; 2010.

Housman TS, Williford PM. Warts (verrucae). In: Rakel RE, Bope ET, eds. *Conn's Current Therapy.* Philadelphia, PA: Saunders, Elsevier, Inc; 2010.

Jacobs AA, Orengo IF. Cancers of the skin. In: Rakel RE, Bope ET, eds. *Conn's Current Therapy.* Philadelphia, PA: Saunders, Elsevier, Inc; 2010.

Katsambas A, Nicolaidou E. Parasitic diseases of the skin. In: Rakel RE, Bope ET, eds. *Conn's Current Therapy.* Philadelphia, PA: Saunders, Elsevier, Inc; 2010.

Kelso RL, Raimer SS. Fungal diseases of the skin. In: Rakel RE, Bope ET, eds. *Conn's Current Therapy.* Philadelphia, PA: Saunders, Elsevier, Inc; 2010.

Kong AS, Williams RL, Smith M, et al. Acanthosis nigricans and diabetes risk factors: Prevalence in young persons seen in southwestern US primary care practices. *Ann Fam Med* 2007;5(3):202-208.

Latenser BA. Burn treatment guidelines. In: Rakel RE, Bope ET, eds. *Conn's Current Therapy.* Philadelphia, PA: Saunders, Elsevier, Inc; 2010.

Lee CS, Koo J. Papulosquamous disorders. In: Rakel RE, Bope ET, eds. *Conn's Current Therapy.* Philadelphia, PA: Saunders, Elsevier, Inc; 2010.

Losi-Sasaki JM, Moore AY. Viral diseases of the skin. In: Rakel RE, Bope ET, eds. *Conn's Current Therapy.* Philadelphia, PA: Saunders, Elsevier, Inc; 2010.

Mason JB. Vitamins, trace minerals and other micronutrients. In Goldman L, Ausiello D, eds. *Cecil Medicine.* 23rd ed. Philadelphia, PA: Saunders, Elsevier, Inc; 2008:1626-1639.

Moore RL, Devere TS. Epidermal manifestations of internal malignancy. *Dermatol Clin.* 2008;26:17-29.

Morelli JG. Cutaneous bacterial infections. In: Kliegman RM, Behrman RE, Jenson HB, et al., eds. *Nelson Textbook of Pediatrics.* Philadelphia PA: Saunders, Elsevier, Inc; 2007a.

Morelli JG. Diseases of the epidermis. In: Kliegman RM, Behrman RE, Jenson HB, Stanton BF, eds. *Nelson Textbook of Pediatrics.* Philadelphia, PA: Saunders, Elsevier, Inc; 2007b.

Morelli JG. Disorders of keratinization. In: Kliegman RM, Behrman RE, Jenson HB, et al., eds. *Nelson Textbook of Pediatrics.* Philadelphia, PA: Saunders, Elsevier, Inc; 2007c.

Morelli JG. Tumors of the skin. In: Kliegman RM, Behrman RE, Jenson HB, et al., eds. *Nelson Textbook of Pediatrics.* Philadelphia, PA: Saunders, Elsevier, Inc; 2007d.

Moses S. Pruritis. In: Rakel RE, Bope ET, eds. *Conn's Current Therapy.* Philadelphia, PA: Saunders, Elsevier, Inc; 2010:31-35.

Nahary L, Tamarkin A, Kayam N, et al., An investigation of antistreptococcal antibody responses in guttate psoriasis. *Arch Dermatol Res* 2008;300(8):441-449.

Physicians' Desk Reference. 63rd ed. Thomson Reuters; 2009.

Piraccini BM, Lorizzo M. Diseases of the nails. In: Rakel RE, Bope ET, eds. *Conn's Current Therapy.* Philadelphia, PA: Saunders, Elsevier, Inc; 2010.

Requena L, Yus ES. Erythema nodosum. *Dermatol Clin.* 2008;26(4):425-438.

Roberts WE. Dermatologic problems of older women. *Dermatol Clin.* 2006; 24:271-280.

Schwartz RA, Janusz CA, Janniger CK. Seborrheic dermatitis: An overview. *Am Fam Physician.* 2007; 75(6):807.

Schwartz RA, Nervi SJ. Erythema nodosum: A sign of systemic disease. *Am Fam Physician.* 2007; 75(5):695-700.

Shah M. Syphilis. In: Rakel RE, Bope ET, eds. *Conn's Current Therapy.* Philadelphia, PA: Saunders, Elsevier, Inc; 2010.

Sharma SK, Mohan A, Sarcoidosis. In: Rakel RE, Bope ET, eds. *Conn's Current Therapy.* Philadelphia, PA: Saunders, Elsevier, Inc; 2010.

Smith MJ. Cat-scratch disease. In: Rakel RE, Bope ET, eds. *Conn's Current Therapy.* Philadelphia, PA: Saunders, Elsevier, Inc; 2010.

Stevens DL, Bacterial diseases of the skin. In: Rakel RE, Bope ET, eds. *Conn's Current Therapy.* Philadelphia, PA: Saunders, Elsevier, Inc; 2010.

Szepietowski JC, Reich A. Pigmentary disorders. In: Rakel RE, Bope ET, eds. *Conn's Current Therapy.* Philadelphia, PA: Saunders, Elsevier, Inc; 2010.

Thomas DR. Pressure ulcers. In: Rakel RE, Bope ET, eds. *Conn's Current Therapy.* Philadelphia, PA: Saunders, Elsevier, Inc; 2008.

Tonneson MG. Erythema multiforme, Stevens-johnson syndrome and toxic epidermal necrolysis. In: Rakel RE, Bope ET, eds. *Conn's Current Therapy.* Philadelphia, PA: Saunders, Elsevier, Inc; 2010.

Weinstein A, Wani S. Lyme disease. In: Rakel RE, Bope ET, eds. *Conn's Current Therapy.* Philadelphia, PA: Saunders, Elsevier, Inc; 2010.

Ziemer M, Eisendle K, Zelger B. New concepts on erythema annulare centrifugum: a clinical reaction pattern that does not represent a specific clinicopathological entity. *Br J Dermatol.* 2009;160(1):119-126.

CHAPTER 4

Endocrinology

Christina M. Robohm, MS, PA-C

DIRECTIONS: Each of the numbered items or incomplete statements is followed by answers or by completion of the statement. Select the ONE-lettered answer or completion that is BEST in each case.

1. A 43-year-old obese man presents for a health maintenance visit. On physical exam, it is noted that his waist circumference is 106 cm and blood pressure is 148/92 mm Hg. Which of the following fasting laboratory levels would suggest a diagnosis of metabolic syndrome (syndrome X) in this patient?

   (A) HDL of 45 mg/dL
   (B) LDL of 180 mg/dL
   (C) triglyceride of 190 mg/dL
   (D) glucose of 100 mg/dL

2. A 36-year-old woman presents to the office complaining of weight loss and a feeling of "nervousness." She also complains of losing hair during the last several weeks. Exam reveals a diffusely enlarged, firm, nontender thyroid gland with an audible bruit. Her eyes have marked proptosis and lid retraction (see Figure 4-1). Her TSH is very low; her free and total thyroid hormone levels are elevated. What is the most likely diagnosis?

   (A) subacute thyroiditis
   (B) Hashimoto thyroiditis
   (C) Graves disease
   (D) multinodular goiter
   (E) Cushing disease

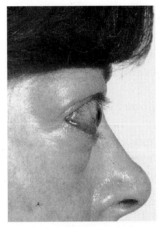

Figure 4-1
(Reproduced, with permission, from Fauci AS, Braunwald E, Kasper DL, et al. Harrison's Principles of Internal Medicine, 17th edition. New York: McGraw-Hill, 2008: 2235.)

3. A 23-year-old woman presents with joint pain, anorexia, amenorrhea, and fatigue. On further questioning, she says that she has been craving salty foods and gets dizzy easily when she stands. Upon physical exam, she is found to have darkened skin over her palms and extensor surfaces and postural hypotension. An 8 AM plasma cortisol level is low. What test is the gold standard to diagnose her condition?

   (A) abdominal CT scan
   (B) rapid ACTH stimulation test
   (C) thyroid stimulating antibody
   (D) urine catecholamines

4. A 44-year-old man has been drinking large quantities of water, up to 12 L/day, for the last week. In addition, he has been passing large quantities of urine. Upon physical exam, there are no remarkable findings except for increased capillary refill time and tacky mucous membranes. Laboratory results show sodium 166 mmol/L, potassium 4.2 mmol/L, chloride 123 mmol/L, and bicarbonate 27 mmol/L. His fasting serum glucose is 80 mg/dL and creatinine 1.2 mg/dL. His serum osmolality is 343 mOsm/kg. Which of the following hormone deficiencies is most likely present in this patient?

    (A) prolactin
    (B) oxytocin
    (C) insulin
    (D) growth
    (E) antidiuretic

5. A 42-year-old woman has experienced recent weight gain, heavy periods, fatigue, cold intolerance, and constipation. She has a rough voice, and her rate of speech is slow. Physical exam is significant for an enlarged thyroid, slow reflexes, and the presence of brittle and coarse hair. She denies any history of bipolar disease or treatment with lithium. Laboratory tests show an elevated TSH and low free T_4. What is the most appropriate treatment for this patient?

    (A) propylthiouracil (PTU)
    (B) levothyroxine
    (C) surgical resection
    (D) radioiodide ablation

6. A 22-year-old man (refer to Figure 4-2) is being evaluated for extremity enlargement unlike anyone in his family. Over the past 2 years, he has noticed that his rings no longer fit and his feet are so wide that he cannot find shoes to fit. He has always been tall for his age, greater than the 95th percentile throughout his teenage years. He has very coarse facial features, macroglossia, and a very deep voice. What is the most likely cause of this patient's condition?

    (A) adrenal neoplasm
    (B) multinodular goiter
    (C) pituitary macroadenoma
    (D) Rathke cleft cyst
    (E) testicular neoplasm

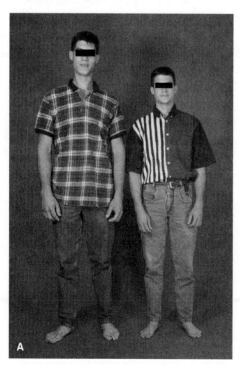
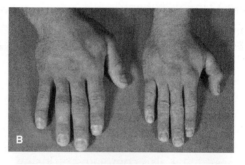
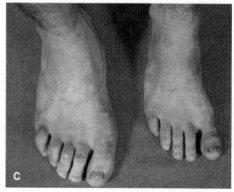

Figure 4-2

7. A 49-year-old man presents to the office complaining of general malaise with muscle aches, anorexia, fever, and severe pain over his anterior neck radiating to his ears. He states that he was ill about 2 weeks ago with a sore throat, but it resolved within a few days. On palpation, the thyroid gland is enlarged and tender. His laboratory workup shows a high T4 level and increased erythrocyte sedimentation rate (ESR). What is the most appropriate therapy for this patient's disease?

   (A) levothyroxine sodium
   (B) PTU therapy
   (C) radioiodine ablation
   (D) surgery
   (E) supportive therapy only

8. A 45-year-old woman presents with weight gain, fatigue, dry skin, and oligomenorrhea. On physical exam, the patient has a palpable thyroid mass over the right lobe. An ultrasound evaluation of the thyroid shows diffuse heterogeneous enlargement of the gland. Which of the following is the most likely diagnosis?

   (A) multinodular goiter
   (B) thyroid carcinoma
   (C) thyroid adenoma
   (D) Hashimoto thyroiditis

9. A 43-year-old woman presents to the emergency department complaining of weakness, abdominal pain, fever, nausea, and vomiting. On evaluation, she is found to have a blood pressure of 82/54 mm Hg, increased serum potassium, decreased serum sodium, and an increased BUN. A cosyntropin stimulation test is unsuccessful. What advice is best for this patient?

   (A) acetaminophen, 500 mg po
   (B) hydrocortisone, 300 mg IV
   (C) flagyl, 500 mg IV
   (D) propranol HCl, 40 mg po
   (E) levothyroxine, 200 μg po

10. A 23-year-old patient with type 1 diabetes mellitus (DM) has been having difficulty sleeping at night. Usually around 3 AM the patient will wake up feeling sweaty, nauseated, and tachycardic. He has recorded the following blood glucose levels:

10 PM	3 AM	7 AM
90 mg/dL	40 mg/dL	200 mg/dL

   What advise is the best for this patient?

   (A) stop eating a bedtime snack
   (B) increase the evening regular dosage
   (C) decrease the evening Lente dosage
   (D) exercise before going to bed at night

11. A 47-year-old woman presents to the office with increased blood pressure, bradycardia, constipation, muscle cramps, and weight gain. What is the best initial laboratory workup for this patient?

   (A) TSH level
   (B) T_3 and T_4
   (C) free T_4 and TSH
   (D) serum thyroglobulin
   (E) RAI uptake and thyroid scan

12. An obese patient with type 2 diabetes mellitus is started on initial therapy to improve glycemic control. Which of the following would be a contraindication for treatment with metformin?

   (A) renal failure
   (B) history of ketoacidosis
   (C) inflammatory bowel disease
   (D) anemia

13. A 45-year-old man with a history of neck irradiation for Hodgkin lymphoma at the age of 15 is found to have a 1.5-cm, nontender, firm thyroid nodule. Upon laboratory evaluation, the patient is found to be euthyroid, and fine needle biopsy reveals malignancy. What histologic type is most likely?

   (A) anaplastic
   (B) follicular
   (C) medullary
   (D) papillary

14. A 25-year-old man presents to the clinic complaining of nocturnal enuresis, weight loss, and blurred vision. On further questioning, he relates that he has increased appetite and thirst. His fasting blood glucose level is 225 mg/dL. Which of the following would also be indicative of type 1 versus type 2 diabetes mellitus?

(A) increased triglycerides
(B) presence of glutamic acid decarboxylase
(C) presence of C-peptide
(D) decreased urine catecholamines

15. A 54-year-old man with type 2 diabetes mellitus has a blood pressure of 146/92 mm Hg and 138/90 mm Hg on two separate occasions. Which of the following treatments offers the best outcomes to reduce cardiovascular complications of disease?

(A) lifestyle modification
(B) calcium channel blockers
(C) diuretics
(D) ACE inhibitors

16. A 68-year-old woman complains of loss of appetite, weakness, fatigue, constipation, and impaired memory. She has a history of two episodes of nephrolithiasis. Laboratory evaluation reveals calcium levels and PTH are high. Which one of the following is a common manifestation of this disease?

(A) anxiety
(B) bone fractures
(C) heart failure
(D) hirsutism
(E) proximal muscle weakness

17. A 63-year-old woman presents with shortness of breath, cough, and proximal muscle weakness of 1-month duration. On clinical exam, she is noted to have a blood pressure of 156/102 mm Hg, facial flushing, mild hirsutism, truncal obesity, marked proximal muscle weakness of both the upper and lower extremity, and hyperpigmentation over the palms and back of the neck. Laboratory exam reveals hypercortisolism

and increased ACTH. Which of the following would be the most likely primary diagnosis in this patient?

(A) lymphoma
(B) ovarian cancer
(C) renal cell carcinoma
(D) small cell lung carcinoma

18. A 54-year-old woman is taking glyburide, a second-generation sulfonylurea, to control her type 2 diabetes mellitus. Which of the following is the most likely mechanism of the therapeutic effect of glyburide on this patient's disease?

(A) increase pancreatic insulin secretion, in part by acting on potassium channels
(B) delay postprandial carbohydrate and glucose absorption
(C) reduce hepatic glucose production by suppressing gluconeogenesis
(D) inhibit cholesterol synthesis and carbohydrate uptake

19. A previously healthy, 28-year-old pregnant woman undergoes a routine prenatal glucose tolerance test. She is found to have increased serum glucose levels at 1 hour and 3 hours following a glucose challenge. What is the most likely consequence of gestational diabetes?

(A) future onset of type 2 diabetes
(B) macrosomic baby
(C) diabetic ketoacidosis
(D) nephropathy

20. A 45-year-old woman presents with weight gain, fatigue, dry skin, constipation, and oligomenorrhea. On physical exam, bradycardia and slow deep tendon reflexes are noted. Her free T_4 is low and TSH is elevated. Which of the following medications may be responsible for her condition?

(A) amiodarone
(B) beta-blockers
(C) levadopa
(D) lithium

21. A 38-year-old man presents to the office following a health fair screening of his cholesterol because he was told that it is high. He watches his diet, plays tennis, exercises three to five times a week, and appears in good physical condition. He is a nonsmoker, and has no family history of cardiovascular disease. His blood pressure today is 106/72 mm Hg. His lipid profile is total cholesterol 202 mg/dL, HDL 65 mg/dL, LDL 128 mg/dL, and triglycerides 145 mg/dL. Following a review of this patient's profile, which of the following would you recommend?

(A) prescribe gemfibrozil
(B) prescribe HMG-CoA reductase inhibitor
(C) prescribe low-dose niacin and slowly increase to achieve 3 g daily
(D) give diet education and continued exercise program

22. A 38-year-old man presents to the emergency department experiencing a severe headache and heart palpitations. He appears to be anxious and perspiring heavily. On exam, he is found to be tachycardic and his blood pressure is 158/102 mm Hg. His urine catecholamines are increased. If imaging were performed, what is the most likely location where a lesion would be found?

(A) pituitary gland
(B) liver
(C) adrenal gland
(D) testicle
(E) kidney

23. A 65-year-old woman presents to the office with decreased hearing, and pain over her sternum, pelvis, and her right tibial tubercle. On x-ray, the involved bones are noted to be expanded and denser than normal. Her serum calcium and phosphorus levels are normal, but serum alkaline phosphatase level is markedly elevated. Which of the following would be the appropriate initial treatment for this patient?

(A) ibuprofen 600 mg po every 6 hours
(B) indomethacin 25 mg po tid
(C) meclizine 25 mg po tid

(D) methotrexate 7.5 mg po qd
(E) tiludronate 400 mg po qd

24. A 40-year-old obese woman presents for her annual physical exam. A fasting blood glucose level drawn with her routine laboratory test is 130 mg/dL. In order to confirm the diagnosis of diabetes mellitus, what would be the most appropriate next step?

(A) glycated hemoglobin
(B) 3-hour glucose tolerance test
(C) repeat fasting blood glucose
(D) insulin level

25. An 11-year-old boy is being seen in the clinic for well-child care. His father inquires whether his son is starting to show physical signs of puberty. Which of the following is the first sign of puberty in males?

(A) change of voice
(B) scrotal and testicular enlargement
(C) gynecomastia
(D) pubic hair development

26. An 8-year-old boy presents with parental concerns that he is the "shortest boy in his class." His growth chart indicates decreased growth velocity falling below the fifth percentile. Laboratory studies show subnormal growth hormone secretion. What additional finding would you expect to see in this child?

(A) inadequate weight gain
(B) delayed skeletal maturation
(C) precocious puberty
(D) normal facies
(E) hypoglycemia

27. A 20-month-old baby girl presents with delayed dental eruption. Upon physical exam, the child is noted to have dry skin and slow deep tendon reflexes. Which of the following laboratory studies is most likely to reveal the cause?

(A) GH
(B) ACTH
(C) TSH
(D) FSH

28. A 67-year-old woman with type 2 diabetes is being treated for dyslipidemia. She does not have additional risk factors. What is the target LDL goal for this patient?

    (A) less than 70 mg/dL
    (B) less than 100 mg/dL
    (C) less than 120 mg/dL
    (D) less than 130 mg/dL
    (E) less than 160 mg/dL

29. A 29-year-old woman presents to the office with complaints of poor sleep, irritability, and nervousness. She appears anxious and restless. You note tachycardia and edematous skin change on the dorsum of the lower legs and feet. She has exophthalmos and a diffusely enlarged thyroid gland on exam. Which of the following findings would be expected on further evaluation?

    (A) low levels of free T_4 level
    (B) high levels of TSH
    (C) low uptake on radioiodine nuclear scan
    (D) high levels of thyroid-stimulating antibodies

30. A 41-year-old woman presents with complaints of weight gain, infrequent menses, and mood changes. You observe her to have moon facies, centripetal fat distribution, and purple striae on her abdomen (see Figure 4-3). Her blood pressure is 152/98 mm Hg. What is the first step in confirming this diagnosis?

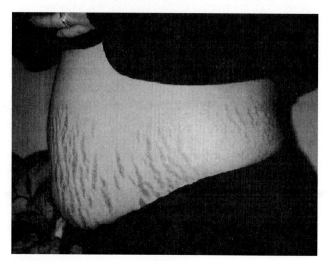

Figure 4-3
(Reproduced, with permission, from Fauci AS, Braunwald E, Kasper DL, et al. Harrison's Principles of Internal Medicine, 17th edition. New York: McGraw-Hill, 2008: 2255.)

    (A) random cortisol level
    (B) overnight dexamethasone suppression test
    (C) thyroid studies
    (D) MRI

31. A 26-year-old woman has decreased appetite, weight gain, cold intolerance, hoarse voice, constipation, and arthralgias. What is the most likely etiology of her condition?

    (A) autoimmune thyroiditis
    (B) congenital hypothyroidism
    (C) dietary iodine deficiency
    (D) surgical resection of the thyroid gland

32. A 28-year-old woman with type 2 diabetes has maintained good control with metformin treatment in addition to diet and exercise. She expresses that she would like to become pregnant. What is the best advice for this patient regarding treatment of her diabetes?

    (A) continue current treatment with metformin
    (B) change oral therapy to rosiglitazone
    (C) change to insulin therapy
    (D) discontinue medical therapy and continue aggressive diet and exercise

33. How often should urine be obtained to screen for microalbuminemia in the management of a type 2 diabetic patient?

    (A) every 6 months
    (B) annually
    (C) every 2 years
    (D) every 5 years

34. A 45-year-old patient presents 2 days postoperatively with a partial thyroidectomy. She has been experiencing vomiting with diarrhea. On physical exam, her temperature is 101°F and jaundice is noted. Her heart rate is irregularly irregular with a rate of 200 bpm. What would be the most appropriate pharmacological intervention?

    (A) radioactive iodine (^{131}I)
    (B) propranolol 80 mg

(C) PTU 600 mg

(D) iopanoic acid 500 mg

35. A 31-year-old woman is being evaluated for irregular, infrequent menstrual periods. On further questioning, she complains of headaches, fatigue, and breast discharge. She takes ibuprofen only occasionally. Which of the following labs would most likely be elevated in this patient?

(A) BUN and creatinine

(B) luteinizing hormone (LH) and follicle-stimulating hormone (FSH)

(C) oxytocin

(D) prolactin

(E) TSH

36. Which of the following oral agents used to treat type 2 diabetes mellitus is effective in lowering fasting blood glucose levels without causing hypoglycemia?

(A) glyburide

(B) metformin

(C) repaglinide

(D) pioglitazone

37. A 75-year-old man with type 2 diabetes presents to the emergency department with a 2-day history of confusion and lethargy. On physical exam, notable dehydration, tachycardia, and confused mental state is noted. Serum sodium, potassium, magnesium, and chloride levels are normal. The arterial blood gases are normal and serum ketones are negative. The abnormal laboratory findings are as follows:

		Normal Reference Range
Glucose	700 (mg/dL)	74–106 (mg/dL)
Osmolality	380 (mOsm/kg)	275–295 (mOsm/kg)

Source: Elin, 2008.

Given this information, what is the most likely diagnosis?

(A) diabetic ketoacidosis

(B) hyperglycemic hyperosmolar state

(C) hypoglycemia

(D) dehydration

38. When treating the dyslipidemia associated with type 2 diabetes, which of the following is the drug class of choice?

(A) bile acid sequestrants

(B) fibrate

(C) fiber supplements

(D) HMG-CoA reductase inhibitors

(E) nicotinic acid derivatives

39. A 28-year-old woman is being treated for hypothyroidism with 200 μg of levothyroxine daily. At a periodic dosage reassessment, her TSH was suppressed at 0.08 mU/L and she is symptomatic. What is the appropriate course of action?

(A) increase her levothyroxine dose

(B) decrease her levothyroxine dose

(C) no change to her levothyroxine dose

(D) change her medication to PTU

40. A 56-year-old woman is being seen for regular assessment and monitoring of her type 2 diabetes mellitus. She has been following a strict diet and exercise plan for 2 years with the addition of metformin 6 months ago for an increased HgA$_{1c}$ level. Her HgA$_{1c}$ at today's visit is 7.1. What is the appropriate management for this patient?

(A) add exenatide to her current therapy

(B) change her oral therapy to rosiglitazone

(C) add insulin to her current therapy

(D) maintain her current therapy and recheck in 6 months

41. A 30-year-old patient presents 2 months post-thyroidectomy. The patient has had symptoms of increased irritability, muscle spasms, and hair loss for the past month. On physical examination, a positive Chovstek sign is noted. Which of the following is the most likely diagnosis?

(A) hypothyroidism

(B) hypopituitarism

(C) hypoparathyroidism

(D) hypogonadism

42. You are treating a 60-year-old man with a history of angina. He has been on the therapeutic lifestyle change (TLC) diet for 12 weeks (with solid effort). This patient has no other medical conditions and takes nitroglycerin as needed and daily enteric-coated aspirin. His fasting lipid panel from last week demonstrates the following:

    > total cholesterol—295 mg/dL
    > low-density lipoproteins—145 mg/dL
    > high-density lipoproteins—48 mg/dL

    What is the most appropriate treatment at this time?

    (A) prescribe colestipol
    (B) prescribe ezetimibe
    (C) prescribe simvastatin
    (D) prescribe niacin
    (E) no pharmacological treatment

43. A patient seen at the prenatal clinic develops Graves disease at 25 weeks' gestation. Which of the following is the most appropriate treatment?

    (A) PTU 100 mg po tid
    (B) methimazole 10 to 30 mg po qd
    (C) propranolol 80 mg po qid
    (D) radioactive iodine therapy (RAI, ^{131}I)
    (E) levothyroxine 0.1 mg po qd

44. You are treating a healthy 50-year-old man with no cardiac risk factors. This patient has no other medical conditions and takes no medications. His fasting lipid panel from last week demonstrates the following:

    > TC—245 mg/dL
    > LDL—155 mg/dL
    > HDL—60 mg/dL

    What is the LDL goal for this patient?

    (A) less than 100 mg/dL
    (B) less than 120 mg/dL
    (C) less than 130 mg/dL
    (D) less than 160 mg/dL
    (E) less than 190 mg/dL

45. You are considering the addition of glipizide therapy to the treatment regimen for a patient with type 2 diabetes mellitus. Which of the following would be a contraindication if present in this patient?

    (A) hypertension
    (B) diabetic retinopathy
    (C) liver impairment
    (D) age less than 85 years
    (E) osteoporosis

46. A 55-year-old man patient presents with tachycardia and heart palpitations. Physical exam shows a multinodular goiter. He does not have obstructive symptoms. He has suppressed TSH and elevated T_3 and T_4, and a thyroid scan shows multiple functioning nodules. What is the treatment of choice for this patient?

    (A) propylthiouracil
    (B) beta-blockers
    (C) ^{131}I ablation
    (D) surgical resection

47. A 12-year-old boy is being seen for concerns of development of breast tissue. Upon physical exam, he is noted to have a firm, slightly tender mass under the left areola. What is the most appropriate action at this time?

    (A) referral to pediatric surgery for resection
    (B) measurement of serum hCG
    (C) measurement of testosterone and estrogen levels
    (D) reassurance and observation

48. A 16-year-old boy is being evaluated for delayed puberty. He is found to have hypogonadism with testes measured at 1.5 cm on the long axis. His face has a juvenile appearance and rounded body type. He has a karyotype of XXY. What is the diagnosis?

    (A) Kallman syndrome
    (B) Klinefelter syndrome
    (C) Marfan syndrome
    (D) myotonic dystrophy

49. Which of the following is the most likely cause of hypercalcemia in an ambulatory patient?

    (A) parathyroid adenoma
    (B) renal insufficiency
    (C) malabsorption
    (D) multiple myeloma

50. A 30-year-old woman presents to the office with polyuria, fatigue, and a chronic white vaginal discharge with vaginal pruritis. She has been having the discharge off and on for the past 6 months with recurrent treatment failures. Which of the following is the most likely diagnosis?

    (A) type 2 diabetes mellitus
    (B) hyperthyroidism
    (C) hypothyroidism
    (D) diabetes insipidus

51. A 26-year-old woman presents to the clinic with a 3-month history of galactorrhea and amenorrhea. Her serum HCG is negative and her serum prolactin is elevated at 220. You suspect a pituitary adenoma. Which of the following physical exam findings is most likely to suggest a macroadenoma versus a microadenoma?

    (A) visual field defects
    (B) significant weight loss
    (C) bilateral nipple discharge
    (D) elevated blood pressure

52. Which of the following drugs can cause syndrome of inappropriate antidiuretic hormone (SIADH)?

    (A) carbamazepine
    (B) glyburide
    (C) lithium carbonate
    (D) metoprolol

53. A 39-year-old woman presents to the office for evaluation of a palpable nodule of 2 years' duration in the neck. She has no other symptoms. She has a history of low-dose chest irradiation for an enlarged thymus gland during infancy. On exam, a firm, nontender 2.5-cm nodule is palpable in the left lobe of the thyroid. Her TSH level is normal. What is the next diagnostic step?

    (A) ultrasound of the neck
    (B) thyroid scan
    (C) MRI of the neck
    (D) fine-needle aspiration of the nodule

Answers and Explanations

1. **(C)** Metabolic syndrome is found in approximately 25% of Americans. It is defined as three or more of the following findings: waist circumference of greater than 102 cm in men or greater than 88 cm in women; serum triglyceride level of at least 150 mg/dL, HDL level of less than 40 mg/dL in men or less than 50 mg/dL in women; blood pressure of at least 130/85 mm Hg; and serum glucose level of at least 110 mg/dL. *(Friedman and Herman-Bonert, 2009, p. 1105).*

2. **(C)** This patient is suffering from Graves disease. Her symptoms are consistent with a hyperthyroid state. Based upon her physical exam, Graves disease is the most likely diagnosis due to the specific associated eye findings of thyroid-associated ophthalmopathy. The lab findings of low TSH and elevated free and total thyroid hormone levels are also consistent with the diagnosis. *(Friedman and Herman-Bonert, 2009, pp. 649-651)*

3. **(B)** Adrenal crisis may present with a history of fatigue, anorexia, weight loss, oligomenorrhea or amenorrhea, joint or back pain, and darkening of the skin. Patients may have postural dizziness, food cravings, hyponatremia, hypoglycemia, hyperkalemia, and prerenal azotemia. The 8 AM plasma cortisol levels may serve as a screening tool for adrenal insufficiency. The gold standard test to diagnose this is an ACTH stimulation test. This test will also differentiate between primary and secondary adrenal insufficiency. *(Nieman, 2008, pp. 660-661)*

4. **(E)** This patient's symptoms and labs are consistent with diabetes insipidus. This condition results from a deficiency of antidiuretic hormone causing polyuria and polydipsia. *(Fitzgerald, 2009, pp. 969-971)*

5. **(B)** This patient's signs and symptoms are consistent with hypothyroidism. Treatment of choice is levothyroxine, which is partially converted in the body to T_3. Significant increases are seen within 1 to 2 weeks, with maximum levels reached in 3 to 4 weeks. *(Friedman and Herman-Bonert, 2009, pp. 652-653)*

6. **(C)** This patient's signs and symptoms are consistent with acromegaly, which is caused by an increased secretion of GH. These are almost always caused by pituitary macroadenomas. The tumors may be locally invasive into the cavernous sinus but are typically not malignant. *(Braunstein, 2009, pp. 971-973)*

7. **(E)** This is subacute, painful thyroiditis. This is a self-limiting disorder that at most requires symptomatic therapy. In mild cases, analgesics (ASA) are sufficient for pain relief and to decrease the inflammation. Prednisone may bring more relief if needed. Transient hypothyroidism should be treated as well. *(Ladenson and Kim, 2008, p. 1708)*

8. **(D)** Hashimoto's thyroiditis is an autoimmune disorder of the thyroid gland. This condition causes hypothyroidism. On physical exam, a goiter may be palpated. In order to distinguish this from other conditions, laboratory and diagnostic studies should be done. When an ultrasound is performed, it will show diffuse heterogeneous enlargement of the gland and not a solitary or multinodular gland. *(Fitzgerald, 2009, pp. 989-990)*

9. **(B)** This patient's symptoms are consistent with adrenal crisis. Immediate treatment with 100 to 300 mg of IV hydrocortisone is indicated, even before serum cortisol results are returned. Because bacterial infection may precipitate acute adrenal crisis, empirical broad-spectrum antibiotic treatment is indicated. *(Fitzgerald, 2009, pp. 1020-1021)*

10. **(C)** The patient has described the Somogyi effect. This effect occurs because the patient is receiving too much intermediate insulin at dinnertime. This occurs when nocturnal hypoglycemia results in counter-regulatory hormones producing hyperglycemia. Either the intermediate insulin dosage can be shifted to a lower dosage at bedtime or the patient can eat a larger snack at bedtime. *(Masharami, 2009, pp. 1074-1075)*

11. **(C)** This patient is displaying symptoms of hypothyroidism. The most appropriate tests to differentiate the cause for this are free T_4 and TSH. Serum T_3 is not a sensitive test for hypothyroidism. *(Fitzgerald, 2009, pp. 977-981)*

12. **(A)** Metformin should not be used in patients with renal insufficiency due to its ability to produce lactic acidosis. Other contraindications include liver disease, severe congestive heart failure, metabolic acidosis, or history of alcohol abuse. *(Masharami, 2009, pp. 1064-1065).*

13. **(D)** Thyroid carcinoma often presents as an asymptomatic thyroid nodule. The most common histologic form is papillary carcinoma, representing more than 80% of cases. *(Ladenson and Kim, 2008, p. 1711)*

14. **(B)** Type 1 diabetes mellitus (DM) is an autoimmune disease. New-onset type 1 diabetic patients have islet cell antibodies. A variety of beta-cell antibodies including insulin and glutamic acid decarboxylase may exist. GAD 65 is present in 70% to 90% of patients with new-onset type 1 DM *(Masharami, 2009, p. 1053)*

15. **(D)** The importance of aggressive blood pressure management in diabetes is important in decreasing cardiovascular and microvascular complications of diabetes. The JNC 7 report has established blood pressure targets of less than 130/85 mm Hg. Beta-blockers and ACE inhibitors have both been effective in reducing cardiovascular and microvascular complications of diabetes. Because of the results of several large trials, ACE inhibitors are recommended as first-line antihypertensive therapy in diabetic patients with hypertension. *(Rizza and Service, 2008, pp. 1759)*

16. **(B)** This patient has hyperparathyroidism. The most common clinical manifestation of disease is nephrolithiasis due to elevated levels of PTH. There is a high rate of bone fractures in patients with PTH due to increased osteoclastic and osteoblastic activity. *(Fitzgerald, 2009, pp. 1007-1012)*

17. **(D)** Tumor cells may secrete hormones that have the same biologic actions as the normal hormone. This patient's symptoms are consistent with adrenocorticoid hyperfunction. The most common cause of ectopic ACTH syndrome is small cell lung carcinoma. This should be suspected in any patient with risk factors for lung cancer. *(Friedman, 2007, pp. 663, 591-592)*

18. **(A)** Sulfonylureas have a principal action of the stimulation of endogenous insulin secretion from pancreatic beta cells. The drug acts to close adenosine triphosphate-dependent potassium channels. *(Inzucchi, 2008, pp. 1753-1754)*

19. **(B)** Gestational diabetes is the presence of glucose intolerance developing during pregnancy. This usually returns to normal following delivery. Screening is routinely performed at 24 and 28 weeks' gestation. The most common complication of gestational diabetes is the delivery of a large for gestational age baby. *(Barnett and Braunstein, 2007, p. 678)*

20. **(A)** Hypothyroidism is reported in up to 10% of patients taking amiodarone, an antiarrhythmic medication. With the high iodine content of the medication and the structural similarities to thyroxine, thyroid abnormalities occur. Common side effects of amiodarone include bradycardia and constipation, so laboratory evaluation for thyroid dysfunction must be used. *(Fitzgerald, 2009, p. 978)*

21. **(D)** Analysis using the Framingham criteria places this patient at a 2% ten-year risk. This

patient does not require pharmacologic treatment at this time. *(Baron, 2009, pp. 1101-1004)*

22. **(C)** Pheochromocytomas produce, store, and secrete catecholamines. They are usually derived from the adrenal medulla, although they may be found in other locations. *(Fitzgerald, 2009, pp. 1031-1034)*

23. **(E)** This patient's signs and symptoms are consistent with Paget disease of bone. Biphosphates have become the treatment of choice for this disease. Tiludronate, taken orally for 3 months, is very effective in treatment of this disease. *(Fitzgerald, 2009, pp. 1018-1020)*

24. **(C)** Diabetes mellitus is confirmed by a fasting serum glucose greater than 126 mg/dL on more than one occasion. Repeating a fasting serum glucose would be the next best step to confirm diabetes in this patient. *(Masharami, 2009, pp. 1056-1057)*

25. **(B)** Scrotal and testicular enlargement is the first sign of puberty in boys. This typically occurs at the average age of 10 to 12 years. *(Kaplan, 2009, pp. 110)*

26. **(B)** Children with growth failure due to growth hormone deficiency have delayed skeletal maturation. This is assessed by left hand/wrist radiographs. These children also often have distinctive facial appearances and truncal obesity. *(Zeitler et al., 2009, p. 935)*

27. **(C)** This child likely has primary hypothyroidism. Laboratory findings include increased TSH and decreased T_3 and T_4 levels. In children, it is important to differentiate central hypothyroidism from intrinsic defects in the thyroid gland. *(Zeitler et al., 2009, pp. 947-949)*

28. **(B)** Type 2 diabetes mellitus is a coronary heart disease (CHD) risk equivalent condition. The LDL goal for these patients is less than 100 mg/dL. Those type 2 DM patients at high risk for CHD should be maintained at or less than 70 mg/dL. *(Masharami, 2009, pp. 308, 1080)*

29. **(D)** This patient's signs and symptoms are consistent with Graves disease. The pathogenesis of

Graves disease involves the formation of autoantibodies that bind to TSH receptors causing the gland to hyperfunction. The disease is often associated with a personal or family history of autoimmune disorders. *(Landenson et al., pp. 1710-1712)*

30. **(B)** This patient's signs and symptoms indicate possible Cushing syndrome. Overnight dexamethasone testing is the most widely used test, with normal results excluding Cushing syndrome. Cortisol levels are not useful because of diurnal variations. *(Molitch, 2008, p. 1686)*

31. **(A)** Auto immune thyroiditis is the most common cause of hypothyroidism in the United States. Dietary iodine deficiency is the most common cause in underdeveloped regions of the world. *(Ladenson and Kim, 2008, p. 1701)*

32. **(C)** Pregnant women should be placed on insulin therapy immediately after conception. Oral hypoglycemic therapy is contraindicated in pregnancy. Second-generation sulfonylureas, specifically glyburide, have been used in pregnancy; however, additional studies are required before approval for use in pregnancy. *(Elliot, 2008, pp. 1846-1847)*

33. **(B)** Screening for proteinuria should be done annually in type 2 diabetic patients starting at the time of diagnosis and yearly in type 1 diabetic patients beginning after 5 years of disease. Approximately 20% to 30% of diabetic patients develop nephropathy. *(Barnett et al., p. 697)*

34. **(C)** This patient is in a thyrotoxic crisis or thyroid storm. She needs to be admitted for monitoring and supportive care. The initial treatment would be PTU 600 mg loading dose followed by 200 to 300 mg every 6 hours given either by nasogastric tube or rectally. *(Fitzgerald, 2009, p. 988)*

35. **(D)** This patient's symptoms are consistent with a pituitary adenoma. Prolactinomas account for about half of all functioning pituitary tumors and may secrete PRL, GH, and ACTH. *(Herman-Bonert, 2007, p. 640)*

36. **(B)** Metformin is considered a "euglycemic" or "antihyperglycemic" drug because it does not

cause a hypoglycemic reaction at therapeutic levels. *(Bonart and Braunstein, 2007, pp. 688-689)*

37. **(B)** A hyperglycemic hyperosmolar state is characterized by dehydration, significant hyperglycemia, and an elevated serum osmolality with an insignificant or negative ketosis. Because of the lack of ketosis, the patient may present with a gradual onset of symptoms, and it can go unnoticed until the dehydration becomes more severe than in ketoacidosis. *(Masharami, 2009, pp. 1084-1085)*

38. **(D)** HMG-CoA reductase inhibitors (statins) are the preferred initial choice for treatment of dyslipidemia in diabetic patients. *(Inzucchi, 2008, p. 1759)*

39. **(B)** It is important to perform regular periodic dosage reassessments for patients with hypothyroidism. Suppressed TSH levels (<0.1 mU/L) may indicate overreplacement with levothyroxine. The dosage should be reduced. *(Fitzgerald, 2009, pp. 980-981)*

40. **(D)** The HgA$_{1c}$ goal for this patient is less than 6.5, with action at a level of greater than 8.0. The appropriate action at this time is to continue her current therapy and reassess in 6 months. *(Barnett et al, pp. 683-694)*

41. **(C)** Hypoparathyroidism commonly presents following thyroidectomy surgery. This patient has classic signs and symptoms of a low calcium level and hypoparathyroidism. Chovestek sign is a physical exam finding that is positive after tapping in front of the ear in the facial nerve region. When doing this, the muscle contracts. When the calcium level is low, this occurs. Hypothyroidism can occur following a thyroidectomy but the symptoms are not the same. *(Fitzgerald, 2009, pp. 1004-1005)*

42. **(C)** This patient's coronary heart disease risk factors and failed TLC diet warrant pharmacological treatment based on his LDL level. Although there are no absolute guidelines for the selection of lipid-modifying medications, an HMG-CoA reductase inhibitor is preferred. *(Semenkovich, 2008, p. 1553)*

43. **(A)** In nonpregnant patients, PTU and methimazole are the drugs of choice for the management of Graves disease. During pregnancy, PTU has a lower incidence of crossing the placental barrier than does methimazole. It also is excreted into breast milk to a lesser degree than is methimazole. Propranolol will help with the symptoms of Graves but not treat it. It can also cause low birth rate in the infant. RAI is contraindicated in pregnancy. Levothyroxine will worsen a Graves patient's hyperthyroidism. *(Elliot, 2008, pp. 1845-1846)*.

44. **(D)** Recommendations of the National Cholesterol Education Program (NCEP) Adult Treatment Panel III Report states the LDL goal for patients with 0 to 1 risk factor to be less than 160 mg/dL. *(Baron, 2009, p. 1101)*

45. **(C)** At least 90% of glipizide is metabolized in the liver to inactive products, and 10% is excreted unchanged in the urine. Because of the short half-life, it is preferable to use glyburide in elderly patients because of lessened risk of hypoglycemia. *(Masharami, 2009, p. 1064)*

46. **(C)** The treatment of choice for multinodular goiter is ^{131}I ablation. In patients with very large thyroid glands with obstructive symptoms, surgical resection may be the best option. *(Herman-Bonert, 2007, p. 651)*

47. **(D)** Type 1 idiopathic gynecomastia in adolescent men presents with a firm mass under the areola ("breast bud") typically during sexual maturation stages (SMR), stages II to III. This is a result of normal estrogen and androgen activity at the breast tissue level. Appropriate action is observation and to reassure the patient that the condition will likely resolve in 1 to 2 years. *(Kaplan, 2009, p. 120)*

48. **(B)** This boy has Klinefelter syndrome. This syndrome occurs in approximately 1:600 male births. It may present at birth with hypotonia and delayed development. It is a common cause of primary gonadal failure. *(Zeitler et al., 2009, p. 1002)*

49. **(A)** The most common cause of hypercalcemia in an ambulatory patient is a primary hyperparathyroid condition. These include parathyroid adenomas and parathyroid malig-

nancies. Both of these account for 90% of the causes of hypercalcemia. Renal insufficiency, malabsorption, and multiple myeloma are all causes of elevated calcium level but they are all secondary causes. *(Fitzgerald, 2009, pp. 1007-1008)*

50. **(A)** Polyuria, polydipsia, and fatigue are all findings that can be consistent with both type 1 and type 2 diabetes. Any woman who presents with a chronic vaginal discharge or chronic vaginal pruritis should be screened for type 2 diabetes. *(Masharami, 2009, p. 1056)*

51. **(A)** Mass effects of an enlarging pituitary tumor are often related to the location of the optic chiasm related to the sella turcica. Expansion of a macroadenoma places pressure on the optic chiasm. Bitemporal hemianopia is the most common visual field abnormality. *(Molitch, 2008, pp. 1678-1679)*

52. **(A)** Many medications can enhance the release or potentiate the effects of ADH. Carbamazepine may increase ADH release. *(Andreoli, 2007, pp. 289-291)*

53. **(D)** The most accurate test to confirm or exclude malignant disease in patients with a thyroid nodule and normal TSH level is a fine-needle aspiration biopsy. Solid nodules larger than 1.0 to 1.5 cm in diameter should be tested. *(Ladenson and Kim, 2008, pp. 1710-1711)*

REFERENCES

Andreoli TE, Safirstein RL. Fluid and electrolyte disorders. In: Andreoli TA, Carpenter CC, Griggs RC, et al., eds. *Cecil Essentials of Medicine.* 7th ed. Philadelphia, PA: WB Saunders; 2007.

Barnett PS, Braunstein GD. Diabetes mellitus. In: Andreoli TA, Carpenter CC, Griggs RC, et al., *Cecil Essentials of Medicine.* 7th ed. Philadelphia, PA: WB Saunders; 2007.

Baron RB. Lipid disorders. In: McPhee SJ, Papadakis MA, eds. *Current Medical Diagnosis and Treatment.* 48th ed. New York, NY: McGraw-Hill; 2009.

Braunstein GD. Male reproductive endocrinology. In: McPhee SJ, Papadakis MA, eds. *Current Medical Diagnosis and Treatment.* 48th ed. New York, NY: McGraw-Hill; 2009.

Elin RJ. Appendix: Reference intervals and laboratory values. In: Goldman L, Ausiello D, eds. *Cecil Textbook of Medicine.* 23rd ed. Philadelphia, PA: WB Saunders; 2008.

Elliot DL. Pregnancy: hypertension and other common medical problems. In: Goldman L, Ausiello D, eds. *Cecil Textbook of Medicine.* 23rd ed. Philadelphia, PA: WB Saunders; 2008.

Fauci AS, Braunwald E, Kasper DL, et al., *Harrison's Principles of Internal Medicine.* 17th ed. http://www.accessmedicine.com/resourceToc.aspx?resourceID=4. Accessed April 28, 2010.

Fitzgerald PA. Endocrine diseases. In: McPhee SJ, Papadakis MA, eds. *Current Medical Diagnosis and Treatment.* 48th ed. New York, NY: McGraw-Hill; 2009.

Friedman TC, Herman-Bonert VS. Thyroid gland. In: McPhee SJ, Papadakis MA, eds. *Current Medical Diagnosis and Treatment.* 48th ed. New York, NY: McGraw-Hill; 2009.

Friedman TC. Adrenal Gland. In: Andreoli TA, Carpenter CC, Griggs RC, et al., eds. *Cecil Essentials of Medicine.* 7th ed. Philadelphia, PA: WB Saunders; 2007.

Herman-Bonert VS. Hypothalamic-pituitary axis. In: Andreoli TA, Carpenter CC, Griggs RC, et al., eds. *Cecil Essentials of Medicine.* 7th ed. Philadelphia, PA: WB Saunders; 2007.

Inzucchi SE, Sherwin RS. Type 2 diabetes mellitus. In: Goldman L, Ausiello D, eds. *Cecil Textbook of Medicine.* 23rd ed. Philadelphia, PA: WB Saunders; 2008.

Kaplan DW, Love-Osborne KA. Adolescence. In: Hay WW, Levin MJ, Sondheimer JM, et al., eds. *Current Pediatric Diagnosis and Treatment.* 19th ed. New York, NY: McGraw-Hill; 2009.

Ladenson P, Kim M. Thyroid. In: Goldman L, Ausiello D, eds. *Cecil Textbook of Medicine.* 23rd ed. Philadelphia, PA: WB Saunders; 2008.

Masharami U. Diabetes mellitus and hypoglycemia. In: McPhee SJ, Papadakis MA, eds. *Current Medical Diagnosis and Treatment.* 48th ed. New York, NY: McGraw-Hill; 2009.

Molitch ME. Anterior pituitary. In: Goldman L, Ausiello D, eds. *Cecil Textbook of Medicine.* 23rd ed. Philadelphia, PA: WB Saunders; 2008.

Nieman LK. Adrenal cortex. In: Goldman L, Ausiello D, eds. *Cecil Textbook of Medicine,* 23rd ed. Philadelphia, PA: WB Saunders; 2008.

Rizza RA, Service FJ. Hypoglycemia/pancreatic islet cell disorders. In: Goldman L, Ausiello D, eds. *Cecil Textbook of Medicine.* 23rd ed. Philadelphia, PA: WB Saunders; 2008.

Semenkovich CF. Disorders of lipid metabolism. In: Goldman L, Ausiello D, eds. *Cecil Textbook of Medicine.* 23rd ed. Philadelphia, PA: WB Saunders; 2008.

Zeitler PS, Travers SH, Hoe F, et al. Endocrine disorders. In: Hay WW, Levin MJ, Sondheimer JM, et al., eds. *Current Pediatric Diagnosis and Treatment.* 19th ed. New York, NY: McGraw-Hill; 2009.

CHAPTER 5

Gastroenterology

Sue M. Nyberg, MHS, PA-C
Anthony A. Miller, MEd, PA-C

DIRECTIONS: Each of the numbered items or incomplete statements in this section is followed by answers or completions of the statement. Select the ONE-lettered answer or completion that is BEST in each case.

1. Patients with chronic gastroesophageal reflux disease (GERD) are at risk for

   (A) candidal esophagitis
   (B) Zenker diverticulum
   (C) Barrett esophagus
   (D) esophageal varices
   (E) achalasia

2. Hepatitis D infection requires coinfection with

   (A) hepatitis A
   (B) hepatitis B
   (C) hepatitis C
   (D) hepatitis E
   (E) hepatitis G

3. Which of the following is a risk factor for non-healing of a duodenal ulcer?

   (A) age greater than 50
   (B) high-fat diet
   (C) cigarette smoking
   (D) chronic stress
   (E) alcohol use

4. Which of the following conditions is associated with perifollicular hemorrhages, ecchymoses of legs, bleeding gums, loose teeth, and gastrointestinal (GI) bleeding?

   (A) Peutz–Jeghers syndrome
   (B) Osler–Weber-Rendu Syndrome
   (C) scurvy
   (D) neurofibromatosis
   (E) Blue Rubber–Bleb Nevus

5. In a patient with chronic hepatitis C infection, which of the following medical conditions would be considered a contraindication to starting the patient on interferon?

   (A) hypertension
   (B) hyperlipidemia
   (C) diabetes
   (D) migraine headaches
   (E) systemic lupus erythematosus

6. A middle-aged woman presents with elevated cholestatic liver enzyme levels. She is not taking any medications, does not drink alcohol, and does not complain of abdominal pain. She has not had any previous biliary tract surgery. Which of the following is the most likely diagnosis?

   (A) primary biliary cirrhosis
   (B) pancreatitis
   (C) cholecystitis
   (D) fatty liver
   (E) primary sclerosing cholangitis

7. An adult patient presents with acute onset of watery, nonbloody, voluminous diarrhea accompanied by nausea and vomiting. Which of the following organisms is the most likely cause?

   (A) *Clostridium difficile*
   (B) enterotoxigenic *Escherichia coli*
   (C) *Salmonella typhi*
   (D) *Shigella flexneri*
   (E) *Campylobacter jejuni*

8. A patient has had problems with prolonged diarrhea. Stool cultures grow out *Cryptosporidium*. It is important to

   (A) test the patient for HIV
   (B) check family members for the organism
   (C) perform a colonoscopy
   (D) perform blood cultures
   (E) isolate the patient

9. Which of the following best describes hepatitis C virus (HCV)?

   (A) the incubation period is 5 to 7 days
   (B) hepatitis C and D infections must be acquired simultaneously
   (C) less likely than hepatitis B to cause chronic hepatitis
   (D) a DNA virus with similarities to rotavirus
   (E) the risk of maternal–neonatal transmission is low

10. Which one of the following is a characteristic finding on computed tomography (CT) of the abdomen in a patient with acute diverticulitis?

   (A) toxic megacolon
   (B) air–fluid levels
   (C) soft tissue inflammation of the pericolic fat
   (D) thinning of the colon wall
   (E) paucity of bowel gas in the colon

11. The Dietary Guidelines for Americans 2005 recommends 2 to 3 servings of protein per day. A 3-oz serving of lean meat is about the size of a

   (A) checkbook
   (B) deck of cards
   (C) paperback book
   (D) matchbook
   (E) legal envelope

12. Which of the following agents is a significant cause of pill-induced esophagitis?

   (A) fluoxetine
   (B) omeprazole
   (C) ibuprofen
   (D) Vitamin D
   (E) ciprofloxacin

13. The most common malignant tumor of the esophagus in the African American male population is

   (A) adenocarcinoma
   (B) leiomyoma
   (C) small cell carcinoma
   (D) squamous cell carcinoma
   (E) granular cell tumor

14. In Western society, diverticulosis most often occurs in which portion of the colon?

   (A) transverse
   (B) sigmoid
   (C) descending
   (D) ascending
   (E) equally common in all parts of the colon

15. Which of the following statements concerning gastroesophageal reflux disease (GERD) is *not* true?

   (A) may exacerbate asthma symptoms
   (B) behavioral interventions include weight loss and eating smaller meals
   (C) mild to moderate symptoms are treated with H_2-receptor agonists (eg, ranitidine or cimetidine) or proton pump inhibitors
   (D) barium esophagography is recommended for most patients

16. What is the most common drug to cause acute liver failure?

    (A) estradiol
    (B) ketoconazole
    (C) lisinopril
    (D) acetaminophen
    (E) methotrexate

17. Which of the following is indicated to confirm the diagnosis of celiac sprue in a patient with positive serologic testing?

    (A) stool for fecal fat
    (B) barium enema
    (C) intestinal biopsy
    (D) antimitochondrial antibodies
    (E) food challenge

18. Mrs. Jones was referred for screening colonoscopy at the age of 50. She has no personal or family history of colorectal cancer. No polyps or lesions were found during the exam. She should be advised that colonoscopy should be repeated in how many years?

    (A) 1 year
    (B) 2 years
    (C) 3 years
    (D) 5 years
    (E) 10 years

19. A nonpenetrating tear of the gastroesophageal junction in association with a history of vomiting is known as

    (A) Boerhaave syndrome
    (B) Plummer–Vinson syndrome
    (C) Peutz–Jeghers syndrome
    (D) Mallory–Weiss syndrome
    (E) Zollinger–Ellison syndrome

20. The treatment of choice for diarrhea caused by *Giardia lamblia* is

    (A) erythromycin
    (B) tetracycline
    (C) quinolones
    (D) metronidazole
    (E) ampicillin

21. Having patients stand straight kneed, 3 then rise from the flat foot, up on to their toes and drop down on to their heels, is a test used to evaluate patients with abdominal pain. It is known as

    (A) Grey Turner sign
    (B) Blumberg sign
    (C) Markle sign
    (D) Psoas sign
    (E) Kernig sign

22. The triad of "dermatitis, diarrhea, and dementia" (pellagra) results from a severe deficiency of which of the following vitamins?

    (A) thiamine
    (B) vitamin K
    (C) riboflavin
    (D) niacin
    (E) pyridoxine

23. An elderly patient is brought in to the emergency department (ED) complaining of incontinence of liquid "like tea water" stool. He is complaining of rectal pressure and lower abdominal pain. The pain is cramping in quality and the patient's abdomen is "bloated." Digital rectal exam reveals hard stool in the rectum. Which of the following should be selected as the initial treatment for this patient?

    (A) passing a nasogastric tube
    (B) milk of magnesia
    (C) opiate analgesics for pain
    (D) oral sodium phosphate
    (E) manual disimpaction

24. The best initial diagnostic modality to diagnose cholelithiasis is which one of the following?

    (A) CT scan of the abdomen
    (B) ultrasound of the abdomen
    (C) oral cholecystogram
    (D) abdominal plain film
    (E) MRI of the abdomen

25. Cullen sign is associated with

    (A) diastasis recti
    (B) ventral hernia
    (C) musculoskeletal injury
    (D) umbilical hernia
    (E) retroperitoneal bleeding

26. Which of the following vitamins helps increase the absorption of calcium in the GI tract?

    (A) A
    (B) B
    (C) C
    (D) D
    (E) E

27. The presence of which of the following risk factors is an important clue in the diagnosis of colitis due to *C difficile?*

    (A) advanced age
    (B) non–insulin-dependent diabetes mellitus
    (C) travel to an underdeveloped country
    (D) recent hospital stay
    (E) attending a daycare or preschool center

28. A 30-year-old woman presents for evaluation of chronic diarrhea. You also note the presence of a papulovesicular rash on her extensor surfaces of the arms and legs, trunk, and neck, which is noted to be pruritic. A diagnosis of dermatitis herpetiformis is made. Which of the following disorders is the most likely cause of her diarrhea?

    (A) irritable bowel syndrome
    (B) celiac disease
    (C) pancreatitis
    (D) diverticulosis
    (E) chronic hepatitis

29. Which of the following clinical profiles is consistent with a diagnosis of Whipple disease?

    (A) 40-year-old woman, right upper quadrant (RUQ) severe pain related to fatty food ingestion and vomiting
    (B) 70-year-old woman, left lower quadrant (LLQ) pain and mass, and fever
    (C) 50-year-old man, fever, arthritis, and malabsorption
    (D) 20-year-old man, abdominal cramps, frequent bloody diarrhea, and anemia

30. Which of the following is more likely to be associated with Crohn disease versus ulcerative colitis?

    (A) anemia
    (B) large bowel involvement
    (C) anal fissure
    (D) bloody diarrhea
    (E) arthritis

31. Regular use of which of the following medications is a significant risk factor for the development of erosive gastropathy?

    (A) acetaminophen
    (B) fluoxetine
    (C) isoniazid
    (D) ibuprofen
    (E) trazodone

32. Which of the following is a complication of Barrett esophagus?

    (A) achalasia
    (B) adenocarcinoma
    (C) diffuse spasm
    (D) varices
    (E) stricture

33. Which of the following antibiotics is the most appropriate treatment for antibiotic-associated colitis?

    (A) oral ciprofloxacin
    (B) intravenous vancomycin
    (C) oral sulfasalazine
    (D) intravenous penicillin
    (E) oral metronidazole

34. A 2-year-old baby girl is brought to the ED with a history of abdominal pain and diarrhea. Mother states that the child was playing

normally and then "doubled over" with what appears to be abdominal pain. The abdomen appears slightly distended and is tender to palpation. While in the ED the child has a bloody, diarrheal bowel movement. Which of the following is the most likely diagnosis?

(A) pyloric stenosis
(B) mesenteric ischemia
(C) Crohn disease
(D) intussusception
(E) Hirschsprung disease

35. Which of the following is required for adequate absorption of vitamin B$_{12}$ from the stomach?

(A) homocysteine
(B) cholecystokinin
(C) intrinsic factor
(D) prostaglandin
(E) folate

36. A 50-year-old woman presents with constipation and crampy abdominal pain for the past 3 months. She is also undergoing a divorce and has had a 15-lb weight loss in the past 3 months. You note mild tenderness to palpation in the left lower quadrant; no masses are noted. Rectal exam result is negative, but her stool tests positive for fecal occult blood. Which of the following is the most appropriate next step to evaluate her symptoms?

(A) keep a food diary for the next 2 weeks
(B) flexible sigmoidoscopy
(C) increase dietary fiber and increase daily water intake
(D) refer for psychologic evaluation to help with stress of her divorce
(E) colonoscopy

37. The best *initial* diagnostic study for a suspected perforated peptic ulcer is which of the following?

(A) abdominal ultrasound
(B) upper GI barium swallow
(C) esophagogastroduodenoscopy (EGD)
(D) upright/decubitus abdominal plain film
(E) colonoscopy

38. Which of the following is the most common cause of traveler's diarrhea in adults?

(A) rotavirus
(B) *E coli*
(C) *Giardia lamblia*
(D) *Vibrio cholera*
(E) *S typhi*

39. A 23-year-old man presents with the complaint of rectal pain and bleeding. The pain is described as "tearing and intense" and occurs only during bowel movements. He notices bright red blood on the toilet paper after defecation but at no other time. Rectal exam is very painful but otherwise negative. His vital signs are within normal limits. Which of the following is the most likely diagnosis?

(A) anal fissure
(B) colon cancer
(C) proctalgia fugax
(D) internal hemorrhoids
(E) anorectal abscess

40. Which of the following is considered the *first-line* medical therapy for mild to moderate ulcerative pancolitis?

(A) cimetidine
(B) metronidazole
(C) sulfasalazine
(D) infliximab
(E) dexamethasone

41. In a patient who presents with hematemesis, which of the following is the most likely etiology?

(A) Meckel diverticulum
(B) diverticulitis
(C) mesenteric ischemia
(D) peptic ulcer
(E) hiatal hernia

42. An ICU patient with sepsis who is being mechanically ventilated due to respiratory failure is at significantly increased risk for which of the following?

(A) esophageal varices
(B) stress ulcer
(C) gastroparesis
(D) Mallory–Weiss tear
(E) volvulus

43. In most cases, the best approach to treatment for acute, mild to moderate, nonbloody diarrhea in an otherwise healthy adult may include all of the following *except*

(A) antibiotics
(B) bland diet
(C) electrolyte replacement by mouth
(D) acetaminophen for fever
(E) bismuth subsalicylate

44. A diet high in nitrates is a significant risk factor for cancer of which of the following?

(A) oropharynx
(B) esophagus
(C) stomach
(D) pancreas
(E) liver

45. A 5-week-old male infant presents with a 1-week history of vomiting which occurs shortly after feeding. The mother describes the vomiting as forceful and the vomitus is occasionally blood streaked; the infant has not had diarrhea. You note that the infant appears slightly dehydrated and has lost weight since a routine check at 2 weeks. Which of the following is the most likely diagnosis?

(A) peptic ulcer disease
(B) viral gastroenteritis
(C) Hirschsprung disease
(D) pyloric stenosis
(E) intussusception

46. A 14-year-old boy presents for evaluation of diarrhea, bloating, and anorexia for the past 3 weeks. He describes four to five episodes of loosely formed stools per day. No one else in his family is sick; he thinks that his symptoms may have started after returning from a camping trip about a month ago. He denies fever, weight loss, or blood in his stools. Which of the following tests would you order next to *confirm* your diagnosis?

(A) stool assay for rotavirus
(B) stool assay for *C difficile*
(C) stool for ova and parasites
(D) stool for fecal leukocytes
(E) stool cultures

47. An elderly man with a long-standing history of cirrhosis is admitted to the hospital with GI bleeding and increasing confusion and lethargy. Which of the following laboratory tests would you include to help you determine if his confusion is the result of hepatic encephalopathy?

(A) blood alcohol
(B) serum sodium
(C) alkaline phosphatase
(D) creatinine
(E) serum ammonia

48. A middle-aged man presents with the acute onset of left upper quadrant (LUQ) and midepigastric pain. He describes the severe pain as constant and gradually worsening over the past couple of hours. In the ED, he has an episode of vomiting. His LUQ and midepigastrium is tender to palpation, and no rebound or masses are noted. The patient appears anxious; his vitals are as follows: temp 100°F, BP 90/40 mm Hg, pulse 120 bpm, respirations 26 per minute. Which of the following is the most likely diagnosis?

(A) cholecystitis
(B) pancreatitis
(C) diverticulitis
(D) appendicitis
(E) gastroenteritis

49. Which of the following conditions is associated with an increase in indirect (unconjugated) bilirubin?

    (A) cholelithiasis
    (B) sclerosing cholangitis
    (C) primary biliary cirrhosis
    (D) Gilbert syndrome
    (E) cholangiocarcinoma

50. Which of the following hernias is most common in men and will typically be palpated below the inguinal ligament?

    (A) obturator
    (B) indirect inguinal
    (C) direct inguinal
    (D) femoral
    (E) ventral

51. The majority of cases of thiamine deficiency in the United States are due to which of the following underlying conditions?

    (A) alcoholism
    (B) pernicious anemia
    (C) celiac disease
    (D) bulimia
    (E) cholestatic liver disease

52. Which one the following symptoms is a "red flag" symptom that suggests a diagnosis other than irritable bowel syndrome?

    (A) passage of mucus in the stool
    (B) hematochezia
    (C) constipation
    (D) abdominal cramping
    (E) watery stools

Answers and Explanations

1. **(C)** Patients with chronic GERD are at risk for Barrett esophagus, which is a metaplasia linked to chronic reflux-induced injury to the squamous epithelium. It may lead to esophageal adenocarcinoma. Therefore, screening endoscopy may be recommended. Candidal esophagitis is likely to be found in immunosuppressed patients, uncontrolled diabetic patients, and those being treated with systemic steroids or antibiotics. A Zenker diverticulum is a protrusion of the pharyngeal mucosa that develops at the pharyngoesophageal junction. Symptoms include dysphagia and regurgitation. It is not a complication of GERD. Esophageal varices develop in patients secondary to portal hypertension. They are associated with cirrhosis and may result in serious upper gastrointestinal bleeding. *(McQuaid, 2009, pp. 516-517)*

2. **(B)** Hepatitis D appears to be a virus infecting a virus. It is a defective RNA virus that can exist only in the presence of hepatitis B. When there is coinfection, the illness produced is more severe than an infection with hepatitis B alone. *(Friedman, 2009, p. 587)*

3. **(C)** Cigarette smoking is known to retard ulcer healing. Alcohol, dietary factors, and stress do not appear to cause or exacerbate ulcer disease. Ulcers occur more frequently in the age range of 30 to 55 years, but age is not implicated in nonhealing. *(McQuaid, 2009, pp. 532, 538)*

4. **(C)** Scurvy is caused by the lack of dietary vitamin C. It will cause perifollicular hemorrhages, ecchymoses of the legs, bleeding gums, loose teeth, and GI bleeding. Melanin spots on the lips, buccal mucosa, and tongue with bleeding polypoid lesions in the small intestines are referred to as Peutz–Jeghers syndrome. Rendu–Osler–Weber is associated with telangiectasias on the face and buccal mucosa and similar lesions in the GI tract. Neurofibromatosis is associated with café au late pigmentation, pedunculated fibromas, and fibromas in the GI tract that may bleed. Rubber-bleb nevus syndrome is associated with cavernous hemangiomas of the skin and similar lesion in the small intestines. *(LeBlond et al., 2009, pp. 607-608)*

5. **(E)** Interferon is contraindicated in patients with autoimmune disease. Interferon is also contraindicated in patients with severe liver disease and history of cardiac arrhythmia. It should be used with caution in patients with major depressive disorders, cytopenia, hyperthyroidism, and severe renal insufficiency. *(Safrin, 2009, pp. 868)*

6. **(A)** Primary biliary cirrhosis affects women typically between ages 40 and 60. It is often discovered incidentally when the serum alkaline phosphatase level is found to be elevated. Many patients do not have pain, which is more common in cholecystitis or pancreatitis. Primary sclerosing cholangitis is more likely to occur in a patient with known inflammatory bowel disease. *(Friedman, 2009, pp. 607-608, 622)*

7. **(B)** Large volume, watery, nonbloody diarrhea accompanied by nausea and vomiting characterizes small bowel diarrhea caused by a toxin-producing bacteria such as *E coli* or a virus. Infection with *Salmonella*, *Shigella*, *C difficile*, and *Campylobacter* results in an inflammatory

diarrhea characterized by small volume, often bloody diarrhea without prominent nausea. *(McQuaid, 2009, pp. 496-497)*

8. **(A)** Chronic diarrhea from cryptosporidiosis may be indicative of underlying immunodeficiency. Patients with a positive culture should be checked for HIV. Rarely do patients with intact immune systems have problems with this organism, so checking family members would not be useful. Isolation also is not indicated. Blood cultures and colonoscopy study would not offer increased information with this diagnosis. *(Rosenthal, 2009, pp. 1336-1337)*

9. **(E)** The maternal–neonatal transmission with hepatitis C is low. Hepatitis C is an RNA virus that is similar to flaviviruses. The incubation period averages 6 to 7 weeks, and is more likely to become chronic than hepatitis B. Coinfection with hepatitis D occurs with hepatitis B, not hepatitis C. *(Friedman, 2009, pp. 587-588)*

10. **(C)** CT findings consistent with diverticulitis include soft tissue thickening of the pericolic fat (98%), diverticula, and thickening of the bowel wall. In immunosuppressed patients, findings may include intraperitoneal and extraperitoneal gases without fluid or abscess formation. *(Travis, 2009, p. 249)*

11. **(B)** A deck of cards or a bar of soap is a good way to help a person visualize a 3-oz portion size of lean meat. A matchboxbook would be about the size of a 1-oz serving and a thin paperback book would represent an 8-oz serving of lean meat. *(Blackburn, 2005, p. 612)*

12. **(C)** The most common causes of pill-induced esophagitis are nonsteroidal medications. Other commonly prescribed medications causing esophageal injury include slow release of potassium chloride, iron sulfate, quinine sulfate, and alendronate sodium. *(McQuaid, 2009, pp. 520-521)*

13. **(D)** Men are more likely than women to get esophageal cancer. The most common esophageal malignancy in the African American population is squamous cell carcinoma. Risk factors include excessive alcohol and tobacco use. Adenocarcinoma is more common in whites and is thought to be a complication of chronic gastroesophageal reflux. Benign tumors such as leiomyomas are rare. *(McQuaid and Rugo, 2009, p. 1441)*

14. **(B)** Diverticulosis may arise anywhere in the large intestine, from the cecum to the end of the sigmoid colon. In Western societies, diverticula most often occur in the sigmoid colon where there is greatest intraluminal pressure. *(McQuaid, 2009, p. 572)*

15. **(D)** Barium esophagography has a limited role in the diagnostic management of patients with GERD. It may be used in patients with severe dysphagia to evaluate the degree of stricture. Asthma, chronic cough, chronic laryngitis, sore throat, and atypical chest pain are increasingly being recognized as atypical manifestations of GERD and reflux may be a causative or exacerbating factor. Behavioral interventions such as those mentioned above (B) as well as avoiding bending after meals have a role in the management of GERD as do the H$_2$-receptor agonists and proton pump inhibitors. *(McQuaid, 2009, p. 525)*

16. **(D)** A number of drugs may cause acute liver failure but acetaminophen toxicity is the most common of acute hepatic failure. Suicide attempts account for a significant portion of acetaminophen-induced hepatic failure. All of the drugs listed can cause acute liver failure. *(Friedman, 2009, p. 591)*

17. **(C)** Intestinal biopsy is the most specific test in establishing the diagnosis of celiac sprue in a patient who has a positive test for IgA endomysial antibody. Classic symptoms of malabsorption are more common in infants but less common in adults. Stool for fecal fat would be a nonspecific finding. Antimitochondrial antibodies are seen in patients with primary biliary cirrhosis. *(McQuaid, 2009, pp. 543-544)*

18. **(E)** In average-risk individuals aged 50 or greater than 50, screening colonoscopy should be repeated every 10 years following an initial

normal exam. If the individual has a first-degree relative with a history of adenomas or colorectal cancer, screening should begin earlier, generally at age 40 or 10 years younger than the age at diagnosis of the youngest affected relative. *(Rugo, 2009, pp. 1452-1453)*

19. **(D)** A mucosal tear of the gastroesophageal junction with a history of prolonged vomiting is known as Mallory–Weiss tear syndrome. Plummer–Vinson is a congenital syndrome associated with anemia and webbing of the esophagus. Boerhaave syndrome is a rare life-threatening problem characterized by a full-thickness tear of the esophageal wall. Zollinger–Ellison syndrome is caused by gastrin-secreting neuroendocrine tumors resulting in acid hypersecretion. *(McQuaid, 2009, pp. 489, 521-522, 541, 576)*

20. **(D)** The treatment of choice for diarrhea caused by *Giardia* is metronidazole 250 to 750 mg po three times per day. Erythromycin can be used to treat *Campylobacter*. Doxycycline or tetracycline can be used to treat cholera. Quinolones can also be used to treat cholera and shigellosis. *(Dipiro, 2008, p. 1888)*

21. **(C)** Markle sign is also known as the jar sign and it may prove superior to rebound tenderness as a localizing sign of peritoneal irritation, especially in the pelvis. It is performed by having the patients go from standing on their toes to dropping quickly down to their heels. When they hit the floor, the location of their abdominal pain should be noted. Blumberg sign is another name for rebound tenderness. It is elicited by pressing the fingers gently into the abdomen and then suddenly withdrawing them. The pain will worsen in a certain area when the fingers are taken away. Succession splash refers to air and fluid in the stomach and the bowel moving and making audible splashing noise. Kernig sign is a test for spinal cord irritation. *(Seidel, 2006, p. 557; LeBlond, 2009, p. 481)*

22. **(D)** Niacin deficiency is known as pellagra. It is rare in the United States and is most often a complication of alcoholism or malabsorption

syndrome. Clinical signs of pellagra are known as the 3 Ds—dermatitis, diarrhea, and dementia. *(Baron, 2009, pp. 1114-1115)*

23. **(E)** Mechanical bowel obstruction in the rectum does not usually respond to oral laxatives. A nasogastric tube would not be used for an obstruction in the distal colon/rectum. One would avoid opiates in fecal impactions and other constipation problems because they tend to be more constipating. This patient needs to be disimpacted. Oral agents are unlikely to be effective against the fecal impaction and may cause complications. *(McQuaid, 2008, p. 481)*

24. **(B)** Ultrasound has replaced oral cholecystograms as the test of choice for diagnosing cholelithiasis. CT is useful in the evaluation of the acute abdomen but the sensitivity for viewing the gallstones is poor. KUB is also not a sensitive study for cholelithiasis. MRI is expensive and not recommended as an initial screening exam for gallstones but can be used if ultrasound is equivocal. *(Paumgartner, 2009, pp. 541-542)*

25. **(E)** A faint blue coloration may occur as a result of retroperitoneal bleeding. This is known as Cullen sign. Diastasis recti occurs when the rectus muscles lack a normal fibrous band that attaches them at the midline. An umbilical calculus is usually the result of poor hygiene. An umbilical hernia will occur when a weakness occurs in the abdominal wall in the area of the umbilicus, and a fistula in that area can tract from various organs causing discharge from the umbilicus. *(LeBlond, 2009, p. 478)*

26. **(D)** Vitamin D increases the absorption of calcium and phosphorus in the GI tract and induces osteoclast activity, which causes an overall increase in serum calcium levels. *(Hutton, 2005, p. 32)*

27. **(D)** Risk factors for the development of *C difficile* include concurrent or recent use of antibiotics as well as a hospital or nursing home stay. *C difficile* colonization is found in approximately 3% of healthy adults. Increasing rates of infection are being noted in hospitalized

patients secondary to transmission by hospital personnel. *(McQuaid, 2009, p. 558)*

28. **(B)** Nearly all patients presenting with dermatitis herpetiformis have histological evidence of celiac disease even if it is not clinically apparent. Less than 10% of patients with celiac disease will also have this dermatologic disorder. Dermatitis herpetiformis is not associated with the other disorders. *(McQuaid, 2009, p. 544)*

29. **(C)** Whipple disease typically occurs in white men in their fourth to sixth decades. It is characterized by seronegative arthritis, fever, lymphadenopathy, weight loss, malabsorption, and diarrhea. Whipple disease is caused by the *Tropheryma whippelii* organism and is diagnosed by polymerase chain reaction (PCR) or endoscopic biopsy of the duodenum. *(McQuaid, 2009, pp. 545-546)*

30. **(C)** Crohn disease and ulcerative colitis are inflammatory conditions affecting the GI tract. Crohn disease primarily involves the small bowel (terminal ileum) and the proximal ascending colon. One-third of cases may have perioral or perianal involvement (fissure, fistula, abscess). Ulcerative colitis affects only the colon, most commonly the distal portion and does not have perianal involvement. Extraintestinal manifestations such as arthritis, arthralgias, and skin rash may occur with both conditions. Both conditions may have bloody diarrhea although it is more common in ulcerative colitis. *(McQuaid, 2009, pp. 562-563, 567-568)*

31. **(D)** One of the most common causes of erosive gastropathy are NSAID medications. Other common causes are alcohol, mechanical ventilation, and stress related to critical illness. *(McQuaid, 2009, p. 529)*

32. **(B)** The most serious complication of Barrett esophagus is esophageal adenocarcinoma, which arises from dysplastic epithelium. Patients with Barrett esophagus have a significantly increased risk compared to those patients who do not. *(Poneros, 2009, pp. 148-150)*

33. **(E)** Oral metronidazole is the drug of choice. Both vancomycin and metronidazole are effective; however, metronidazole is less expensive and there is less of a concern for vancomycin resistance. *(Dipiro, 2008, p. 1863)*

34. **(D)** Intussusception is the most frequent cause of intestinal obstruction in the first 2 years of life. The patient develops paroxysms of pain followed by bloody bowel movements. Pyloric stenosis typically presents prior to the age of 6 months with vomiting but not with diarrhea. Hirschsprung disease results from an absence of ganglion cells in the colon and typically presents early in life with failure to pass meconium, followed by vomiting and abdominal distension. The typical age of onset is later in adolescence in Crohn disease and in the elderly in mesenteric ischemia. *(Sondheimer, 2007, pp. 607-608, 612, 617, 634)*

35. **(C)** After ingestion, vitamin B_{12} binds to intrinsic factor, which is secreted by gastric parietal cells. Vitamin B_{12} is involved in the conversion of homocysteine to methionine. Cholecystokinin is secreted by cells of the small intestine and stimulates contraction of the gallbladder. Absorption of iron occurs in the stomach, duodenum, and upper jejunum. Folate absorption occurs along the entire GI tract. *(Linker, 2009, pp. 427, 433-434)*

36. **(E)** Any symptomatic adult with a positive fecal occult blood test should undergo colonoscopy to rule out colorectal cancer. A flexible sigmoidoscopy will allow for only partial visualization of the colon. *(McQuaid, 2009, p. 507)*

37. **(D)** The presence of free intraperitoneal air on an upright or decubitus film in the majority of patients with peptic ulcer perforation. This finding along with a classic history of sudden onset of severe abdominal pain and a rigid, quiet abdomen should establish the diagnosis in most cases without the need for further studies. Barium studies are contraindicated in patients with a possible perforation. *(McQuaid, 2009, p. 540)*

38. **(B)** Bacteria cause 80% of cases of traveler's diarrhea, with enterotoxigenic *E. coli*, *Shigella* species, and *C jejuni* being the most common pathogens. Viruses such as rotavirus are the most common cause of acute gastroenteritis in children. *(Sondheimer, 2007, pp. 621-622; Trier, 2009, pp. 50-56)*

39. **(A)** Anal fissure is thought to be due to trauma to the anal canal during defecation. Patients will complain of severe pain during defecation with occasional blood noted on the surface of the stool or on the toilet paper. Proctalgia fugax presents with acute, severe rectal pain but without bleeding. Internal hemorrhoids may have bleeding but are typically painless. Colorectal cancer more typically presents with a change in bowel habits or obstructive symptoms. Anorectal abscess typically manifests as continuous, throbbing perianal pain. *(McQuaid, 2009, pp. 580-581; Rugo, 2009, p. 1450)*

40. **(C)** 5-ASA products such as sulfasalazine or mesalamine are generally considered initial treatment agents for patients with mild to moderate colitis. Topical therapy with 5-ASA products or hydrocortisone may be effective for patients with distal colitis. Immunomodulating agents such as infliximab are generally reserved for patients with severe or unresponsive disease. Oral antibiotics such as metronidazole and ciprofloxacin are used in the treatment of active Crohn with little evidence for effectiveness. *(McQuaid, 2009, pp. 564-569)*

41. **(D)** Approximately 50% of episodes of upper GI bleeding are due to peptic ulcers. Meckel diverticulum, diverticular disease, and mesenteric ischemia may present with lower GI bleeding. Hiatal hernias usually cause no symptoms. *(McQuaid, 2009, pp. 502, 515, 532)*

42. **(B)** Stress-related ulcers develop in a majority of critically ill patients within 72 hours of admission. Additional factors that place the patient at risk for significant bleeding are mechanical ventilation for greater than 72 hours and coagulopathy. Additional risk factors for development of stress ulcers are severe burns, trauma, and sepsis. Mallory–Weiss tears usually with hematemesis usually follow a prolonged period of retching/vomiting. Volvulus or a twisting of the bowel is most frequently due to adhesions or redundant colon in adults. Gastroparesis is a chronic condition with multiple etiologies including endocrine and neurologic conditions such as diabetes and multiple sclerosis. *(McQuaid, 2009, pp. 529, 551)*

43. **(A)** Most mild diarrhea will not lead to dehydration if the patient takes adequate oral fluids containing carbohydrates and electrolytes. "Resting" the bowel by avoiding high-fiber foods, fats, and caffeine may be helpful. Loperamide and bismuth subsalicylate may also be safely used to reduce symptoms and acetaminophen to reduce a low-grade fever. Empiric antibiotic treatment of all patients with diarrhea is not indicated. Antibiotic treatment is typically considered only if the patient presents with moderate to severe fever, tenesmus, and bloody diarrhea. *(McQuaid, 2009, pp. 497-499)*

44. **(C)** In addition to chronic *H pylori* infections, dietary nitrates are a significant risk factor for gastric cancer. *(Rugo, 2009, pp. 1443-1444)*

45. **(D)** Pyloric stenosis usually presents with forceful/projectile vomiting between 2 and 4 weeks of age. There is a 4:1 male predominance; dehydration and failure to thrive may develop. Peptic ulcer disease can occur at any age and commonly affects more men but is more common from 12 to 18 years of age. Intussusception is more common in men but presents with colicky abdominal pain with subsequent development of vomiting and bloody diarrhea. *(Sondheimer, 2007, pp. 607-610, 616)*

46. **(C)** Giardiasis, caused by *Giardia lamblia*, typically presents with chronic diarrhea, anorexia, malabsorption, and weight loss. Giardiasis is the most common intestinal protozoal infection in children in the United States and is diagnosed by finding the parasite in the stool or detecting *Giardia* antigen in feces. *(Weinberg, 2007, p. 1228)*

47. **(E)** One of the causes of hepatic encephalopathy manifesting as CNS dysfunction is the liver's failure to remove toxic byproducts of

digestion such as ammonia in an advanced state of liver disease, cirrhosis, or severe hepatitis. Bleeding into the GI tract may also significantly increase the level of proteins in the bowel and precipitate encephalopathy. One symptom of hyponatremia is confusion, but this would not be specific to hepatic encephalopathy as there are many causes of hyponatremia. *(Friedman, 2009, p. 605)*

48. **(B)** The classic presentation of acute pancreatitis is the typically sudden onset of severe, deep epigastric or LUQ pain, which often radiates to the back or left shoulder. Fever, nausea, vomiting, and signs of hypovolemic shock may be present. Cholecystitis, diverticulitis, appendicitis would typically present with pain in different quadrants; low-grade fever and hypovolemic signs would be uncommon. Gastroenteritis would present with nausea, vomiting, and possibly low-grade fever but without abdominal pain or hypovolemia. *(Friedman, 2009, pp. 617-618, 623-624; Seidel et al., 2006, p. 552)*

49. **(D)** Elevations of unconjugated (indirect) bilirubin result from hemolysis or inability to conjugate bilirubin in the liver as in Gilbert syndrome. Conjugated (direct) bilirubinemia results from impaired excretion of bilirubin from the liver due to hepatocellular disease such as hepatitis or obstruction of the bile ducts from conditions such as cholelithiasis, sclerosing cholangitis, and cancer of biliary ducts (cholangiocarcinoma). *(Fischbach, 2000, p. 387; Friedman, 2009, pp. 582-583)*

50. **(D)** The femoral nerve, artery, and vein lie lateral and inferior to the inguinal ligament. Just medial to the vein is the femoral canal through which a hernia may bulge. Direct and indirect inguinal hernias are typically palpated above the inguinal ligament. Obturator hernias are rare and typically occur in elderly women. *(LeBlond, 2009, p. 524)*

51. **(A)** Most cases of thiamine deficiency in the United States are due to chronic alcoholism. Patients with chronic alcoholism have poor dietary intake as well as impaired thiamine absorption and metabolism. *(Baron, 2009, p. 1113)*

52. **(B)** Typical symptoms of irritable bowel syndrome include abdominal pain relieved by defecation, constipation, loose or watery stools, mucus in the stools, and a feeling of abdominal bloating. The presence of blood in the stools, hematochezia, is not a feature of irritable bowel syndrome and warrants further investigation. *(McQuaid, 2009, pp. 554-555)*

REFERENCES

Baron RB. Nutritional disorders. In: McPhee SJ, Papadakis MA, eds. *Current Medical Diagnosis and Treatment.* 48th ed. New York, NY: McGraw-Hill; 2009.

Blackburn GL, Waltman BA. Physician's guide to the new 2005 dietary guidelines: how best to counsel patients. *Cleve Clin J Med.* 2005; 72(7):609-617.

Dipiro JT, Talbert RL, Yee GC, et al., *Pharmacotherapy: A Pathophysiologic Approach.* 7th ed. New York, NY: McGraw-Hill; 2008.

Fischbach F. *A Manual of Laboratory and Diagnostic Tests.* 6th ed. Philadelphia, PA: Lippincott; 2000.

Friedman LS. Liver, biliary tract, and pancreas disorders. In: McPhee SJ, Papadakis MA, eds. *Current Medical Diagnosis and Treatment.* 48th ed. New York, NY: McGraw-Hill; 2009.

Hutton E. Evaluation and management of hypercalcemia. *JAAPA.* 2005; 18(6):30-35.

LeBlond RF, Brown DD, DeGowin RL. *DeGowin's Diagnostic Examinnation.* New York: McGraw-Hill; 2009.

Linker CA. Blood disorders. In: McPhee SJ, Papadakis MA, eds. *Current Medical Diagnosis and Treatment.* 48th ed. New York, NY: McGraw-Hill; 2009.

McQuaid KR, Rugo HS. Esophageal cancer. In: McPhee SJ, Papadakis MA, eds. *Current Medical Diagnosis and Treatment.* 48th ed. New York, NY: McGraw-Hill; 2009.

McQuaid KR. Gastrointestinal disorders. In: McPhee SJ, Papadakis MA, eds. *Current Medical Diagnosis and Treatment.* 47th ed. New York, NY: McGraw-Hill; 2008.

McQuaid KR. Gastrointestinal disorders. In: McPhee SJ, Papadakis MA, eds. *Current Medical Diagnosis and Treatment.* 48th ed. New York, NY: McGraw-Hill; 2009.

Paumgartner G, Greenberger NJ. Gallstone disease. In: Greenberger NJ, ed. *Current Diagnosis & Treatment: Gastroenterology, Hepatology, & Endoscopy.* New York, NY: McGraw-Hill; 2009.

Poneros JM. Barrett esophagus. In: Greenberger NJ, ed. *Current Diagnosis & Treatment: Gastroenterology, Hepatology, & Endoscopy.* New York, NY: McGraw-Hill; 2009.

Rosenthal PJ. Protozoal & helminthic infections. In: McPhee SJ, Papadakis MA, eds. *Current Medical Diagnosis and Treatment.* 48th ed. New York, NY: McGraw-Hill; 2009.

Rugo HS. Cancer. In: McPhee SJ, Papadakis MA, eds. *Current Medical Diagnosis and Treatment.* 48th ed. New York, NY: McGraw-Hill; 2009.

Safrin S. Antiviral agents. In: Katzung BG, Masters SB, Trevor AJ, eds. *Basic and Clinical Pharmacology.* 11th ed. New York, NY: McGraw-Hill; 2009.

Seidel HM, Ball JW, Dains JE, et al. *Mosby's Guide to Physical Examination.* 6th ed. St. Louis, MO: Mosby; 2006.

Sondheimer JM. Gastrointestinal tract. In: Hay WW, Levin MJ, Sondheimer JM, eds. *Current Diagnosis and Treatment in Pediatrics.* 18th ed. New York, NY: McGraw-Hill; 2007.

Travis AC, Blumberg RS. Diverticular disease of the colon. In: Greenberger NJ, eds. *Current Diagnosis & Treatment: Gastroenterology, Hepatology, & Endoscopy.* New York, NY: McGraw-Hill; 2009.

Trier JS. Acute diarrheal disorders. In: Greenberger NJ, ed. *Current Diagnosis & Treatment: Gastroenterology, Hepatology, & Endoscopy.* New York, NY: McGraw-Hill; 2009.

Weinberg A, Levin MJ. Infections: parasitic & mycotic. In: Hay WW, Levin MJ, Sondheimer JM, Deterding RR, eds. *Current Diagnosis and Treatment in Pediatrics.* 18th ed. New York, NY: McGraw-Hill; 2007.

CHAPTER 6

Hematology/Oncology

Maura Polansky, MS, PA-C

DIRECTIONS: Each of the numbered items or incomplete statements in this section is followed by answers or by completion of the statement. Select the ONE lettered answer or completion that is BEST in each case.

1. A 32 year-old African-American asymptomatic woman presents to her gynecologist's office for a physical examination. She has no medical history. She mentions that she has recently become engaged and that she is aware that her fiancée's family has suffered from sickle cell disease, although he is "healthy." They are planning a honeymoon to the mountains. Which of the following issues would be MOST appropriate to discuss?

   (A) The risk of infertility for her husband, if he carries the sickle cell gene.
   (B) Reassure her of the low risk of illness for her children, given her and her future husband's lack of apparent sickle cell disease.
   (C) Offer to refer her for genetic counseling.
   (D) Advise against travel to high-altitude regions for her husband.
   (E) Counseling regarding the increased risk of sexually transmitted infections for those with sickle cell trait.

2. Which of the following is true of iron deficiency anemia?

   (A) It is most commonly due to acute blood loss.

   (B) It does not frequently occur from the typical American diet.
   (C) The primary cause during pregnancy is increased red blood cells destruction.
   (D) Confirmation by bone marrow aspiration is required.
   (E) Treatment with long-term iron replacement is typically greater than 1 year.

3. Which of the following are consistent with lead poisoning?

   (A) profound anemia
   (B) complaints of severe fatigue and persistent muscle weakness
   (C) acute difficulty concentrating after exposure
   (D) basophilic stippling
   (E) treatment with chelating agent is always required

4. A 48-year-old previously healthy, African-American man presents to his local emergency center with dyspnea on exertion while mowing the grass. He has no significant medical history. Laboratory studies reveal a WBC of 6.1, Hgb of 9.7, Hct of 29, mean corpuscle volume (MCV) of 68, and platelet count of 254,000. What diagnosis is most likely causing his symptoms?

   (A) sickle cell anemia
   (B) thalassemia
   (C) iron deficiency
   (D) hemolytic anemia
   (E) TTP

5. Which of the following is true of macrocytic anemias?

   (A) Causes include poor absorption of vitamin B_{12} in the stomach due to prior gastrectomy.
   (B) Schilling test is used to diagnose folate deficiency.
   (C) Folate supplementation should be started empirically to prevent worsening anemia, while further studies are being performed.
   (D) When associated with loss of taste and atrophy of the tongue mucosa, it suggests vitamin B_{12} deficiency.
   (E) Strict vegetarians are at risk of folate deficiency and may need chronic supplementation.

6. One day, while covering the internal medicine floor, you evaluate a 74 year-old woman patient who was admitted for pneumonia from the nursing home where she lives. Upon reviewing the routine laboratory studies ordered for that day, you note that the patient has developed an anemia. The chemistry profile reveals a total bilirubin of 2.6 with an elevated lactate dehydrogenase (LDH). Other labs, including additional chemistries and coagulation panel, are normal. The most likely cause of both her anemia and hyperbilirubinemia is

   (A) malaria
   (B) medication
   (C) folate deficiency
   (D) iron deficiency
   (E) disseminated intravascular coagulopathy (DIC)

7. When using tamoxifen in the treatment of malignancy, one must keep which of the following toxicities in mind.

   (A) impotence
   (B) peripheral neuropathy
   (C) secondary malignancy
   (D) pulmonary fibrosis
   (E) thromboembolic disease

8. Which tumor marker may be used in the screening of patients for cancer?

   (A) prostatic acid phosphate
   (B) carcinoembryonic antigen
   (C) cancer antigen 19–9
   (D) alpha-fetoprotein
   (E) cancer antigen 125

9. Thalassemia

   (A) is a rare cause of normocytic, normochronic anemia
   (B) is most common in those of European descent
   (C) may result in few problems, except during stress states
   (D) may be diagnosed by peripheral smear
   (E) may be an acquired or hereditary disease

10. A 76 year-old woman presents to the emergency department (ED) after experiencing severe pain in the left hip, worse upon standing or walking. She denies any falls or trauma precipitating the pain. Physical examination reveals enlarged suboccipital and cervical lymph nodes. Electrophoresis studies are positive for serum IgM. Subsequent urinalysis was positive for Bence-Jones proteins. Which of the following additional findings would be consistent with the most probable diagnosis?

    (A) hypercalcemia
    (B) jaundice
    (C) osteoblastic lesions on x-ray
    (D) splenomegaly
    (E) hypotension

11. A 16 year-old girl presented with an enlarged lymph node at the back of her neck. After an ultrasound of the lymph node, she was told that it was "benign." Two weeks later, another node appeared in the same general region and it was mildly tender. Upon questioning, she stated she does have cats but does not remember being scratched prior to the first enlarged lymph node. The patient was placed on azithromycin without resolution. A complete blood cell count (CBC) was obtained, which

revealed hematocrit of 31.8 and WBC of 152.4 with a differential of 26% neutrophils (normal 48%–55%), 69% lymphocytes (normal 7%–33%), 3% monocytes (normal 2%–7%), 1% eosinophils (normal 1%–4%), and 1% basophils (normal 0%–1%). Given the patient's age and presentation, the probable diagnosis is

(A) cat-scratch disease

(B) chronic myelogenous leukemia (CML)

(C) chronic lymphocytic leukemia (CLL)

(D) aplastic anemia

(E) acute lymphocytic leukemia (ALL)

12. A 68-year-old man presents with a 10-week history of fatigue, anorexia, and a 10-lb weight loss. During the last 2 days he has had increasing shortness of breath and bleeding of the gingivae. He is found to be profoundly anemic and thrombocytopenic. Total white blood cell count is 15,000/uL. What diagnostic evaluation is promptly indicated to confirm your suspected diagnosis?

(A) chest x-ray

(B) lumbar puncture

(C) blood cultures

(D) bone marrow biopsy

(E) genetic testing

13. Disseminated intravascular coagulopathy

(A) is a common complication of perioperative blood loss.

(B) when diagnosed promptly is often self-limiting, resulting in low mortality.

(C) frequently causes thrombotic complications.

(D) is often idiopathic.

(E) should not be managed with fresh frozen plasma (FFP) and platelets, as both are contraindicated.

14. Common complications of external beam irradiation may include

(A) myelosuppression

(B) cancer growth

(C) fatigue

(D) worsening bone pain during treatment of bone metastasis

(E) generalized hair loss

15. Choose the correct statement regarding the condition known as Christmas disease.

(A) is a deficiency of factor XI.

(B) is similar to factor VIII deficiency and may be treated with factor VIII concentrates.

(C) may result in both easy bleeding and clotting.

(D) another name for this disease is Hemophilia A.

(E) is a x-linked recessive disease, affecting primarily men.

16. A 44-year-old 80-kg Caucasian man presents to the emergency department with slurred speech and right arm numbness for 1 hour. He had a history of a similar episode 6 months prior, without residual effect. He also had a myocardial infarction at age 40 and deep venous thrombosis (DVT) of the right leg with no history of hypertension or diabetes. Which of the following should be included in his work-up to determine the cause of his condition?

(A) myelogram

(B) lupus anticoagulant

(C) hemoglobin electrophoresis

(D) platelet function assay

(E) d-dimer

17. What is a common cause of intravascular hemolytic anemia?

(A) blood transfusion reaction

(B) lead poisoning

(C) thrombotic thrombocytopenic purpura (TTP)

(D) sickle cell anemia

(E) DIC

18. A 28-year-old woman presented to her primary care physician for her annual examination reporting that she had noticed recently that when she took her normal dose of two aspirin for menstrual cramps, she subsequently experienced a small amount of nose bleeding. She was concerned because she had been told that her family had "problems with bleeding." She was found to have a prolonged bleeding time and a reduced level of VIII antigen. Considering the patient's age, the most appropriate initial tests would include

(A) plasma von Willebrand factor (vWF) concentration

(B) factor VIII:C level

(C) factor IX coagulant activity

(D) vitamin K level

(E) folate

19. A 44-year-old woman presents to the emergency department after receiving a puncture wound to the foot by a rusty nail, while working in the yard. On examination, she is found to have splenomegaly. What signs or symptoms may be helpful in identifying the underlying cause of her splenomegaly?

(A) petechiae

(B) spider angiomas

(C) LUQ (lower upper quadrant) fullness

(D) reflux

(E) early satiety

20. In which situation should you most likely consider referring a patient for genetic counseling?

(A) personal history of breast cancer at age 52

(B) family history of a mother with primary brain tumor at age 3

(C) family history of maternal grandmother with breast cancer at age 52, maternal grandfather with prostate cancer diagnosed at age 78, and paternal grandfather with lung cancer diagnosed at age 64

(D) family history of a sister with colon cancer at age 29

(E) personal history of several skin cancers and three prior colonic polyps, now with colon cancer at age 58

21. Heparin-induced thrombocytopenia (HIT)

(A) typically occurs within 24 hours of first exposure to heparin.

(B) is more common with low-molecular-weight heparin.

(C) is frequently associated with severe bleeding complications.

(D) is treated with steroids, which may allow for continuation of heparin when medically necessary.

(E) can result in complications, such as pulmonary embolus.

22. When encountering a patient with petechiae noted on physical examination,

(A) a platelet count of 204,000 suggests evolving thrombocytopenia as the cause.

(B) a platelet count of 204,00 in a patient on clopidogrel (Plavix) suggests this agent is not therapeutic in its antiplatelet effect.

(C) with a platelet count of 45,000, a bleeding time should be performed.

(D) hepatic dysfunction should be in the differential diagnosis.

(E) suspected overdose of coumadin should be considered in those on that agent.

23. A 40-year-old woman presents to her primary care provider for an annual evaluation. Routine laboratory studies include a CBC with a hemoglobin of 11.2 (normal 12–14) and MCV of 82 (normal 82–98). Because of the low hemoglobin, the patient is asked to return to the lab for additional studies. These include the following:

Serum iron 57 (normal 49–181)	Ferritin 193 (normal 22–322)
TIBC 545 (normal 250–450)	Folate 40.4 (normal 1.5–22)
B_{12} 260 (normal 211–911)	Reticulocyte count 0.9 (normal 0.5–1.5)

The results suggest that the low hemoglobin is caused by

(A) normal variation in hemoglobin level

(B) anemia of chronic disease

(C) pernicious anemia

(D) iron deficiency anemia

(E) sickle cell trait

24. A 33-year-old man presents after passing out at the gym. His wife states he had been feeling fine but had recently experienced some gingival bleeding while brushing his teeth. There is no past medical history in this previously healthy young man. The only medication he uses is a nonsteroidal anti-inflammatory agent. On examination, he is noted to be slightly pale; otherwise the examination is completely normal. His blood counts are as follows: hemoglobin of 8.2, hematocrit of 15.6, MCV of 90, platelet count of 20,000, and white blood cell count of 1.3 with a normal differential. What is the most likely diagnosis?

(A) Hodgkin's disease

(B) aplastic anemia

(C) chronic lymphocytic lymphoma

(D) lupus

(E) idiopathic thrombocytopenic purpura

25. What is the most frequent cause of anemia in cancer patients?

(A) iron deficiency

(B) intrinsic factor deficiency

(C) inadequate erythropoietin

(D) pernicious anemia

(E) hemolysis

26. A 68-year-old woman with a history of ovarian cancer presents to your emergency department with fever. She is undergoing neoadjuvant chemotherapy prior to a planned resection in a couple months. What is the most important diagnostic test to order in determining how best to evaluate and manage this patient?

(A) CA 125

(B) computed tomography (CT) scan

(C) bone marrow aspirate

(D) complete blood cell count

(E) bacterial and fungal blood cultures

27. A 52-year-old man presents complaining of early satiety and mild fatigue for the last 5 months. He has no other complaints and no significant medical history, other than a tonsillectomy at age 6 and well-controlled hypertension. On examination, there is no lymphadenopathy or hepatomegaly, but his spleen is palpable. A blood smear shows a hemoglobin of 13.9, hematocrit of 42.0, platelet count of 580,000, and a white blood cell count of 85,000 with some immature cells but only 1% blasts. A bone marrow performed the next day shows a hypercellular sample with essentially a normal differential, and again, only 1% blasts. Chromosome analysis shows presence of the Philadelphia chromosome (t(9;22)). What is the most likely diagnosis?

(A) acute lymphocytic leukemia

(B) acute myelogenous leukemia

(C) chronic myelogenous leukemia

(D) chronic lymphocytic leukemia

(E) Burkitt lymphoma

28. A 33-year-old woman presents complaining of profound fatigue for the past 6 weeks, necessitating her quitting her job. She looks pale and is tachycardic at 110 bpm, but otherwise her exam is normal. A blood smear shows a hemoglobin of 4.5, hematocrit of 13.4, platelet count of 19,000, and white blood cell count of 3.1 with 21% blasts that have Auer rods. The most likely diagnosis is

(A) Hodgkin's disease

(B) non-Hodgkin's lymphoma

(C) chronic myelogenous leukemia

(D) acute myelogenous leukemia

(E) hemolytic anemia

29. On routine exam of an 18-year-old man entering college, bilateral nontender, supraclavicular lymphadenopathy is noted. The patient denies any pain on palpation. Which of the following specific symptoms is most concerning for your suspected diagnosis?

(A) hoarseness

(B) fever

(C) pharyngeal erythema

(D) hair loss

(E) early satiety

30. A 55-year-old African-American man recently presented to the clinic with severe back pain, constipation, and confusion. Laboratory studies revealed anemia, hypercalcemia, and renal failure. Plain radiographs revealed a pathological fracture involving T5–T6 vertebrae. Osteolytic lesions were also present in the skull and fifth rib. What is the most likely diagnosis?

    (A) vitamin D deficiency
    (B) primary hyperparathyroidism
    (C) multiple myeloma
    (D) large cell lymphoma
    (E) Paget disease of bone

31. A 25-year-old woman presented with reddish purple spots on the upper and lower extremities. She had no complaints other than menorrhagia. Blood work was Hgb 11.2, WBC 8.2 with normal differential, platelets 32,000. No blast cells were present. What is the most likely diagnosis?

    (A) acute leukemia
    (B) idiopathic thrombocytopenia purpura
    (C) Sweets syndrome
    (D) aplastic anemia
    (E) DIC

32. Which of the following is true regarding Vitamin K deficiencies?

    (A) It may result in abnormal platelet function.
    (B) In the United States, it is most commonly due to inadequate intake.
    (C) It should be suspected in patients with prolongation of the partial thromboplastin time (PTT).
    (D) Treatment with fresh frozen plasma is typically required.
    (E) It occurs in primary biliary cirrhosis.

33. Decreased platelet production may be observed in which of the following conditions?

    (A) hypersplenism
    (B) DIC
    (C) Henoch–Schonlein disease

    (D) aplastic anemia
    (E) alcoholism

34. A 15-year-old boy presents to your clinic for a routine physical examination prior to joining the football team. A CBC reveals an Hgb of 10.1 with a MCV of 72. Ferritin, serum iron, total iron-binding capacity (TIBC), and iron saturation studies are all normal. A reticulocyte count is 2.3. Which test would be most appropriate to perform?

    (A) hemoglobin electrophoresis
    (B) Schilling test
    (C) bone marrow biopsy
    (D) folate level
    (E) direct and indirect Coombs test

35. Which of the following is true of Hodgkin's disease?

    (A) It is associated with a high mortality rate of >50% within the first 2 years.
    (B) A common presenting symptom is tender lymphadenopathy.
    (C) Most patients present with B symptoms (fever, night sweats, and weight loss).
    (D) Malignant cells present in this disease are the Reed-Sternberg cells.
    (E) Lymphadenopathy on presentation is typically subdiaphragmatic.

36. Glucose-6-phosphate dehydrogenase (G6PD) deficiency

    (A) is a rare form of hemolytic anemia.
    (B) is an autosomal dominant disorder.
    (C) is typically diagnosed within the first two decades of life.
    (D) results in hepatomegaly.
    (E) may be precipitated by antibiotics.

37. Which of the following is true of idiopathic thrombocytopenic purpura (ITP)?

    (A) It is almost always chronic.
    (B) It is commonly precipitated by severe bleeding.

(C) The primary treatment involves transfusion of platelets until bleeding is controlled.

(D) It may be associated with lupus.

(E) It rarely occurs in children.

38. While working in the hospital emergency center, a 34-year-old, otherwise healthy woman presents with acute onset of anxiety, shortness of breath, and right-sided chest pain. She is found to be tachypneic and hypoxemic. A diagnosis of pulmonary embolism is confirmed by CT angiogram. What additional tests are indicated?

(A) d-dimer

(B) ventilation-perfusion scan

(C) protein C

(D) pulmonary venogram

(E) bleeding time

39. Which of the following is true regarding thrombotic thrombocytopenic purpura?

(A) It is typically associated with prolonged PT and PTT.

(B) It can be distinguished from hemolytic anemia by finding a normal hemoglobin.

(C) It is typically self-limited and usually does not require treatment.

(D) Schistocytes may be found on peripheral blood smear.

(E) It is more common in men.

40. Which of the following is true concerning heparin-induced thrombocytopenia?

(A) Aspirin may be used for the treatment of pulmonary embolus.

(B) Aspirin is indicated for prevention of venous thrombosis.

(C) Low-molecular-weight heparin can be used in patients with heparin-induced thrombocytopenia.

(D) Platelet transfusion should be used to prevent bleeding in patients with platelet counts of less than 100,000.

(E) Bleeding is not a hallmark of HIT.

Answers and Explanations

1. **(C)** Sickle cell disease (hemoglobin S disease) is an autosomal dominant hemoglobinopathy. The homozygous form (SS), sickle cell anemia, results in sickling of erythrocytes, occurring when oxygen levels decrease at the tissue level. This results in impedance of blood flow to organs. Hemolysis often accompanies these abnormal erythrocytes. Although sexual and growth maturation are often delayed, most patients with the disease are fertile. Sickle cell crises are often precipitated by infection and those with sickle cell disease are at increased risk of infections from encapsulated organisms. Given the apparent good health of this woman's fiancée, he likely does not have sickle cell disease but may carry the trait. Those heterogenous (AS) for the gene are referred to as having sickle cell trait. The risk of carrying the trait is approximately 8% for those of African decent in the United States. Therefore, those with family histories of the disease likely carry the trait and genetic testing should be offered before childbearing. Given the strong family history of this man and the woman being of African descent, testing should be offered as they both may carry the gene. Those with sickle cell trait are typically asymptomatic with mild or absent anemia. Although sickle cell crises may occur at high altitudes for those with the disease, sickle cell crises are rare in those who are only carriers. The risk of sexually transmitted diseases is not increased for those with the trait or disease. (*Benz, 2008, pp. 635-640*)

2. **(B)** Iron deficiency anemia is most commonly due to chronic blood loss. In the United States, dietary deficiency is uncommon (except during pregnancy) and should not be presumed unless potential sources of blood loss have been excluded. However, dietary deficiency often occurs in pregnancy because of increased production of erythrocytes. Supplementation during pregnancy is routinely recommended. In mild to moderate iron deficiency, the reticulocyte count is mildly elevated although the corrected reticulocyte count is usually low. Low reticulocyte counts are seen in more severe forms of the disease. Elevated TIBC and low levels of iron, ferritin, and transferritin in the setting of microcytic anemia confirm the diagnosis. Although diminished iron stores are noted on bone marrow aspiration, this is not routinely needed to confirm the diagnosis. Once the diagnosis of iron deficiency anemia is made, the underlying cause must be found and treated. Iron replacement may be needed in moderate to severe cases and is typically accomplished within 6 to 12 months. Once iron stores have been replaced, iron supplementation should be stopped to prevent iron toxicity or mask further blood loss. (*Adamson, 2008, pp. 628-633*)

3. **(D)** Lead poisoning is a common occurrence, usually resulting in a mild anemia. Patients often have vague complaints including fatigue, abdominal pain, difficulties with concentration, and muscle weakness. The most common severe complication of the disease is the development of episodic paralytic ileus. Mild anemia and the presence of basophilic stippling are often seen. Lead levels should be checked in anyone presenting with these complaints and at risk, including children and adults with an occupational/environmental exposure. Primary treatment is to remove the source of

lead. Chelating agents may be needed for those who are symptomatic or with very high levels. *(Luzzatto, 2008, pp. 659; Bird and Miller, 2008, p. 2548; Brown, 2008, p. 2574)*

4. **(C)** Anemia may be the result of a wide variety of causes. Once a patient is found to be anemic, the next step is determining the underlying etiology. Anemia may be divided into microcytic, normocytic, and macrocytic on the basis of the MCV of the erythrocytes. Once this has been determined, the differential diagnosis may be narrowed and appropriate adjuvant tests can be ordered. Microcytic anemia is most commonly seen in the presence of iron deficiency. Thalassemia will also result in a microcytic anemia but is less common in the United States. Both lead poisoning and anemia of chronic illness may result in a mildly lower MCV, but a normocytosis is more commonly seen. In addition, patients with chronic illnesses often have more than one contributing factor for their anemia; and therefore, the MCV may be low, high, or normal. In a previously healthy individual with microcytic anemia, and with normal WBC and platelet counts, iron deficiency should be suspected. *(Adamson, 2008, pp. 628-633)*

5. **(D)** Vitamin B_{12} and folate deficiencies are the common forms of macrocytic anemia. Vitamin B_{12} is found in animal products and is generally available in typical American diets. Intrinsic factor is secreted in the stomach to allow absorption of B_{12} in the small intestine. Those with prior gastrectomy are at high risk of B_{12} deficiency anemia and therefore commonly need monthly replacement. B_{12} deficiency results in neurologic injury and atrophy of the tongue along with loss of taste sensation. A Schilling test may be used to determine the cause of B_{12} deficiency. A 24-hour urine sample is collected after radiolabeled cyanocobalamin is taken orally. If absorbed normally, at least 7% of the isotope will be excreted in the urine. If less than 7% is excreted, the cause of malabsorption will be determined by administering intrinsic factor along with oral cyanocobalamin. If an intrinsic factor deficiency exists, this will correct the B_{12} deficiency. If the deficiency is not corrected, the problem is due to poor absorption in the small bowel. The Shilling test is not commonly used in the United States, having been largely replaced by serum B_{12} level direct measurement. Folate (folic acid) is found in vegetables, and deficiencies are more commonly seen in the United States. It is important to confirm the cause of macrocytic anemia prior to beginning folate replacement. Folate supplementation in a patient deficient in B_{12} may help to correct the anemia but will mask B_{12} deficiency and could result in permanent neurologic impairment. *(Hoffbrand, 2008, pp. 643-651)*

6. **(B)** Anemia associated with hyperbilirubinemia and elevated LDH suggests hemolytic anemia. There are many causes of hemolytic anemia. In hospitalized patients, the differential may include DIC, idiopathic thrombocytopenia purpura, thrombotic thrombocytopenia purpura, drug reactions, and blood incompatibility. Drug reactions may also develop in the setting of G6PD deficiency. Although malaria is not commonly seen in this country, some regions do report cases. In addition, frequent travel and immigration necessitate consideration of additional infectious causes of illness when evaluating patients. A travel history should be obtained in patients with unexplained hemolytic anemia. Folate deficiency and iron deficiency (typically due to blood loss) does not result in hemolysis and; therefore, elevated bilirubin and LDH levels would not be expected. Given the lack of other indicators of DIC, this is less likely. *(Luzzatto, 2008, pp. 652-662)*

7. **(C)** Anticancer therapy often results in complications that may be mild to severe, acute, and chronic. Many chemotherapeutic agents share similar side effects including alopecia, nausea, vomiting, diarrhea, mucositis, fatigue, and myelosuppression. The frequency and severity of these common toxicities vary with each drug and dosage. Tamoxifen use has been shown to increase the risk of uterine malignancies. Although this risk remains relatively low, it must be considered and discussed with patients when considering its use in treatment and prevention of malignancy. *(Sausville and Longo, 2008a, pp. 521-524)*

8. **(D)** Tumor markers are biochemical abnormalities, which are often elevated in particular malignancies. They are typically measured in the blood but may sometimes be analyzed in urine or tumor tissue. Tumor markers are often present at low levels in healthy individuals and levels may occasionally be elevated in nonmalignant conditions. Although tumor markers are often quite helpful in monitoring patients with known cancer, they are rarely sensitive enough to allow for screening of the disease. Prostate-specific antigen (PSA) is the most commonly used tumor marker for cancer screening (eg, prostate cancer). Prostatic acid phosphate level may be elevated in prostate cancers, particularly when metastatic disease is present, but is much less sensitive than PSA and should not be used for screening. Carcinoembryonic antigen (CEA) levels may be elevated in a variety of malignancies, most commonly colon cancer, while cancer antigen 19–9 (CA 19–9) levels may be elevated in pancreatic cancer. Unfortunately, neither CEA nor CA 19–9 is sensitive enough for cancer screening. Alpha feta protein is recommended in screening for hepatocellular carcinoma in those considered at increased risk, including those with chronic hepatitis B and C and those with cirrhosis from all causes. The role of CA 125 is currently under investigation for screening of ovarian cancer but to date it is not considered standard of care. *(Haynes, 2008, pp. 774-780; Longo, 2008a, p. 483; Mayer, 2008, p. 583)*

9. **(C)** Thalassemia is a group of genetic disorders affecting one or more of the subunits of the hemoglobin chain resulting in a microcytic, hypochromic anemia. It is most common in those of African descent. Presentation may occur early or later in life, depending upon the affected subunit and number of genetic abnormalities involved. The most common form (Thalassemia minor) results in only mild disease, often goes undiagnosed and requires no treatment; other forms are life-threatening. Diagnosis is made by Hb electrophoresis, which should be ordered when the disease is suspected. *(Benz, 2008, pp. 636-642)*

10. **(A)** This patient has multiple myeloma which is confirmed by serum electrophoresis. Multiple myeloma is a malignancy of plasma cells arising from a single clone. These plasma cells secrete immunoglobin, resulting in a clone spike on electrophoresis. Plasma cells proliferate bones, resulting in osteolytic lesions (not osteoblastic). Bone pain and fractures as well as hypercalcemia are the most common findings. Hypercalcemia can result in renal impairment or failure. Associated infiltration of the bone marrow results in anemia, neutropenia, and thrombocytopenia. Hypotension would not be expected in such a patient unless she presented with a neutropenic infection resulting in shock (which is not consistent with the clinical scenario). Splenomegaly does not occur with multiple myeloma. *(Munshi et al., 2008, pp. 701-705)*

11. **(E)** The initial suspected diagnosis of cat-scratch fever, Bartonella infection, is typically self-limited but may be treated with azithromycin. The presence of a significant leukocytosis with associated lymphocytosis suggests leukemia as a probable diagnosis. ALL is the most common childhood leukemia. Although most patients present with symptoms such as fatigue, frank bleeding, or shortness of breath, others may present with more subtle complaints. Bone marrow biopsy is necessary to confirm the diagnosis. *(Longo, 2008b, pp. 687-700; Spach and Darby, 2008, pp. 987-990)*

12. **(D)** This patient's history and presentation is most consistent with acute myelogenous leukemia, which typically presents later in life. A prompt diagnosis, with bone marrow biopsy, is essential to guide additional evaluation and allow for prompt treatment. Although other tests such as chest x-ray, lumbar puncture, and cultures may be necessary, these will not be diagnostic of the patient's leukemia *(Wetzler et al., 2008, pp. 677-683)*

13. **(C)** DIC is a systemic disorder resulting from abnormal and excessive activation of the clotting cascade. Underlying causes may include sepsis, trauma, obstetric complications, and other causes of shock. Treatment of the underlying cause is the most important consideration, given the high mortality of 30% to 80%. The disease results in both excessive bleeding

and clotting, often resulting in organ damage such as renal impairment. The condition may be life-threatening and rapid treatment of the underlying disease is critical for survival. Replacement factors such as platelets, FFP, and cryoprecipitate should be used if needed; however, they could result in worsening organ damage because of increased clotting. Heparin is sometimes used for treatment of the disease with the goal to reduce thrombosis formation; however, heparin therapy remains controversial since it also has the potential of worsening bleeding. *(Arruda and High, 2008, pp. 728-730)*

14. **(C)** External beam irradiation is a common modality of anticancer therapy. In previous years, it had been used to treat benign conditions including thyroid disorders and acne. Complications may include local damage to tissues/organs, including delayed wound healing, and fatigue. Myelosuppression may occur if bone marrow is involved in the radiation field. However, significant myelosuppression is not typical. Radiation therapy is often used to palliate pain for patients with metastatic disease to the bone. It may produce relief of pain within a few days of initiation of treatment. Worsening bone pain is not expected but may signal a complication of the disease, such as a pathologic fracture. *(Lawrence et al., 2008, pp. 331-332)*

15. **(E)** Christmas disease, also known as hemophilia B and factor IX (not factor XI) hemophilia, is a hereditary bleeding disorder. Abnormal thrombosis does not occur. It is managed with factor IX concentrates or FFP. It is necessary to distinguish between hemophilia A and hemophilia B, since both diseases present similarly but require appropriate factor replacement. *(Arruda and High, 2008, pp. 725-726)*

16. **(B)** This patient's history suggests some form of coagulopathy, resulting in an increased incidence of thrombotic events. Although a myelogram may be helpful in evaluating peripheral neuropathy, in the setting of concurrent slurred speech, a central cause should be suspected. Hemoglobin electrophoresis is used in evaluation of hemoglobinopathies,

such as sickle cell disease. Although sickle cell disease may result in microthrombotic events, macrothrombotic events such as DVT would not occur. Sickle cell disease occurs most commonly in those of African descent and should be diagnosed earlier in life. Platelet function assays are helpful in the evaluation of platelet functional defects. With the clinical information, there is no sign of any chronic platelet abnormalities. Lupus anticoagulant, an antibody against phospholipids, may occur in autoimmune diseases and results in increased thrombotic events. *(Rosendaal and Buller, 2008, pp. 731-735; Konkle, 2008a, pp. 365-369)*

17. **(A)** Hemolysis may occur in a variety of settings and is associated with both acute and chronic illness. Distinguishing intravascular and extravascular hemolysis will assist in determining the underlying cause. Testing for hemoglobinemia and hemoglobinuria will make this distinction. Causes of intravascular hemolysis include transfusion reactions, malaria, and mechanical heart valves. Extravascular hemolysis may occur with drugs such as antibiotics and antimalarial agents, DIC, TTP, and sickle cell anemia. Lead poisoning results in inhibition of heme synthesis and injury to red cell membranes, resulting in a mild to moderate microcytic anemia. It is not typically associated with hemolysis. *(Luzzatto, 2008, pp. 652-661)*

18. **(A)** von Willebrand factor is found in both plasma and platelets. Deficiencies may manifest with variable degrees of easy bleeding. von Willebrand disease is the most common inherited bleeding disorder and should be considered first in someone with abnormal bleeding. Factor VIII:C level should be measured in evaluation for hemophilia A, while factor IX results in hemophilia B. Vitamin K deficiencies typically occur in those with chronic disease and would be unlikely in an otherwise healthy young woman. *(Arruda and High, 2008, pp. 725-728)*

19. **(B)** Splenomegaly may be associated with LUQ fullness, pain, early satiety, and reflux. Because of sequestration of platelets, petechiae are often found on exam. Splenomegaly may be caused

by various illnesses including infectious, oncologic, and inflammatory. Splenomegaly frequently is a result of hepatic parenchymal or veno-occlusive disease and patients presenting with unexplained splenomegaly should be examined for the presence of findings to suggest portal hypertension. Additional symptoms and signs should be sought to help in narrowing a differential diagnosis. The presence of physical findings of liver disease may be identified to include spider angiomas, caput medusa, palmar erythema, gynecomastia, and with more advanced disease, ascites, jaundice, and asterixis. Lymphadenopathy suggests possible infectious or malignant causes of splenomegaly in this patient. *(Henry and Longo, 2008, pp. 372-375)*

20. **(D)** Genetic testing has become increasingly available for various genetic mutations, although there is much work to be done in this field. Since cancer is a primary cause of death in the United States, virtually all patients will have some family history of the disease. Personal and family histories, which may raise concern for a possible hereditary disease, include multiple family members with malignancy and the diagnosis of malignancy at a young age (i.e., younger than expected for the particular disease). Consideration of genetic susceptibility is most important when screening tests for the disease are available and when risk reduction strategies are available. For these patients, referral to a genetics counselor should be considered. Risk factors for hereditary cancer syndromes include early age of onset, multiple family members with the same cancer, and clustering of cancers known to be caused by a single gene mutation. *(Morin et al., 2008, pp. 494-495)*

21. **(E)** Heparin-induced thrombocytopenia (HIT) is an immune-mediated disease resulting in the formation of immune complex binding of platelets, which results in typically mild to moderate thrombocytopenia. These platelet complexes can result in thrombotic complications. HIT may occur after prior exposure to heparin and typically develops within the first few days following exposure. It is more common with unfractionated heparin, as opposed to low-molecular-weight heparin. Management is primarily withdrawal of the agent and further exposure to heparin is contraindicated. *(Konkle, 2008b, p. 721)*

22. **(D)** Petechiae is typically a sign of thrombocytopenia. It does not usually occur with other disorders of the coagulation cascade. It would not be expected in patients who receive excess coumadin, in the absence of a platelet abnormality. Antiplatelet medications affect platelet function but should not result in thrombocytopenia. Platelet function may be evaluated by performing a bleeding time. In patients with a normal platelet count and petechiae on exam, this test should be ordered. Various conditions may result in thrombocytopenia, including immune, infectious, oncologic, and hepatic or splenic dysfunction. *(Konkle, 2008b, pp. 718-725)*

23. **(D)** In the presence of a mild anemia and normocytosis, various causes must be considered to include iron, vitamin B_{12}, and folate deficiencies. Although this patient has a normal serum iron and ferritin level, her total iron-binding capacity is mildly elevated. Once the iron saturation level (30%–50%) is calculated (iron $\times$ 100/TIBC), one sees that the patient's labs do reflect an iron deficiency. Appropriate evaluation for the underlying cause of iron deficiency should be pursued. Of note, this patient's serum folate is high, which is often seen in those taking vitamin supplements. *(Adamson, 2008, pp. 628-632)*

24. **(B)** Profound pancytopenia, with a normocytic anemia and few signs or symptoms (except for bleeding), is characteristic for aplastic anemia. A bone marrow aspiration and biopsy must be performes to confirm—it will be hypocellular. This is a typical presentation of aplastic anemia, in this case, probably caused by chronic medication use. Management includes discontinuation of the offending drugs, providing supportive care (transfusions, rapid treatment of any infection), and close observation to determine whether the marrow recovers spontaneously. If it does not, then therapeutic intervention is needed. Hodgkin's disease does not

usually present in this manner and often the blood smear is normal, except in advanced disease when the bone marrow is affected. CLL may present in a similar manner; however, the white blood cell count must be elevated for the diagnosis of CLL to be made, with an absolute lymphocytosis of more than 10,000/mL. CLL is rare in this age group. Significant anemia and leukopenia are extremely rare in idiopathic thrombocytopenic purpura (ITP), with presentations typically acute in onset, and patients manifest bleeding, with or without splenomegaly. *(Young, 2008, pp. 663-667)*

25. **(C)** Anemia in cancer patients is quite common. Patients may have acute or chronic bleeding, malabsorption of iron, B_{12}, or folate, or even hemolysis. However, the most common cause is anemia of chronic illness, with low or ineffective erythropoietin hormone. Erythropoietin therapy may be beneficial in the treatment of anemia in these patients, but careful evaluation of other potential causes is essential prior to beginning therapy. *(Young, 2008, pp. 633-634)*

26. **(D)** When cancer patients undergoing chemotherapy develop fever, neutropenic infection must be considered. Prompt medical attention is critical in reducing mortality from neutropenic fever. These patients should undergo careful evaluation for possible sources of infection. However, for many patients, an infectious source may not be identified. Prompt treatment with broad-spectrum antibiotics is critical for all patients with neutropenic infection, regardless of an identifiable source. Therefore, patients with fever need initial evaluation with a CBC to determine if neutropenia does or does not exist. If the patient is found to be nonneutropenic, more directed treatment of possibly infectious causes should be provided. Additional evaluation of those with neutropenic fever includes chest x-ray and urine and blood cultures. CT scan may be indicated for suspected infections such as an abscess. Fungal infection would be suspected in patients with profound and prolonged neutropenia, which is not consistent with this clinical scenario. *(Sausville and Longo, 2008, pp. 529-530)*

27. **(C)** The myeloproliferative disorder CML is the most likely diagnosis here. Early satiety is a common manifestation of splenomegaly; fatigue is a general complaint with a single cause often never found (other than the disease). Causes of leukemias are rarely identified, although radiation is considered a cause of some leukemias, of which CML is one. Often, splenomegaly is the only physical finding in a newly diagnosed CML patient. An elevated white blood cell count might be the only abnormality on a blood smear. If there were more blasts (>30%), this would be correctly diagnosed as an acute leukemia. Bone marrow analysis is necessary for diagnosis. The Philadelphia chromosome is characteristic of CML, although it also occurs in approximately 25% of patients with ALL. The presence of the Philadelphia chromosome in AML is exceedingly rare. CLL is a lymphoproliferative disorder; the Philadelphia chromosome abnormality does not occur in CLL or in Burkitt lymphoma. Typical chromosomal translocations in Burkitt lymphoma are t(8;14) and t(8;22). *(Wetzler et al., 2008, pp. 683-686)*

28. **(D)** Auer rods are pathognomonic of acute leukemia, especially AML. This presentation is typical for AML. Lymphomas do not present with profound pancytopenias. CML could be in the differential; however, the high number of blasts rules out the chronic phase of CML. There would be no thrombocytopenia and no blasts (definitely no Auer rods) if hemolytic anemia was the cause of this woman's fatigue. Therefore, acute leukemia is the most likely diagnosis. Auer rods are eosinophilic needle-like inclusions in the cytoplasm, seen in AML. Hodgkin's and non-Hodgkin's lymphomas can present with anemia but rarely are abnormal platelet counts involved nor are Auer rods present. CML and CLL usually present with high WBC counts but no Auer rods. *(Wetzler et al., 2008, pp. 677-682)*

29. **(E)** Nontender adenopathy in an otherwise healthy appearing patient is suspicious for lymphoma. Hodgkin's lymphoma has a bimodal age distribution, with the first peak in the 20s. The presence of B symptoms (weight loss, fatigue,

fevers) are nonspecific but should raise your clinical suspicion while many patients may be asymptomatic. Early satiety and abdominal pain often occur in the presence of splenomegaly, which is present with advancing stages of lymphoma. Hoarseness may occur with some upper respiratory diseases but is not typical in patients with lymphoma. Hair loss may be associated with various illnesses but is not typically seen in patients with untreated lymphoma. *(Henry and Longo, 2008, pp. 370-372)*

30. **(C)** Multiple myeloma is a clonal malignancy of the plasma cells. It is seen more commonly in African-Americans and typically presents with bone pain. Radiographs reveal the presence of osteolytic lesions commonly found in the axial skeleton, skull, long bones, spine, and ribs. Various other conditions may result in bone pain. Vitamin D deficiency, due to inadequate sun exposure, malnutrition, or malabsorption, can also be associated with bone pain as well as proximal muscle weakness. Primary hyperparathyroidism is associated with an adenoma of the parathyroid gland resulting in increased PTH levels and hypercalcemia. Large cell lymphoma is a type of non-Hodgkin lymphoma that presents with painless adenopathy and is associated with B symptoms of fever, night sweats, or unintentional weight loss. Less commonly, it can affect the lymphatic system, the central nervous system, or any organ including the bone. Paget disease is often asymptomatic, but may produce bone pain usually of the skull, femur, tibia, pelvis, or humerus. In this patient, the presence of anemia, hypercalcemia, and renal failure suggest multiple myeloma as the cause of his bone pain. *(Munshi et al., 2008, pp. 701-706)*

31. **(B)** Idiopathic (immune) thrombocytopenia purpura is an acquired disease, often presenting in young, otherwise healthy, patients. As the name implies, no known cause is identified in this condition of isolated thrombocytopenia. Because of the resulting bleeding, such as menorrhagia, patients may have associated anemia. In conditions such as DIC, acute leukemia, aplastic anemia, or Sweets syndrome

(a rare cutaneous form of myelodysplastic syndrome) other symptoms or laboratory abnormalities would be expected. *(Konkle, 2008b, pp. 721-722)*

32. **(E)** Vitamin K is a fat-soluble vitamin that is stored in the liver. It is critical in the clotting cascade and deficiencies result in prolongation of the prothrombin time. With severe or prolonged deficiencies, prolongation of the PTT may also occur. Deficiencies may occur from dietary deficiencies, malabsorption, and most commonly, chronic liver disease, such as cirrhosis. Treatment is with parenteral administration of vitamin K, with monthly injections in those with chronic deficiencies. FFP may be needed if patients have active hemorrhage. *(Konkle, 2008a, p. 368, Russell, 2008, p. 448)*

33. **(D)** Various conditions may result in thrombocytopenia. Many are due to a reduction in the number of circulating platelets in the setting of adequate production. These include DIC (due to consumption of platelets during abnormal clotting), hypersplenism resulting in sequestration of platelets, and Henoch–Schonlein purpura (a systemic vasculitis with typical manifestations of palpable purpura, abdominal pain, and hematuria). Alcoholism may result in cirrhosis, particularly in the presence of hepatitis C or other chronic liver disease. Cirrhosis results in portal hypertension, splenomegaly, and thrombocytopenia. Platelet production may be reduced in malignant conditions involving the bone marrow such as leukemia or in the setting of marrow failure with aplastic anemia. Alternatively, essential thrombocytosis is a rare myeloproliferative disorder that is identified by an elevated platelet count caused by abnormal proliferation of megakaryocytes in the bone marrow. Therefore, increased risk of thrombosis is a complication and may occur in small veins such as the mesenteric, hepatic, or portal venous system. *(Konkle, 2008b, pp. 718-723)*

34. **(A)** Microcytic anemia is most commonly caused by iron deficiency. However, thalassemia and lead poisoning may also result in microcytosis. In patients with normal iron

studies, including iron saturation levels, consideration of these differential diagnoses is necessary. Although thalassemia is not common, it may be found in patients with microcytic anemia by serum electrophoresis. Thalassemia may result is severe anemia in childhood (beta-thalassemia major) while those with thalassemia trait (thalassemia minor) may have only mild anemia. Thalassemia syndromes are inherited disorders of alpha- or beta-globin synthesis. *(Benz, 2008, pp. 640-641)*

35. **(D)** Hodgkin's disease is a group of cancers. They are usually characterized by Reed-Sternberg cells, which are necessary, but NOT sufficient, for a diagnosis of Hodgkin's disease. Patients can experience fever, severe night sweats, and weight loss, but these classic symptoms occur in only about one-third of patients. Patients typically present with painless supra-diaphragmatic lymphadenopathy, although some patients will complain of discomfort if the lymph nodes are "bulky." The vast majority of patients with localized disease will be cured, while even those with more advanced disease may have a long-term disease-free survival. *(Longo, 2008b, pp. 698-699)*

36. **(E)** Glucose-6-phosphate dehydrogenase (G6PD) deficiency is the most common cause of hemolytic anemia. It is a genetic disorder, being x-linked with several mutant forms. Many patients carry this deficiency and may go undiagnosed until a precipitating illness develops later in life. Hemolysis is typically precipitated by oxidant drugs or stress situations, such as infection, although it may go unrecognized as it is often self-limited. As with all types of hemolysis, splenomegaly may result, although typically not hepatomegaly. *(Luzzatto, 2008, pp. 656-658)*

37. **(D)** Idiopathic (immune) thrombocytopenia purpura is an acquired disease, often presenting in young, otherwise healthy patients. As the name implies, no known cause is identified in this condition of isolated thrombocytopenia. It is typically acute in children, while more chronic for adults. It may be associated with infections or autoimmune disorders such as systemic lupus erythematosis. Because of the resulting bleeding, such as menorrhagia or gastrointestinal bleeding, patients may have associated anemia. Treatment is indicated in those with several thrombocytopenia and significant bleeding. Treatment may include prednisone or Rh0 immune globulin therapy. *(Konkle, 2008b, pp. 721-722)*

38. **(C)** Patients who present with unexplained thromboembolic events (such as pulmonary embolus) should be evaluated for possible hypercoagulable states to include checking protein C to evaluate for possible deficiency. D-dimer and ventilation-perfusion scans are used in the diagnosis of pulmonary embolus and are not indicated once the diagnosis is confirmed by gold standard, CT angiogram. Bleeding times are checked in patients with suspected prolonged bleeding. *(Rosendaal and Buller, 2008, pp. 731-734)*

39. **(D)** Thrombotic thrombocytopenic purpura (TTP) is a disorder characterized by thrombocytopenia, microangiopathic hemolytic anemia, and microvascular thrombosis. It occurs more frequently in women than men. Evidence of hemolysis may be evident by anemia, schistocytes, elevated bilirubin, and elevated LDH. It is not associated with prolonged bleeding times. It is a disease that must be treated promptly by plasma exchange. *(Konkle, 2008b, pp. 722-723)*

40. **(E)** Heparin-induced thrombocytopenia (HIT) can occur after exposure to unfractionated heparin or low-molecular-weight heparin. HIT is not typically associated with bleeding but often results in thrombosis. Platelet transfusion is therefore not indicated. Aspirin is not indicated for treatment or prophylaxis of thrombosis. *(Konkle, 2008b, pp. 720-721)*

REFERENCES

Adamson JW. Iron deficiency and other hypoproliferative anemias. In: Fauci AS, Braunwald E, Kasper DL, et al., eds. *Harrison's Principles of Internal Medicine.* 17th ed. New York, NY: McGraw-Hill; 2008.

Arruda V, High KA. Coagulation disorders. In: Fauci AS, Braunwald E, Kasper DL, et al., ed. *Harrison's Principles of Internal Medicine.* 17th ed. New York, NY: McGraw-Hill; 2008.

Benz EJ. Disorders of hemoglobin. In: Fauci AS, Braunwald E, Kasper DL, et al., eds. *Harrison's Principles of Internal Medicine.* 17th ed. New York, NY: McGraw-Hill; 2008.

Bird TD, Miller BL. Dementia. In: Fauci AS, Braunwald E, Kasper DL, et al., eds. *Harrison's Principles of Internal Medicine.* 17th ed. New York, NY: McGraw-Hill; 2008.

Brown RH. Amyotrophic lateral sclerosis and other motor neuron diseases. In: Fauci AS, Braunwald E, Kasper DL, et al., eds. *Harrison's Principles of Internal Medicine* 17th ed. New York, NY: McGraw-Hill; 2008.

Haynes DF. Specialized techniques in cancer management-biomarkers. In: DeVita VT, Lawrence TS, Rosenberg SA, eds. *DeVita, Hellman, and Rosenberg's Cancer Principles & Practice of Oncology.* 8th ed. Philadelphia, PA: Lippincott Williams & Wilkins; 2008.

Henry PA, Longo DL. Enlargement of lymph nodes and spleen. In: Fauci AS, Braunwald E, Kasper DL, et al., eds. *Harrison's Principles of Internal Medicine.* 17th ed. New York, NY: McGraw-Hill; 2008.

Hoffbrand AV. Megaloblastic anemias. In: Fauci AS, Braunwald E, Kasper DL, et al., eds. *Harrison's Principles of Internal Medicine.* 17th ed. New York, NY: McGraw-Hill; 2008.

Konkle BA. Bleeding and thrombosis. In: Fauci AS, Braunwald E, Kasper DL, et al., eds. *Harrison's Principles of Internal Medicine.* 17th ed. New York, NY: McGraw-Hill; 2008a.

Konkle BA. Disorders of platelets and vessel wall. In: Fauci AS, Braunwald E, Kasper DL, et al., eds. *Harrison's Principles of Internal Medicine.* 17th ed. New York, NY: McGraw-Hill; 2008b.

Lawrence TS, Haken RKT, Giaccia A. Principles of radiation oncology. In: DeVita, VT, Lawrence TS, Rosenberg SA, et al., *DeVita, Hellman, and Rosenberg's Cancer Principles & Practice of Oncology.* 8th Ed. Philadelphia, PA: Lippincott Williams & Wilkins; 2008.

Longo DL. Approach to the patient with cancer. In: Fauci AS, Braunwald E, Kasper DL, et al., eds. *Harrison's Principles of Internal Medicine.* 17th ed. New York, NY: McGraw-Hill; 2008a.

Longo DL. Malignancies of lymphoid cells. In: Fauci AS, Braunwald E, Kasper DL, et al., eds. *Harrison's Principles of Internal Medicine* 17th ed. New York, NY: McGraw-Hill; 2008b.

Luzzatto L. Hemolytic anemias and anemia due to acute blood loss. In: Fauci AS, Braunwald E, Kasper DL, et al., eds. *Harrison's Principles of Internal Medicine.* 17th ed. New York, NY: McGraw-Hill; 2008.

Mayer RJ. Gastrointestinal tract cancer. In: Fauci AS, Braunwald E, Kasper DL, et al., eds. *Harrison's Principles of Internal Medicine.* 17th ed. New York, NY: McGraw-Hill; 2008.

Morin PJ, Trent JM, Collins FS, et al., Cancer genetics. In: Fauci AS, Braunwald E, Kasper DL, et al., eds. *Harrison's Principles of Internal Medicine.* 17th ed. New York, NY: McGraw-Hill; 2008.

Munshi NC, Longo DL, Anderson KC. Plasma cell disorders. In: Fauci AS, Braunwald E, Kasper DL, et al., eds. *Harrison's Principles of Internal Medicine.* 17th ed. New York, NY: McGraw-Hill; 2008.

Rosendaal FD, Buller HR. Venous thrombosis. In: Fauci AS, Braunwald E, Kasper DL, et al., eds. *Harrison's Principles of Internal Medicine.* 17th ed. New York, NY: McGraw-Hill; 2008.

Russell RM, Suter PM. Vitamin and trace mineral deficiency and excess. In: Fauci AS, Braunwald E, Kasper DL, et al., eds. *Harrison's Principles of Internal Medicine* 17th ed. New York, NY: McGraw-Hill; 2008.

Sausville EA, Longo DL. Principles of cancer treatment. In: Fauci AS, Braunwald E, Kasper DL, et al., eds. *Harrison's Principles of Internal Medicine.* 17th ed. New York, NY: McGraw-Hill; 2008.

Spach DH, Darby E. Bartonella infections, including cat-scratch disease. In: Fauci AS, Braunwald E, Kasper DL, et al., eds. *Harrison's Principles of Internal Medicine.* 17th ed. New York, NY: McGraw-Hill; 2008.

Wetzler M, Byrd JC, Bloomfield CD. Acute and chronic myeloid leukemia. In: Fauci AS, Braunwald E, Kasper DL, et al., eds. *Harrison's Principles of Internal Medicine.* 17th ed. New York, NY: McGraw-Hill; 2008.

Young, NS. Aplastic anemia, myelodysplasia, and related bone marrow failure syndromes. In: Fauci AS, Braunwald E, Kasper DL, et al., eds. *Harrison's Principles of Internal Medicine.* 17th ed. New York, NY: McGraw-Hill; 2008.

CHAPTER 7

HIV-AIDS

Rebecca Lovell Scott, PhD, PA-C

DIRECTIONS: Each of the numbered items or incomplete statements in this section is followed by answers or by completion of the statement. Select the ONE-lettered answer that is BEST in each case.

1. The two major risk factors for human immunodeficiency virus (HIV) infection in American women are intravenous drug use and which of the following?

   (A) history of blood transfusion
   (B) needle stick injuries
   (C) pelvic inflammatory disease
   (D) sexual contact with an infected male
   (E) use of oral contraceptives

2. Of the following sexual practices, which poses the greatest risk of HIV transmission when practiced with an infected partner but without the use of a reliable barrier method of prophylaxis?

   (A) insertive anal intercourse
   (B) insertive vaginal intercourse
   (C) receptive anal intercourse
   (D) receptive fellatio with ejaculation
   (E) receptive vaginal intercourse

3. Which of the following patients, without laboratory evidence of HIV, meets the Centers for Disease Control and Prevention case definition for acquired immunodeficiency syndrome (AIDS)?

   (A) 29-year-old man with pulmonary tuberculosis

   (B) 32-year-old man with Kaposi sarcoma
   (C) 35-year-old woman with invasive cervical cancer
   (D) 36-year-old man with recurrent *Salmonella septicemia*
   (E) 40-year-old woman with recurrent pneumonia

4. A 28-year-old man has a positive HIV ELISA and Western Blot but has never had an opportunistic infection. Of the following laboratory parameters, which, if present, is consistent with a diagnosis of AIDS in this man?

   (A) CD4 lymphocyte count of 175/mL
   (B) HHV-8 titer of 1:160
   (C) HSV-2 titer of 1:80
   (D) platelet count of 10,000/mL
   (E) total white blood cell count of 1500/mL

5. A 35-year-old patient with AIDS has had unintended weight loss of nearly 30 lb over the past 6 months. This loss has been primarily in muscle mass. He has little appetite but no nausea, diarrhea, or evidence of oral candidiasis. He reports interest in resuming his former weight-training regimen. Which of the following is the most appropriate pharmacologic agent to help him gain weight?

   (A) dronabinol
   (B) megestrol acetate
   (C) odansetron
   (D) prochlorperazine
   (E) testosterone enanthate

6. A 42-year-old man who is HIV positive develops fever of 38.8°C, mild nonproductive cough, and shortness of breath. He takes no medications other than a multivitamin tablet, does not smoke cigarettes, or use alcohol or illicit drugs. Of the following findings on diagnostic studies, which is most consistent with a diagnosis of *Pneumocystic jiroveci* pneumonia in this man?

   (A) apical infiltrates on chest radiography
   (B) bronchiolar consolidation on computed tomographic (CT) scan
   (C) CD4 count of 300 cells/mL
   (D) PO$_2$ of 54 mm Hg
   (E) serum lactate dehydrogenase (LDH) level of 54 units/L

7. A 33-year-old man with HIV infection is brought in by his partner for evaluation of altered mental status. The partner has noticed waxing and waning periods of confusion throughout the day, difficulty in performing tasks such as balancing a checkbook, and deterioration of handwriting. The patient reports no fever or headache. What is the most likely diagnosis?

   (A) AIDS dementia complex
   (B) central nervous system lymphoma
   (C) cryptococcal meningitis
   (D) progressive multifocal leukoencephalopathy (PML)
   (E) toxoplasmosis

8. A 38-year-old man with HIV infection has had fever and a severe generalized headache for the past several hours. On examination, he is noted to be alert and oriented and gives a coherent history that is corroborated by his partner. He has no papilledema or meningismus. What is the most likely diagnosis?

   (A) AIDS dementia complex
   (B) central nervous system lymphoma
   (C) cryptococcal meningitis
   (D) progressive multifocal leukoencephalopathy
   (E) toxoplasmosis

9. A 32-year-old man who is HIV positive has a seizure. On presentation to the emergency department (ED) he is confused and unsure of what happened. His partner reports that he had been complaining of headache in the days preceding the event. CT scanning of the head demonstrates five peripheral contrast-enhancing lesions. What is the most likely diagnosis?

   (A) AIDS dementia complex
   (B) central nervous system lymphoma
   (C) cryptococcal meningitis
   (D) progressive multifocal leukoencephalopathy
   (E) toxoplasmosis

10. A 42-year-old man with AIDS has had gradual onset of "my feet always going to sleep on me." This tingling and burning keeps him awake much of the night and he "can't cope much longer" because of the sleep deprivation. He drinks no alcohol nor does he use any illicit drugs. His physical examination reveals no gross motor or sensory deficits. His thyroid function tests and vitamin B$_{12}$ levels are within normal limits and syphilis screening is negative. Of the following, what is the recommended initial therapy?

    (A) didanosine
    (B) gabapentin
    (C) ibuprofen
    (D) stavudine

11. A 28-year-old man who is HIV positive has developed stringy vertical white lesions on the lateral aspects of his tongue. While not painful, they bother him for cosmetic reasons. On examination, these lesions are noted to be raised and appear corrugated. They adhere to the tongue when gently scraped with a tongue depressor. What is the most likely cause of these lesions?

    (A) *Candida albicans* infection
    (B) Epstein–Barr virus infection
    (C) herpes simplex virus infection
    (D) iron deficiency
    (E) vitamin B$_{12}$ deficiency

12. A 28-year-old woman who is HIV positive presents with substernal discomfort and painful swallowing for the past week. Her physical examination is unremarkable, but on endoscopy she has extensive adherent yellowish plaques on the esophageal mucosa. What is the most likely diagnosis?

    (A) candidal esophagitis
    (B) cytomegalovirus (CMV) esophagitis
    (C) gastroesophageal reflux disease (GERD)
    (D) herpetic esophagitis

13. A physician assistant student suffers a needlestick injury while caring for an HIV-positive patient whose viral load is currently undetectable. Of the following, which is the most appropriate management for the student?

    (A) no drug treatment unless HIV testing performed immediately and at 6 weeks, 3 months, and 6 months results become positive
    (B) administration of zidovudine and lamivudine until results of baseline testing are received
    (C) administration of zidovudine and lamivudine for 4 weeks
    (D) administration of zidovudine, lamivudine, and indinavir for 4 weeks

14. A surgical physician assistant suffers a deep puncture wound during surgery on an HIV-positive patient. The patient, who is on a multidrug regimen, has a viral load of 120,000 copies. Which of the following drugs is contraindicated for the physician assistant because of its potential for hepatotoxicity in the setting of HIV prophylaxis?

    (A) abacavir
    (B) indinavir
    (C) lamivudine
    (D) nevirapine
    (E) zidovudine

15. A 24-year-old woman with HIV is diagnosed with *Mycobacterium avium* complex infection. She is started on a treatment regimen of clarithromycin with ethambutol. She needs to be educated that which of the following is a potential complication of this therapy?

    (A) anemia
    (B) azotemia
    (C) methemoglobinemia
    (D) mucositis
    (E) optic neuritis

16. Which one of the following tests is most appropriate for monitoring the success of antiretroviral therapy in a patient with HIV?

    (A) absolute CD4 lymphocyte count
    (B) CD4 lymphocyte percentage
    (C) HIV enzyme-linked immunosorbent assay
    (D) serum viral load
    (E) Western blot

17. An HIV-positive man develops elevated cholesterol and triglyceride levels while taking an antiretroviral cocktail that includes two nucleoside analogs and a protease inhibitor. Which of the following cholesterol-lowering therapies is contraindicated in this patient because of its interactions with protease inhibitors?

    (A) atorvastatin
    (B) gemfibrozil
    (C) lovastatin
    (D) pravastatin

18. A 29-year-old man who is taking combination antiretroviral therapy develops severe right-sided flank pain and dysuria. He is also nauseated, which he attributes to the severity of the pain. He is unable to sit still and paces about the examination room. Dipstick urine is remarkable for 3+ hematuria. Which of the following drugs is most likely to be responsible for this clinical picture?

    (A) abacavir
    (B) delavirdine
    (C) didanosine
    (D) indinavir
    (E) nelfinavir

19. A 26-year-old African-American man with HIV infection has a CD4 lymphocyte percentage of 12%. Prior to beginning prophylactic therapy for *Pneumocystis jiroveci* pneumonia, which of the following drugs requires testing for G6PD deficiency?

    (A) aerosolized pentamidine
    (B) atovaquone
    (C) dapsone
    (D) trimethoprim-sulfamethoxazole

20. A 25-year-old gravida 1 woman who is HIV positive arrives at the hospital in early labor. Membranes are intact and the cervix is 50% effaced and 3 to 4 cm dilated. Fetal heart rate is 150 beats/min. Which of the following procedures is contraindicated during labor?

    (A) amniotomy
    (B) augmentation of labor with oxytocin
    (C) external monitoring
    (D) operative delivery
    (E) use of fetal scalp electrodes

21. A 25-year-old woman with HIV disease delivers a 6-lb infant at 39 and 1/2 weeks' gestation. She received three-drug prophylaxis during her pregnancy. Of the following, what is the most appropriate course of action regarding the infant?

    (A) combination therapy for 1 to 2 weeks
    (B) indefinite therapy with zidovudine alone
    (C) no additional prophylaxis is needed
    (D) treat only if two separate HIV-PCR test results are positive

22. An infant is born to an HIV-positive mother who received three-drug treatment during pregnancy. Which of the following, if positive, indicates HIV infection in the infant?

    (A) HIV ELISA and Western Blot on cord blood
    (B) HIV ELISA and Western Blot at 1 month of age
    (C) HIV ELISA and Western Blot at 6 months of age

    (D) HIV ELISA and Western Blot at 12 months of age
    (E) HIV ELISA and Western Blot at 24 months of age

23. A woman who has had no prenatal care presents to the emergency department in active labor. She has a history of exchanging sexual intercourse for intravenous drugs. An HIV rapid antibody test result performed in the ED is positive. In addition to management of labor, what is the next step in her care?

    (A) determine CD4 lymphocyte percentage
    (B) initiate antiretroviral therapy immediately
    (C) perform standard HIV testing with ELISA and Western Blot
    (D) test for HIV viral load

24. At how many months of age should an asymptomatic HIV-positive infant receive her first measles–mumps–rubella (MMR) vaccine?

    (A) 12
    (B) 15
    (C) 18
    (D) 24
    (E) 60

25. Pediatric patients in which age group are most likely to experience rapid progression of HIV infection?

    (A) infants
    (B) toddlers
    (C) elementary aged
    (D) pubescent
    (E) adolescents

26. A 3-year-old boy who is HIV positive begins preschool. He is toilet trained and is not known to bite other children or have any open skin lesions. What is the most effective means of preventing transmission to the other children in his class?

    (A) having the child use a separate toilet
    (B) excluding the child from activities likely to cause sweating

(C) reminding the staff to use blood precautions with all children

(D) requiring the child to stay home if he has gastrointestinal symptoms

(E) using disposable plates and flatware for this child

27. How often should HIV-positive men who have sex with men (MSM) be screened for syphilis?

(A) every 3 months

(B) every 6 months

(C) every 12 months

(D) only upon diagnosis of HIV disease

(E) when their CD4 cell count drops below 200/mcL

28. Which of the following vaccines is contraindicated in a person with HIV infection and a low CD4 count?

(A) herpes zoster

(B) inactivated influenza

(C) measles

(D) pneumococcal

(E) tetanus-diphtheria

29. A 29-year-old man who is HIV positive has developed dark purple papular nonblanching lesions between the toes of his right foot. He has no other symptoms. Careful examination shows that this is the only area of involvement. His CD4 count is 150 cells/mL. Of the following, what is the most appropriate treatment?

(A) alpha interferon

(B) chemotherapy with daunorubicin, bleomycin, and vinblastine

(C) intralesional vinblastine

(D) liposomal doxorubicin

(E) radiation

30. A 28-year-old woman has recently been diagnosed with HIV infection. She has no evidence of opportunistic infection and her CD4 count is >200. She has had Pap smears every year for the past 5 years and they have all been normal. In how many months should she have another Pap and pelvic examination?

(A) 3

(B) 6

(C) 12

(D) 24

(E) 36

31. A 4-week-old baby whose mother is HIV positive is started on *Pneumocystis* prophylaxis with trimethoprim–sulfamethoxazole (TMP–SMX). Two weeks later, the TMP–SMX is discontinued when the baby develops a rash over much of her body. What is the most appropriate next step regarding prophylaxis?

(A) administer monthly intravenous immune globulin instead

(B) discontinue prophylaxis unless the CD4 count drops below 500/mL

(C) reintroduce TMP–SMX when the rash resolves

(D) substitute dapsone or atovaquone for TMP–SMX

32. The American College of Obstetricians and Gynecologists (ACOG) recommends which of the following regarding delivery to prevent HIV transmission to the infant?

(A) cesarean delivery only for those women who have not received HAART during pregnancy

(B) cesarean delivery if the infant has not been delivered within 3 hours of membrane rupture

(C) determination of type of delivery based on maternal viral load

(D) scheduled cesarean section at 38 weeks' gestation

33. Which of the following tests should an HIV-positive pregnant woman undergo in each trimester of pregnancy?

(A) CD4+ lymphocyte count

(B) cytomegalovirus serology

(C) postpartum depression with controls

(D) shielded chest radiography

(E) venereal disease research laboratory (VDRL)

34. Which of the following is an antiretroviral drug which acts by binding to the viral envelope protein, thereby interfering with HIV fusion with the host cell plasma membrane?

(A) atazanavir

(B) didanosine

(C) enfuvirtide

(D) lopinavir

(E) nevirapine

35. What class of antiretroviral drugs is most likely to affect serum lipid profiles?

(A) entry inhibitors

(B) integrase inhibitors

(C) nonnucleoside reverse transcriptase inhibitors

(D) nucleoside/nucleotide reverse transcriptase inhibitors

(E) protease inhibitors

Answers and Explanations

1. **(D)** The major risk factors for HIV infection in American women are intravenous drug use (33%) and heterosexual contact with an infected partner (65%). Thanks to universal blood donor screening using the HIV ELISA, antigen, and viral load testing, the risk for any person contracting HIV from a screened unit of blood is only 1:1,000,000. The risk for any person following a needle-stick injury is about 1:300 with deeper sticks, hollow bore needles, visible blood on the needle, and advanced stage of disease in the source increasing the risk. HIV infection puts a woman at increased risk for gynecologic complications such as pelvic inflammatory disease. Unlike the use of latex condoms, the use of oral contraceptives does not protect against HIV transmission, but is not, per se, a risk factor for HIV infection. *(Katz and Zolopa, 2009, p. 1178)*

2. **(C)** In unprotected intercourse with an infected partner, receptive anal intercourse carries a risk of HIV transmission between 1:100 and 1:30. Insertive anal intercourse, receptive vaginal intercourse, and fellatio with ejaculation each carry a risk of about 1:1000. Insertive vaginal intercourse carries a risk of 1:10,000. *(Katz and Zolopa, 2009, p. 1178)*

3. **(B)** The Centers for Disease Control and Prevention AIDS case definition includes the following diseases that, with or without laboratory evidence of HIV infection, constitute a definitive diagnosis of AIDS: candidiasis of the esophagus, trachea, bronchi, or lungs; extrapulmonary cryptococcosis; cryptosporidiosis with diarrhea persisting more than 1 month; cytomegalovirus disease of an organ other than liver, spleen, or lymph nodes; herpes simplex virus infection causing a mucocutaneous ulcer that persists longer than 1 month or causing bronchitis, pneumonitis, or esophagitis; Kaposi sarcoma in a patient younger than 60; lymphoma of the brain in a patient younger than 60; disseminated *Mycobacterium avium* complex or *Mycobacterium kansasii* disease; *Pneumocystis jiroveci* pneumonia; progressive multifocal leukoencephalopathy; or toxoplasmosis of the brain. Other conditions in the case definition require laboratory evidence of HIV infection. *(Katz and Zolopa, 2009, p. 1177)*

4. **(A)** Persons with a CD4 count less than 200/mL or a CD4 percentage below 14% are now included in the Centers for Disease Control and Prevention category of "definitive AIDS diagnoses with laboratory evidence of HIV infection." Persons with HIV-AIDS may have positive herpes titers or depressed platelet or white blood cell counts, but these are not diagnostic of AIDS in the absence of symptoms. *(Katz and Zolopa, 2009, p. 1177)*

5. **(E)** Anabolic steroids, most commonly testosterone enanthate or cypionate, increase lean body mass in patients with AIDS, particularly those who do weight training. Dronabinol, an antiemetic, and megestrol acetate, a progestational agent, are used to increase appetite and assist in weight gain but have little effect on lean muscle mass. Odansetron and prochlorperazine are both used to treat weight loss caused by nausea of unclear origin in patients with AIDS and are given prior to meals. *(Katz and Zolopa, 2009, p. 1181)*

6. **(D)** Severe hypoxemia is a common finding in *Pneumocystis* pneumonia even when symptoms are not severe. The characteristic chest radiograph findings are diffuse or perihilar infiltrates. Apical infiltrates are more likely to be seen in patients who have been receiving aerosolized pentamidine prophylaxis. High-resolution chest CT scanning would most likely demonstrate interstitial lung disease. This pneumonia is rare unless the CD4 count is less than 250. An elevated LDH is found in about 95% of patients, but this is not specific. *(Katz and Zolopa, 2009, pp. 1183, 1361)*

7. **(A)** AIDS dementia complex is the most common cause of mental status changes in patients with HIV infection. The deterioration of handwriting is often an early manifestation. Difficulty in performing cognitive tasks and diminished motor speed are typical, as is the waxing and waning of manifestations of dementia. Patients with central nervous system lymphoma and toxoplasmosis present with headache, focal neurologic deficits, seizures, and/or altered mental status. Patients with cryptococcal meningitis have, most typically, headache and fever, but fewer than 20% have meningismus. They also usually have normal mental status. Patients with PML have primarily focal neurologic deficits such as aphasia, hemiparesis, and cortical blindness. *(Katz and Zolopa, 2009, p. 1183)*

8. **(C)** Patients with cryptococcal meningitis have, most typically, headache and fever, but fewer than 20% have meningismus. They also usually have normal mental status. AIDS dementia complex is characterized by difficulty in performing cognitive tasks, diminished motor speed, and waxing and waning of manifestations of dementia. Patients with central nervous system lymphoma and toxoplasmosis present with headache, focal neurologic deficits, seizures, and/or altered mental status. Patients with progressive multifocal leukoencephalopathy primarily have focal neurologic deficits such as aphasia, hemiparesis, and cortical blindness. *(Katz and Zolopa, 2009, p. 1183)*

9. **(E)** The most common space-occupying CNS lesion in patients with HIV is toxoplasmosis. This condition may present with headache, focal neurologic deficits, seizures, and/or mental status changes. The typical appearance on brain imaging is that of multiple contract-enhancing lesions in the periphery, particularly the basal ganglia. CNS lymphoma is more typically a single lesion. AIDS dementia complex presents a diagnosis of exclusion, without a characteristic appearance on imaging. The diagnosis of cryptococcal meningitis is made by examination of the spinal fluid, while PML imaging shows nonenhancing white matter lesions without mass effect. *(Katz and Zolopa, 2009, p. 1183)*

10. **(B)** It is not unusual for persons with HIV infection to develop peripheral neuropathies. Recommended initial treatment is gabapentin, which provides symptomatic relief for neuropathic pain. Since this is not an inflammatory process, ibuprofen is not indicated. Didanosine and stavudine are the most common causes of peripheral neuropathy. *(Katz and Zolopa, 2009, pp. 1183-1184)*

11. **(B)** The lesions described are hairy leukoplakia, caused by the Epstein–Barr virus. *Candida* usually causes uncomfortable lesions that may be either removable white plaques or red friable plaques. Herpes simplex virus causes painful ulcerations. Both iron and vitamin B_{12} deficiencies can cause pain and the tongue appears smooth and beefy. *(Katz and Zolopa, 2009, p. 1184)*

12. **(A)** The most common symptoms of infectious esophagitis in immunocompromised persons are dysphagia and odynophagia. Endoscopic evaluation is highly accurate. Candidal esophagitis is characterized by the yellow-white plaques described. CMV esophagitis is characterized by a few large, shallow, superficial ulcerations while herpetic esophagitis has many small deep ones. About half of patients with GERD will have erosions or ulcers distally at the squamocolumnar junction. *(Katz and Zolopa, 2009, p. 520)*

13. **(C)** After a needle-stick injury, a health-care worker should have baseline testing with follow-up testing at 6 weeks, 3 months, and 6 months. Risk of seroconversion is approximately 1:300. Administration of antiviral therapy decreases this risk by 79%, so the worker should be offered treatment with zidovudine and lamivudine as soon as possible after the injury, for a total of 4 weeks. However, workers with a high-risk exposure (source patient with advanced disease, a viral load >50,000, or with resistant organisms) should have a protease inhibitor added to the prophylactic regimen. *(Katz and Zolopa, 2009, p. 1192)*

14. **(D)** Nevirapine should be avoided for HIV prophylaxis as reports have linked it to hepatotoxicity in the prophylactic setting. Abacavir may cause rash and fever, indinavir kidney stones, lamivudine rash and peripheral neuropathy, and zidovudine anemia, neutropenia, nausea, malaise, headache, insomnia, and myopathy. *(Katz and Zolopa, 2009, p. 1192)*

15. **(E)** Optic neuritis is associated with the use of ethambutol. Anemia is associated with many of the drugs used to treat AIDS-related opportunistic infections, including trimethoprim-sulfamethoxazole, pentamidine, amphotericin B, ganciclovir, and valganciclovir. Amphotericin B is associated with azotemia and trimethoprim with methemoglobinemia. Trimetrexate can cause mucositis. *(Katz and Zolopa, 2009, p. 1193)*

16. **(D)** As the goal of antiretroviral therapy is to suppress viral replication, the most appropriate test for monitoring therapy is the viral load in the serum. The CD4 count and percentage are useful in deciding when to initiate prophylaxis for opportunistic infections. The ELISA and Western Blot tests are used to diagnose HIV infection. *(Katz and Zolopa, 2009, p. 1197)*

17. **(C)** Lovastatin and simvastatin should be avoided in patients taking protease inhibitors because of drug interactions. In general, patients should be started on atorvastatin or pravastatin. Gemfibrozil is used for patients who have very high triglyceride levels that do

not respond to dietary modification. *(Katz and Zolopa, 2009, pp. 1198-1199)*

18. **(D)** A common side effect of indinavir is the development of kidney stones. Abacavir is associated with rash and fever. Delavirdine is associated with rash; didanosine is associated with peripheral neuropathy, pancreatitis, dry mouth, and hepatitis. Diarrhea is the most common side effect of nelfinavir. *(Katz and Zolopa, 2009, p. 1195)*

19. **(C)** Patients with G6PD deficiency are at increased risk for developing hemolytic anemia if treated with dapsone. In all patients, adverse effects associated with dapsone include anemia, nausea, and methemoglobinemia. Risks associated with aerosolized pentamidine include bronchospasm and, rarely, pancreatitis. Those associated with trimethoprim-sulfamethoxazole include rash, neutropenia, hepatitis, and Stevens-Johnson syndrome. Atovaquone is used only in those patients who cannot tolerate the other treatments. Adverse effects include rash, nausea, vomiting, diarrhea, fever, and abnormal liver function. *(Katz and Zolopa, 2009, p. 1203)*

20. **(E)** Use of fetal scalp electrodes and scalp sampling is contraindicated in the HIV-positive woman because it increases the risk of vertical transmission of the human immunodeficiency virus to the infant. While ruptured membranes for more than 4 hours is associated with an increased risk of vertical transmission, amniotomy per se is not contraindicated. Augmentation of labor, external monitoring, and operative delivery are not contraindicated and, in fact, may be indicated in specific instances for the well-being of the infant and/or mother. *(Ainbinder et al., 2007, p. 693)*

21. **(A)** Zidovidine or other antiretroviral prophylaxis during pregnancy with additional prophylaxis for the infant during the first 1 to 2 weeks of life decreases vertical transmission to less than 1%. No evidence exists to show that indefinite zidovudine therapy is useful. If the infant is HIV positive, as shown by two separate HIV-PCR tests, HIV cultures, or HIV

antigen tests, treatment should commence according to current guidelines. *(McFarland, 2009, p. 1115)*

22. **(E)** The median age at which infants no longer show the maternal antibody for HIV is 10 months; by 18 months, they all do not. HIV ELISA and Western blot are not appropriate for testing pediatric patients until after that age. HIV nucleic acid, RNA in plasma, or DNA in blood cells can be detected earlier. Tests for these include polymerase chain reaction (PCR), branched DNA chain assay (bDNA), and nucleic acid sequence-based amplification (NASBA). *(McFarland, 2009, p. 1114)*

23. **(C)** The HIV rapid antibody test is a screening test that produces results in 1 to 20 minutes. A positive test result must, however, be confirmed with standard testing (ELISA and Western Blot). Should these results be positive, it is appropriate to obtain CD4 lymphocyte percentage and viral load prior to initiating anti-retroviral therapy. *(Katz and Zolopa, 2009, p. 1188).*

24. **(A)** HIV-positive children should receive most standard pediatric vaccines at the usually scheduled times. However, the measles-mumps-rubella (MMR) vaccine should be given at 12 months rather than the usual 15, with a booster 1 month later. The risk of measles is considered greater than the risk of the vaccine in children who are not symptomatic. However, titers decrease over time and with increased immunodeficiency, so an immunized infant who is exposed to measles should receive immune globulin. *(McFarland, 2009, p. 1119)*

25. **(A)** In the pediatric population, the risk of progression varies with age; therefore, age-specific guidelines for treatment are important. Infants are most likely to undergo rapid disease progression in the first year of life compared with older children and adolescents. *(McFarland, 2009, p. 1117)*

26. **(C)** The HIV-positive child who is well should receive the same treatment as other children. Unless contaminated with gross blood, other body fluids (saliva, tears, urine, stool) are not contagious. All schools and daycares should have written policies and training regarding precautions to prevent blood-borne illness. *(McFarland, 2009, p. 1121)*

27. **(B)** All MSM, whether HIV infected or not, should undergo syphilis screening with a rapid plasma regain or VDRL every 6 months due to the recent resurgence of syphilis in MSM. *(Katz and Zolopa, 2009, p. 1191)*

28. **(A)** The herpes zoster is contraindicated in HIV-positive persons who have evidence of immune suppression. The inactivated influenza vaccine should be given annually. Although measles is a live vaccine, it appears to be appropriate for an HIV-positive person who has no protection against measles. The pneumococcal and tetanus-diphtheria vaccines form an important part of health-care maintenance for HIV-positive persons. *(Katz and Zolopa, 2009, p. 1191)*

29. **(C)** Kaposi sarcoma that is in a limited area of the skin may be treated with intralesional vinblastine or by simply observing it over time. Liposomal doxorubicin and alpha interferon are used for extensive or aggressive skin disease, while combination chemotherapy is used for visceral disease. *(Katz and Zolopa, 2009, p. 1194)*

30. **(B)** Semiannual Pap smears are recommended for all HIV-infected women. Quarterly Paps are appropriate for any woman in the first year following treatment for human papilloma virus infection. For uninfected women with no risk factors, annual Paps are recommended during the reproductive years. Some groups recommend alternate or every third year Pap testing following three normal annual smears in a low-risk woman. *(Katz and Zolopa, 2009, p. 1187)*

31. **(D)** The Centers for Disease Control and Prevention recommendations are that babies of HIV-positive mothers receive prophylaxis against infection with *Pneumocystis jiroveci* pneumonia because this infection has its highest incidence during the first year of life. Prophylactic treatment should be continued until 12 months of age if the infant becomes HIV positive but may be discontinued at 3 to

4 months if testing is negative. Appropriate agents include TMP–SMX, dapsone, atovaquone or, for older children, aerosolized pentamidine. Monthly immune globulin is effective in reducing other bacterial infections and hospitalizations in babies not receiving *Pneumocystis jiroveci* pneumonia prophylaxis. *(McFarland, 2009, p. 1121)*

32. **(D)** ACOG recommends a scheduled cesarean for all HIV positive women at 38 weeks' gestation for the prevention of vertical transmission. *(Ainbinder et al., 2007, p. 693)*

33. **(A)** HIV-positive pregnant women should undergo CD4+ serology each trimester. Early in the pregnancy, they should undergo shielded chest radiography, CMV baseline testing, and tuberculosis testing with controls. Syphilis testing should be completed initially and as

usually recommended later in pregnancy. *(Ainbinder et al., 2007, p. 693)*

34. **(C)** Enfuvirtide and maraviroc are entry inhibitors that prevent the virus from getting into the host cell. Atazanavir and lopinavir are protease inhibitors; didanosine is a nucleoside/nucleotide reverse transcriptase inhibitor; and nevirapine is a nonnucleoside reverse transcriptase inhibitor. *(McFarland, 2009, p. 1119)*

35. **(E)** The protease inhibitors are most likely to increase cholesterol and triglycerides; thus, lipid profiles should be monitored carefully in persons taking them. The entry, integrase, and nonnucleoside reverse transcriptase inhibitors require no special monitoring, while some of the nucleoside/nucleotide reverse transcriptase inhibitors require monitoring for neuropathies. *(Katz and Zolopa, 2009, p. 1195)*

REFERENCES

Ainbinder SW, Ramin SM, DeCherney AH. Sexually transmitted diseases and pelvic infections. In: DeCherney AH, Nathan L, Goodwin TM, Laufer N, eds. *Current Obstetric and Gynecologic Diagnosis and Treatment.* 10th ed. New York, NY: McGraw-Hill; 2007.

Katz MH, Zolopa AR. HIV infection. In: McPhee SJ, Papadakis MA, eds. *Current Medical Diagnosis and Treatment.* 48th ed. New York, NY: McGraw-Hill; 2009.

McFarland EJ. Human immunodeficiency virus (HIV) infection. In: Hay WW, Hayward AR, Levin MJ, Sondheimer JM, et al., eds. *Current Pediatric Diagnosis and Treatment.* 19th ed. New York, NY: McGraw-Hill; 2009.

CHAPTER 8

Infectious Disease

Brenda L. Quincy, MPH, PA-C

DIRECTIONS: Each of the numbered items or incomplete statements is followed by answers or by completion of the statement. Select the ONE lettered answer or completion that is BEST in each case.

1. A 33-year-old woman presents with an itchy vaginal discharge for the past 2 days. She has been healthy other than a recent sinus infection for which she took a 10-day course of amoxicillin. Her husband is her only sexual partner and he has no symptoms. On examination, the vulva is noted to be slightly erythematous and swollen with some evidence of excoriation. Discharge is white and clumpy. Provided the most likely diagnosis is confirmed on microscopy, first-line therapy is

   (A) metronidazole 500 mg i po bid for 1 week
   (B) metronidazole 500 mg 4 tablets po at HS × 1 night
   (C) fluconazole 150 mg i po × 1 day
   (D) rocephin 250 mg IM × 1 dose

2. A patient with known human immunodeficiency virus (HIV) infection presents with the gradual onset of a cough, shortness of breath on exertion, and a feeling of a "catch" on inspiration. The chest X-ray reveals a lobar infiltrate. His O_2 sat is 95% and purified protein derivative (PPD) is negative. CD4 cell count is 500. What is the most likely etiology?

   (A) herpes simplex
   (B) mycobacterium
   (C) *Streptococcus pneumoniae*
   (D) *Pneumocystis jiroveci*
   (E) *Toxoplasmosis gondii*

3. An HIV positive patient with CD4 count of 225 cells/mL should receive prophylaxis for which of the following opportunistic infections?

   (A) *Pneumocystis jiroveci*
   (B) toxoplasmosis
   (C) candidiasis
   (D) *Mycobacterium avium*
   (E) cytomegalovirus

4. A 35-year-old HIV positive woman presents to the office for routine follow-up. She has not received antiretroviral therapy to date. She has been essentially asymptomatic other than recently experiencing more fatigue than usual. Her physical examination is unremarkable and her laboratory results return with a CD4 count of 150 (down from 250 6 months ago). The best recommendation for treatment at this point is

   (A) no ART (antiretroviral) recommended
   (B) two NNRTIs (nonnucleoside reverse transcriptase inhibitors) and one PI (protease inhibitor)
   (C) two NNRTIs and one NRTI (nucleoside reverse transcriptase inhibitor)
   (D) two NRTIs and one PI
   (E) three NNRTIs

5. A 55-year-old man with a history of chronic renal failure, 6 months status post renal transplant, presents with chest pain, productive cough, and low-grade fever. He reports generalized malaise as well. Current medications include only those related to the transplant. He has no known allergies. Examination reveals a temperature of 102°F, unremarkable HEENT (head, ears, eyes, nose, throat), and few crackles anteriorly in the upper right lung field. Chest X-ray reveals a solitary nodule in the right upper lobe. The most likely etiology for his symptoms is

(A) *Streptococcus pneumoniae*
(B) *Pneumocystis jiroveci*
(C) cryptococcosis
(D) Candida
(E) influenza A

6. Which of the following infectious agents is most likely to be found in a rural Kentucky farmer or in someone who is responsible for clearing bats out of the local caverns before the tourist season begins?

(A) cryptococcosis
(B) histoplasmosis
(C) psittacosis
(D) Candidal species

7. An 8-year-old girl is brought in to the emergency department with abdominal cramps, nausea, and vomiting since early this morning. She has had two loose stools but denies melena or hematochezia. She has had a low-grade fever. In the past hour, her vision has become blurry and she feels increasingly weak. Her mother has had similar but milder symptoms. Twenty-four hour dietary recall includes only chicken broth today. Last night for dinner they had meatloaf (fully cooked), mashed potatoes, and green beans. Her mother cans all their vegetables. Her medical history is unremarkable. She takes no medications. No known drug allergies. Examination reveals a temperature of 99°F, clear lungs, and mildly tachycardic heart with no murmur audible. Abdomen-bowel sounds present, soft with mild diffuse tenderness, no guarding. Neurologic examination is significant for decreased visual acuity and

decreased motor strength (2/5) in the upper and lower extremities. The most likely etiology is

(A) enterotoxic *E coli*
(B) cholera species
(C) pinworms
(D) *Clostridium botulinum*

8. A 21-year-old bodybuilder presents with complaints of diarrhea, cramps, and low-grade fever × 24 hours. He has been training for a competition, eating large amounts of protein, and supplementing with shakes made with raw eggs. He reports three loose stools today, but he says he has been able to eat and take fluids. He only came in today because the blood in the commode alarmed him. On examination, he is noted to be a well-muscled man in no apparent distress; lungs and heart unremarkable; abdomen, mildly hyperactive bowel sounds with no tenderness or organomegaly; no evidence of hemorrhoid or fissure, no masses, and no stool present for hemoccult. The most appropriate first-line management is

(A) ciprofloxacin 500 mg po bid × 1 week
(B) metronidazole 500 mg po bid × 1 week
(C) trimethoprim sulfamethoxazole DS po bid × 1 week
(D) fluconazole 200 mg po qd × 1 week
(E) supportive care

9. Which of the following foodborne infectious illnesses may cause seizures in pediatric patients?

(A) salmonellosis
(B) shigellosis
(C) cholera
(D) campylobacter

10. Which of the following foodborne illnesses is most likely to be acquired through eating raw oysters?

(A) salmonellosis
(B) shigellosis
(C) cholera
(D) giardia
(E) hookworms

11. A 3-year-old African immigrant woman is brought into the emergency department with congestion and a sore throat. Her family has been in the United States for only 1 month. They were "rescued" from a refugee camp by a private relief organization. This is her first medical evaluation. On examination, she is noted to have a low-grade fever; tympanic membranes are pearly gray without injection or visible air fluid levels. Throat is erythematous with enlarged tonsils covered by a grayish membrane. Tonsillar nodes are tender. Lungs are clear to auscultation. Rapid strep screen is negative. The most likely etiologic agent is

    (A) *Bordetella pertussis*
    (B) *Corynebacterium diphtheriae*
    (C) *Streptococcal pyogenes*
    (D) *Hemophilus influenza*

12. A 23-year-old woman presents with complaints of pelvic discomfort and a vaginal discharge for the past 3 days. She finished her period last week. She is taking oral contraceptives as directed. Her medical history is significant for a therapeutic abortion with no other hospitalizations or pregnancies. She has had three sexual partners in the past 6 weeks and does not use condoms. Her most recent partner reported that he was treated recently for gonorrhea. On examination, she has a mucopurulent discharge with "strawberry" cervix on speculum examination. After collecting the appropriate specimens, the best therapeutic option for this patient is

    (A) ofloxacin 400 mg i po × 1 dose plus azithromycin 250 mg iiii po × 1 dose
    (B) fluconazole 150 mg i po × 1 dose
    (C) metronidazole 500 mg iiii po × 1 dose
    (D) ceftriaxone 250 mg IM × 1 dose

13. Which of the following organisms causes dysentery and has a cystic form that contaminates the water supply through poor handling of human sewage and can be spread through anal intercourse in homosexual men?

    (A) *Vibrio cholera*
    (B) *Entamoeba histolytica*
    (C) hookworm
    (D) salmonella
    (E) giardia

14. The organism shown in Figure 8-1 usually enters the body from infected soil through a break in the skin of the feet. It then is carried to the lungs, travels to the mouth, and is swallowed. Once in the gastrointestinal (GI) tract, it attaches to the wall and induces bleeding, leading to an iron deficiency anemia. Associated GI symptoms are uncommon. Additional symptoms include swelling and intense itching at the site in which the larva penetrates the skin. Which of the following organisms best fits this clinical picture and the organism shown in Figure 8-1?

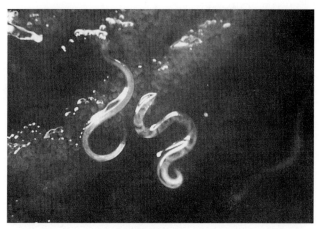

Figure 8-1
(*Courtesy of Centers for Disease Control and Prevention, National Center for Infectious Diseases, Division of Parasitic Diseases.*)

    (A) Strongyloides
    (B) whipworms
    (C) pinworms
    (D) hookworms

15. The most common cause of fever of unknown origin, with other symptoms including nausea, vomiting, abdominal pain, myalgias, and arthralgias, severe enough to require hospitalization in the returning traveler is

    (A) malaria
    (B) dengue
    (C) enteric fever
    (D) leptospirosis

16. A 16-year-old boy presents to the office with complaints of a rash, low-grade fever, headache, and malaise. Symptoms began yesterday after he spent most of his free time in the past 4 days deer hunting in the woods around his house. He reports that he does check himself for ticks every night. He often finds them but has not noticed any this season that were latched on to his skin. On examination, his temperature is noted to be 99.9°F, his HEENT is unremarkable, and he has 1 to 2 mm red macules over wrists and ankles with remainder of skin clear. Heart, lungs, and abdomen unremarkable. The most likely diagnosis in this patient is

   (A) Lyme disease
   (B) Rocky Mountain spotted fever
   (C) ehrlichiosis
   (D) Q fever

17. Which of the following causes an opportunistic infection in those with HIV when the CD4 count drops below 100 and is associated with esophagitis, encephalitis, and peripheral neuropathies and has prophylaxis available for retinitis when CD4 counts drop below 50?

   (A) *Cytomegalovirus*
   (B) *Toxoplasma gondii*
   (C) *Mycobacterium avium*
   (D) *Pneumocystis jiroveci*

18. Which of the following childhood exanthems is characterized by a 10-day incubation period followed by 3 days of fever, runny nose, and conjunctivitis giving way to a maculopapular rash starting on the head, progressing to the trunk, and accompanied by white spots on the buccal mucosa?

   (A) herpes simplex infection
   (B) coxsackie virus
   (C) measles
   (D) rubella

19. Which of the following viral infections often begins with a mild or asymptomatic course in childhood followed by a period of latency in which the virus remains in the trigeminal ganglia and reactivates later?

   (A) herpes simplex 1 virus
   (B) parvovirus
   (C) herpesvirus 6
   (D) varicella zoster

20. A 6-year-old child with leukemia presents with a very painful vesicular rash as seen in Figure 8-2. This is the only dermatologic manifestation but is accompanied by fever and malaise. His medical history is significant for the leukemia, tonsillectomy, and adenoidectomy at age 3 and chicken pox 4 months later. He has had all his other childhood immunizations. The most likely diagnosis in this case is

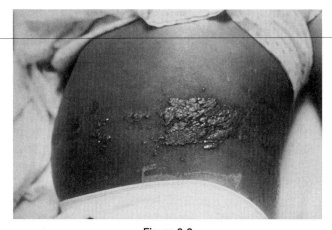

Figure 8-2
(Courtesy of Centers for Disease Control and Prevention, National Immunization Program.)

   (A) measles
   (B) roseola
   (C) recurrent chicken pox
   (D) zoster
   (E) molluscum contagiosum

21. A 7-year-old girl is brought in by her mom for evaluation of a rash. She has had a fever for a few days and woke up this morning looking like she had been slapped on both cheeks. Other than supportive care, which instruction below represents the best patient education for this patient?

(A) She should remain out of school because she is contagious until the rash resolves.

(B) She may return to school but stay out of physical education class to avoid splenic injury.

(C) It spreads by the fecal–oral route, so she should wash her hands after using the bathroom.

(D) She may resume normal activities as her energy level improves.

22. A 22-year-old sexually active woman presents for her annual gynecologic evaluation. She reports one partner for the past 6 months and takes oral contraceptive pills as directed. Her periods have been regular. Her examination is unremarkable and her Pap smear returns with atypical squamous cells of undetermined significance and positive for human papillomavirus-16. The next most appropriate step for this patient is to

(A) proceed with colposcopy

(B) repeat Pap smear in 12 months

(C) repeat Pap smear in 24 months

(D) schedule her for a loop electrosurgical excision procedure (LEEP)

23. A 55-year-old woman presents for a preemployment physical for a nursing home where she will begin working as a certified nursing assistant. This is her first time working in a health care facility. She wonders about vaccines, specifically measles, mumps, and rubella (MMR). She does not think she has ever received any component of this vaccine but does remember having measles as a child. The first step in management of this case is to

(A) tell the patient she does not need the vaccine at her age

(B) draw titers of each component of the vaccine

(C) give two MMR doses today regardless of titer

(D) give one dose today, return in 1 month for the second dose, delay employment 1 month

24. A 25-year-old man presents for evaluation of diarrhea. He is generally healthy and reports he finished a 4-day hike about 2 weeks ago. He does mention that he ran out of water on day 3 and did not have a filter with him. Today he reports that he does not feel too badly but he has had 24 hours of abdominal bloating, increased flatulence, and loose stools. He denies melena or hematochezia. His physical examination is unremarkable but stool ova and parasite examination reveal ova and trophozoites. The most appropriate antimicrobial agent for this patient is

(A) no medicine needed; this is self-limiting and will resolve in 24 hours

(B) ciprofloxacin

(C) amphotericin

(D) metronidazole

25. Which of the following viral exanthems includes a fever followed by a diffuse maculopapular rash that spares the face and resolves in about 2 days?

(A) measles

(B) erythema subitum

(C) erythema infectiosum

(D) rubella

26. For an uncomplicated soft tissue infection with community-acquired methicillin-resistant *Staphylococcus aureus*, the preferred therapy is

(A) high-dose Augmentin × 7 days

(B) Clindamycin orally for 2 weeks

(C) incision and drainage alone

(D) incision and drainage plus high-dose amoxicillin

27. The most common cause of community-acquired bacterial pneumonia in the United States is

(A) *Streptococcus pyogenes*

(B) *Streptococcus pneumoniae*

(C) *Legionella pneumophila*

(D) *Staphylococcus aureus*

(E) *Haemophilus influenzae*

28. Which of the following purified protein derivative (PPD)-tested patients should receive antituberculosis prophylaxis?

(A) PPD of 13 mm in a person with no risk factors

(B) PPD of 8 mm in a foreign-born person from a country with a high prevalence of tuberculosis

(C) PPD of 3 mm in an HIV-positive person

(D) PPD of 6 mm in a Native American person

(E) PPD of 12 mm in an inmate at a correctional institution

29. A patient with no history of treatment for primary syphilis presents with symptoms and signs consistent with secondary syphilis. The most common sign of secondary syphilis is

(A) generalized lymphadenopathy

(B) aseptic meningitis

(C) alopecia

(D) generalized maculopapular rash

(E) superficial painless gummas

30. A 30-year-old man presents to the office for follow-up on an endoscopically diagnosed gastric ulcer. At endoscopy, he was found to have a *Helicobacter pylori* infection and now he has completed appropriate therapy. He has another refill available on the proton-pump inhibitor. He is currently asymptomatic. What is the most appropriate follow-up on the infection?

(A) Because he is asymptomatic, no further testing is required.

(B) Check urea breath test or fecal antigen today.

(C) Repeat endoscopy with histologic testing for *H. pylori.*

(D) Check *H. pylori* serology today.

(E) Collect stool specimen for culture.

31. An adult male, not previously vaccinated for rabies, presents to the emergency department after being bitten by an aggressive stray dog. The dog was captured, and declared "probably rabid" by a local veterinarian. Which of the fol-

lowing treatment options should you select for this patient?

(A) administer human rabies immune globulin only

(B) administer equine rabies antiserum only

(C) administer human rabies immune globulin and equine rabies antiserum

(D) administer human rabies immune globulin and equine rabies antiserum and human diploid cell rabies vaccine

(E) administer human rabies immune globulin and human diploid cell rabies vaccine

32. An otherwise healthy, immunocompetent health care worker converts to a positive PPD. Which of the following drugs is optimal therapy for this person?

(A) rifampin

(B) pyrazinamide

(C) ethambutol

(D) streptomycin

(E) isoniazid

33. In the treatment of peptic ulcer disease (PUD) of infectious etiology, which of the following drug combinations will provide the most efficacious therapy?

(A) metronidazole and omeprazole

(B) bismuth subsalicylate and omeprazole and sucralfate

(C) amoxicillin and bismuth subsalicylate and antacid

(D) omeprazole and amoxicillin and clarithromycin

(E) clarithromycin and metronidazole and sucralfate

34. An adult with a high risk for bacterial endocarditis is scheduled for a dental extraction. The patient has a history of penicillin allergy. Which of the following is an appropriate oral prophylactic drug to give this patient?

(A) amoxicillin

(B) vancomycin

(C) clindamycin

(D) doxycycline

(E) gentamicin

35. Septic arthritis in adults younger than 30 years is usually caused by

(A) *Neisseria gonorrhea*

(B) *Staphylococcus aureus*

(C) *Pseudomonas aeruginosa*

(D) *Streptococcus pyogenes*

(E) *Salmonella* species

36. A 30-year-old woman presents with 2 weeks of arthralgias, migrating from distal to proximal joints. It began with increased warmth and erythema in her right ankle and left knee. She has a low-grade fever and reports a history of sore throat and swollen glands about 1 month ago. Antistreptolysin O titer is positive. The most likely explanation for her joint pain is

(A) new-onset rheumatoid arthritis

(B) rheumatic fever

(C) gonococcal arthritis

(D) gram-positive septic arthritis

(E) osteoarthritis

37. A sexually active 19-year-old woman presents with clusters of painful vesicles on an erythematous base on the vulva and cervix, accompanied by temperature of 100°F and mild malaise. She reports a history of a similar outbreak last month, which resolved in 10 days. Microscopic examination of cells from the basement of a blister treated with Giemsa stain is likely to reveal

(A) multinucleated giant cells

(B) gram-positive cocci in clusters

(C) gram-positive cocci in chains

(D) gram-negative rods

(E) hyphae and buds

38. Which of the following characteristics is most helpful in distinguishing *Mycoplasma pneumoniae* as the etiologic agent in community-acquired pneumonia from other bacteria and viruses?

(A) Mycoplasma has an incubation period that averages 28 days compared to weeks for most viruses.

(B) Mycoplasma is more common in the elderly.

(C) Sputum Gram stain often shows increased white blood cell counts (WBCs) with little or no bacteria.

(D) Sputum culture is the gold standard for diagnosis.

(E) Mycoplasma often follows exposure to cockroach infestation.

39. Which of the following treatments is first-line therapy for sputum culture-positive Legionnaire's pneumonia in an immunocompetent patient?

(A) ampicillin/sulbactam

(B) erythromycin

(C) ceftriaxone

(D) vancomycin

(E) clindamycin

40. Koplik spots are a differentiating diagnostic feature of which of the following viral exanthems?

(A) rubella

(B) rubeola

(C) varicella

(D) parvovirus

(E) Kawasaki disease

41. A 16-year-old girl presents to the office complaining of a very sore throat, swollen lymph nodes, fever, and general malaise. Her examination reveals a temperature of 102.2°F, enlarged exudative tonsils, tender cervical lymphadenopathy, and borderline enlarged spleen. Rapid strep screen is negative. Which of the following laboratory findings best supports the most likely diagnosis?

(A) decreased white blood cell count

(B) increased monocytes on white cell differential

(C) thrombocytosis

(D) decreased levels of antibody to Epstein-Barr viral capsid antigen

(E) increased atypical lymphocytes on white blood cell differential

42. Which of the following viruses is rodent-borne and the cause of hemorrhagic fever and a pulmonary syndrome, which begins with a fever and may rapidly progress to shock and adult respiratory distress syndrome?

(A) human T-cell lymphotropic virus (HTLV)
(B) Flavivirus
(C) Hantavirus
(D) Filovirus
(E) coronavirus

43. Which of the following patients may receive an influenza immunization?

(A) 12-year-old with hypersensitivity to chicken eggs
(B) otherwise healthy male on concomitant warfarin therapy
(C) 21-year-old with Guillain–Barré syndrome
(D) 55-year-old with thrombocytopenia
(E) 4-year-old with acute febrile illness

44. Severe acute respiratory syndrome (SARS) is an atypical pneumonia caused by

(A) West Nile virus
(B) Flavivirus
(C) coronavirus
(D) Hantavirus
(E) respiratory syncytial virus

45. A 4-year-old boy presents with 5 days of fever, conjunctivitis, strawberry tongue, red lips, and injected throat. He has large, swollen, slightly tender lymph nodes in his neck and a peeling rash in the palms and soles. The most likely cause is

(A) Kawasaki syndrome
(B) respiratory syncytial virus
(C) coxsackievirus
(D) fifth disease

46. A 25-year-old woman presents not feeling well 1 week after returning from a trip to central Africa. She has had steadily increasing fever, abdominal distention, and diarrhea. She also has rashes on her abdomen, chest, and back, which are characterized by 3-mm pink papules, which blanch with pressure. Heart rate is 60 beats/min. Blood culture is positive but final identification is pending. Most likely diagnosis is

(A) typhoid fever
(B) yellow fever
(C) malaria
(D) hepatitis
(E) shigellosis

47. In a patient with high fever, malaise, and severe myalgias, which of the following additional pieces of history would raise the index of suspicion for plague?

(A) history of tick bite in the northeastern United States
(B) exposure to wild rats in Southern California
(C) history of drinking stream water while hiking in the Appalachian mountains
(D) history of raising sheep in Wyoming
(E) exposure to exotic birds in upper Midwest

48. A 14-year-old girl presents 1 week after the neighbor's cat bit her hand. In the first 3 days after the bite she developed a shallow ulcer at the bite site. Because her parents knew the cat was up to date on shots, they treated the ulcer with topical antibiotics and did not seek medical care. Now, the patient has low-grade fever and headache and feels tired. Axillary nodes on the affected side are swollen. The ulcer on the hand is nearly healed. The best treatment option is

(A) doxycycline 100 mg bid × 21 days
(B) Augmentin 500 mg po bid × 10 days
(C) azithromycin 500 mg po qd × 7 days
(D) acyclovir 400 mg po bid × 10 days
(E) no therapy required

49. A 27-year-old woman presents with 3 days of fever, chills, headache, and a deep dry cough. She has been working at a pet store for the past month and thinks that one of the parakeets that came in 10 days ago may be sick. On examination, she has dullness to percussion of the right lung base and right-sided coarse crackles. The most likely diagnosis is

    (A) sarcoidosis
    (B) tularemia
    (C) psittacosis
    (D) brucellosis
    (E) listeriosis

50. A 35-year-old forest ranger presents with a rash on his back. It started 4 days ago as a red maculopapular lesion about 2 cm in diameter. Now it is 14 cm in diameter with an area of central clearing. In addition to the rash, he has had a headache, fever, chills, and muscle aches. The most likely diagnosis is

    (A) cellulitis
    (B) wasp sting
    (C) Rocky Mountain spotted fever
    (D) poison ivy
    (E) Lyme disease

51. Pregnant women should avoid contact with cat feces because of the potential harmful sequelae of congenital transmission of

    (A) toxoplasmosis
    (B) schistosomiasis
    (C) leishmaniasis
    (D) brucellosis
    (E) echinococcosis

52. Which of the following is the appropriate treatment for acute *Clostridium tetani* infection?

    (A) tetanus immune globulin, tetanus toxoid, and metronidazole
    (B) tetanus immune globulin and penicillin
    (C) tetanus toxoid and penicillin
    (D) tetanus immune globulin, tetanus toxoid, and penicillin
    (E) tetanus immune globulin and tetanus toxoid

53. A 73-year-old man is hospitalized for a prolonged period because his prostate surgery was complicated by pneumonia. After 10 days of broad-spectrum antibiotics, he developed fever, leukocytosis, and dysentery. Colonoscopy reveals pseudomembranes in his colon. Stool cultures are pending. The most likely etiology for his diarrhea is

    (A) Norwalk virus
    (B) *Clostridium difficile*
    (C) *Clostridium perfringens*
    (D) Enterobacteriaceae
    (E) *Pseudomonas aeruginosa*

54. Which of the following forms of anthrax is most common?

    (A) inhalational
    (B) hematogenous
    (C) cutaneous
    (D) gastrointestinal
    (E) congenital

Answers and Explanations

1. **(C)** The clinical presentation is consistent with vulvovaginal candidiasis. The recent oral antibiotic use increased her risk for developing the infection. The white clumpy discharge and relatively benign bimanual examination support the diagnosis, which is confirmed by 10% potassium hydroxide wet mount of the secretions. Treatment for an uncomplicated case may include topical or oral antifungals. Oral fluconazole in the one dose regimen is effective, convenient, and likely to increase compliance. The metronidazole regimens are appropriate for bacterial vaginosis and trichomoniasis, respectively. Rocephin is an option for gonococcal infection and would likely worsen the candidiasis. *(Nyirjesy, 2008, p. 642)*

2. **(C)** Patients with HIV infections are at increased risk for ordinary bacterial pneumonias as their immune system begins to decline in function. When CD4 counts are in the 200 to 500 cells/mm^3 range, their risk for pneumococcal pneumonia is 3 to 4 times greater than that of the immunocompetent patient. The clinical picture and lobar infiltrate on X-ray are consistent with typical pneumonia, most often caused by *Streptococcus pneumoniae*. *Pneumocystis jiroveci* pneumonia is unlikely until the CD4 count drops below 200 cells/mm^3. Mycobacterial pneumonia would likely be associated with a more chronic cough and the others are not likely to cause pulmonary disease. *(Carpenter et al., 2007, p. 1005)*

3. **(A)** Prophylaxis against opportunistic infections is an important part of management in the HIV-infected patient. Prophylaxis for PCP with trimethoprim sulfamethoxazole is the only one in the list indicated when the CD4 count is >200 cells/mm^3. Toxoplasma prophylaxis with trimethoprim sulfamethoxazole is recommended when the CD4 count drops below 100 cells/mm^3. *Mycobacterium avium* prevention with clarithromycin and cytomegalovirus retinitis prevention are considered when the CD4 count drops below 50 cells/mm^3. *(Carpenter et al., 2007, p. 1000)*

4. **(D)** The timing of initial therapy with antiretroviral agents is a clinical challenge. The patient and health care provider should make the decision together and carefully, particularly in the asymptomatic patient. In this case, the rapid decline in CD4 count to a level below 200 cells/mm^3 is a reason to begin therapy. Therapeutic decisions should be made individually on the basis of patient factors including comorbid illness and drug side effects. Therapeutic classes of antiretroviral agents include nucleoside/nucleotide reverse transcriptase inhibitors (NRTIs), nonnucleoside/nucleotide reverse transcriptase inhibitors (NNRTIs), protease inhibitors (PIs), and viral entry inhibitor. The most studied combinations for initial therapy include one NNRTI + two NRTIs or one PI plus two NRTIs. *(Carpenter et al., 2007, pp. 998-999)*

5. **(C)** Cryptococcal species are opportunistic organisms responsible for infections in immune-compromised hosts. With the rise of HIV infections in the past few decades in the United States, cryptococcosis is becoming increasingly prevalent. It is also a common infection in those who have undergone solid organ transplantation. The two most common

areas for infection are the lungs and the central nervous system. Pulmonary involvement includes fever, productive cough, chest discomfort, and weight loss. Pleural effusions, lymphadenopathy, and solitary or multiple nodules can all be seen on chest x-ray. Central nervous system manifestations include meningitis and meningoencephalitis. Diagnosis is confirmed with India ink prep of cerebrospinal fluid showing yeast or histologic stains of tissue from the involved organs. Treatment is with oral or parenteral antifungal agents. *(Chayakulkeeree and Perfect, 2006, pp. 507-544)*

6. **(B)** Histoplasmosis is found throughout the continental United States with greater concentration in the Ohio and Mississippi river valleys. It is found in soil, particularly in areas with large quantities of decaying wood or bird droppings. Bats also carry histoplasma. Cryptococcus is most likely in people exposed to pigeons and is also found in soil enriched by bird droppings or in cockroach-infested environments. Parrots, parakeets, ducks, and turkeys are the usual hosts and most commonly infected species for psittacoccal infections as well. It is less common in humans. *(Kleigman, 2007, p. 1288; McCoy and Aronoff, 2007, pp. 1316-1318; Flood and Aronoff, 2007, p. 1310)*

7. **(D)** Clostridium botulinum produces a neurotoxin that can lead to life-threatening illness including respiratory paralysis. Botulism infection is caused by the spore-forming bacteria that lives in soil and can be foodborne. In the latter case, home-canned foods are often the cause. After a 12-hour to 3-day incubation period, botulism begins with classic symptoms of abdominal pain, nausea, vomiting, and mild diarrhea and, if unchecked, evolves into a progressive neurologic disorder marked by double vision, motor weakness, and ptosis. Respiratory muscle involvement may occur ultimately and result in death. Because of the virulence of the neurotoxin it has been used as an agent of bioterrorism. Cholera and enterotoxigenic *E. coli* cause a foodborne diarrheal illness that can result in significant morbidity and mortality, but they do not have neurologic manifestations. Pinworm infection is usually

found among younger children, is marked by severe anal itching, and fecal-oral transmission. *(Armitage and Salata, 2007, p. 1019; Pigott, 2008, pp. 488-489, 492)*

8. **(E)** Salmonella infection, caused by consuming raw eggs, is the most likely diagnosis in this case. The most common salmonella serotypes in the United States include Typhimurium and Enteritidis. Infection is characterized by fever, abdominal cramps, diarrhea (sometimes with blood) following a 12- to 72-hour incubation period. Most cases are self-limited, resolving within a week. For this reason, they are usually managed with supportive care only. In the rare case in which sepsis occurs, the patient should be hospitalized and treated with trimethoprim sulfamethoxazole or a fluoroquinolone. *(Pigott, 2008, pp. 485-486)*

9. **(B)** Shigella, salmonella, and campylobacter infections all include fever, cramping, and bloody diarrhea but only shigella is known to progress to seizures in children. Salmonella is generally self-limited and resolves with supportive care. Campylobacter may cause an overwhelming sepsis in the immune-compromised. Cholera is a waterborne infection with large volume diarrhea and associated dehydration and also has the potential to result in sepsis. *(Pigott, 2008, pp. 486-489)*

10. **(C)** Cholera infection is most often caused by *Vibrio cholerae, Vibrio vulnificus,* or *Vibrio parahaemolyticus.* Although cholera infection can be transmitted through wounds, the most often reported cause is eating undercooked shellfish. The clinical picture most often includes a watery diarrhea that can lead to dehydration. In the immune compromised host, overwhelming sepsis is possible. It is most often treated with doxycycline plus a third-generation cephalosporin or by a fluoroquinolone alone. Salmonella infection is associated with consumption of raw eggs and undercooked chicken or beef. Shigella is transmitted by the fecal–oral route, often because of poor hygiene. Giardia is waterborne and hookworms are found in the soil. *(Weller, 2008, p. 1311; Weller and Nutman, 2008, pp. 1320-1321; Pigott, 2008, pp. 484-486, 489)*

11. **(B)** The clues to the etiology of this presentation include the gray pseudomembranes on the tonsils and the lack of medical care resulting in missed childhood vaccines. *Corynebacterium diphtheriae* causes a respiratory and posterior pharyngeal infection with little likelihood of sepsis. However, the case fatality rate is high with mortality from neurologic impairment increasing the longer treatment is delayed. Because it releases a toxin into the local tissue in the throat, a tough gray colored pseudomembrane over the tonsils is the classic clinical finding. Although culture on special medium of a specimen collected from beneath the membrane confirms the diagnosis, therapy should be started based on clinical suspicion and includes parenteral penicillin or erythromycin. Vaccination with diphtheria toxin is preventive. *Bordetella pertussis* infection is marked by the characteristic whooping cough. *Streptococcus pyogenes* usually manifests with tonsillar exudate without membranes and palatal petechiae and in this case is ruled out by the negative rapid strep test. Hemophilus influenza in a 3-year-old may result in an epiglottitis, ear infection, or pneumonia. *(Simberkoff, 2007, pp. 2223-2225; Sutter, 2007, p. 2192; Stevens, 2007, p. 2176; Hewlett, 2007, p. 2259)*

12. **(A)** Clinical presentation is consistent with cervicitis in a young woman with risk factors for sexually transmitted infection. She has likely been exposed specifically to *Neisseria gonorrhea*. Coinfection with *Chlamydia trachomatis* is common. While test results are pending, the Centers for Disease Control and Prevention in its 2006 Guidelines for STD treatment recommend treating for both with single doses (improved compliance) of ofloxacin and azithromycin first-line. In areas with quinolone resistance, intramuscular ceftriaxone is an option but coverage for Chlamydia is still necessary. Metronidazole is the appropriate therapy for trichomoniasis and fluconazole for vaginal candidiasis. *(CDC, 2006, pp. 39, 43)*

13. **(B)** *Entamoeba histolytica* has two stages in its life cycle. In the active stage in the human intestine, it causes symptoms of dysentery, abdominal pain, stool mucus, and tenesmus. In the dormant stage, the cystic form is excreted in the stool and in developing nations frequently contaminates the supply of drinking water. When the amoeba is in the dormant stage, the cystic form can be excreted in the stool and, in the case of food handlers with poor personal hygiene, be transmitted to others. In addition, because of the cystic stage, individuals engaging in anal intercourse can transmit the infection unknowingly. Diagnosis is made by microscopic evaluation of a stool wet prep and confirmed by serology. Treatment includes agents such as metronidazole or tinidazole. *(Schuster and Glaser, 2007, pp. 2404-2405)*

14. **(D)** As described, hookworms generally enter through the skin and travel to the lungs. There they migrate to the mouth, are swallowed, and reproduce in the gut. Females lay thousands of eggs, which are subsequently excreted in the feces and mature in soil. The adult worms attach to the intestinal wall, causing bleeding and a subsequent anemia. They can also affect absorption, leading to nutritional deficiencies. Diagnosis is made through microscopic evaluation of a stool specimen and treatment is with albendazole. Whipworms (*Trichuris trichiura*) also lay eggs in the stool, which then reside in the soil. Many whipworm infections are asymptomatic. Strongyloides is different from other nematodes in that it can reproduce inside the intestine and persist for years. Pinworms (enterobiasis) are very small worms that exit the anus at night to lay eggs, causing intense itching and promoting the fecal-oral transmission. *(Weller and Nutman, 2008, pp. 1322-1324; Kazura, 2007, pp. 2425-2431)*

15. **(A)** Malaria is the most common cause of fever and hospitalization in travelers returning to the United States. Those with no history of exposure develop the most severe cases. There are four species of Plasmodium causing human infections in the United States, with *P. falciparum* and *P. vivax* being the most common and *P. falciparum* causing the most severe disease. Most U.S. travelers contract malaria in West Africa. *P falciparum* has a shorter incubation period (up to 30 days). Symptoms are variable but may include fever, nausea, vomiting,

abdominal pain, myalgias, and arthralgias. On physical examination, some will have increased heart rate with decreased blood pressure progressing to changes in mental status. Complete blood cell count may show decreases in red cells and platelets and increased atypical lymphocytes on peripheral smear. Confirmation is obtained with Giemsa-stained peripheral smears. Treatment includes oral quinine for less severe cases or intravenous quinine for the more severe. Doxycycline or clindamycin are added to either regimen. Prophylaxis for malaria for travelers to endemic areas is very effective, relatively safe, and easy to take and should be encouraged. Dengue is the second most common cause of fever in returning travelers and has a much shorter incubation period. Clinical presentation usually includes fever, chills, headache, lymphadenopathy, and myalgias. Severe back pain may occur as well. It is generally self-limited. Enteric fevers include typhoid and paratyphoid and are more common in those returning from the Indian subcontinent. Symptoms are constitutional and physical examination may include organomegaly. On complete blood cell count, all cell lines are down. Liver transaminase levels are often elevated. The organisms may be cultured from blood, urine, stool, or bone marrow. Treatment is with fluoroquinolones. Leptospirosis is much less common. Transmission is through contact with infected animals' urine or body tissue. Cases have been reported in those who swam in infected water. Clinical pattern is often biphasic with two periods of fever and constitutional symptoms. Diagnosis is confirmed with serology or culture and treatment is with doxycycline or amoxicillin. (*Speil et al., 2007, pp. 1100-1106*)

16. **(B)** Rocky Mountain spotted fever (RMSF) is a rickettsial infection caused by *Ricketsia ricketsii*. The organism is transmitted to humans through the bite of the dog tick and is more common among those who spend time outdoors in a wooded area. The illness begins with generalized symptoms of fever, headache, nausea, vomiting, malaise, and myalgias. The rash of RMSF begins as a macular rash and progresses to nonblanching petechiae. The rash begins over the wrists and ankles and progresses to the arms, legs, and trunk. Untreated, it can progress to respiratory failure and/or central nervous system involvement. Serologic confirmation is not usually valid until 7 to 10 days after clinical symptoms begin so treatment is often begun empirically. Drug of choice is doxycycline 100 mg po bid until the patient is afebrile and clinically better for 2 to 3 days. Lyme disease is distinguished from RMSF by the pattern of the rash. Lyme disease is characterized by the classic erythema chronicum migrans rash, usually on the trunk. Ehrlichiosis usually does not manifest with a rash. It begins with the same general symptoms but can progress to a toxic shock syndrome. Q fever can be transmitted by ticks, but it is often acquired through contact with sheep, cattle, and goats. It has similar generalized symptoms but can progress to a cough and pneumonia. It is usually without rash. All of these illnesses respond to doxycycline. (*Walker et al., 2008, pp. 1061-1067; Steere, 2008, p. 1055*)

17. **(A)** Cytomegalovirus is an opportunistic agent that causes clinical symptoms in a number of systems. CMV esophageal ulcers can occur when the CD4 count drops below 100 and usually respond well to IV ganciclovir. CMV can also cause encephalitis with altered level of consciousness. In addition to central nervous system impairment, CMV infection can lead to a peripheral polyradiculopathy. The retinitis associated with CMV usually does not develop until the CD4 count drops below 50. Prophylaxis is available, but the benefits must outweigh the risks of the medicine. Toxoplasmosis prophylaxis begins when CD4 count drops below 100. *Pneumocystis jiroveci* primarily causes pneumonia and *mycobacterium avium* causes fever and gastrointestinal symptoms rather than neurologic. (*Carpenter et al., 2007, pp.1000-1007*)

18. **(C)** The description best fits that of measles. It has a 7- to 10-day incubation period followed by 3 days of coryza, fever, and conjunctival involvement. The prodrome dissipates as the characteristic rash develops first on the head and face and then the trunk. Koplick spots are

the pathognomonic white spots that occur on the buccal mucosa in measles' infection. Herpes simplex infection can present as painful vesicles on the mouth and lips (HSV-1) or genitalia (HSV-2). It is preceded by fever and a tingling or burning sensation at the site where the vesicle will develop. Coxsackievirus causes hand, foot, and mouth disease with lesion distribution in those three areas. Rubella has a longer incubation period (2 to 2.5 weeks) and is less contagious than measles. It is sometimes asymptomatic or produces a milder course than measles. *(Ruocco et al., 2007, pp. 671-672)*

19. **(A)** The description best fits that of herpes simplex 1. The infection is usually acquired in childhood and may be asymptomatic or severe enough to produce a painful stomatitis. Subsequent outbreaks may be triggered by fever, other infection, stress, or excess sun exposure and are characterized by orolabial outbreak along the trigeminal nerve producing a painful vesicle which over 10 to 14 days crusts over and resolves. Treatment with topical or oral antifungals (such as acyclovir) shortens the course and lessens the severity if started early. Parvovirus and herpesvirus 6 do not have a period of latency. Varicella zoster does have a latency period but often in a spinal nerve or the opthalmic branch of the trigeminal with rare orolabial involvement. *(Ruocco et al., 2007, pp. 669-673)*

20. **(D)** Varicella zoster outbreak (shingles) most often occurs in an elderly patient years after experiencing chicken pox as a child or who have received the immunization. The virus lies dormant in the spinal nerve root and later manifests as a very painful, skin-sensitive vesicular rash in a dermatomal distribution. Unlike chicken pox, a postherpetic neuralgia pain can persist for years and is at times, debilitating. Although most common in the elderly, zoster can occur in children in immunocompromised states such as those with malignancy or human immunodeficiency virus infection. Molluscum contagiosum presents with flesh colored, umbilicated papules and is typically not painful. Measles and roseola are maculopapular rashes. *(Ruocco et al., 2007, p. 673)*

21. **(D)** The "slapped cheek" appearance to the rash is consistent with a Parvovirus B19 etiology for erythema infectiosum. It is a droplet infection that is no longer contagious once the rash breaks out. It generally has a benign course and patients recover fully with supportive care. Splenic involvement is not typically a part of the course, so she may resume activities as she feels able. *(Servey et al., 2007, p. 373)*

22. **(A)** Human papillomavirus subtypes 6, 11, 16, and 18 increase risk for the development of cervical cancer. In a young woman over 21 years old with atypical squamous cells of undetermined significance and positive HPV 16 subtype, the next step in evaluation is the colposcopic evaluation. Alternatively, she could be followed with Pap smears at 6 and 12 months. The LEEP procedure is indicated for those with recurrent histologic finding of cervical intraepithelial neoplasm grade 2 or 3. *(Warren et al., 2009, pp. 140-142)*

23. **(B)** Adults born before 1957 are generally considered immune to measles and mumps. In this case, the patient has a history of clinical measles but no proof of mumps. Because she is becoming a health care worker and has no evidence of immunity to mumps, it is recommended that she receive one dose of MMR for the mumps benefit with a second dose given in an outbreak. Rubella vaccine also should be given if there is lack of laboratory evidence of immunity. In the case of this patient who is past childbearing age, testing for immune status for measles, mumps, and rubella is a logical first step with one dose of MMR given in the event the titers do not demonstrate immunity. A second dose could then be given if she becomes exposed to an outbreak situation. *(Centers for Disease Control and Prevention, 2008)*

24. **(D)** The clinical picture is consistent with infection with *Giardia lamblia*, a parasite that can be picked up from contaminated water and infects the small intestine. It can be difficult to diagnose because it may be clinically asymptomatic. Nevertheless, an infected person passes the cysts in the stool and they can survive for weeks in cold water. Infection can also be

transmitted by direct fecal–oral route, especially among small children and their caregivers. Clinical symptoms vary but often include bloating, loose stools or diarrhea, belching, and possibly weight loss. The course can be episodic. Diagnosis is made with stool specimen examined for ova and parasites or by stool antigen immunoassay. First-line therapy is metronidazole 250 mg po tid for 5 days. Tinidazole is an effective alternative. *(Weller, 2008, pp. 1311-1313)*

25. **(B)** Erythema subitum or roseola is caused by the human herpesvirus 6 and presents clinically as described. The fever resolves when the rash begins and the entire process is self-limiting with usual full recovery with supportive care. The key to this question is that the rash spares the face. Erythema infectiosum (fifth disease), rubella, and measles also begin with a febrile prodrome, but each of the associated rashes starts on the head or face before progressing to other parts of the body. *(Kaye and Kaye, 2008, p. 122)*

26. **(C)** In recent years, the prevalence of community-acquired methicillin-resistant *Staphylococcus aureus* (CA-MRSA) infection has increased. CA-MRSA can manifest in a variety of ways but soft tissue abscess is among the more common. Controversy around treatment options exists but currently, for an uncomplicated abscess, incision and drainage alone is recommended. In prospective studies to date, adding antibiotics provided no additional benefit. In the event that antibiotics are to be used, sensitivity reports are key and doxycycline or trimethoprim sulfamethoxazole are the preferred oral choices. *(Wallin et al., 2008, p. 438)*

27. **(B)** Pneumococcal pneumonia, caused by *Streptococcus pneumoniae*, is the most commonly occurring pneumonia worldwide. In the United States, it is the leading cause of community-acquired bacterial pneumonia, responsible for two-thirds of the cases with a bacterial cause. Pneumococcal vaccine confers excellent protection against the most common serotypes that cause the disease. *(Chesnutt et al., 2009, pp. 237-241)*

28. **(E)** Recommendations by the Advisory Committee for the Elimination of Tuberculosis indicate that the following high-risk groups should receive preventive chemotherapy if their tuberculin skin test (PPD) is >10 mm: 1. Foreign-born persons from high-prevalence countries. 2. Medically underserved, low-income populations, including high-risk racial or ethnic minority populations 3. Residents and employees of facilities for long-term care (eg correctional facilities, nursing homes) 4. Injection drug users who are HIV negative 5. Children younger than 4 years or children and adolescents in contact with high-risk adults 6. Lab employees working in mycobacteriology. *(Chesnutt et al., 2009, p. 247)*

29. **(D)** Secondary syphilis generally manifests itself a month or two after appearance of the primary chancre. Patients will complain of headache, fever, sore throat, and malaise and will exhibit generalized lymphadenopathy along with a maculopapular rash that begins at the sides of the trunk and later spreads over the rest of the body. The skin lesions may coalesce in warm moist areas, such as the perineum, and form large, flat-topped, pale papules termed *condyloma lata*. Skin and mucosal lesions are the most common signs of secondary syphilis. Aseptic meningitis and alopecia may also occur in secondary syphilis. Formation of granulomatous nodules (*gummas*) is not a feature of secondary disease, but rather is the hallmark of tertiary syphilis. *(Philip and Jacobs, 2009, pp. 1301-1302)*

30. **(D)** *Helicobacter pylori* is a spiral, Gram-negative rod that resides in the gastric mucosa, where it causes PUD. It may be diagnosed by rapid urease test or by histology when endoscopy is performed. Noninvasive *H pylori* testing options include the urease breath test, fecal antigen testing, and serology. Serological and fecal antigen tests are the most cost-effective methods. All three noninvasive tests have sensitivities and specificities greater than 90%. Proton-pump inhibitor therapy should be discontinued 1 to 2 weeks prior to the fecal antigen or breath tests because PPIs may increase the number of false negatives. In this case, serology is the least invasive, most cost-effective, and

least likely to be invalidated by the proton-pump inhibitor therapy. *(McQuaid, 2009, pp. 531-538)*

31. **(E)** Transmission of rabies to this patient must be seriously considered, and postexposure immunization should begin immediately by the administration of human rabies immune globulin (HRIG; 40 units/kg). About half the HRIG should be infiltrated around the bite wound, and the remainder injected intramuscularly. Human diploid cell rabies vaccine (HDCV) should also be given (1 mL IM in the deltoid), and again on days 3, 7, 14, and 28. HDCV should be delivered in a different syringe and administered at a different site than HRIG. *(Shandera and Corrales-Medina, 2009, p. 1225)*

32. **(E)** The drug of choice for prophylaxis of tuberculosis is isoniazid (INH), given at a daily dose of 300 mg/day for 9 months (children: 10 to 14 mg/kg/day). The major risk of INH prophylaxis is drug-induced hepatitis, especially in the elderly. Therefore, periodic monitoring of liver function tests during the course of INH treatment is recommended for persons aged 35 and older. Minor transferase elevations (up to three times normal) are not indications to discontinue therapy. *(Chesnutt et al., 2009, p. 251)*

33. **(D)** Combination therapy is recommended for eradication of *Helicobacter pylori*–associated PUD. Administration of a proton-pump inhibitor (omeprazole or lansoprazole) and two antibiotics (clarithromycin and either amoxicillin or metronidazole) achieves eradication rates of over 80%. However, emerging resistance of *H pylori* to metronidazole makes amoxicillin preferable for combination therapy. Regimens using bismuth compounds require higher dosing and linkage with antibiotics, plus a proton-pump inhibitor, to enhance efficacy. Also, bismuth regimens are associated with a higher incidence of side effects than are proton-pump inhibitor regimens. Antacids and sucralfate are outmoded as primary therapy for PUD. *(McQuaid, 2009, pp. 535-536)*

34. **(C)** The American Heart Association recommends that patients who are at moderate to high risk for bacterial endocarditis receive antibiotic prophylaxis prior to undergoing oral/dental, respiratory tract, or esophageal procedures. Amoxicillin 2.0 g orally 1 hour before the procedure is the standard regimen. Patients who have a history of amoxicillin/penicillin allergy may be given clindamycin, cephalexin, azithromycin, or clarithromycin. For adults, clindamycin is given at a dose of 600 mg po 1 hour before the procedure. *(Schwartz and Chambers, 2009, pp. 1272-1273)*

35. **(A)** In patients younger than 30 years, gonococcus is the most common cause of septic arthritis. When all patients are considered, *Staphylococcus aureus* is the most common cause. Patients with prevalent joint disease and intravenous drug users are especially susceptible to *Staphylococcus*. *Pseudomonas* is also a common cause of septic arthritis in intravenous drug users. *Salmonella* is not a common cause of joint infection. *(Lange and Lederman, 2007, p. 966)*

36. **(B)** Rheumatic fever is an immune-mediated process occurring in response to prior infection with Group A *Streptococcus*. The arthritis often moves from joint to joint in an asymmetrical pattern. In some cases there may be cardiac symptoms, skin rash (erythema marginatum), and subcutaneous nodules. Antistreptolysin O titer is often positive. It is important to quickly diagnose rheumatic fever because it requires long-term prophylaxis against *Streptococcus*. *(Litman, 2007, p. 95)*

37. **(A)** The clinical presentation is consistent with herpes simplex. The appropriate microscopic study is a Tzanck smear, prepared by staining cells from the floor of a vesicle using Papanicolau, Giemsa, or Wright methods. The Tzanck smear will show multinucleated giant cells. It has a sensitivity of 60% to 70% and as a result should be confirmed by viral culture. Gram-positive cocci are consistent with staphylococcal or streptococcal infection and gram-negative rods are usually enteric pathogens. Hyphae and buds are seen on KOH prep with candidal infection. *(Whitley, 2007, p. 2501)*

38. **(C)** The incubation period for mycoplasma is actually longer than that of most viruses (weeks

vs. days). Mycoplasma is much more common in adolescents and young adults than in the elderly. Sputum culture will grow mycoplasma but it is of limited clinical utility because the mycoplasma organism persists in the sputum for months after the illness has resolved. Exposure to insects is associated with Q fever or tularemia, rather than mycoplasma. Sputum gram stain can be helpful because it will show the WBCs consistent with an inflammatory process but very few or no bacteria. The WBCs are predominantly polymorphonuclear cells or lymphocytes. *(Baum, 2007, pp. 2270-2275)*

39. **(B)** First-line therapy for legionella pneumonia (mild to moderate) in the immunocompetent host is erythromycin 500 mg to 1 g IV qid or 500 mg po qid for 14 to 21 days. Another option for first-line therapy is doxycycline 200 mg IV or po once daily for 14 to 21 days. Alternatives include levofloxacin 500 mg IV or po q day for 7 to 10 days or azithromycin 500 mg IV or po q day for 3 days. Severe infection or treatment in the immunocompromised patient is levofloxacin or azithromycin. *(Edelstein, 2007, pp. 2264-2265)*

40. **(B)** Koplik's spots, white lesions on the buccal mucosa, are characteristic of rubeola. The rash in rubeola usually presents as a red–brown rash starting with the head and moving caudally. It follows a 3- to 4-day prodrome consisting of fever, nasal drainage, conjunctivitis, and cough. Varicella may also present with mucosal lesions but they are vesicular on an erythematous base. Parvovirus, rubella, and Kawasaki disease generally do not have mucosal involvement. *(Shandera and Carrales-Medina, 2009, p. 1217)*

41. **(E)** With a negative rapid strep screen, the most likely explanation for this presentation is acute infectious mononucleosis. The fever, fatigue, tonsillar hypertrophy, and splenomegaly are all classic symptoms and signs. Laboratory evaluation often includes an elevated total white blood cell count with increased atypical lymphocytes on differential. Platelets may be decreased. Initially, IgM antibodies for the Epstein-Barr virus, and viral capsid antigen (VCA) levels will be elevated. Later, the IgG

levels increase and IgM normalizes. *(Shandera and Corrales-Medina, 2009, p. 1213)*

42. **(C)** Hantavirus has a rodent vector and usually manifests in either hemorrhagic fever or Hantavirus pulmonary syndrome, which can be fatal. In the United States, outbreaks are usually in the southwest. There have been 300 cases since 1993. HTLV is a lymphotropic oncovirus associated with lymphoma. Dengue and yellow fever are both caused by Flaviviridae, which is carried by mosquitoes. Filoviruses cause Ebola fever and Marburg fever. The vector is unknown. Coronavirus is the etiologic agent in severe acute respiratory syndrome. During the 2002–2003 epidemic that began in Southeast Asia, it was postulated that it was carried by the masked palm civet. *(Shandera and Corrales-Medina, 2009, pp. 1233-1234)*

43. **(B)** Influenza vaccine is an important adjunct to clinical and public health practice. The vaccine is produced from different components and is recommended yearly in the fall for adults older than 50 years; people with chronic heart or lung disease, renal disease, diabetes, or immuno-compromise; nursing home residents, health care workers, and children 6 months to 18 years. It is contraindicated in those with hypersensitivity to the vaccine or eggs and in patients with Guillain–Barré syndrome, low platelets, or fever. Patients on steroids or warfarin are able to take it if they have no other contraindication. *(Shandera and Corrales-Medina, 2009, p. 1238)*

44. **(C)** SARS was first identified in 2003 in Guangdong province in China. It appears to be transmitted when mucous membranes are contacted by respiratory droplets or fomites. SARS has been identified in people of all ages. It has an incubation period of less than 1 week and presents with symptoms consistent with atypical pneumonia, including fever, cough, dyspnea, headache, sore throat, myalgias and, in some, watery diarrhea. Rales and rhonchi may be heard on physical examination. None of the symptoms or physical examination findings is diagnostic. Several laboratory studies may return abnormal results including decreased WBCs and platelets. Liver functions

and coagulation studies may also be abnormal. Arterial oxygen saturation is often low. Chest CT may show ground-glass opacifications. The etiologic organism is the coronavirus. *(Shandera and Corrales-Medina, 2009, pp. 1241-1242)*

45. **(A)** Kawasaki syndrome occurs throughout the world, primarily in children. It is thought to be infectious but the etiologic agent has never been isolated. The syndrome is composed of fever and four of five of the following symptoms: bilateral conjunctivitis, some type of mucous membrane change, a peripheral extremity change, transverse grooves on the nails, a polymorphous rash, and cervical lymph nodes >1.5 cm. It can be complicated by arteritis. Treatment may include aspirin, immune globulin, plasmapheresis, or corticosteroids. *(Shandera and Corrales-Medina, 2009, pp. 1254-1255)*

46. **(A)** Typhoid fever is caused by *Salmonella typhus.* It is contracted by contaminated food or water. There are several endemic areas throughout Africa. Symptoms and signs may be nonspecific but often include blanchable, pink, papular rash over the trunk and fever that increases in stepwise fashion. Blood culture is positive in 80% of cases in the first week. Abdominal symptoms may include distention and constipation, initially, followed by diarrhea and, possibly, splenomegaly. Prevention is accomplished by multidose oral or single-dose vaccine. *(Schwartz and Chambers, 2009, pp. 1279-1281)*

47. **(B)** The etiology of plague is the *Yersinia pestis* bacterium. Plague is transmitted by direct contact with wild rodents or fleabites by fleas that have bitten the rodents. Droplet transmission is also possible with exposure to an infected human host. Symptoms include high fever, increased heart rate, malaise, and headache. There may be signs of meningitis in addition to axillary, cervical, and inguinal adenopathy. Lymph nodes are very swollen and may drain purulent material. Central nervous system changes can progress to coma, and in "black plague," purpura are visible on the skin. Blood and aspirate cultures confirm the diagnosis. Treatment is with streptomycin or gentamycin.

Yersinia pestis must also be considered as a possible agent of bioterrorism. *(Schwartz and Chambers, 2009, pp. 1285-1286)*

48. **(E)** The history and course of illness are consistent with cat-scratch fever. It is caused by infection with *Bartonella henselae.* Cat scratch or bite transmits it to humans. Clinical course usually begins with papule or ulcer at the site within a few days of the bite. Fever, headache, and malaise develop 7 to 21 days later. Lymph drainage of the site may result in swollen, tender, and/or suppurative nodes. Clinical diagnosis is the norm but special cultures or biopsy is possible. The symptoms usually resolve spontaneously with no specific therapy required. Complications may include encephalitis or disseminated disease in immunocompromised patients. *(Schwartz and Chambers, 2009, p. 1288)*

49. **(C)** The key piece of history in this question is the new exposure to parakeets. The symptoms and signs, including atypical pneumonia, are consistent with psittacosis but are not pathognomonic. Sarcoidosis is an illness of unknown cause. Listeriosis has been linked to exposures to contaminated food, particularly dairy products and hot dogs. Brucellosis can be caused by exposure to hogs, cattle, or goats. Tularemia is associated with contact with rabbits, other rodents, and biting arthropods. *(Schwartz and Chambers, 2009, p. 1296)*

50. **(E)** The description of the rash is consistent with the erythema chronicum migrans rash of Lyme disease. Lyme disease is caused by the spirochete, *Borrelia burgdorferi,* which is transmitted by tick bite. The course of Lyme disease usually involves progression through three stages. In stage 1, 80% to 90% of patients develop the rash, usually within a week of a tick bite. The rash begins with a maculopapular red lesion at the site. Over several days, the lesion can become much larger and develop central clearing. It is often described as looking like a bull's-eye. In addition to the rash, half of the patients will develop fever, chills, and myalgias. Stage 1 symptoms usually resolve within a month without treatment.

Stage 2 is characterized by disseminated symptoms, generally involving the skin, central nervous system, and musculoskeletal system. Symptoms may include headaches, stiff neck, and joint pains. Arrhythmias and heart block are also possible. Bell's palsy, personality changes, forgetfulness, peripheral neuropathy, and conjunctivitis can all manifest in stage 2 as well. Months to years after the bite, untreated patients can develop stage 3 symptoms, including arthritis and synovitis and permanent disability. Further neurologic symptoms may develop, along with a diffuse fasciitis. Treatment for Lyme disease is doxycycline 100 mg po bid for 2 to 3 weeks in stage 1. Central nervous system involvement requires intravenous therapy. Alternative antibiotics are amoxicillin or cefuroxime. *(Philip and Jacobs, 2009, pp. 1309-1313)*

51. **(A)** Cats are the definitive host for the parasite *Toxoplasma gondii*. It can exist in three forms but it is the oocyst that is found in cat feces. These oocysts can remain infective in soil for years. Human infections are frequently asymptomatic. In an otherwise healthy individual, symptoms resemble infectious mononucleosis. They may include swollen lymph nodes, malaise, arthralgias, headache, sore throat, and rash. Up to 1% of women have been found to be infected during pregnancy. Fetal effects are more severe if maternal infection occurs in the first trimester. Less than 15% of births among infected mothers result in severe brain or eye damage at birth but more than 85% manifest brain or eye effects later in their lives. Diagnosis can be made with serological tests. Treatment of pregnant women includes spiramycin 1g tid until delivery. Spiramycin does not cross the placenta and so if the fetus is infected, sulfadiazine, pyrimethamine, and folinic acid should be used. *(Rosenthal, 2009, pp. 1330-1332)*

52. **(A)** *Clostridial tetani* infection is a vaccine-preventable disease that results in approximately 50 cases/yr in the United States. Even with modern medical resources, one of four or one of five patients with generalized tetanus dies. Almost all cases occur in individuals who are not properly immunized. Sixty percent of cases occur in older adults for whom immunity has waned. Tetanus presents in different forms including generalized, localized, cephalad, and neonatal. Generalized is the most common and symptoms include mood changes, trismus, diaphoresis, dysphagia, and drooling. Later symptoms include painful flexion and adduction of the arms and pain with extension of the legs. Convulsions and spasms are possible, along with a variety of autonomic symptoms. Treatment includes airway protection, benzodiazepines for muscle spasm, tetanus immune globulin immediately, and three doses of tetanus toxoid given by the standard schedule. Metronidazole has been demonstrated to be the most effective antimicrobial. Labetalol may be used for catecholamine-induced hypertension but the patient must also be monitored for hypotension and bradycardia. *(Bartlett, 2007, pp. 2205-2207)*

53. **(B)** Pseudomembranous colitis is caused by the toxin-producing *Clostridium difficile*. It usually presents as fever, elevated WBC count, abdominal pain, and diarrhea (possibly bloody) following antibiotic therapy. It is thought that *C. difficile*, which is generally harmless when colonized, overgrows when the normal balance of gut flora is altered by antibiotic use. In addition to making the diagnosis on colonoscopy, *C. difficile* can be cultured or the toxins detected by immunoassay. It can be treated by cessation of antibiotics and fluid replacement but most often an antibiotic targeted at the organism is employed. Metronidazole, oral or intravenous, is usually the first choice. Vancomycin has better evidence but is more expensive and the risk for resistance exists so metronidazole is still often used first. *(Bartlett, 2007, pp. 2202-2203)*

54. **(C)** *Bacillus anthrax* is one of the biological agents that has been used in acts of terrorism. Anthrax infection manifests in three forms: cutaneous, gastrointestinal, and inhalational. The cutaneous form occurs in 95% of cases. The incubation period can last up to a week. The initial manifestation is papular and evolves over days to an ulcer. The ulcer is surrounded by swelling and redness and eventually becomes an eschar. The eschar falls off in 7 to

14 days. The cutaneous lesions are usually painless. Gastrointestinal anthrax is caused by eating infected meat. It is very uncommon and can be highly lethal. Inhalational anthrax happens when spores are inhaled. The incubation period may be up to 2 months. The symptoms may include fever, fatigue, body aches, chest discomfort, and, later, shortness of breath, shock, and death. First-line therapy is ciprofloxacin or doxycycline. Two months of therapy is the standard prevention after exposure. (*Bradsher, 2007, pp. 1027-1028*)

REFERENCES

Armitage KB, Salata RA. Infectious diseases of travelers: protozoal and helminthic infections. In: Andreoli TE, Carpenter CCJ, Griggs RC, et al., eds. *Andreoli and Carpenter's Cecil Essentials of Medicine.* 7th ed. Philadelphia, PA: Saunders Elsevier; 2007.

Bartlett JG. Clostridial infections. In: Goldman L, Ausiello D, eds. *Cecil Medicine.* 23rd ed. Philadelphia, PA: Saunders Elsevier; 2007.

Baum SG. Mycoplasma infections. In: Goldman L, Ausiello D, eds. *Cecil Medicine.* 23rd ed. Philadelphia, PA: Saunders Elsevier; 2007.

Bradsher RW. Bioterrorism. In: Andreoli TE, Carpenter CCJ, Griggs RC, et al., eds. *Andreoli and Carpenter's Cecil Essentials of Medicine.* 7th ed. Philadelphia, PA: Saunders Elsevier; 2007.

Carpenter CCJ, Beckwith CG, Rodriguez B, et al., Human immunodeficiency virus infection and acquired immunodeficiency syndrome. In: Andreoli TE, Carpenter CCJ, Griggs RC, et al., eds. *Andreoli and Carpenter's Cecil Essentials of Medicine.* 7th ed. Philadelphia, PA: Saunders Elsevier; 2007.

Centers for Disease Control and Prevention. Sexually transmitted diseases treatment guidelines. *Morbidity and Mortality Weekly Report;* 2006.

Centers for Disease Control and Prevention. Recommended Adult Immunization Schedule. 2008. http://www.cdc.gov/vaccines/recs/schedules/downloads/adult/07-08/adult-schedule.pdf. Accessed March 10, 2009.

Chayakulkeeree M, Perfect JR. Cryptococcus. *Infect Dis Clin N Am.* 2006;20:507-544.

Chesnutt MS, Murray JA, Prendergast TJ. Pulmonary disorders. In: McPhee SJ, Papadakis MA, eds. *Current Medical Diagnosis and Treatment.* 48th ed. New York, NY: McGraw-Hill; 2009.

Edelstein PH. Legionella infections. In: Goldman L, Ausiello D, eds. *Cecil Medicine.* 23rd ed. Philadelphia, PA: Saunders Elsevier; 2007.

Flood RG, Aronoff SC. Cryptococcus neoformans. In: Kliegman RM, ed. *Nelson Textbook of Pediatrics.* 18th ed. Philadelphia, PA: Saunders Elsevier; 2007.

Hewlett EL. Whooping cough and other Bordetella infections. In: Goldman L, Ausiello D, eds. *Cecil Medicine.* 23rd ed. Philadelphia, PA: Saunders Elsevier; 2007.

Kaye ET, Kaye KM. Fever and rash. In: Fauci AS, Braunwald E, Kasper DL, et al., eds. *Harrison's Principles of Internal Medicine.* 17th ed. New York, NY: McGraw-Hill; 2008.

Kazura JW. Nematode infections. In: Goldman L, Ausiello D, eds. *Cecil Medicine.* 23rd ed. Philadelphia, PA: Saunders Elsevier; 2007.

Kleigman RM. *Nelson Textbook of Pediatrics.* 18th ed. Philadelphia, PA: Saunders Elsevier; 2007.

Lange C, Lederman MM. Infections involving bones and joints. In: Andreoli TE, Carpenter CCJ, Griggs RC, et al., eds. *Andreoli and Carpenter's Cecil Essentials of Medicine.* 7th ed. Philadelphia, PA: Saunders Elsevier; 2007.

Litman SE. Acquired valvular heart disease. In: Andreoli TE, Carpenter CCJ, Griggs RC, et al., eds. *Andreoli and Carpenter's Cecil Essentials of Medicine.* 7th ed. Philadelphia, PA: Saunders Elsevier; 2007.

McCoy ACS, Aronoff SC. Histoplasmosis (*Histoplasma capsulatum*). In: Kliegman RM, ed. *Nelson Textbook of Pediatrics.* 18th ed. Philadelphia, PA: Saunders Elsevier; 2007.

McQuaid KR. Gastrointestinal disorders. In: McPhee SJ, Papadakis MA, eds. *Current Medical Diagnosis and Treatment.* 48th ed. New York, NY: McGraw-Hill; 2009.

Nyirjesy P. Vulvovaginal candidiasis and bacterial vaginosis. *Infect Dis Clin N Am.* 2008;22:637-652.

Philip SS, Jacobs RA. Spirochetal infections. In: McPhee SJ, Papadakis MA, eds. *Current Medical Diagnosis and Treatment.* 48th ed. New York, NY: McGraw-Hill, 2009.

Pigott DC. Foodborne illness. *Emerg Med Clin N Am.* 2008;26:484-489, 492.

Rosenthal PJ. Protozoal and helminthic infections. In: McPhee SJ, Papadakis MA, eds. *Current Medical Diagnosis and Treatment.* 48th ed. New York, NY: McGraw-Hill; 2009.

Ruocco E, Donnarumma G, Baroni A, et al. Bacterial and viral skin diseases. *Dermatol Clin.* 2007;25:663-676.

Schuster FL, Glaser CA. Amebiasis. In: Goldman L, Ausiello D, eds. *Cecil Medicine.* 23rd ed. Philadelphia, PA: Saunders Elsevier; 2007.

Schwartz BS, Chambers HF. Bacterial and chlamydial infections. In: McPhee SJ, Papadakis MA, eds. *Current Medical Diagnosis and Treatment.* 48th ed. New York, NY: McGraw-Hill; 2009.

Servey JT, Reamey BV, Hodge J. Clinical presentations of parvovirus B19 infections. *Am Fam Physician.* 2007;75: 373-376.

Shandera WX, Corrales-Medina VF. Viral & rickettsial infections. In: McPhee SJ, Papadakis MA, eds. *Current Medical Diagnosis and Treatment.* 48th ed. New York, NY: McGraw-Hill; 2009.

Simberkoff MS. Haemophilus and moraxella infections. In: Goldman L, Ausiello D, eds. *Cecil Medicine.* 23rd ed. Philadelphia, PA: Saunders Elsevier; 2007.

Speil C, Mushtaq A, Adamski A, et al. Fever of unknown origin in the returning traveler. *Infect Dis Clin N Am.* 2007;21:1091-1113.

Steere AC. Lyme B. In: Fauci AS, Braunwald E, Kasper DL, et al., eds. *Harrison's Principles of Internal Medicine.* 17th ed. New York, NY: McGraw-Hill; 2008.

Stevens DL. Streptococcal infections. In: Goldman L, Ausiello D, eds. *Cecil Medicine.* 23rd ed. Philadelphia, PA: Saunders Elsevier; 2007.

Sutter RW. Diphtheria and other corynebacteria infections. In: Goldman L, Ausiello D, eds. *Cecil Medicine.* 23rd ed. Philadelphia, PA: Saunders Elsevier; 2007.

Walker DH, Dumler JS, Marrie T. In: Fauci AS, Braunwald E, Kasper DL, et al., eds. *Harrison's Principles of Internal Medicine.* 17th ed. New York, NY: McGraw-Hill; 2008.

Wallin TR, Hern HG, Frazee BW. Community-acquired methicillin-resistant *Staphylococcus aureus. Emerg Med Clin N Am.* 2008;26:431-455.

Warren JB, Gullet H, King VJ. Cervical cancer screening and updated pap guidelines. *Prim Care.* 2009;36: 131-149.

Weller PF. Protozoal intestinal infections and trichomoniasis. In: Fauci AS, Braunwald E, Kasper DL, et al., eds. *Harrison's Principles of Internal Medicine.* 17th ed. New York, NY: McGraw-Hill; 2008.

Weller PF, Nutman TB. Intestinal nematodes. In: Fauci AS, Braunwald E, Kasper DL, et al., eds. *Harrison's Principles of Internal Medicine.* 17th ed. New York, NY: McGraw-Hill; 2008.

Whitley RJ. Herpes simplex virus infections. In: Goldman L, Ausiello D, eds. *Cecil Medicine.* 23rd ed. Philadelphia, PA: Saunders Elsevier; 2007.

CHAPTER 9

Nephrology

Carla J. Moschella, PA-C, MS, RD

DIRECTIONS: Each of the numbered items or incomplete statements in this section is followed by answers or by completion of the statement. Select the ONE-lettered answer or completion that is BEST in each case.

1. The earliest sign of chronic kidney disease (CKD) is

   (A) microscopic hematuria
   (B) hypertension (HTN)
   (C) proteinuria
   (D) abnormal creatinine
   (E) hyperkalemia

2. Assuming that a patient has maintained a normal baseline creatinine of 1.0 mg/dL with a normal glomerular filtration rate (GFR) of 100 mL/min, which of the following indicates a more significant change in the GFR?

   (A) increase in creatinine from 1.0 to 2.0 mg/dL
   (B) increase in creatinine from 2.0 to 4.0 mg/dL
   (C) increase in creatinine from 4.0 to 8.0 mg/dL
   (D) increase in creatinine from 8.0 to 16.0 mg/dL

3. How often should patients with diabetes mellitus be screened for microalbuminuria?

   (A) once a month
   (B) every 3 months
   (C) every 6 months
   (D) once a year
   (E) there is no specific timetable

4. Which of the following urinary findings is suggestive of acute glomerulonephritis?

   (A) red cells and red cell casts
   (B) white cells and white cell casts
   (C) renal tubular epithelial cells
   (D) oval fat bodies
   (E) hyaline casts

5. In patients with known chronic kidney disease, which of the following is an absolute indication to initiate dialysis?

   (A) proteinuria >3 g/24 h
   (B) GFR <10 mL/min
   (C) hyperkalemia >5.0 mEq/L
   (D) seizures
   (E) hyperphosphatemia >6.5 mg/dL

6. A renal ultrasound would be most beneficial for diagnosing which of the following?

   (A) nephrotic syndrome
   (B) polycystic kidney disease
   (C) glomerulonephritis
   (D) acute tubular necrosis
   (E) lupus nephritis

7. Which of the following types of renal calculi is associated with an infectious cause?

   (A) struvite
   (B) uric acid
   (C) calcium oxalate
   (D) cystine
   (E) calcium phosphate

8. Which of the following is diagnostic of nephrotic syndrome?

   (A) hypoalbuminemia, hypolipidemia, proteinuria >10 g/24 h
   (B) hypoalbuminemia, hyperlipidemia, proteinuria >1 g/24 h
   (C) hypoalbuminemia, hyperlipidemia, proteinuria >2 g/24 h
   (D) hypoalbuminemia, hyperlipidemia, proteinuria >3.5 g/24 h
   (E) normal albumin, hyperlipidemia, proteinuria >10 g/24 h

9. Prolonged, heavy use of nonsteroidal anti-inflammatory drugs (NSAIDs) causes which type of kidney damage?

   (A) glomerular
   (B) tubulointerstitial
   (C) autoimmune
   (D) macrovascular

10. A 16-year-old girl is referred for a sports physical. Her blood pressure is 170/92 mm Hg. Urinalysis (UA) reveals 2+ protein. The girl's mother reports multiple episodes of urinary tract infections (UTIs) throughout childhood that were never investigated. The most likely diagnosis is

    (A) obstructive uropathy
    (B) orthostatic proteinuria
    (C) chronic reflux nephropathy
    (D) nephrotic syndrome
    (E) exercise-induced proteinuria

11. Which of the following best describes the mechanism of action of angiotensin-converting enzyme (ACE) inhibitors in controlling blood pressure and preventing or slowing kidney damage?

    (A) They result in systemic vasodilation.
    (B) They increase renal tubular excretion of sodium.
    (C) They result in dilation of the efferent arteriole, reducing glomerular pressure.
    (D) They block the angiotensin II receptor on the cell membrane.
    (E) They reduce production of angiotensinogen, the precursor to angiotensin I.

12. In which of the following settings would the use of an ACE inhibitor be contraindicated?

    (A) diabetic nephropathy
    (B) hypertensive nephrosclerosis
    (C) lupus nephritis
    (D) polycystic kidney disease
    (E) significant renal artery stenosis

13. Which of the following is most useful in diagnosing renal artery stenosis?

    (A) magnetic resonance angiography (MRA)
    (B) computed tomography (CT) scanning
    (C) captopril renal scan
    (D) renal artery biopsy
    (E) intravenous pyelogram (IVP)

14. Abnormal urinary protein excretion is defined as

    (A) >30 mg/24 h
    (B) >150 mg/24 h
    (C) >300 mg/24 h
    (D) >1 g/24 h
    (E) >3.5 g/24 h

15. Which type/class of medications is useful to treat renal calculi due to hypercalciuria?

    (A) calcium channel blockers
    (B) colchicine
    (C) allopurinol
    (D) potassium citrate
    (E) thiazide diuretics

16. Glucose will spill into the urine when the serum glucose reaches what level?

    (A) >126 mg/dL
    (B) 150 to 175 mg/dL
    (C) 180 to 200 mg/dL
    (D) >250 mg/dL
    (E) >400 mg/dL

17. Which of the following is MOST indicative of UTI?

    (A) positive nitrite on dipstick
    (B) positive leukocyte esterase on dipstick
    (C) 2 to 3 white blood cells (WBCs) per high power field (HPF) on urine dipstick
    (D) urine culture revealing 10,000 to 20,000 colonies of *Lactobacillus*
    (E) positive nitrite and leukocyte esterase on dipstick

18. A unilateral small kidney on ultrasound would suggest which of the following etiologies?

    (A) polycystic kidney disease
    (B) hypertensive nephrosclerosis
    (C) diabetic nephropathy
    (D) renal artery stenosis
    (E) malignancy

19. Which of the following statements about postinfectious glomerulonephritis is TRUE?

    (A) It is most commonly due to an immunologic reaction to a streptococcal antigen.
    (B) It is a process that will inevitably result in renal failure.
    (C) It occurs in 50% of people with a history of streptococcal pharyngitis.
    (D) It is a disease that results only from infection with *Streptococcus*.
    (E) Treatment of the streptococcal infection with antibiotics will prevent its development.

20. Which of the following treatments for hyperkalemia works by redistributing potassium from the blood into the cell?

    (A) sodium polystyrene sulfonate po
    (B) insulin and D5W IV
    (C) low potassium diet
    (D) calcium gluconate IV
    (E) hemodialysis

21. Complications associated with hyperkalemia include

    (A) hyperventilation
    (B) nausea and vomiting
    (C) ventricular arrhythmias
    (D) diarrhea
    (E) seizures

22. Which of the following signals a good prognosis for recovery from acute renal failure (ARF)?

    (A) maintenance of normal urine output as creatinine increases
    (B) low blood urea nitrogen level
    (C) the etiology of the ARF is sepsis
    (D) the etiology of the ARF is pregnancy
    (E) aggressive use of furosemide to stimulate urine output

23. A 72-year-old man is transported via ambulance to the emergency department with severe chest pain and shortness of breath. Electrocardiogram (ECG) reveals ST-segment elevation in leads II, III, and aVF. While in the emergency department, he loses consciousness and is found to be in ventricular fibrillation. Resuscitation is successful, and a pulse is restored within 3 minutes. He is taken to the cardiac catheterization laboratory, where he undergoes two-vessel stenting. Two days later, his creatinine has increased from a baseline of 1.1 to 2.2 mg/dL. The next day, the creatinine is 3.9 mg/dL. Fractional excretion of sodium is ordered. You would expect this to be

    (A) <1
    (B) >1
    (C) unchanged from baseline
    (D) undetectable
    (E) equal to the serum creatinine level

24. When initially screening for CKD, which of the following would be ordered?

    (A) 24-hour urine collection
    (B) blood pressure measurement, serum creatinine level, spot urine protein measurement
    (C) renal ultrasound
    (D) abdominal CT scan
    (E) renal angiogram

25. A 32-year-old construction worker presents to the emergency department after being involved in an accident at a job site. His left thigh was pinned under a 100-lb cement block. He is in moderate pain on presentation, and there is swelling and a large ecchymosis over the entire anterior thigh. Urine is rust-colored. Urine dip is positive for blood and protein, negative for glucose, ketones, nitrite, and leukocyte esterase. Urine sediment is negative for cells, organisms, and casts. What is the most likely cause of the positive urine dip for blood?

    (A) hemoglobin due to hematoma formation
    (B) contamination of the urine sample
    (C) myoglobin due to rhabdomyolysis
    (D) red cell casts due to glomerulonephritis
    (E) UTI

26. Which of the following statements about anemia associated with CKD is TRUE?

    (A) Iron and folic acid by mouth are the most effective treatments.
    (B) Transfusion of packed red blood cells monthly is the most effective treatment.
    (C) IM erythropoietin given monthly is the most effective treatment.
    (D) It is due to the inability of the kidney to transform erythropoietin into its physiologically active form.
    (E) It occurs early in the course of CKD.

27. Which of the following best describes the pathophysiologic mechanism of distal renal tubular acidosis?

    (A) a defect in the ability of the distal renal tubule to excrete hydrogen ion

    (B) a defect in the ability of the distal renal tubule to reabsorb bicarbonate
    (C) a defect in the ability of the proximal renal tubule to excrete hydrogen ion
    (D) a defect in the ability of the proximal renal tubule to reabsorb bicarbonate
    (E) inadequate aldosterone production

28. What is the most common complication of hemodialysis?

    (A) hypokalemia
    (B) hyperglycemia
    (C) hypotension
    (D) infection
    (E) anemia

29. Most UTIs are caused by

    (A) Gram-positive bacteria
    (B) *Pseudomonas aeruginosa*
    (C) *Staphylococcus aureus*
    (D) *Escherichia coli*
    (E) *Candida albicans*

30. Which of the following statements about urinary tract infections (UTIs) in patients with chronic indwelling catheters is true?

    (A) Leukocytes in the urine are always indicative of an acute UTI.
    (B) The most likely etiologic agent is *Escherichia coli.*
    (C) All positive findings of WBCs in the urine should be treated with antibiotics.
    (D) All positive findings of bacteriuria should be treated with antibiotics.
    (E) The etiology is likely to be polymicrobial.

31. Which of the following is a potential complication of acute pyelonephritis?

    (A) perinephric abscess
    (B) renal vein thrombosis
    (C) allergic interstitial nephritis
    (D) struvite stones
    (E) hepatic failure

32. Large numbers of epithelial cells on urine sediment indicate

    (A) UTI
    (B) acute tubular necrosis
    (C) sample contamination
    (D) vaginitis in women
    (E) prostatitis in men

33. Which of the following patients would require the LONGEST antibiotic treatment course for a UTI?

    (A) a 32-year-old woman with a history of one UTI 3 years ago
    (B) a 79-year-old woman with a history of renal calculi but no previous history of UTI
    (C) an 8-year-old girl with no previous history of UTI
    (D) a 42-year-old man with no significant past medical history
    (E) a 41-year-old woman with history of cervical diaphragm use for birth control

34. A 17-year-old boy high school wrestler is brought into the emergency department after he collapsed at a wrestling match. He spent time fully clothed in a hot sauna prior to the match to try to "make weight." Labs are ordered, and results come back as follows:

Sodium	162 mEq/L	Glucose	108 mg/dL
Potassium	3.8 mEq/L	BUN	30 mg/dL
Chloride	121 mEq/L	Creatinine	2.0 mg/dL
Carbon dioxide	29 mEq/L	Urine sodium	<10 mEq/L
Weight	70 kg	Urine osmolality	428 mOsm/kg

    Which IV fluid regimen would most effectively treat this patient's hypernatremia?

    (A) quarter normal (hypotonic) saline
    (B) half-normal saline
    (C) isotonic (normal) saline
    (D) dextrose 5% in water
    (E) lactated Ringer's

35. The most common cause of nephrotic syndrome in children is

    (A) post–streptococcal glomerulonephritis
    (B) minimal change disease
    (C) diabetes mellitus
    (D) NSAIDs
    (E) polycystic kidney disease

36. You are asked to see a diabetic patient with retinopathy and hypertension. On examination, the patient's blood pressure is noted to be 180/90 mm Hg. Urinalysis shows microalbumin of 300 mg/dL. Labs: blood urea nitrogen 22 mg/dL, creatinine 1.5 mg/dL. Which of the following classes of antihypertensive medications would be best to prescribe in this setting?

    (A) calcium channel blocker
    (B) loop diuretic
    (C) alpha blocker
    (D) thiazide diuretic
    (E) ACE inhibitor

37. Which of the following diuretics results in potassium wasting?

    (A) triamterene
    (B) amiloride
    (C) hydrochlorothiazide
    (D) spironolactone
    (E) eplerenone

38. When adjusting medication dosing for patients with CKD, which of the following factors is the LEAST important?

    (A) serum blood urea nitrogen (BUN) level
    (B) serum creatinine level
    (C) age
    (D) weight
    (E) gender

39. The organism responsible for most cases of peritonitis in patients on peritoneal dialysis is

(A) *Candida albicans*

(B) *Escherichia coli*

(C) *Streptococcus pneumoniae*

(D) *Pseudomonas aeruginosa*

(E) *Staphylococcus aureus*

40. The most serious consequence of rapid correction of hyponatremia is

(A) brainstem herniation

(B) central pontine myelinolysis

(C) muscle cramps

(D) hypernatremia

(E) fluid overload

41. Based upon the following laboratory values, what is the patient's estimated serum osmolality?

Sodium	Glucose	BUN
132 mEq/L	167 mg/dL	15 mg/dL

(A) 279 mOsm/kg

(B) 285 mOsm/kg

(C) 292 mOsm/kg

(D) 301 mOsm/kg

(E) 315 mOsm/kg

42. What is the most common electrolyte abnormality seen in hospitalized patients?

(A) hypokalemia

(B) hyperkalemia

(C) hyponatremia

(D) hypernatremia

(E) hypomagnesemia

43. A 66-year-old man with a medical history of aortic stenosis is admitted to the hospital with increasing shortness of breath. Physical examination reveals a regular pulse of 120 beats/min, blood pressure of 95/50 mm Hg, and a respiratory rate of 32 breaths/min. The estimated jugular venous pressure (JVP) is greater than 15 cm, rales are heard halfway up the lung fields bilaterally, and a holosystolic murmur is heard at the apex. There is a tender enlarged liver with hepatojugular reflux and 2+ pretibial and pedal edema. Plain film of the chest reveals cardiomegaly and pulmonary edema. ECG is suggestive of left ventricular hypertrophy. Admission laboratory studies include the following:

Sodium	128 mEq/L	Potassium	3.6 mEq/L
Chloride	93 mEq/L	Bicarbonate	27 mEq/L
BUN	45 mg/dL	Creatinine	1.0 mg/dL
Urine sodium	12 mEq/L	Glucose	75 mg/dL

What type of hyponatremia does this patient most likely have?

(A) hypovolemic hypotonic

(B) hypervolemic hypotonic

(C) hypovolemic isotonic

(D) hypervolemic hypertonic

(E) hypovolemic hypertonic

44. A 17-year-old boy high school wrestler is brought into the emergency department after he collapsed at a wrestling match. He spent time fully clothed in a hot sauna prior to the match to try to "make weight." Labs are ordered, and results come back as follows:

Sodium	162 mEq/L	Glucose	108 mg/dL
Potassium	3.8 mEq/L	BUN	30 mg/dL
Chloride	121 mEq/L	Creatinine	2.0 mg/dL
Carbon dioxide	29 mEq/L	Urine sodium	<10 mEq/L
Weight	70 kg	Urine osmolality	428 mOsm/kg

What is this patient's estimated free water deficit?

(A) 2.1 L

(B) 3.3 L

(C) 5.1 L

(D) 6.6 L

(E) 7.2 L

45. A 22-year-old woman presents to the emergency department after spending a week in Cancun for spring break. She noted onset of significant diarrhea about 3 days ago, accompanied by mild nausea but no vomiting. She hoped it would resolve on its own, but she is starting to feel worse with weakness and lightheadedness. You order labs with the following results:

Sodium	138 mEq/L	pH	7.32
Potassium	2.2 mEq/L	P_{CO_2}	16 mm Hg
Chloride	119 mEq/L	BUN	68 mg/dL
Bicarbonate	8 mEq/L	Creatinine	2.0 mg/dL

What is the nature of the acid–base disturbance?

(A) respiratory acidosis

(B) respiratory alkalosis

(C) metabolic alkalosis

(D) high anion gap metabolic acidosis

(E) nonanion gap metabolic acidosis

46. What is the most likely etiology of the acid-base disturbance in the patient scenario above?

(A) diarrhea

(B) hypokalemia

(C) vomiting

(D) acute renal failure

(E) alcohol (EtOH) intoxication

47. You have just received labs back on a 42-year-old woman with severe vomiting and no oral intake in the last 3 days. You note a metabolic alkalosis, based on her arterial blood gases. You also note that compensatory changes are present. Which of the following best represents these changes? (Normal P_{CO_2} = 35–45 mm Hg, normal HCO_3 = 24–31 mEq/L)

(A) P_{CO_2} = 32 mm Hg

(B) P_{CO_2} = 38 mm Hg

(C) P_{CO_2} = 47 mm Hg

(D) HCO_3 = 38 mEq/L

(E) HCO_3 = 24 mEq/L

48. A 65-year-old woman with diabetes mellitus and peripheral vascular disease is about to undergo a diagnostic radiographic procedure involving the use of intravenous (IV) contrast dye. Her serum creatinine is 1.9 mg/dL. An appropriate action prior to the procedure would be to

(A) start an ACE inhibitor

(B) administer a 1,000 cc bolus of normal saline and acetylcysteine po

(C) administer a 1,000 cc bolus of normal saline only

(D) administer an intravenous diuretic

(E) no specific preprocedure treatment is needed

49. A 46-year-old man with a history of EtOH abuse is brought to the emergency department in the morning by his wife. She has noted that he has developed tremors in both arms, and he seems mildly confused to her. He complains of feeling weak, with some cramping in the legs. On physical examination, his blood pressure is noted to be 162/95 mm Hg, and his heart rate is 108 beats/min. There is no asterixis. Which of the following electrolyte disorders are you likely to find in this patient?

(A) hypercalcemia

(B) hypocalcemia

(C) hypermagnesemia

(D) hypomagnesemia

(E) hyperphosphatemia

50. Your 65-year-old patient with a history of tobacco abuse was recently diagnosed with stage III lung cancer. He has not started treatment yet and presents to his oncologist with complaints of nausea, anorexia, and increasing fatigue over the last several days. He has been eating less than usual but has been able to maintain a normal fluid intake. His wife reports that he has been more forgetful and confused than usual. His medical history includes hypertension, for which he has been taking 25 mg of hydrochlorothiazide for 12 years, and gastroesophageal reflux disease (GERD), for which he takes omeprazole. He has no history of significant side effects from his medications. You order labs, and the calcium level is elevated at 11.9 mg/dL. What is the most likely etiology of his hypercalcemia?

(A) malignancy

(B) hyperparathyroidism

(C) thiazide diuretic use

(D) dehydration

(E) vitamin D toxicity

51. Your 65-year-old patient with a history of tobacco abuse was recently diagnosed with stage III lung cancer. He has not started treatment yet and presents to his oncologist with complaints of nausea, anorexia, and increasing fatigue over the last several days. He has been eating less than usual but has been able to maintain a normal fluid intake. His wife reports that he has been more forgetful and confused than usual. His medical history includes hypertension, for which he has been taking 25 mg of hydrochlorothiazide for 12 years, and GERD, for which he takes omeprazole. He has no history of significant side effects from his medications. You order labs, and the calcium level is elevated at 11.9 mg/dL. How would you treat this patient's hypercalcemia?

(A) increase thiazide diuretic dose
(B) bisphosphonate
(C) does not need to be treated
(D) encourage fluid intake
(E) initiate hemodialysis

52. A 32-year-old woman presents for a routine physical examination. She feels well with no specific complaints. On physical examination, her blood pressure is noted to be 154/92 mm Hg. You note slight fullness to the abdomen on palpation without tenderness or obvious mass. Routine labs are ordered, including a UA, with the following results:

BUN 12	Creatinine 0.8

UA and sediment analysis: 2+ blood, trace protein, negative leukocyte esterase, negative nitrite; 10 to 20 red blood cells (RBCs) per high power field (HPF), no leukocytes, bacteria, or other cells; rare granular cast

What is the most likely cause of the hematuria?

(A) urinary tract infection
(B) glomerulonephritis
(C) renal calculi
(D) urinary sample contamination
(E) polycystic kidney disease

53. A 73-year-old man with type II diabetes mellitus was diagnosed with CKD 4 years ago. At this time, his creatinine is 1.9 mg/dL, with an estimated GFR of 72 mL/min. What stage of kidney disease has this patient reached?

(A) Stage I
(B) Stage II
(C) Stage III
(D) Stage IV
(E) Stage V

54. Which of the following complications are associated with Stage III kidney disease?

(A) no notable complications
(B) acid–base abnormalities
(C) hypertension only
(D) anemia, disorders of calcium and phosphorus metabolism
(E) fluid and electrolyte abnormalities

55. A 65-year-old man with a history of smoking, hypertension, and peripheral vascular disease was admitted 3 days earlier for unstable angina. He underwent a cardiac catheterization and three-vessel coronary bypass grafting 48 hours prior to your call from the intern. His postoperative course was complicated by a subendocardial infarction but was otherwise unremarkable until yesterday when his urine output began to drop (150 cc in 24 hours). His serum creatinine was noted to be 3.5 mg/dL (1.2 mg/dL on admission). The patient is intubated and can give no history. Medications include digoxin, lasix, enalapril, IV nitroglycerin, atenolol, and perioperative cefazolin. For which type(s) of acute renal failure is this patient MOST at risk?

(A) prerenal and intrarenal
(B) intrarenal only
(C) postrenal
(D) not at risk for acute renal failure
(E) cannot be determined from the information provided

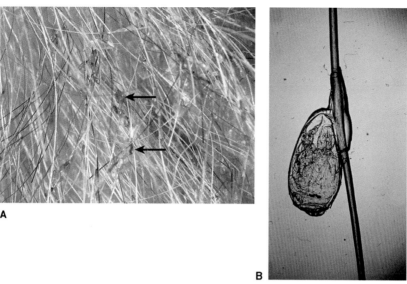

Figure 3-4. Reproduced with permission from Fitzpatrick, Johnson, Wolff, et al. Dermatology in General Medicine, 4th ed. McGraw-Hill, Inc., 1993, with permission.

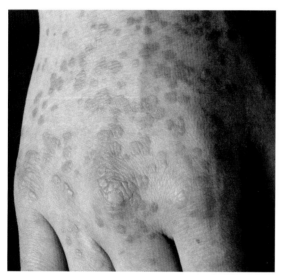

Figure 3-5. Reproduced, with permission, from Wolff K, Johnson RA, Suurmond D. Fitzpatrick's Color Atlas & Synopsis of Clinical Dermatology. 5th ed. New York: McGraw-Hill, 2005:781.

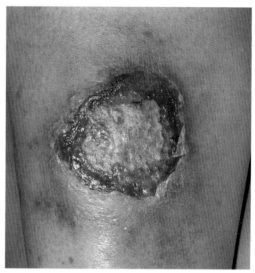

Figure 3-6. Reproduced, with permission, from Wolff K, Johnson RA, Suurmond D. Fitzpatrick's Color Atlas & Synopsis of Clinical Dermatology. 5th ed. New York: McGraw-Hill, 2005:594.

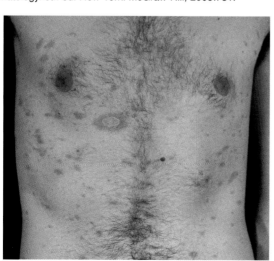

Figure 3-7. Reproduced, with permission, from Wolff K, Johnson RA, Suurmond D. Fitzpatrick's Color Atlas & Synopsis of Clinical Dermatology. 5th ed. New York: McGraw-Hill, 2005:119.

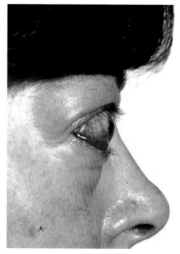

Figure 4-1. Reproduced, with permission, from Fauci AS, Braunwald E, Kasper DL, et al. Harrison's Principles of Internal Medicine, 17th edition. New York: McGraw-Hill, 2008: 2235.

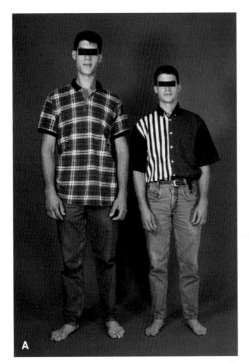

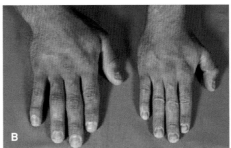

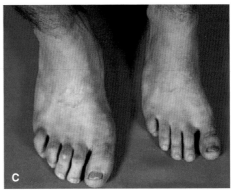

Figure 4-2. Reproduced, with permission, from Gagel R, McCutcheon IE. N Engl J Med, 1999;340:524. Copyright © 1999 Massachusetts Medical Society. All rights reserved.

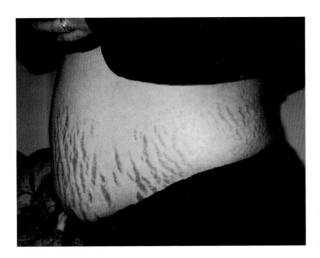

Figure 4-3. Reproduced, with permission, from Fauci AS, Braunwald E, Kasper DL, et al. Harrison's Principles of Internal Medicine, 17th edition. New York: McGraw-Hill, 2008: 2255.

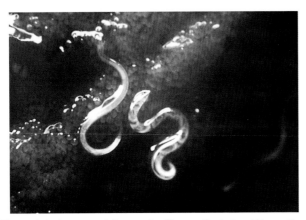

Figure 8-1. Courtesy of Centers for Disease Control and Prevention, National Center for Infectious Diseases, Division of Parasitic Diseases.

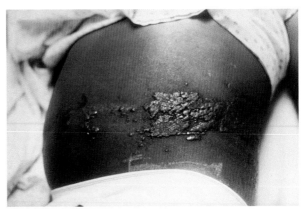

Figure 8-2. Courtesy of Centers for Disease Control and Prevention, National Immunization Program.

56. Hyperphosphatemia is associated with stage III CKD. Which of the following is the appropriate treatment for mild hyperphosphatemia in this patient population?

(A) magnesium oxide 250 to 500 mg po tid

(B) calcium carbonate 0.5 to 1.5 g po qd on an empty stomach

(C) calcium carbonate 0.5 to 1.5 g po tid on an empty stomach

(D) calcium carbonate 0.5 to 1.5 g po tid with meals

(E) no treatment indicated for mild hyperphosphatemia

Answers and Explanations

1. **(C)** Injury to the nephron results in excessive protein leak and decreased protein reabsorption from the tubules. This occurs long before the creatinine becomes abnormal and 5 to 10 years before overt proteinuria, detectable by routine dipstick, develops. Persistent proteinuria eventually will result in an abnormal creatinine but, in the case of CKD, years later. Therefore, proteinuria, best assessed by the protein-to-creatinine ratio from a urine specimen, is considered the earliest marker of CKD. Microscopic hematuria can result from many processes, some transient, including infection, malignancy, calculi, acute glomerulonephritis, and IgA nephropathy, and is not, in and of itself, an indicator of permanent kidney damage. Hypertension, if not the cause of the CKD, can occur early in the course of CKD, but proteinuria usually occurs before hypertension develops. Chronic hyperkalemia develops later in the course of CKD, generally when glomerular filtration rate is <30 mL/min. (*NKF-K/DOQI Guidelines, 2002, pp. 48-49*)

2. **(A)** GFR describes the amount of blood passing through the kidneys per minute. There is an inverse relationship between GFR and serum creatinine. In a patient with normal renal function, doubling of the serum creatinine represents a loss of approximately 50% of GFR. Using this information, the loss of GFR can be estimated from changes in the serum creatinine. For example, assume normal creatinine levels of 1.0 mg/dL and normal GFR of 100 mL/min. A doubling of the serum creatinine from 1.0 mg/dL to 2.0 mg/dL represents an approximate reduction in GFR from 100 mL/min to 50 mL/min (50% of GFR has been lost). Each additional doubling of the creatinine decreases the remaining GFR by approximately one half. When renal function is severely impaired, large increases in the creatinine (ie, from 8.0 to 16.0 mg/dL) represent only small decreases in GFR (from about 12 to 6 mL/min). This example emphasizes the importance of detecting increases in serum creatinine early. However, serum creatinine level does not become abnormal until ~25% of renal function is lost. Therefore, other methods of estimating GFR are more useful in detecting early decreases in GFR. (*Levey, 1999; Stevens and Perrone, 2008*)

3. **(D)** The American Diabetes Association (ADA) recommends checking urine for microalbumin 5 years after the diagnosis is made and once a year thereafter to screen for diabetic nephropathy in patients with type I diabetes mellitus. For patients with type II diabetes mellitus, the ADA recommends checking the urine at the time of the diagnosis and yearly thereafter. (*American Diabetes Association, 2009, p. 533*)

4. **(A)** Casts in the urine indicate a pathologic process, with the exception of the presence of the rare hyaline cast (1 to 2/HPF). The acute inflammatory process of glomerulonephritis is characterized by red cells and red cell casts in the urine. White cells and white cell casts occur with an allergic or infectious process, such as acute interstitial nephritis or pyelonephritis, respectively. Renal tubular epithelial cells indicate damage to the renal tubules, as with acute tubular necrosis. Oval fat bodies result from renal tubular cells that have absorbed fats or monocytes and macrophages that have ingested fats. (*Post and Rose, 2008*)

5. **(D)** The development of seizures due to uremia is an absolute indication to begin hemodialysis. The waste products of urea metabolism must be removed to abort the seizure activity. Proteinuria is never an indication to begin hemodialysis. Proteinuria is a sign of kidney damage, poses no immediate threat to life (although the underlying process causing it might), and hemodialysis will not correct it. Calculations of GFR are used to assess kidney function, predict when complications of CKD and ESRD (end-stage renal disease) will occur, and guide treatment plan but not to indicate when to initiate hemodialysis. Rather, the decision to initiate renal replacement therapy is a clinical one, based upon clinical assessment of functioning and physical manifestations of ESRD. A potassium level of >5.0 mEq/L does not represent an immediate threat to the patient and can be treated medically. Cardiac abnormalities associated with hyperkalemia generally occur at levels >6.5 mEq/L, and conservative measures to correct hyperkalemia generally are initiated when the serum level is >5.5 mEq/L, although this varies with practice. Hyperphosphatemia is best treated with phosphate binders, such as calcium carbonate and calcium acetate, and a low phosphorus diet. *(Watnick and Morrison, 2009, pp. 800-801)*

6. **(B)** Renal ultrasound is useful for assessing kidney size and thickness of the cortex, and for the presence of masses, cysts, obstruction, and hydronephrosis. Intrinsic disease is best assessed by establishing the clinical context, analyzing the urine for protein, cells, and casts, and possibly by doing a biopsy. Loss of cortical thickness is a nonspecific finding, and ultrasound does not establish an etiology. *(Bazari, 2008, pp. 810-811; Watnick and Morrison, 2009, p. 805)*

7. **(A)** Struvite stones form when urea-splitting organisms, such as *Proteus*, *Klebsiella*, *Pseudomonas*, and *Staphylococcus*, are present in the urinary tract. Ammonia is formed when urease breaks down urea. This results in an alkaline urine, which decreases the solubility of struvite, favoring the production of stones. Calcium stones result from hyperabsorption of calcium in the intestine, impaired renal tubular reab-sorption of calcium, primary hyperparathyroidism, intestinal hyperabsorption of oxalate, and hypocitraturia. Uric acid stones are due to hyperuricosuria or a urinary pH <5.5, which causes uric acid to dissociate. They are also the only radiolucent calculi. Cystinuria, an inborn error of metabolism, results in cystine stones. *(Stoller et al., 2009, pp. 833-837)*

8. **(D)** Nephrotic syndrome is defined as proteinuria >3.5 g/24 h resulting in hypoalbuminemia (<3.0 g/dL), hyperlipidemia (total cholesterol >250 mg/dL), and edema, probably due to increased renal tubule permeability. Causes include diabetic nephropathy, HIV nephropathy, chronic hepatitis B and C, amyloidosis, systemic lupus erythematosus, constrictive pericarditis, Hodgkin's disease, minimal change disease, and many medications, including phenytoin and NSAIDs. *(Watnick and Morrison, 2009, pp. 815-817)*

9. **(B)** Analgesic nephropathy results from ingestion of at least 1 g of analgesics per day for at least 3 years. NSAIDs are also one of the most common causes of acute interstitial nephritis. The pathophysiologic mechanism of injury appears to be tubulointerstitial inflammation and papillary necrosis. *(Watnick and Morrison, 2009, p. 822)*

10. **(C)** Retrograde flow of urine from the bladder damages the renal interstitium, causing inflammation and fibrosis. If untreated, irreversible damage to the kidneys will occur. Because this is a tubulointerstitial process, the urinalysis will be negative for protein in the early stages of damage. Most damage is done before age 5, but if undetected, glomerular damage will occur and protein will appear in the urine eventually. Hypertension develops as the GFR decreases. *(Watnick and Morrison, 2009, p. 822)*

11. **(C)** ACE inhibitors prevent the conversion of angiotensin I to angiotensin II, thereby interrupting the renin–angiotensin–aldosterone system, which regulates blood pressure. The glomerular efferent arteriole dilates, given the decreased stimulus from angiotensin II to constrict. This lowers pressure in the glomerulus

by lowering resistance to outflow. This effectively results in a decrease in GFR, resulting in increased serum creatinine and potassium levels. However, these changes are not necessarily indications to discontinue the ACE inhibitor. Usually, the creatinine increases 0.2 to 0.4 mg/dL and then levels out. Monitoring serum creatinine and potassium levels is indicated. If only mild increases occur and stabilize, or if there are no changes, the ACE inhibitor can, and should, be continued so that the patient derives the beneficial effect of the decline in pressure within the glomerulus, which will slow down the progression of CKD. *(Benowitz, 2007, pp. 175-176)*

12. **(E)** Among other mechanisms of action, ACE inhibitors interfere with vasoconstriction of the efferent arteriole, thereby decreasing pressure within the glomerulus. If significant blockage is present in the renal artery, blood flow to the glomerulus is already compromised, resulting in lowered glomerular pressure. If pressure within the glomerulus is lowered further because of the vasodilating effect of the ACE inhibitor on the efferent arteriole, blood flow is further compromised. Ischemia and acute renal failure can result. *(Benowitz, 2007, pp. 175-176)*

13. **(A)** Magnetic resonance angiography, enhanced with gadolinium, is 99% to 100% sensitive and 71% to 96% specific for diagnosing renal artery stenosis (RAS). This study has largely replaced the captopril renal scan and contrast-enhanced arteriography in diagnosing RAS. The principle behind the captopril renal scan is that ACE inhibitors lower GFR. In a kidney with already-compromised blood flow due to RAS, administration of the ACE inhibitor further decreases GFR in the affected kidney despite maintenance of adequate plasma volume. GFR in the contralateral kidney remains normal. Subsequent injection of a radionuclide reveals delayed uptake in the compromised kidney. Although arteriography provides the most definitive diagnosis, it carries its own risks of contrast-induced injury and bleeding. MRA is a low-risk procedure due to its noninvasive nature. Renal artery biopsy would not

yield this diagnosis. IVP is utilized to visualize the anatomical structure of the urinary tract in situations such as urinary tract trauma and outflow obstruction, although increasingly it too is being replaced by noninvasive testing, such as ultrasound, CT scanning, and MRI. It remains a useful test to pinpoint the location of a calculus in the urinary tract. *(DuBose and Santos, 2008, pp. 892-893; Watnick and Morrison, 2009, p. 810)*

14. **(C)** The normal glomerulus filters a small amount of low-molecular-weight proteins, which are reabsorbed in the tubules, generally at a rate of <150 mg/24 h. However, up to 300 mg/24 h can be accepted as normal. High-molecular-weight proteins, such as albumin, are not filtered by the normal kidney, and therefore, albumin's appearance in the urine at >30 mg/24 h is considered abnormal. Standard urine dipsticks will react in the presence of all proteins, including glycoproteins, gamma-globulins, Tamm–Horsfall mucoproteins, Bence–Jones proteins, and albumin. However, they generally cannot detect protein until it reaches an excretion level of >200 to 300 mg/24 h. This will produce a urine dipstick reading of 1+ (equivalent to about 30 mg of protein in that sample). Contamination of the urine specimen with blood, semen, pus, vaginal discharge, and mucous can result in false-positive readings. Specific reagent strips designed to detect microalbuminemia, defined as 30 to 300 mg/24 h, have been developed and are the preferred strips to use when testing for early signs of diabetic nephropathy. Expressed another way, a protein level of >300 mg/24 h or a microalbumin level of >30 mg/24 h is defined as abnormal. A random spot urinary albumin-to-creatinine ratio is also a good screening test for early nephropathy, with normal results defined as 17 to 250 mg/g in men and 25 to 355 mg/g in women. *(Graff, 1983, pp. 27-30; NKF-K/DOQI Guidelines, 2002, p. 21; Watnick and Morrison, 2009, pp. 794-795)*

15. **(E)** In patients with hypercalciuria, thiazide diuretics can lower urinary calcium levels, reducing the risk of nephrolithiasis. An episode of nephrolithiasis mandates a metabolic

workup, including blood work to check serum levels of creatinine, parathyroid hormone (PTH), calcium, phosphorus, and uric acid, and a 24-hour urine collection to measure pH, total volume, sodium, calcium, phosphorus, oxalate, citrate, cystine, and uric acid. *(Stoller et al., 2009, pp. 834-835)*

16. **(C)** Because glucosuria does not occur until serum glucose levels are ≥180 mg/dL, urine testing is not considered an adequate screening tool for diagnosing diabetes mellitus. *(Delmez and Windus, 2001, p. 1347)*

17. **(E)** Nitrite is formed when organisms that produce nitrate reductase, that is, *Escherichia coli*, *Klebsiella*, *Proteus*, and *Enterobacter*, are present in the urine. The enzyme reduces nitrate to nitrite. However, the urine has to be present in the bladder at least 4 hours for this to occur. Leukocyte esterase is produced by various WBCs, including polymorphonuclear neutrophils, monocytes, eosinophils, and basophils. The enzyme can appear in the urine with the presence of any of these WBCs and not just as the result of bacterial infection, although UTI is the most common cause of positive leukocyte esterase in the urine. Other causes are vaginal and perineal contamination. The combination of urinary nitrite and leukocyte esterase has a sensitivity and specificity of 85% and 75%, respectively, and therefore, provides more information than either alone. WBCs can occur in the urine as the result of infection, an inflammatory process, such as interstitial nephritis, or vaginal or perineal contamination, and levels <3 to 5 WBCs/HPF are not considered indicative of infection. Infection is strongly indicated when WBCs reach 4 to 6/HPF. Urine culture is considered positive for infection at >100,000 colonies. *(Bastani, 2001, p. 1367; McBride, 1998, pp. 70-71)*

18. **(D)** Renal artery stenosis causes compromised blood flow to the kidney, resulting in atrophy. Frequently, the contralateral kidney will hypertrophy in an attempt to compensate for the declining GFR. Polycystic kidney disease results in enlarged kidneys due to growth of multiple cysts. Hypertensive nephrosclerosis and diabetic nephropathy affect both kidneys equally and would result in bilateral, not unilateral, cortical atrophy. Malignancy would not result in atrophy. *(Watnick and Morrison, 2009, pp. 805, 810)*

19. **(A)** Renal biopsies done on patients with postinfectious glomerulonephritis (GN) show deposition of immune complexes and proliferation of inflammatory cells. The most common cause of postinfectious GN is Group A beta-hemolytic *Streptococci*, but other organisms, such as *Staphylococcus aureus*, can cause it as well. Antibiotic treatment for the underlying infection has no impact on the development of postinfectious GN because the kidney has already been exposed to the microbial antigen before treatment was initiated. About 25% of those infected with nephritogenic strains will develop postinfectious GN, but not all people are infected with these strains. Most patients recover spontaneously, and progression to renal failure is extremely rare. *(Watnick and Morrison, 2009, pp. 802, 811-812)*

20. **(B)** Hyperkalemia can be treated by three mechanisms: antagonizing the effect on the cell membrane, which can be achieved by infusing calcium gluconate 10 to 30 mL of 10% solution IV; redistributing potassium from the blood into the cell, which can be accomplished by infusing sodium bicarbonate 44 to 132 mEq IV or regular insulin along with glucose (5–10 g of glucose per unit of insulin); or removing it by giving sodium polystyrene sulfonate (Kayexalate) po or via retention enema or by initiating hemo- or peritoneal dialysis. Insulin acts to drive potassium into the cell but must be given with glucose to avoid significant hypoglycemia. *(Cho et al., 2009, pp. 775-776)*

21. **(C)** Hyperkalemia is defined as serum potassium level greater than 5.0 mEq/L. ECG changes (tall, peaked T waves and shortening of the QT interval) start to occur at 5.5 mEq/L. At serum levels of ≥6.5 mEq/L, the QRS will widen, the PR interval will be prolonged, and then the P wave will disappear. Nodal and ventricular arrhythmias can start to occur. A sine wave pattern precedes asystole at a serum level of ~10 mEq/L. *(McMillan, 2007)*

22. **(A)** Maintenance of normal urine output as the serum creatinine level increases, so-called nonoliguric ARF, has a better prognosis for recovery than oliguric ARF. Oliguria is defined as urine output <500 mL/24 h. Anuria is absence of urine output. A low BUN level does not indicate the degree of renal damage because the blood urea nitrogen level can be affected by other factors, such as an elevated rate of catabolism, dietary protein intake, and gastrointestinal bleeding. Poor outcome is associated with ARF, due to sepsis and pregnancy. Administration of furosemide has not been shown to favorably affect the outcome of ARF. *(McMillan, 2007)*

23. **(B)** Intrinsic ARF results in alterations in the kidneys' ability to respond to changes in hemostasis. When the integrity of the kidneys remains intact, sodium is conserved when GFR declines in an attempt to reestablish volume and perfusion, resulting in a fractional excretion of sodium (FENa) of <1. However, when the glomeruli are injured, the kidneys lose the ability to reabsorb sodium as the GFR decreases, and the FENa will be >1. The etiology of this patient's renal failure is most likely contrast-induced acute tubular necrosis following an ischemic episode, which is intrinsic ARF. *(Cho et al., 2009, p. 798)*

24. **(B)** Screening for the presence of chronic kidney disease involves checking a serum creatinine level, checking blood pressure for the presence of hypertension, checking urinary protein for evidence of glomerular injury, and obtaining a history to check for the presence of risk factors, such as hypertension, diabetes mellitus, autoimmune disease, infection, or family history. Initial screening would not include a 24-hour urine collection. This is a cumbersome, inconvenient, more expensive test than the spot urinary protein reading and would not provide additional information. Renal ultrasound and abdominal CT scan would not be indicated in the initial stages of the work-up. These would be done only after laboratory studies were done and only if indicated. *(NKF-K/DOQI Guidelines, 2002, p. 31)*

25. **(C)** Urine reagent strips are suffused with an indicator dye that changes color when oxidized by peroxidase in hemoglobin, indicating the presence of blood in the urine. However, myoglobin also has peroxidase activity, and therefore, the indicator for blood on the dipstick will turn positive in the presence of myoglobin without hemoglobin. Myoglobin can appear in the urine as the result of rhabdomyolysis due to crush injuries, surgery, ischemia, hyperthermia, significant exercise, seizures, electric shock, illicit drug use, and muscle-wasting diseases. A positive urine dip for blood, with a negative urinary sediment for red cells, mandates a workup for diseases/injuries resulting in myoglobinuria. *(Graff, 1983, p. 52; McBride, 1998, p. 68)*

26. **(D)** Anemia associated with CKD is the result of inadequate erythropoietin synthesis by the kidneys. This hormone signals the bone marrow to synthesize red blood cells. A deficiency will result in anemia. In the absence of erythropoietin, iron would not be of use since red blood cell synthesis is inadequate. Folic acid would also not be of use and does not play a role in the etiology of this type of anemia. Transfusion is a tempering measure only, used to increase oxygen-carrying capacity in the case of symptomatic ischemia. Anemia due to erythropoietin deficiency generally does not occur until the GFR decreases to <60 mL/min, or approximately 50% of normal. Intramuscular administration of erythropoietin is the only effective treatment to induce red blood cell production. Depending on the formulation used, this can be given once a week or once every 2 weeks. Oral iron supplementation is needed to produce adequate hemoglobin for the increased de novo red cell production. *(Guyton and Hall, 2006, p. 376; NKF-K/DOQI Guidelines, 2002, p. 51)*

27. **(A)** Renal tubular acidosis is classified into subtypes: Type I is characterized by an inability of the distal renal tubule to excrete hydrogen ion. Type II is characterized by overexcretion of HCO_3^- into the urine. Type III is no longer used, as it is considered a subtype of Type I, where there is a distal acidification defect and

a proximal bicarbonate leak. Type IV is caused by either aldosterone deficiency or an inability of the distal tubule to respond to aldosterone. *(Cho et al., 2009, p. 788)*

28. **(C)** Hypokalemia can occur rarely as a complication of hemodialysis (HD) if excessive potassium is removed during the treatment. Hyperglycemia can result from peritoneal dialysis, since the dialysate contains dextrose. Infection occurs rarely, given meticulous maintenance of sterile technique. Anemia is a result of CKD and can be worsened by hemodialysis if significant bleeding occurs due to heparin administered during HD. However, hypotension remains the most common complication due to excessive removal of volume during treatment. *(Tolkoff-Rubin, 2008, p. 938)*

29. **(D)** Eighty-five percent of uncomplicated UTIs are caused by *E. coli*. Other common etiologic agents are the gram-negative bacteria *Proteus*, *Klebsiella*, and *Enterobacter*. *(Norrby, 2008, pp. 2138-2139)*

30. **(E)** Patients with indwelling catheters are at risk for UTIs due to multiple organisms, including *Pseudomonas aeruginosa*, *Acinetobacter baumannii*, *Serratia marcescens*, *Stenotrophomonas maltophilia*, *Proteus mirabilis*, and *Escherichia coli*, which accounts for less than 50% of cases. Asymptomatic leukocyturia or bacteriuria need not be treated since this can result in increased incidence of antibiotic resistance. The patient should be observed for any signs or symptoms of UTI. If treatment is indicated, the best antibiotic choice is a beta-lactam/beta-lactamase inhibitor combination, possibly including vancomycin. *(Bonomo and Johnson, 2004, p. 349; Norrby, 2008, p. 2139)*

31. **(A)** Because pyelonephritis is an infectious disease, the most likely complication is a perinephric abscess, which occurs as the result of inadequate therapy. Since it is not vascular in origin, renal vein thrombosis would not occur. Allergic interstitial nephritis is caused by an antigen–antibody reaction, which does not occur with acute pyelonephritis. Struvite stones

are due to chronic infection with urease-producing organisms, such as *Proteus* and *Pseudomonas*, not to an acute infection. Hepatic failure can be a complication of acute renal failure, but not acute pyelonephritis. *(Stoller et al., 2009, p. 830)*

32. **(C)** Squamous epithelial cells line the distal portion of the urethra in men and the entire urethra in women. They appear in the urine due to inadequate cleaning of the external urinary meatus prior to obtaining the sample and indicate that the sample is contaminated. In women, the source is usually vaginal/perineal. Uncircumcised men commonly have squamous epithelial cells in the urine sample. *(McBride, 1998, p. 103)*

33. **(D)** Men and pregnant women require the longest course of treatment for UTI—generally 7 to 10 days. Some advocate single-dose treatment of an uncomplicated UTI, although in practice, this is rare. Most are treated for 3 to 5 days with trimethoprim–sulfamethoxazole (TMP–SMZ) or a fluoroquinolone. Treatment with ampicillin, amoxicillin, and first-generation cephalosporins alone is infrequent given the widespread incidence of resistant organisms, as well as their decreased effectiveness in eliminating vaginal and periurethral colonization compared with TMP–SMZ. Remote history of UTI, history of renal calculi, and UTI in young girls are not indications to prolong antibiotic treatment course. Young, sexually active women are at higher risk for developing UTIs because of the risk of bacterial contamination into an anatomically short urethra, and those who use a diaphragm or spermicides are at highest risk. However, using these types of birth control does not indicate a need for a prolonged antibiotic course. *(Bastani, 2001, pp. 1369-1370)*

34. **(C)** The patient presents with a combination of inadequate fluid intake and excessive losses due to perspiration, resulting in hypovolemia and hypernatremia. The most common causes of hypernatremia are inadequate fluid intake resulting in hemoconcentration and diabetes insipidus (DI), resulting in excessive renal fluid

losses. Normal urine osmolality is 500 to 850 mOsm/kg but can range from 50 to 1,200 mOsm/kg depending on the patient's fluid intake. Urine osmolality >400 mOsm/kg indicates that the renal fluid-conserving mechanism is intact, as the kidneys are working to preserve volume. A lower urine osmolality would be consistent with DI, characterized by a lack of response to anti-diuretic hormone (ADH), resulting in excessive urinary losses of water with worsening hypernatremia. Treatment is directed at the cause. If the patient is dehydrated, restoring fluid volume is the goal. If the patient has DI, treating the underlying disease will lower the serum sodium level. For this dehydrated patient, the treatment would be to administer isotonic (normal) saline, which contains 0.9% sodium, because of the large free water deficit. Quarter-normal saline contains 0.25% sodium, half-normal saline contains 0.45% sodium, and lactated Ringer's solution is similar to half-normal saline in its sodium content. Dextrose 5% in water (D5W) contains no electrolytes. Isotonic saline is the appropriate choice because it treats not only the volume deficit but the serum osmolality as well. Its osmolality (308 mOsm/kg) is often lower than the plasma osmolality because of the hypovolemic state and, therefore, helps restore normal serum osmolality. Once serum osmolality becomes more normal, the isotonic saline can be replaced by D5W to replace the remaining free water deficit. If the free water deficit were less dramatic, initial IV fluid treatment could be half-normal saline, followed by D5W. (*Cho et al., 2009, pp. 771-772; Graff, 1983, p. 19*)

35. **(B)** The most common cause of nephrotic syndrome in children is minimal change disease. Diffuse injury to the capillaries is the underlying cause, resulting in significant proteinuria, edema, hypoalbuminemia, and hyperlipidemia. It accounts for 65% of cases of nephrotic syndrome in children; however, 10% of adults with nephrotic syndrome have minimal change disease. Treatment is with corticosteroids for 2 to 4 weeks, dietary sodium restriction, and sometimes diuretics to reduce the edema. Relapse and lack of response to corticosteroids can occur. If the latter occurs, renal biopsy is indicated to rule out other causes of the nephrotic syndrome, such as focal glomerulosclerosis and membranoproliferative glomerulonephritis. (*Appel, 2008, p. 868; Kumar et al., 2007, pp. 549-550*)

36. **(E)** ACE inhibitors are the drug of choice in this setting. Control of systemic blood pressure can reduce renal vascular damage. In diabetic patients, ACE inhibitors are especially beneficial because of the added effect of reducing intraglomerular pressure and decreasing proteinuria. Current target blood pressure in patients with diabetic nephropathy is <130/80 mm Hg. Calcium channel blockers and diuretics do not offer renoprotective benefits but may be used to control hypertension. (*American Diabetes Association, 2009, p. S28; JNC 7 Report, 2003; NKF-K/DOQI Guidelines, 2002, pp. 79-80; Watnick and Morrison, 2009, p. 819*)

37. **(C)** The thiazide diuretics, including hydrochlorothiazide, block sodium reabsorption in the terminal portion of the loop of Henle and the proximal portion of the distal convoluted tubule. This leads to loss of both sodium and potassium in the urine. Triamterene, amiloride, spironolactone, and eplerenone are potassium-sparing diuretics. Triamterene and amiloride act to reduce potassium secretion in the distal tubule. Spironolactone and eplerenone are aldosterone receptor blockers. (*Ives, 2007, p. 246*)

38. **(A)** Because many drugs are excreted in the urine, knowledge of the renal function is important when dosing medication, especially in patients with abnormal GFR. Drug toxicity or adverse side effects may occur if the drug is dosed improperly. Estimation of the creatinine clearance can help in making the proper drug adjustment for the degree of CKD. In a steady state (ie, stable creatinine), the Cockcroft–Gault equation can be used to estimate creatinine clearance. The formula is

$$\text{Creatinine clearance (mL/min)} = \frac{(140 - \text{age}) \times \text{weight (kg)}}{\text{serum creatinine} \times 72}$$

In female patients, the result is multiplied by 0.85 because of smaller muscle mass.

Appropriate medication adjustments can be made based on the estimated creatinine clearance. The MDRD (modification of diet in renal disease) equation is the most accurate indicator of GFR, utilizing serum creatinine level, age, gender, and race, and it also eliminates the need for a 24-hour urine collection, which is cumbersome and inconvenient. The equation can be accessed online at www.kdoqi.org. The blood urea nitrogen is not a reliable index, because several factors may alter tubular reabsorption of, or generation of, urea. These include the patient's hydration status, protein intake, and degree of catabolic activity occurring. *(Levey, 1998, p. 23; Watnick and Morrison, 2009, p. 796)*

39. **(E)** *S. aureus* is the organism responsible for most cases of peritonitis in patients on peritoneal dialysis. Overall, gram-positive organisms are responsible for 50% of cases, and gram-negative organisms cause 15% of cases. Four percent of cases are polymicrobial in nature. Improper technique by the patient in making catheter connections during dialysis exchanges is the reason for bacterial inoculation in most cases. Abdominal pain, fever, and cloudy dialysis fluid are the presenting symptoms and signs. *(Burkart, 2008)*

40. **(B)** Hyponatremia is defined as a serum sodium concentration of <130 mEq/L. Common causes include dehydration, diarrhea, vomiting, overuse of diuretics, syndrome of inappropriate ADH, postoperative state, hypothyroidism, congestive heart failure (CHF), liver disease, and pulmonary disease. Rapid correction of hyponatremia can result in severe brain damage, including central pontine myelinolysis. For this reason, the serum sodium concentration in those patients displaying neurological symptoms should be increased by no more than 1 to 2 mEq/L/h and no more than 25 to 30 mEq/L in the first 2 days. Once neurological symptoms improve, the rate of increase should be decreased to 0.5 to 1 mEq/L/h. *(Cho et al, 2009, pp. 767-770)*

41. **(A)** The following formula can be used to estimate serum osmolality when an actual lab value is not available:

$$2(Na^{2+}) + \frac{glucose}{18} + \frac{BUN}{2.8}$$

Utilizing this formula, the estimated serum osmolality would be

$$2(132) + \frac{167}{18} + \frac{15}{2.8} = 279$$

Normal serum osmolality is 285 to 295 mOsm/kg. Serum osmolality is the measure of the total concentration of solutes in the blood. It is helpful to be able to estimate serum osmolality for various reasons, including to help determine the cause of serum sodium abnormalities and to determine whether inactive metabolites, such as methanol, ethylene glycol, and salicylates, may be present in the blood. A low serum osmolality in the presence of hyponatremia suggests volume overload. *(Cho et al., 2009, pp. 766-767)*

42. **(C)** Hyponatremia affects approximately 20% of hospitalized patients and is the most common electrolyte abnormality found in this population. The incidence of hypokalemia is less well-documented but has been estimated by one source to be approximately 13%. *(Fukagawa et al., 2008, p. 758; Lederer et al., 2007)*

43. **(B)** Most often, hyponatremia is due to excessive water retention rather than a true sodium deficiency. The first step in evaluating hyponatremia is to determine serum osmolality. Knowing whether the serum is isotonic (normal osmolality), hypotonic (low osmolality), or hypertonic (high osmolality) can help determine the etiology of the hyponatremia, and therefore, treatment. The most common causes of isotonic hyponatremia are hyperproteinemia and hyperlipidemia. The most common causes of hypertonic hyponatremia are hyperglycemia, presence of radiocontrast agents, and the presence of inactive metabolites, that is, mannitol, sorbitol, glycerol, and maltose. Treatment is aimed at correcting the underlying disorder. Most commonly, hyponatremia occurs in the setting of low osmolality (hypotonic). To further evaluate the etiology of the hyponatremia, it must be determined if the patient is hypovolemic, euvolemic, or hypervolemic. Hypovolemic hyponatremia is usually due either to extrarenal or intrarenal sodium losses. Extrarenal losses occur from dehydration, diarrhea, and vomiting.

Urinary sodium measures <10 mEq/L (normal, >20 mEq/L), as the kidneys are avidly retaining sodium in an attempt to restore volume. Treatment is directed at restoring volume. Intrarenal sodium losses occur from the use of diuretics and ACE inhibitors, nephropathies, and mineralocorticoid deficiency. Urinary sodium measures >20 mEq/L. Treatment is directed at reversing the underlying cause. The most common causes of euvolemic hyponatremia are SIADH, postoperative hyponatremia, hypothyroidism, psychogenic polydipsia, and endurance exercise. In these cases, electrolyte-free water is retained, which results in a true physiologic hyponatremia. Treatment is directed at correcting the underlying abnormality and replacing sodium losses. Hypervolemic hyponatremia is caused by congestive heart failure, liver disease, nephrotic syndrome, and advanced CKD in general, anything that causes fluid retention. Treatment is directed at treating the underlying disease, restricting water intake, and facilitating excretion of water. The first step in characterizing this patient's hyponatremia is to determine the serum osmolality, which is 276 mOsm/kg. This is low, so we know that this is hypotonic. Second, we have to determine the volume status. Urinary sodium is 12 mEq, which does not indicate either intrarenal or extrarenal losses of sodium and is not consistent with hypovolemia. Given the elevated JVP, extensive edema, and hepatojugular reflux, this patient is presenting with a clinical picture of fluid overload, or hypervolemia. This patient has hypervolemic hypotonic hyponatremia due to CHF. *(Cho et al, 2009, pp. 767-771)*

44. **(D)** Approximately 60% of body weight is water: 20% of body weight is in the extracellular spaces and 40% in the intracellular spaces. Free water deficit can be calculated by using the following formula:

Volume in liters to be replaced =

$$[\text{current wt (kg)} \times 0.6] \times \frac{[Na^{2+}] - 140}{140}$$

Utilizing this formula, the patient's water deficit is approximately 6.6 L. *(Cho et al., 2009, pp. 766, 772)*

45. **(E)** This patient's pH is acidemic, with a low HCO_3, suggesting a metabolic acidosis. The P_{CO_2} of 16 mm Hg represents appropriate pulmonary compensation for the acidosis, as the respiratory rate increases to expire more CO_2. When evaluating a metabolic acidosis, the anion gap should be calculated to help determine the etiology. Calculation of the anion gap is done as follows: $Na^{2+} - (Cl^{2-} + HCO_3)$. A normal anion gap is 8 to 12 mEq/L. This patient's anion gap is 138 − (119 + 8) = 138 −127 = 11, which is normal. Causes of a normal anion gap metabolic acidosis include diseases/disorders that cause a loss of HCO_3, including diarrhea, losses from an ileostomy, and carbonic anhydrase inhibitors. Disorders that cause losses of chloride, such as renal tubular acidosis, also cause a nonanion gap metabolic acidosis. *(Cho et al, 2009, pp. 784-788)*

46. **(A)** This patient has been having significant diarrhea for several days, which is the most likely cause of the metabolic acidosis. *(Cho et al, 2009, pp. 787-788)*

47. **(C)** With any acid–base disorder, the body tries to compensate to restore pH to normal. By definition, an alkalosis is characterized by a pH of >7.45. This patient has sustained losses of acid (HCl, NaCl, KCl) through vomiting. In addition, volume contraction results in a decrease in GFR, which causes avid sodium and bicarbonate reabsorption, further worsening the alkalosis. The body has two ways to increase serum levels of acid to try to decrease the pH to normal: the lungs slow the respiratory rate to retain CO_2 and/or the kidneys reabsorb chloride and hydrogen ion $[H^+]$ and increase excretion of bicarbonate (HCO_3). The lungs can respond more quickly (within minutes) and, therefore, P_{CO_2} will rise before serum HCO_3 will drop (over hours to days). Normal P_{CO_2} levels are 35 to 45 mm Hg. This patient's P_{CO_2} is 47 mm Hg, which indicates that her respiratory rate is slowing, and she is retaining CO_2. Levels of 32 mm Hg and 38 mm Hg are low and normal, respectively, and, therefore, would not be appropriate compensation for the alkalosis. Normal serum bicarbonate levels are 24 to 31 mEq/L. An HCO_3 level of 38 mEq/L would not be appropriate compensation, as this would increase the pH.

A HCO_3 level of 24 mEq/L is at the lower end of normal. Given that this patient's symptoms have been present for 3 days, one would expect the HCO_3 level to be lower at this time as the kidneys have had time to adjust and increase excretion of HCO_3. *(Cho et al, 2009, pp. 790-792)*

48. **(B)** This patient has CKD with an elevated creatinine level of 1.9 mg/dL. Her kidney function can worsen if exposed to any nephrotoxins, including contrast dye and some medications, such as aminoglycosides, amphotericin B, NSAIDs, cisplatin, and cyclosporine. The mechanism of injury from contrast dye is thought to be due to renal vasoconstriction, possibly mediated by alterations in the amount of nitric oxide and/or endothelin present, which results in ischemia. In addition, there are also direct toxic effects of the contrast agents on the renal cells. A byproduct of the renal injury is oxygen-free radicals, which are important modulators of renal perfusion and GFR. Maintaining adequate hydration protects the glomeruli in the presence of vasoconstriction, therefore, providing a preprocedure fluid bolus of 1 L is appropriate. In addition, acetylcysteine has been found to have a potentially protective effect as well. *N*-Acetylcysteine is a precursor for glutathione synthesis. It improves endothelin-dependent vasomotor function in the coronary and peripheral circulation and is also a potent antioxidant that may result in scavenging of free radicals. Therefore, it improves renal hemodynamics and prevents direct oxidative tissue damage. The recommended dose of acetylcysteine is 600 mg po every 12 hours twice before and after a dye load. Contrast nephropathy is the third-leading cause of new ARF in the hospitalized population, with the injury usually occurring 24 to 48 hours after the study. Administering a diuretic and/or ACE inhibitor may worsen the risk of nephropathy. *(Briguori et al., 2002; Watnick and Morrison, 2009, pp. 799-801)*

49. **(D)** Hypomagnesemia is a common finding in the patient who abuses alcohol. Other leading causes include diarrhea, diuretics, aminoglycosides, and amphotericin B. The etiology of hypomagnesemia in the patient with a history of alcohol abuse is thought to be a combination of malabsorption and inadequate dietary intake, possibly with alcohol exerting an antagonistic effect on absorption. Signs and symptoms are those of neuromuscular and central nervous system hyperirritability, including weakness and muscle cramps, tremors, nystagmus, a positive Babinski response, confusion, and disorientation. Hypertension, tachycardia, and ventricular arrhythmias may develop. *(Fukagawa et al, 2008, pp. 774-775)*

50. **(A)** Primary hyperparathyroidism and malignancy account for 90% of all cases of hypercalcemia. Ten to twenty percent of patients with cancer develop hypercalcemia, most commonly because of breast, lung, kidney, head and neck carcinomas, and multiple myeloma and lymphoma. Given this patient's history of lung cancer, this is the most likely etiology of his hypercalcemia. Although it is possible that the patient's symptoms could be due to hyperparathyroidism, this is a relatively rare disorder, affecting only about 0.1% of the population, making malignancy a much more likely etiology. He is taking a low dose of hydrochlorothiazide, which has been stable for years; therefore, this is unlikely to be causing excessive fluid losses and dehydration with hemoconcentration. However, this medication could be exacerbating the hypercalcemia. He is not taking vitamin D, so there is nothing to suggest vitamin D toxicity. *(Cho et al., 2009, pp. 778-780; Fitzgerald, 2009, pp. 1007-1009; Rugo, 2009, pp. 1483-1484)*

51. **(B)** When hypercalcemia becomes symptomatic, it must be treated to prevent neurologic and muscular dysfunction. Principles of treatment include establishing euvolemia since hypercalcemia can result in volume depletion. Since excretion of sodium is accompanied by excretion of calcium, intravenous saline (0.45% or 0.9%), followed by IV furosemide, will replete volume and promote natriuresis. Once calcium levels have normalized, the treatment of choice is bisphosphonates for hypercalcemia associated with malignancy. IV administration of zoledronic acid 4 mg over 15 minutes normalizes serum calcium levels in less than 3 days in 80% to 100% of patients. Doses can be repeated as necessary. *(Cho et al., 2009, pp. 779-780)*

52. **(E)** Polycystic kidney disease (PKD) is an autosomal dominant disorder that affects approximately 500,000 patients in the United States, occurring in about 1 in 800 live births. Fifty percent of patients will reach ESRD by age 60, and PKD accounts for approximately 10% of hemodialysis patients. It is the most common hereditary disorder to result in ESRD. Family history is positive in 75% of cases, but genetic mutations can occur spontaneously, and patients can present without a family history. Signs and symptoms of PKD include abdominal fullness due to enlarged kidneys, abdominal pain due to bleeding into cysts, microscopic or gross hematuria, depending on the extent of the disease, and hypertension. Patients are often asymptomatic, and the first signs of the disease may be hypertension, microscopic hematuria, and mild proteinuria. Abdominal fullness and pain occur later in the disease, as the number and size of cysts increase. Ultrasound is the diagnostic test of choice to detect PKD: three or more cysts in patients younger than 30, three or more cysts in each kidney in patients 30 to 59 years of age, and five or more cysts in each kidney in patients older than 60 are the diagnostic criteria. Complications include pain, gross hematuria from a ruptured cyst, infected cysts, nephrolithiasis, HTN, and cerebral aneurysms (10% to 15% of patients have arterial aneurysms in the Circle of Willis). There is no effective treatment. Good control of blood pressure and a low protein diet may slow disease progression. There are two distinct genotypes of PKD—PKD1 and PKD2. The disease progresses more slowly in the latter. Urinary tract infection would not fit this patient scenario, as she has no dysuria, and UA is negative for leukocytes, leukocyte esterase, nitrites, and bacteria. Renal calculi would not cause abdominal fullness and hypertension and would be symptomatic on presentation. The urine sample is not contaminated as there are no squamous epithelial cells reported. In the absence of RBC casts and clinical signs and symptoms, this would not be glomerulonephritis. *(Watnick and Morrison, 2009, pp. 824-825)*

53. **(B)** Kidney disease is characterized by five stages, based upon GFR. Specific complications are associated with each stage, and specific treatments are recommended based upon the complication. Stage I: GFR >90 mL/min; patient has a history of previous kidney damage; no specific complications; avoid nephrotoxins, control cardiovascular risk factors. Stage II: GFR 60 to 89 mL/min; no specific complications; evaluate rate of decline in GFR, avoid nephrotoxins, control cardiovascular risk factors. Stage III: GFR 30 to 59 mL/min; complications include anemia, HTN, malnutrition, disorders of calcium and phosphorous metabolism, reduced functioning and well-being, neuropathy; screen for and treat complications as appropriate, avoid nephrotoxins, control cardiovascular risk factors, adjust doses of renally excreted medications. Stage IV: GFR 15 to 29 mL/min; complications include all of those in stage III, in addition to fluid, electrolyte, acid–base abnormalities; screen for and treat complications as appropriate, begin planning for ESRD with transplant or dialysis, avoid nephrotoxins, control cardiovascular risk factors, adjust doses of renally excreted medications. Stage V: GFR <15 mL/min; initiate dialysis or transplant when appropriate. *(NKF-K/DOQI Guidelines, 2002, pp. 26, 45-66; Watnick and Morrison, 2009, pp. 803-810)*

54. **(D)** Stage III: GFR 30 to 59 mL/min; complications include anemia, HTN, malnutrition, disorders of calcium and phosphorous metabolism, reduced functioning and well-being, neuropathy; screen for and treat complications as appropriate, avoid nephrotoxins, control cardiovascular risk factors, adjust doses of renally excreted medications. *(NKF-K/DOQI Guidelines, 2002, pp. 51-52, 62)*

55. **(A)** Acute renal failure can be classified as prerenal, intrarenal, or postrenal. The most common causes of prerenal ARF are diseases and disorders that (a) cause a decline in effective circulating volume, such as hemorrhage, GI losses, dehydration, excessive diuresis, burns, trauma, and peritonitis; (b) cause a change in systemic vascular resistance, such as sepsis, anesthesia, anaphylaxis; some medications such as ACE inhibitors and NSAIDs; and renal artery stenosis; or (c) cause a decline in cardiac output, such as

CHF and shock. Intrarenal causes of ARF include diseases and disorders that cause acute tubular necrosis (ATN) (toxins such as aminoglycosides, contrast media, chemotherapy, massive hemolysis, rhabdomyolysis, hyperuricemia; or intrarenal vasoconstriction due to seizures, cocaine, and alcohol), AIN (some medications, such as penicillin, cephalosporins, sulfonamides, diuretics, NSAIDs, phenytoin, and allopurinol; some infections such as cytomegalovirus (CMV), histoplasmosis, Rocky Mountain Spotted Fever; and some diseases such as systemic lupus erythematosus (SLE), Sjogren's syndrome, and sarcoidosis), and glomerulonephritis (autoimmune disorders, malignant HTN, thrombotic thrombocytic purpura (TTP), and hemolytic uremic syndrome (HUS)). Postrenal causes are the least common etiology of ARF and include obstruction due to benign prostatic hypertrophy (BPH), mass, or bilateral renal calculi. This patient has several risk factors for developing ARF: recent cardiac arrest with a period of decreased effective circulating volume, recent administration of contrast dye during the cardiac catheterization and anesthesia during the bypass surgery, and he is on an ACE inhibitor and a diuretic. All of these place him at risk for either prerenal or intrarenal ARF, most likely ATN. Since he is at risk for both, the best way to determine the cause is to analyze the urine, specifically looking for cells and casts, the specifics of which will help determine the etiology. He is at negligible risk for postrenal ARF as he has no history of BPH. Bilateral obstructing renal calculi would be extremely rare and, though possible, a mass is unlikely to be causing his ARF given the preponderance of other risk factors. In ARF, the serum creatinine increases about 1 to 2 mg/dL/day. *(McMillan, 2007; Watnick and Morrison, 2009, pp. 797-801)*

56. **(D)** Hyperphosphatemia develops in patients with CKD because of impaired renal excretion as GFR declines. Consequently, this results in downregulation of some phosphate transporters, a decrease in vitamin D production due to inhibition of an enzyme system that activates vitamin D, and an increase in PTH production. Also, as synthesis of 1,25-$(OH)_2D$ declines in the kidney, calcium absorption decreases further. Excess phosphorus complexes with calcium in the blood, decreasing ionized calcium levels, which results in hypocalcemia. As a result, PTH is further stimulated in an attempt to increase serum calcium levels. This eventually results in secondary hyperparathyroidism, renal osteodystrophy as calcium is drawn out of the bones to maintain a normal serum level, and extraosseous calcification of soft tissues due to calcium–phosphorus complexes. Treatment should be initiated early to prevent these long-term complications. Calcium carbonate binds phosphorous in the intestine before it can be absorbed and decreases serum levels. This must be taken with meals to bind dietary phosphorous. A synthetic phosphate binder, sevelamer hydrochloride, can also be utilized. The most effective regimen is 0.5 to 1.5 g po taken at the start of each meal. *(Cho et al., 2009, p. 782; Guyton, 2006, p. 344; Lederer et al., 2007)*

REFERENCES

American Diabetes Association. Diabetes care. *Diabetes Care.* 2009;32:S13-S61.

Appel GB. Glomerular disorders and nephrotic syndromes. In: Goldman L, Ausiello D, eds. *Cecil Medicine.* 23rd ed. Philadelphia, PA: Saunders; 2008.

Bastani B. Urinary tract infections. In: Noble J, ed. *Textbook of Primary Care Medicine.* 3rd ed. St. Louis, MO: Mosby; 2001.

Bazari H. Approach to the patient with renal disease. In Goldman L, Ausiello D, eds. *Cecil Medicine.* 23rd ed. Philadelphia, PA: Saunders; 2008.

Benowitz NL. Antihypertensive agents. In: Katzung BG, ed. *Basic and Clinical Pharmacology.* 10th ed. New York, NY: McGraw-Hill; 2007.

Bonomo RA, Johnson MA. Common infections. In: Landefeld CS, Palmer RM, Johnson MA, Johnston CB, et al., eds. *Current Geriatric Diagnosis and Treatment.* New York, NY: McGraw-Hill; 2004.

Briguori C, Manganelli F, Scarpato P, et al. Acetylcysteine and contrast agent-associated nephrotoxicity. *J Am Coll Cardiol.* 2002;40:298-303.

Burkart JM. Microbiology and therapy of peritonitis in continuous peritoneal dialysis. In: Rose BD, ed. 2008. http://*www.uptodate.com*, version 16.3.

Cho K, Fukagawa M, Kurokawa K. Fluid and electrolyte disorders. In: Tierney LM, McPhee SJ, Papadakis MA, eds. *Current Medical Diagnosis and Treatment.* 48th ed. New York, NY: McGraw-Hill; 2009.

Delmez JA, Windus DW. Generalist's guide to diagnostic tests. In: Noble J, ed. *Textbook of Primary Care Medicine.* 3rd ed. St. Louis, MO: Mosby; 2001.

DuBose TD, Santos RM. Vascular disorders of the kidney. In: Goldman L, Ausiello D, eds. *Cecil Medicine.* 23rd ed. Philadelphia, PA: Saunders; 2008.

Fitzgerald PA. Endocrine disorders. In: Tierney LM, McPhee SJ, Papadakis MA, eds. *Current Medical Diagnosis and Treatment.* 48th ed. New York, NY: McGraw-Hill; 2009.

Fukagawa M, Kurokawa K, Papadakis M. Fluid and electrolyte disorders. In: Tierney LM, McPhee SJ, Papadakis MA, eds. *Current Medical Diagnosis and Treatment.* 47th ed. New York, NY: McGraw-Hill; 2008.

Graff L. *A Handbook of Routine Urinalysis.* Philadelphia, PA: Lippincott Williams & Wilkins; 1983.

Guyton AC, Hall JE. *Textbook of Medical Physiology.* 11th ed. Philadelphia, PA: Saunders; 2006.

Ives HE. Diuretic agents. In: Katzung BG, ed. *Basic and Clinical Pharmacology.* 10th ed. New York, NY: McGraw-Hill; 2007.

Kumar V, Abbas AK, Fausto N, et al. *Robbins Basic Pathology.* 8th ed. Philadelphia, PA: Saunders; 2007.

Lederer E, Ouseph R, Yazel L. Hypokalemia. *eMedicine Nephrology;* March 20, 2007.

Lederer E, Ouseph R, Yazel L. Hyperphosphatemia. *eMedicine Nephrology;* April 5, 2007.

Levey AS. Clinical evaluation of renal function. In: Greenberg A, Coffman TM, Cheung AK, et al., eds. *Primer on Kidney Disease.* 2nd ed. San Diego, CA: Academic Press; 1998.

Levey AS. Bosch JP, Lewis JB, et al. A more accurate method to estimate glomerular filtration rate from serum creatinine: a new prediction equation. *Ann Intern Med.* 1999;130:461-470.

McBride L. *Textbook of Urinalysis and Body Fluids.* Philadelphia, PA: Lippincott Williams & Wilkins; 1998.

McMillan J. Merck Manual On-line, www.merck.com/ mmpe 2006-2008.

NKF-K/DOQI Clinical Practice Guidelines for Chronic Kidney Disease: Executive Summary. New York, NY: National Kidney Foundation; 2002.

Norrby SR. Approach to the patient with urinary tract infection. In: Goldman L, Ausiello D, eds. *Cecil Medicine* 23rd ed. Philadelphia, PA: Saunders; 2008.

Post TW, Rose BD. Urinalysis in the diagnosis of renal disease. In Rose BD, ed. *www.uptodate.com*, version 16.3; 2008.

Rugo HS. Cancer. In: Tierney LM, McPhee SJ, Papadakis MA, eds. *Current Medical Diagnosis and Treatment*, 48th ed. New York, NY: McGraw-Hill; 2009.

The seventh report of the Joint National Committee on Prevention, Detection, Evaluation, and Treatment of High Blood Pressure: the JNC 7 Report. *JAMA.* 2003; 289:2560-2572.

Stevens L, Perrone RD. Assessment of kidney function: serum creatinine; BUN; and GFR. In: Rose BD, ed. 2008. *http://www.uptodate.com*, version 16.3.

Stoller ML, Kane CJ, Meng MV. Urology. In: Tierney LM, McPhee SJ, Papadakis MA, eds. *Current Medical Diagnosis and Treatment.* 48th ed. New York, NY: McGraw-Hill; 2009.

Tolkoff-Rubin N. Treatment of irreversible renal failure. In: Goldman L, Ausiello D, eds. *Cecil Medicine.* 23rd ed. Philadelphia, PA: Saunders; 2008.

Watnick S, Morrison G. Kidney. In: Tierney LM, McPhee SJ, Papadakis MA, eds. *Current Medical Diagnosis and Treatment.* 48th ed. New York, NY: McGraw-Hill; 2009.

CHAPTER 10

Neurology

Mark E. Archambault, DHSc, PA-C

DIRECTIONS: Each of the numbered items or incomplete statements in this section is followed by answers or by completion of the statement. Select the ONE-lettered answer or completion that is BEST in each case.

1. A 6-year-old boy is struck by a car while riding his bicycle. He is reported to be unconscious for 2 minutes following the accident. He is conscious and alert upon arrival to the emergency department, but within 45 minutes he begins to vomit and shortly thereafter he becomes completely unresponsive. Which of the following most likely explains this child's injury?

   (A) spinal cord transection
   (B) chronic subdural hematoma
   (C) acute epidural hematoma
   (D) acute subarachnoid hemorrhage
   (E) grade III concussion

2. A 75-year-old man is involved in a motor vehicle accident and strikes his forehead on the windshield. He complains of neck pain and severe burning in his shoulders and arms. His physical examination reveals weakness of his upper extremities. What type of spinal cord injury does this patient have?

   (A) anterior cord syndrome
   (B) central cord syndrome
   (C) Brown–Séquard syndrome
   (D) complete cord transection
   (E) cauda equina syndrome

3. A 41-year-old woman presents to the emergency department complaining of a sudden onset of the "worst headache of my life." A stat computed tomography (CT) scan of her head is found to be normal. The next appropriate step in the diagnosis of this patient would be

   (A) outpatient magnetic resonance imaging (MRI) of the brain
   (B) complete blood cell count (CBC) with differential
   (C) injection of sumatriptan (Imitrex)
   (D) lumbar puncture
   (E) repeat CT scan in 48 hours

4. A 45-year-old woman with a known seizure disorder has been noncompliant with her anticonvulsant medication due to side effects she has been experiencing. While in your office, she starts convulsing at a frequency that does not allow consciousness. Which of the following is the most appropriate initial drug treatment?

   (A) lorazepam
   (B) phenytoin
   (C) phenobarbital
   (D) valproic acid

5. While performing a routine history and physical examination on a 70-year-old man, you note a right carotid bruit. He denies any symptoms suggestive of a transient ischemic attack (TIA) or cerebrovascular accident. A carotid Doppler ultrasound shows a 50% stenosis of the right common carotid artery. The next most appropriate step would be

   (A) stat carotid arteriogram
   (B) initiate antiplatelet therapy with aspirin
   (C) anticoagulate with warfarin
   (D) intra-arterial tissue plasminogen activator (t-PA)
   (E) carotid endarterectomy

6. A cerebrospinal fluid analysis reveals the following results: opalescent color, increased protein, decreased glucose, and increased polymorphonuclear white blood cells (WBCs). The most likely diagnosis would be

   (A) subarachnoid hemorrhage
   (B) bacterial meningitis
   (C) viral meningitis
   (D) multiple sclerosis
   (E) encephalitis

7. A 45-year-old man presents to the office with a 24-hour history of right facial droop, slurred speech, and drooling from the right side of his mouth. On examination, the patient is found to have a right facial droop, and he is unable to close his right eye and raise his right eyebrow. The remainder of the physical examination is completely normal. What would be the most appropriate therapy at this time?

   (A) prednisone for 1 week and reevaluate in office
   (B) stat CT scan of the head and neurology consult
   (C) obtain Lyme disease titers
   (D) aspirin

8. A 30-year-old man presents complaining of back pain radiating down his right leg. On examination, you note that his knee jerk reflex is absent on the right. This finding suggests compression of which spinal nerve root?

   (A) L1–L2
   (B) L3–L4
   (C) S1–S2
   (D) T11–T12
   (E) C5–C6

9. A 62-year-old obese woman presents with progressive numbness and tingling in her feet for the past 3 months. On physical examination, the patient is found to have decreased sensation to pinprick and vibration, absence of ankle reflexes, and difficulty with tandem walking. Which is the most common etiology of her symptoms?

   (A) diabetes mellitus
   (B) alcoholism
   (C) vitamin B_{12} deficiency
   (D) spinal cord tumor
   (E) rheumatoid arthritis

10. A 19-year-old woman presents to the emergency department complaining of headache. The headaches are generalized and increasing in intensity. They have not responded to over-the-counter (OTC) medications. She complains of approximately 1 week of blurred vision, intermittent diplopia, and vague dizziness. Her medical history includes obesity and acne. She takes Accutane and oral contraceptives. She is found to have bilateral papilledema, visual acuity of 20/30 on physical examination, and a normal MRI of the brain. The next most appropriate step would be

    (A) CT scan of the head
    (B) lumbar puncture
    (C) therapy with high-dose prednisone
    (D) stat cerebral arteriogram
    (E) reassurance and follow-up in the office in 6 months

11. A 12-year-old, left-hand dominant girl is being evaluated for "spells" that she has been experiencing. According to her parents, she was born following an uncomplicated pregnancy and was a healthy child until last year when she was struck by a drunk driver when she was walking home from a friend's house. The

episodes begin by her complaining of an upset stomach and then she appears confused, turns her head to the left, and raises her left arm in the air. Each episode lasts for about 30 to 60 seconds, after which she is very tired for another hour. This scenario best describes which type of seizure disorder?

(A) absence
(B) tonic–clonic
(C) simple partial
(D) complex partial
(E) pseudoseizures

12. A 65-year-old man presents to the emergency department with an acute ischemic stroke. His CT scan is normal. His blood pressure is 180/100 mm Hg. What is the most appropriate treatment for his hypertension?

(A) labetalol (Normodyne) 20 mg IV
(B) nifedipine (Procardia) 10 mg po
(C) nitroprusside (Nipride) drip at 1 mg/kg/min
(D) clonidine (Catapres) 0.1 mg po
(E) no antihypertensive at this time

13. A 78-year-old woman presents to the office complaining of a constant left-sided headache for 2 months. She has tried various over-the-counter (OTC) medications without relief. The patient admits to vision loss of her left eye last night for 10 minutes. The patient states that her vision then returned to normal. She denies pain in her eye. On review of systems, she relates several months of muscle aches and weight loss. On physical examination, she is found to have a tender, nonpulsatile superficial temporal artery. Her sedimentation rate is elevated at 90 mm/h. What is the next most appropriate step in the evaluation of this patient?

(A) stat MRI/MRA of the brain and cranial vessels
(B) aspirin therapy
(C) high-dose prednisone

(D) lumbar puncture
(E) sumatriptan (Imitrex) injection

14. A 28-year-old man presents with a complaint of new-onset headache. The pain awakens him early in the morning and is described as a sharp, lancinating pain around his right eye, which is 9 out of 10. When he looks in the mirror he notices tearing of his right eye as well as redness and a different sized pupil compared to the left. The pain lasts only for a few minutes but can recur later in the morning. This has happened for the past several days. The patient has a history of recurrent headaches that follow this pattern and usually last for 5 to 7 days. Prior to this occurrence it has been 4 years since his last episode. Which of the following is the most appropriate preventive treatment the patient should be offered at this time?

(A) sumatriptan (Imitrex)
(B) dihydroergotamine
(C) verapamil (Calan)
(D) oral corticosteroids
(E) oxygen

15. An otherwise healthy 16-year-old girl presents to your office with a complaint of headache. Reportedly, this is the second time she has experienced such a headache, the last time being last month. The pain builds up over several hours to 9 out of 10 and can last into the next day. It is holocephalic and throbs when she moves. She has to stop what she is doing to go lay down in a dark and quiet room or she vomits. No over-the-counter medications that she tried have worked. Her history is consistent with which of the following?

(A) migraine with aura
(B) cluster headache
(C) tension-type headache
(D) migraine without aura
(E) medication withdrawal headache

16. A 20-month-old boy is brought into the emergency department by his parents. They state he has not been feeling well for 2 days and this morning noted he was "shaking all over" and was not responding to commands. This went on for less than 10 minutes and has never happened before. His current rectal temperature is 100.7°F. The seizures are characteristic of

    (A) absence seizures
    (B) Lennox–Gastaut syndrome
    (C) febrile seizures
    (D) infantile spasms
    (E) juvenile myoclonic epilepsy

17. After a carotid endarterectomy, a patient experienced a unilateral small pupil, mild ptosis with normal response to light and accommodation. This abnormality is called

    (A) Adie pupil
    (B) Argyll Robertson pupil
    (C) Horner syndrome
    (D) Marcus Gunn pupil
    (E) light-near dissociation

18. A previously healthy, 27-year-old woman experiences an episode of vision loss in her left eye. She states it developed over hours and was like she was "looking through fog." The vision in her right eye was never affected. She denies any paresthesia, weakness, or bladder dysfunction. The sight in her left eye improved after several days but has not returned to baseline. Which of the following is the most likely diagnosis?

    (A) diabetic retinopathy
    (B) pseudotumor cerebri
    (C) amaurosis fugax
    (D) multiple sclerosis
    (E) carotid artery dissection

19. A 73-year-old man is brought into your office by his adult children with a concern of memory loss. They report their father's memory has been declining since the death of their mother a few months ago but are now concerned because he is losing weight, sleeping during the daytime, and is not keeping up with current events like he usually does. This type of behavior is most associated with which of the following?

    (A) Pick disease
    (B) Creutzfeldt–Jakob disease
    (C) depression
    (D) Alzheimer disease
    (E) vitamin B_{12} deficiency

20. A postural tremor that occurs at rest and may be exacerbated by fear, anxiety, excessive physical activity, or sleep deprivation is consistent with which of the following?

    (A) Wilson disease
    (B) intention tremor
    (C) asterixis
    (D) physiologic tremor
    (E) hemiballismus

21. Which of the following is the most appropriate initial disease-modifying treatment for a patient diagnosed with multiple sclerosis?

    (A) beta-interferon
    (B) methylprednisone
    (C) methotrexate
    (D) natalizumab

22. A 62-year-old man presents to the emergency department with aphasia and right lower extremity weakness that started about 4 hours ago. He now has progressing right upper extremity weakness, worsening right lower extremity weakness, and decreased sensation throughout his right side. This cerebral ischemia is best characterized as

    (A) transient ischemic attack
    (B) stroke in evolution
    (C) completed stroke
    (D) subarachnoid hemorrhage
    (E) global cerebral ischemia

23. A 58-year-old man presents to your office with a complaint of tremor in his right hand. Upon questioning, you discover that the tremor is

getting worse and he is having trouble eating with a fork and buttoning his shirt. On your physical examination, you notice bradykinesia, rigidity, and a shuffling gait. What is your initial assessment?

(A) essential tremor

(B) Wilson disease

(C) Huntington disease

(D) Parkinson disease

(E) progressive supranuclear palsy

24. A 55-year-old right-hand dominant man presents with a 4-hour history of weakness and tingling of his right hand and numbness of the right side of his mouth. Mild difficulty was noted with word finding. His symptoms have improved since onset but have not fully resolved. There is no significant medical history. Physical examination revealed flat right nasolabial fold, subjective numbness of the right hand, right pronator drift, clumsiness of finger tapping on the right hand, increased deep tendon reflexes on the right, as well as a present Babinski. What is the most likely etiology for this patient's problem?

(A) migraine headache

(B) peripheral neuropathy

(C) syncope

(D) transient ischemic attack

(E) seizure

25. A 65-year-old man is brought to the clinic by his family because he has taken to wandering the streets. For the past 6 months he has been increasingly forgetful of names and places. He has become listless and has lost interest in his usual hobbies. Recently, his decline has accelerated. This patient is most likely experiencing

(A) depression

(B) delirium

(C) hypothyroidism

(D) normal pressure hydrocephalus

(E) Alzheimer dementia

26. A 52-year-old male bus driver presents to the clinic with a chief complaint of intense, shooting pains in his left cheek, each lasting for only a few seconds. He avoids touching certain parts of his face and has started to chew food only on the right side of his mouth because he is afraid he will set off an attack of pain. In between attacks, the patient feels well. What is the most likely diagnosis?

(A) cluster headache

(B) tension-type headache

(C) trigeminal neuralgia

(D) giant cell arteritis

(E) dental abscess

27. A 22-year-old woman, with no previous medical problems, suddenly cried out, fell to the ground, extended her legs, flexed her arms, and jerked her extremities for 30 seconds. There was associated tongue biting and urinary incontinence. She awoke slowly over a 10-minute period and recalled nothing about the episode. She remained lethargic for several hours but the rest of her neurologic examination was normal. What is the most likely etiology for this episode?

(A) epilepsy

(B) hyperventilation

(C) cardiac arrhythmia

(D) seizure

(E) stroke

28. The physical examination test of placing a vibrating tuning fork in the middle of a patient's forehead to test for sensorineural hearing loss is called

(A) Rinne

(B) Tinel

(C) Dix-Hallpike

(D) Babinski

(E) Weber

29. A 36-year-old auto mechanic presents to the emergency department after hurting his back on the job. While lifting an object, he experienced sudden pain in his lower back with radiation to the right buttock. He was initially treated for muscle strain with a nonsteroidal anti-inflammatory drug (NSAID) after x-rays of his lumbosacral spine demonstrated no pathology. He continued to complain of this low back pain now radiating posteriorly down his left leg to the mid-thigh. Physical examination is unremarkable. The most likely diagnosis is

    (A) lumbosacral strain
    (B) left S1 radiculopathy
    (C) cauda equina syndrome
    (D) L5–S1 disc herniation
    (E) lateral femoral cutaneous neuropathy

30. A 35-year-old woman presents with a 4-month history of dysarthria and muscle fatigue. She works as a nurse and at the end of her workday she notices profound difficulty enunciating her words and producing a full smile. These symptoms resolve after rest. On physical examination, you notice ptosis of the left eyelid on prolonged upgaze and progressive dysarthria while speaking. What is the most likely diagnosis?

    (A) multiple sclerosis
    (B) amyotrophic lateral sclerosis
    (C) herpes zoster
    (D) myasthenia gravis
    (E) Guillain–Barré syndrome

31. A 48-year-old woman presents with new-onset headache that she describes as nonspecific, worse on awakening, intermittent throughout the day but can worsen with bending over or coughing. Her husband reports that she has not been herself since the headaches started about 4 to 6 weeks ago. Which of the following tests would be best for determining the etiology of her presenting symptoms?

    (A) noncontrast head CT scan
    (B) lumbar puncture
    (C) contrast-enhanced brain MRI

    (D) noncontrast brain MRI
    (E) cerebral angiography

32. An 18-year-old woman is transferred to your emergency department from a local college infirmary. She presented yesterday with a complaint of headache but became confused and is now febrile. You notice a petechial rash on physical examination and her cerebrospinal fluid comes back with increased WBCs, increased protein, and decreased glucose. What is the most likely organism responsible for her meningitis?

    (A) *Haemophilus influenzae*
    (B) cytomegalovirus
    (C) *Neisseria meningitidis*
    (D) *Mycobacterium tuberculosis*
    (E) coxsackievirus B

33. Huntington disease is a movement disorder characterized by involuntary writhing of muscle groups. It consists of a clinical triad that includes the following:

    (A) progressive dementia, chorea, and a pattern of inheritance
    (B) progressive dementia, tremor, and a pattern of inheritance
    (C) depression, tremor, and a pattern of inheritance
    (D) depression, chorea, and a pattern of inheritance

34. An otherwise healthy 20-year-old man has been given the accurate diagnosis of migraine. His frequency of attack is about one per month. He has never experienced adequate relief with any over-the-counter analgesics. Which of the following would be appropriate to try next?

    (A) verapamil 120 mg once daily
    (B) amitriptyline 25 mg once nightly
    (C) codeine/acetaminophen 15 mg prn
    (D) rizatriptan 10 mg at onset, may repeat once in 2 hours
    (E) oxygen at 7 L/min inhaled via nonrebreather mask

35. Which of the following is the most common etiology for a subarachnoid hemorrhage?

(A) trauma

(B) ruptured aneurysm

(C) bleeding arteriovenous malformation

(D) embolic stroke

(E) primary intracerebral hemorrhage

36. A 34-year-old man presents to your office with the complaint of pain and fatigue in his right wrist. He states that the pain can sometimes wake him up at night and feels as if his thumb is falling asleep. He reports the problem started since he has been writing a book. On physical examination, you note a positive Tinel sign but no response to a Phalen maneuver. While sending him for a nerve conduction study, you tell him the most likely diagnosis is

(A) ulnar nerve compression

(B) radial nerve compression

(C) thoracic outlet syndrome

(D) median nerve compression

(E) peroneal nerve compression

37. A 63-year-old woman with a medical history of type II diabetes, hypertension, obesity, and dyslipidemia presents to the clinic complaining of burning pain in her feet bilaterally. Neurological examination is normal except for hyperesthesia and loss of vibratory sensation bilaterally in her feet. Which of the following is the preferred treatment for managing this patient's pain?

(A) amitriptyline

(B) celecoxib (Celebrex)

(C) oxycodone (OxyContin)

(D) vitamin D

(E) ibuprofen (Motrin)

38. A 43-year-old woman presents complaining of a "pins and needles" sensation that started bilaterally in her feet 2 days ago. The sensation now extends up to her mid-thighs. On physical examination, she is noted to have mild sensory loss, weakness, and absent reflexes bilaterally in her legs. Which of the following is the most likely diagnosis?

(A) diabetic peripheral neuropathy

(B) Guillain–Barré syndrome

(C) multiple sclerosis

(D) myasthenia gravis

(E) hypothyroidism

39. A 53-year-old man presents to the emergency department because of fever, headache, and confusion. On physical examination, you note an obtunded man who appears acutely ill with temperature of 104°F, blood pressure of 128/76 mm Hg, pulse of 98, and respiratory rate of 20. The patient has stomatitis, nuchal rigidity, and a positive Kernig sign. CSF examination shows increased opening pressure, 80 WBC/mL (normal < 10/mL), mildly elevated protein, and normal glucose. Which of the following tests would confirm the most likely causative organism?

(A) CT of the head

(B) polymerase chain reaction test for herpes simplex virus

(C) blood culture for herpes simplex virus

(D) serum IgG for herpes simplex virus

(E) MRI of the head

40. A 62-year-old man is brought to the emergency department after being found unresponsive in his car. On physical examination, his pupils are noted to be 7 mm on the right and 3 mm on the left. Which of the following diagnostic tests is most likely to identify the cause of the patient's signs and symptoms?

(A) CBC with differential

(B) serum electrolytes

(C) MRI with contrast

(D) liver function tests

(E) skull X-rays

41. A 38-year-old woman presents with a history of frequent headaches that begin behind her right eye and are associated with a visual aura, photophobia, and phonophobia. She feels her headaches are worse due to job-related stress and insomnia. She is having six to eight instances of headache a month. Her medical history is remarkable for exercise-induced asthma. Which of the following agents is the best prophylactic agent for this patient?

    (A) amitriptyline (Elavil)
    (B) celecoxib (Celebrex)
    (C) propranolol (Inderal)
    (D) sumatriptan (Imitrex)
    (E) butalbital/caffeine (Midrin)

42. An 11-year-old boy is diagnosed with a new onset of absence seizures. Which of the following medications is the best initial treatment option for this patient?

    (A) carbamazepine (Tegretol)
    (B) phenytoin (Dilantin)
    (C) phenobarbital
    (D) valproic acid (Depakote)
    (E) topiramate (Topamax)

43. A 3-year-old girl is being followed by the neurologist to evaluate her motor spasticity that resulted from anoxia during labor and delivery. Which of the following is the most likely cause of this patient's spasticity?

    (A) cerebral palsy
    (B) congenital hypothyroidism
    (C) meningitis
    (D) multiple sclerosis

44. During physical examination, a 58-year-old man is instructed to hold his hands up as if he were attempting to stop traffic. After about 20 seconds of observation his wrists intermittently flex and return to extension. This physical examination sign is known as

    (A) asterixis
    (B) Brudzinski sign
    (C) clonus
    (D) stereognosis

45. A 16-year-old girl presents to the clinic complaining of strong desires to sleep at inappropriate times. She is very concerned because she "felt paralyzed" while falling asleep on the couch last night. Which of the following is the best diagnostic test to confirm this patient's diagnosis?

    (A) CT of the head
    (B) multiple sleep latency test
    (C) Tensilon test
    (D) thyroid stimulating hormone
    (E) polysomnography

46. A 12-year-old boy presents to the clinic for follow-up regarding his recently diagnosed partial seizures. He reports no seizures or side effects since starting carbamazepine (Tegretol) 1 month ago. What study should be ordered to monitor this patient's treatment?

    (A) blood glucose
    (B) complete blood cell count
    (C) electroencephalogram
    (D) vitamin B_{12}
    (E) urinalysis

47. Which of the following findings is consistent with a lower motor neuron deficit?

    (A) aphasia
    (B) dysdiadochokinesia
    (C) sensory loss
    (D) weakness
    (E) hyperreflexia

48. A 78-year-old woman with a medical history of diabetes and hypertension presents to the emergency department complaining of left hand weakness and slurred speech. Which of the following tests is most likely to determine the source of an arterial thrombus?

    (A) carotid ultrasound
    (B) CT of the brain
    (C) erythrocyte sedimentation rate
    (D) magnetic resonance angiography (MRA) of the vertebral arteries

Answers and Explanations

1. **(C)** This is the classic history of an epidural hematoma. The typical presentation is that of a child who sustains a hard blow to the head and experiences a brief loss of consciousness, followed by a lucid interval, when the child is awake and alert. As the hematoma expands, the patient experiences a headache followed by vomiting, lethargy, and hemiparesis and may progress to coma if left untreated. This injury usually results from a temporal bone fracture with a laceration of the middle meningeal artery or vein and less often a tear in a dural venous sinus. Epidural hematomas are treated with surgical evacuation of the clot and ligation of the bleeding vessel. Spinal cord transection should not present initially as a loss of consciousness and will affect distal motor and sensory function. Chronic subdural hematomas present more than 20 days after the trauma. Subarachnoid hemorrhage typically presents as a generalized headache without associated trauma. A grade III concussion usually involves continued improvement after consciousness is gained. The lucid period followed by worsening symptoms in this question is worrisome of more severe intracranial pathology. *(Aminoff et al., 2005, p. 329)*

2. **(B)** The central cord syndrome involves loss of motor function that is more severe in the upper extremities than in the lower extremities, and is more severe in the hands. There is typically hyperesthesia over the shoulders and arms. Anterior cord syndrome presents with paraplegia or quadriplegia, loss of lateral spinothalamic function with preservation of posterior column function. Brown–Séquard syndrome consists of weakness and loss of posterior column function on one side of the body distal to the lesion with contralateral loss of lateral spinothalamic function one to two levels below the lesion. Complete cord transection would affect motor and sensory function distal to the lesion. Cauda equina syndrome typically presents as low back pain with radiculopathy. *(Hauser and Ropper, 2008, p. 2580)*

3. **(D)** The hallmark of a subarachnoid hemorrhage is the very sudden onset of a severe headache. The headache is often described as the "worst headache of my life." A CT scan will detect a subarachnoid hemorrhage in more than 95% of cases. When the history suggests subarachnoid hemorrhage and the CT scan fails to detect bleeding, a lumbar puncture is mandatory. The lumbar puncture will yield bloody cerebrospinal fluid in subarachnoid hemorrhage. Outpatient MRI or repeat CT scan in 48 hours would create a potentially harmful delay in diagnosis. CBC with differential may be ordered but will not confirm the suspected diagnosis. Treatment with Imitrex is contraindicated in the presence of a potential cerebrovascular syndrome. *(Hemphill and Smith, 2008, p. 1728)*

4. **(A)** Status epilepticus, defined as a continuous seizure or repeated seizures in which interval consciousness is not obtained, is a medical emergency. An intravenous infusion of a longer acting benzodiazepine, such as lorazepam, has been shown to be effective in terminating a seizure. If the seizures persist, then other potential agents to use after the initial lorazepam infusion include fosphenytoin (phenytoin) or valproic acid (phenobarbital). *(Lowenstein, 2008, p. 2511)*

5. **(B)** The patient exhibits an asymptomatic carotid bruit. The most appropriate step would be to initiate antiplatelet therapy with daily aspirin. Arteriography would not be indicated for an asymptomatic carotid bruit. Anticoagulation with warfarin (Coumadin) should be limited to symptomatic bruits manifested as multiple TIAs. Carotid endarterectomy is reserved for carotid stenosis that is greater than 70% in patients who have had recurrent TIAs on medical therapy. *(Aminoff et al., 2005, pp. 308-310)*

6. **(B)** The cerebrospinal fluid (CSF) analysis in bacterial meningitis includes a cloudy appearance with a markedly elevated protein and white cell content. The white cells are predominantly polymorphonuclear leukocytes (polys). Bacterial utilization of CSF glucose causes it to be low. Gram stain may or may not be positive for bacteria. The diagnosis of bacterial meningitis requires a culture of the CSF. CSF pressures at the time of the lumbar puncture are elevated in 90% of cases. In viral meningitis, the CSF white count is usually 1,000/mL. The cell types are lymphocytes or monocytes but early in the disease polys may predominate. CSF glucose is normal in viral meningitis and protein is elevated. Gram stain will be negative and the culture will show no growth. The CSF in multiple sclerosis may have a mild lymphocytosis with an increased protein concentration. CSF protein electrophoresis in multiple sclerosis shows discrete bands of IgG called *oligoclonal bands*. These oligoclonal bands are present in 90% of patients with multiple sclerosis. The CSF in subarachnoid hemorrhage is grossly bloody. Because bleeding can be caused by a traumatic puncture, the red blood cell (RBC) count should be done on the first and last tubes and the counts compared. In subarachnoid hemorrhage, the RBC count will be the same, whereas in a traumatic lumbar puncture, the RBCs will not be present in the last tube that is collected. The CSF in subarachnoid hemorrhage may reveal xanthochromia. This is a yellow appearance in the centrifuged CSF supernatant caused by the degradation of RBCs in the CSF. The CSF becomes xanthochromic after it has been exposed to blood for several hours. *(Aminoff et al., 2005, p. 12)*

7. **(A)** This is a typical presentation of Bell's palsy. Bell's palsy is an idiopathic facial nerve palsy that results in unilateral weakness or paralysis of the facial muscles. This results in facial drooping, slurred speech, drooling, as well as an inability to close the eye and to raise the affected eyebrow. Facial weakness caused by a stroke does not affect the ability to close the affected eye or to move the forehead. This weakness is characteristic of peripheral seventh nerve palsy. In a stroke, there are often other abnormalities beyond the facial nerve. Bell's palsy is often preceded or accompanied by pain around the ear. It is more common in pregnancy and diabetes. It is believed that starting prednisone within 5 days of the onset of symptoms increases the number of patients who recover completely. The weakness or paralysis is usually maximal between 2 and 5 days. Eighty percent of patients recover in several weeks. In some cases, it may take up to 2 months to resolve. Improvement in facial motor function within the first 5 to 7 days is the most favorable prognostic sign. A CT scan of the head and neurologic consult are not indicated in this patient. Lyme disease would be a rare cause of facial nerve paralysis and is not part of the routine evaluation for it. Aspirin is not indicated, since this is not caused by cerebrovascular disease. *(Aminoff et al., 2005, p. 182)*

8. **(B)** Absence of the knee jerk reflex suggests compression of the L3–L4 spinal nerve root. The four most commonly tested deep tendon reflexes are the Achilles (ankle jerk) reflex, quadriceps (knee jerk) reflex, triceps reflex, and the biceps reflex. The nerve roots that each tests in ascending order are 1 and 2, 3 and 4, 5 and 6 (biceps), and 7 and 8 (triceps). One only needs to remember that the ankle jerk is a sacral nerve root, the knee jerk is a lumbar nerve root, and the biceps and triceps are cervical nerve roots. *(Aminoff et al., 2005, p. 367)*

9. **(A)** Peripheral neuropathy is a syndrome that is manifested by muscle weakness, paresthesias, decreased deep tendon reflexes, and autonomic disturbances most commonly in the hands and feet, such as coldness and sweating. There are many causes of peripheral neuropathy ranging

from metabolic conditions to malignant neoplasm, rheumatoid arthritis, and drug and alcohol use. The increase in non-insulin–dependent diabetes mellitus due to obesity in the American population has increased the incidence of associated disease states. *(Aminoff et al., 2005, pp. 213-214)*

10. **(B)** The presence of headache associated with papilledema raises the concern for a brain tumor. The MRI excluded a mass lesion, raising a strong suspicion of pseudotumor cerebri. This is also known as *benign intracranial hypertension*. It is not a benign condition, however, since it causes severe headache and may result in visual loss. It is particularly frequent in obese adolescent girls and young women. The etiology is unknown but may be associated with the use of oral contraceptives, vitamin A, and tetracycline. The presentation consists of headaches caused by an increase in intracranial pressure and blurring of vision. There may be diplopia, but the remainder of the neurologic examination is unremarkable. Papilledema is virtually always part of the presentation. The mental status is normal. The differential diagnosis includes venous sinus thrombosis, sarcoidosis, and tuberculosis or carcinomatous meningitis. The last two are excluded by lumbar puncture. An abnormal cerebrospinal fluid is not consistent with pseudotumor cerebri. The diagnosis is made by excluding mass lesions with CT scan or MRI and demonstrating markedly increased intracranial pressure by lumbar puncture. The treatment involves weight loss, diuretics, and steroids. Repeat lumbar punctures to remove cerebrospinal fluid and decrease intracranial pressure are effective. In cases that are unresponsive to these measures, lumbar-peritoneal shunting is effective, as is unilateral optic nerve sheath fenestration. Effective treatment can improve headaches and prevent vision loss. *(Horton, 2008, p. 188)*

11. **(D)** Complex partial seizures are usually preceded by some type of sensory aura. This is followed by an impairment of consciousness but not total loss of consciousness along with an involuntary motor activity. The seizure will resolve in about 30 minutes and is followed by postictal confusion. Simple partial seizures have no alteration of consciousness. Absence and tonic–clonic seizures are generalized seizure disorders in which consciousness is lost. Absence seizures are characterized by staring spells without motor involvement, whereas tonic–clonic seizures involve strong muscle extension and contraction in many major muscle groups. Pseudoseizures are a diagnosis of exclusion. All tests results including an electroencephalogram (EEG) are normal, and the seizures may be a manifestation of an underlying psychiatric disturbance. *(Aminoff et al., 2005, pp. 267-278)*

12. **(E)** Blood pressure is typically elevated at the time of presentation in acute ischemic stroke. It will decline without medication in the first few hours to days. Aggressively lowering blood pressure in an acute ischemic stroke may decrease the blood flow to the ischemic but salvageable brain tissue. This potentially salvageable brain tissue is referred to as the *penumbra*. Decreasing blood flow to the ischemic penumbra by acutely lowering blood pressure may result in eventual infarction of this brain tissue. Treatment of previously undiagnosed hypertension should be deferred for several days. Blood pressure should be treated if there are other indications, such as angina or heart failure. Control of blood pressure is appropriate in patients who are receiving tissue plasminogen activator (t-Pa) for their stroke. Blood pressure should be lowered cautiously to a systolic of less than 185 mm Hg and a diastolic of less than 110 mm Hg. This is thought to decrease the incidence of intracerebral hemorrhage in these patients. *(Wells et al., 2009, p. 158)*

13. **(C)** The diagnosis is temporal arteritis. This is an arteritis of the temporal branch of the external carotid artery characterized by unilateral or bilateral headaches that may be localized to a tender temporal artery. The temporal artery may be thickened and tender and may be thrombosed and nonpulsatile late in the disease. Many patients present with malaise and have anemia and a low-grade fever. Fifty percent of patients report generalized muscle aches consistent with polymyalgia rheumatica.

The most severe complication of temporal arteritis is blindness resulting from thrombosis of the ophthalmic artery. In some cases, this may be preceded by previous episodes of amaurosis fugax before the blindness becomes irreversible. Once blindness occurs in one eye, it may be prevented in the other by initiating treatment. The diagnosis is based on recognizing the clinical picture and obtaining a temporal artery biopsy. Treatment should not be delayed pending the biopsy. Early treatment with prednisone may prevent irreversible blindness. The efficacy of treatment can be measured with serial sedimentation rates. MRI and MRA have no value in establishing the diagnosis of temporal arteritis. Antiplatelet therapy would not be inappropriate but is inadequate for this diagnosis. The potentially unilateral headache should not be confused with a migraine for which Imitrex therapy would be appropriate. In addition, lumbar puncture has no role in establishing this diagnosis. *(Langford and Fauci, 2008, p. 2127)*

14. **(D)** Oral corticosteroids started immediately will often force a cluster cycle into remission and prevent future headaches. The infrequent recurrence pattern of the cluster headaches does not support the chronic use of verapamil. Sumatriptan, dihydroergotamine, and oxygen are very useful abortive agents but do not work on stopping the cluster cycle. Both sumatriptan and dihydroergotamine have maximum daily doses and may not be used for all attacks during the day as some cluster patients may have multiple attacks throughout the day. *(Aminoff et al., 2005, pp. 90-91)*

15. **(D)** The history is consistent with migraine without aura. Migraine is a headache that is defined by a pain that is usually unilateral, is pounding or will take on a pounding quality with activity, can be made worse with physical activity, is associated with both light and sound sensitivity, and is associated with nausea and/or vomiting. If the headache is preceded by an abnormal sensory experience such as a visual disturbance that lasts no longer than 60 minutes and totally remits, it is classified as a migraine with aura. Cluster headaches are usually unilateral as well but tend to be periorbital and are of shorter duration but greater intensity, often described as a stabbing pain. In addition, patients may experience ipsilateral autonomic symptoms such as lacrimation, rhinorrhea, and ptosis. Tension-type headaches are mostly due to contraction of cranial and cervical muscles and are described as bilateral, tight, or squeezing in nature, and are sometimes relieved by physical activity. Medication withdrawal headaches typically present as daily, constant headaches. *(Aminoff et al., 2005, pp. 85-92)*

16. **(C)** Febrile seizures can occur in children younger than 5 years when accompanied by a fever. They are characterized by a brief generalized motor seizure. Absence seizures are generalized seizures characterized by a loss of consciousness without motor involvement, typically seen in older children. Lenox–Gastaut syndrome presents in childhood as well but is usually associated with developmental delay and seizures of akinetic and myoclonic nature (referred to as drop attacks). Infantile spasms occur without relation to systemic illness and are massive myoclonic events with bending at the waist. Juvenile myoclonic epilepsy evolves in the teenage years and is characterized by repeated episodes of myoclonic seizure activity. *(Aminoff et al., 2005, p. 265)*

17. **(C)** Horner syndrome is defined by a unilateral, small pupil with mild ptosis in which pupillary response to light and accommodation is preserved. It may also be associated with ipsilateral anhydrosis. It is usually caused by some interruption in the oculosympathetic pathway. An Adie pupil is characterized by a unilateral dilated pupil that is sluggish to direct light stimuli. An Argyll Robertson pupil usually affects both eyes, is irregular in shape, and is poorly reactive to light. A Marcus Gunn pupil constricts slower to direct light stimulation than to the consensual stimulation. Light-near dissociation is usually bilateral and consists of preserved constriction to accommodation but impaired response to light. *(Aminoff et al., 2005, pp. 138-139)*

18. **(D)** Multiple sclerosis is a demyelinating disease that is thought to have an autoimmune

pathophysiology. The presenting symptoms of multiple sclerosis are highly variable but can include focal weakness, paresthesia, or visual disturbance. Once the patient experiences a set of symptoms, they may improve but will not return to baseline function. The visual loss associated with diabetic retinopathy is usually bilateral. Pseudotumor cerebri is often accompanied by headache and presents as diplopia. Amaurosis fugax is unilateral but will resolve over 10 to 20 minutes and is caused by an embolic source. Carotid artery dissection can also cause unilateral vision loss but is usually total and followed by other, more severe, neurologic deficits. (*Aminoff et al., 2005, pp. 164-167, 293*)

19. **(C)** This patient's symptoms are most consistent with situational depression over the loss of his spouse. Transient memory problems can be a component of depression as a result of decreased attention and interest. Dementia is a progressive impairment of higher cognitive function, and initially, the patient's social graces are preserved. It has many causes, of which Pick disease, Creutzfeldt–Jakob disease, and Alzheimer disease are irreversible. Vitamin B_{12} deficiency can cause reversible form of cognitive impairment, in which the elderly are susceptible, so serum analysis of vitamin B_{12} should be performed in diagnostic evaluations of dementia in this population. (*Aminoff et al., 2005, pp. 44-51*)

20. **(D)** Physiologic tremor is a postural tremor that may be exacerbated by the factors outlined in this question. Both asterixis and intention tremor are also postural tremors; however, asterixis is seen in the context of metabolic encephalopathy and intention tremor during activity. Wilson disease occurs with other abnormal cerebellar findings. Hemiballismus is a choreiform movement disorder and not an oscillatory movement. (*Aminoff et al., 2005, pp. 234-236*)

21. **(A)** The goal of the treatment of multiple sclerosis is to reduce the frequency and severity of recurrent attacks. Most data agree that the use of beta-interferons as early as possible in the diagnosis of multiple sclerosis is the treatment of choice for attaining this goal. Corticosteroids may be used to lessen the severity of an acute attack but have not been shown to be effective in suppressing further attacks. Methotrexate and natalizumab are not first-line agents. The use of amantadine and physical therapy can help with energy and mobility issues. (*Hauser and Goodin, 2008, pp. 2618-2619*)

22. **(B)** During a stroke in evolution, symptoms will worsen or new symptoms will appear. A completed stroke is one in which neurologic symptoms have stabilized, whereas a transient ischemic attack produces deficits that resolve over time. This patient's symptoms do not match those of an acute subarachnoid hemorrhage. Global cerebral ischemia as seen in sudden cardiac arrest would involve loss of consciousness. (*Aminoff et al., 2005, pp. 286-297*)

23. **(D)** The symptoms of tremor, bradykinesia, and rigidity are classic for Parkinson disease. Difficulty with activities of daily living will usually prompt a patient to seek medical attention. Essential tremor and Wilson disease are postural tremors with different characteristics than the tremor seen in Parkinson disease. Huntington disease produces choreiform movements and has a much earlier age of onset. Progressive supranuclear palsy is characterized by an ophthalmoplegia in addition to tremor. (*Aminoff et al., 2005, pp. 241-250*)

24. **(D)** Three key features of a transient ischemic attack include sudden onset and complete reversal of symptoms within 24 hours, usually within 15 minutes. The symptoms are usually in the anatomical distribution of a single blood vessel. This patient's history is not suggestive of migraine or syncope. His physical examination findings do not correlate with peripheral neuropathy or seizure. (*Aminoff et al., 2005, p. 286*)

25. **(E)** This presentation is classic for Alzheimer dementia. There is a global decrease in mentation, which is chronic yet relatively stable. His symptoms are not fluctuating as is usually seen in delirium. There is no history of urinary incontinence, which would suggest normal

pressure hydrocephalus. Depression is a possibility along with his dementia. There are no other historical or examination findings suggestive of hypothyroidism. *(Aminoff et al., 2005, pp. 47-49)*

26. **(C)** Trigeminal neuralgia is characterized by sharp, brief pain often described as "shooting, jabbing, electric shock, or stabbing." The history given for cluster headache (typically ipsilateral ocular headaches with tearing, and lasting for 2 hours) and tension-type headache is not at all like this patient's. The history for temporal arteritis is generally different, as it typically includes ocular symptoms, but it may be worth getting a sedimentation rate just to be sure. This location pain pattern is different than that of a focal dental problem. *(Beal and Hauser, 2008, pp. 2583)*

27. **(D)** This event represents a well-demarcated episode affecting some combination of consciousness, motor, and/or sensory function consequent to abnormal electrical discharges in the brain. This is consistent with the definition of a seizure. Epilepsy refers to multiple, recurrent seizures. This history is not consistent with hyperventilation, stroke, or cardiac arrhythmia, which would typically include chest pain, shortness of breath, dyspnea on exertion, or focal neurological deficits. *(Aminoff et al., 2005, p. 265)*

28. **(E)** The test described is the Weber. Rinne is also used to assess sensorineural hearing loss but is performed by placing a vibrating tuning fork on the mastoid process. Once the patient states the noise is no longer heard, the examiner places the tuning fork by the ipsilateral ear. The patient should still hear the vibratory noise. Tinel is a test for nerve compression where the examiner taps over the nerve to elicit paresthesia. Dix-Hallpike is a maneuver to test for positional vertigo. Babinski is a pathological response to the superficial reflex of the foot, indicating an upper motor neuron lesion. *(Aminoff et al., 2005, p. 103)*

29. **(A)** Low back pain is one of the more common presenting neurologic complaints to a primary care provider. Most acute pain syndromes are benign, self-limiting conditions, with pain arising from myofascial sources. Patients with back pain and normal neurologic examinations are unlikely to have any serious underlying pathology and further diagnostic testing is usually unrevealing. *(Engstrom, 2008, p. 110)*

30. **(D)** Myasthenia gravis is an immune-mediated disorder in which there are circulating antibodies against the postsynaptic nicotinic acetylcholine receptors at the neuromuscular junction of skeletal muscle cells. It has a bimodal age-related onset in the second or third decade in women and in the sixth or seventh decade in men. Characteristically, weakness becomes more severe with repeated use of a muscle or during the course of the day. Herpes viruses are a potential cause of Bell's palsy, but this condition does not involve just the facial nerve. Guillain-Barré syndrome typically presents as an ascending polyneuropathy with areflexia. Multiple sclerosis is less likely than myasthenia gravis in this case due to the description of muscle fatigue. Amyotrophic lateral sclerosis produces muscle weakness, but this patient lacks the upper motor neuron findings that are indicative of amyotrophic lateral sclerosis. *(Aminoff et al., 2005, p. 184)*

31. **(C)** This patient has an intracranial mass until proven otherwise. Headaches starting later in life and accompanied by other neurologic or cognitive problems should raise a high suspicion of a tumor. Obtaining a contrast-enhanced MRI of the brain will demonstrate an intracranial mass lesion. The contrast will follow blood flow distribution and help in determining possible tumor type. Some lesions are difficult to see without contrast enhancement. MRI scans have a much higher resolution for soft tissue over CT scans and are preferred for looking at brain parenchyma. Prior to the advent of CT and MRI, cerebral angiography was used to look for intracranial masses. Vascular tumors have characteristic blush patterns, and if a mass effect is present, it will distort the position of the blood vessels. *(Aminoff et al., 2005, pp. 82-83)*

32. **(C)** *Neisseria meningitidis* and *Streptococcus pneumoniae* are the most common etiologic agents

for bacterial meningitis in this patient's age group. So much so that many colleges and universities require a vaccine for students who live in dormitories. Her fever and the cerebrospinal fluid values are consistent with a bacterial and not a viral infectious source for the meningeal irritation. *(Aminoff et al., 2005, pp. 20-30)*

33. **(A)** Huntington disease is characterized by progressive dementia, which may start by subtle changes in cognitive functioning, and by choreiform movements, which may start slightly appearing as restlessness and progressing to expansive, dance-like movements in multiple limbs; it is an autosomal dominant disorder. Tremor is not a component of Huntington disease. Depression may occur comorbidly in patients with Huntington disease but is not a component of the clinical triad of inheritance, dementia, and choreiform movements. *(Aminoff et al., 2005, p. 249-250)*

34. **(D)** Rizatriptan, like the other 5-HT receptor agonists, is an extremely effective medication for the acute treatment of migraine. This patient has tried over-the-counter analgesics, which can work for mild forms of migraine, and so the use of a migraine-specific abortive agent is appropriate. Narcotic analgesics should be avoided not only because of the possibility of dependence but more importantly because they are not as effective as other analgesics for targeting the neurochemical causes of migraine. With a frequency of about 1 attack per month, a preventive agent such as verapamil or amitriptyline is not needed. Oxygen can be useful as an acute treatment for cluster headache but has not been shown to be useful for migraine. *(Aminoff et al., 2005, pp. 88-89)*

35. **(B)** Up to 75% of subarachnoid hemorrhages can be attributed to the rupture of an intracranial aneurysm. Because of cerebrovascular anatomy, the blood is usually confined to the subarachnoid space. Blood from a ruptured arteriovenous malformation can be intraparenchymal and cause focal neurologic symptoms. Trauma is more likely to cause epidural or subdural hematoma. *(Aminoff et al., 2005, pp. 74-76)*

36. **(D)** Median nerve compression can be precipitated by repetitive use of the wrist or hand or by compression of the median nerve within the carpal tunnel at the wrist from inflammation or trauma. Characteristic fatigue and pain, especially at night, may be accompanied by paresthesia in the median nerve distribution. The pain may be reproduced on examination by performing either the Tinel or Phalen maneuver but electrophysiology studies will usually confirm the entrapment. *(Aminoff et al., 2005, pp. 221-222)*

37. **(A)** The patient most likely is suffering from diabetic peripheral neuropathy (pending further testing to rule out other causes). Amitriptyline is effective in some cases of diabetic neuropathy. Celecoxib and Ibuprofen should not be used in this patient who has significant cardiovascular risk factors and whose renal function is unknown. Oxycodone would not be used as initial treatment of this potentially chronic condition, and vitamin D is not closely associated with peripheral neuropathy. Gabapentin is starting to emerge as the best first-line therapy, but awaiting further controlled trial results. *(Aminoff et al., 2005, pp. 211-212)*

38. **(B)** The pattern of sensory, motor, and reflex findings occurring over an acute time period is consistent with Guillain-Barré Syndrome. Diffuse diabetic peripheral neuropathy develops more insidiously than this case scenario. Multiple sclerosis presents with central nervous system (CNS) lesions that are unlikely to occur in this pattern. Myasthenia gravis causes intermittent motor symptoms without sensory involvement. Hypothyroidism may cause weakness and delayed reflexes, but is not the single best answer for this question. *(Aminoff et al., 2005, p. 212)*

39. **(B)** The patient's presentation is consistent with viral meningitis with potential encephalitis. The presence of active stomatitis indicates herpes simplex virus as the most likely causative organism. A CT of the head could be considered prior to performing a lumbar puncture and may show temporal lobe abnormalities that support a diagnosis of herpes virus

encephalitis, but like an MRI will not identify the causative organism and has limited sensitivity. Of the three herpes tests described, the PCR technique is the most likely to identify the herpes simplex virus as the causative organism in the CSF due to its high sensitivity and specificity. Serum IgG indicates prior infection from herpes simplex virus but does not confirm the causative organism of the patient's encephalitis. Viral blood cultures for herpes simplex would likely show no growth even in the presence of herpes simplex virus encephalitis. *(Aminoff et al., 2005, p. 30)*

40. **(C)** The patient's unilateral symptoms are best explained by a local anatomical cause (e.g., tumor) that would be detected with an imaging study (MRI). An MRI is preferred over skull X-rays to assess directly for intracranial pathology. CNS abnormalities arising from systemic causes are more likely to be symmetric. *(Aminoff et al., 2005, p. 138)*

41. **(A)** Amitriptyline would be an appropriate prophylactic agent that may also treat her insomnia. Celecoxib and sumatriptan are common abortive agents that also have a limited role as prophylactic agents. They are inappropriate choices for this patient due to the frequency of her headaches and ill-defined pattern. Propranolol is contraindicated because of her history of exercise-induced bronchospasm. Butalbital/caffeine is not indicated for use as a prophylactic agent. *(Wells et al., 2009, p. 609)*

42. **(D)** Only two anti-epileptic drugs have FDA approval for absence seizures: valproic acid and ethosuximide. Carbamazepine and phenobarbital are known to exacerbate absence seizures and should not be prescribed to this patient. Topiramate is currently an alternative for generalized tonic–clonic seizures, but it is still not a first-line agent. Phenytoin is an alternative if valproic acid is contraindicated. *(Wells et al., 2009, p. 582)*

43. **(A)** Cerebral palsy is caused by perinatal injury to the nervous system and results in motor spasticity. The history of perinatal anoxia is consistent with cerebral palsy. Congenital

hypothyroidism is typically asymptomatic at birth and diagnosed through routine screening tests. Neonatal meningitis may result in anoxia, but this patient's anoxia is attributed to the birthing process. Multiple sclerosis is caused by inflammation, demyelination, and scarring. *(Sudarsky, 2008, p. 151)*

44. **(A)** The test described is known as asterixis, and its finding is associated with metabolic encephalopathy. Brudzinski sign is performed by passively flexing the neck of a supine patient. Clonus is assessed by rapid passive plantar-dorsiflexion of the ankle followed by sustained dorsiflexion. Stereognosis is assessed by having the patients recognize a familiar object placed in their hand. *(Bickley, 2009, p. 704)*

45. **(B)** Narcolepsy is characterized by hypersomnolence, loss of muscle tone prior to sleep, hallucinations upon initiating or arising from sleep, and episodes of sleep paralysis. The diagnostic test that is used in conjunction with clinical history to establish the diagnosis is the multiple sleep latency test. The Tensilon test is utilized to assess for the presence of myasthenia gravis. Polysomnography can be useful in excluding other sleep disorders, but it does not assess sleep latency time necessary to support the diagnosis of narcolepsy. *(Czeisler et al., 2008, pp. 177-178)*

46. **(B)** Carbamazepine is an anti-epileptic drug that potentially causes blood dyscrasias and requires CBC monitoring. Disorders of carbohydrate metabolism, vitamin B_{12} deficiency, or renal toxicity are not commonly reported. EEG is used to help establish a diagnosis of a seizure disorder. *(Aminoff et al., 2005, pp. 275-277)*

47. **(D)** Weakness is one potential finding of a lower motor neuron process. Aphasia results from injury to the speech pathways within the brain. Sensory loss arises from many causes, but it is not a motor issue. Dysdiadochokinesia is consistent with cerebellar pathology. Hyperreflexia is typically a signal of upper motor neuron disease. *(Bickley, 2009, p. 662)*

48. **(A)** The patient's symptoms are consistent with pathology arising from the anterior cerebral

circulation including the carotid arteries. A CT should be ordered to rule out acute hemorrhage and an erythrocyte sedimentation rate may be useful if giant cell arteritis were suspected. An MRA of the vertebral arteries would likely show deficits but is not likely to demonstrate the etiologic location of this stroke. *(Aminoff et al., 2005, pp. 287-291)*

REFERENCES

Aminoff MJ, Greenberg DA, Simon RP. *Clinical Neurology.* 6th ed. New York, NY: McGraw-Hill; 2005.

Beal MF, Hauser SL. Trigeminal neuralgia, Bell's palsy and other cranial nerve disorders. In: Fauci AS, Braunwald E, Kasper DL, et al., eds. *Harrison's Textbook of Medicine.* 17th ed. New York, NY: McGraw-Hill; 2008.

Bickley LS. *Bates' Guide to Physical Examination and History Taking.* 10th ed. Philadelphia, PA: Lippincott, Williams and Wilkins; 2009.

Czeisler CA, Winkelman JW, Richardson GS. Sleep disorders. In: Fauci AS, Braunwald E, Kasper DL, et al., eds. *Harrison's Textbook of Medicine.* 17th ed. New York, NY: McGraw-Hill; 2008.

Engstrom JW. Back and neck pain. In: Fauci AS, Braunwald E, Kasper DL, et al., eds. *Harrison's Textbook of Medicine.* 17th ed. New York, NY: McGraw-Hill; 2008.

Hauser SL, Goodin DS. Multiple sclerosis and other demyelinating diseases. In: Fauci AS, Braunwald E, Kasper DL, et al., eds. *Harrison's Textbook of Medicine.* 17th ed. New York, NY: McGraw-Hill; 2008.

Hauser SL, Ropper AH. Diseases of the spinal cord. In: Fauci AS, Braunwald E, Kasper DL, et al., eds. *Harrison's Textbook of Medicine.* 17th ed. New York, NY: McGraw-Hill; 2008.

Hemphill JC, Smith WS III. Neurologic critical care, including hypoxic-ischemic encephalopathy and subarachnoid hemorrhage. In: Fauci AS, Braunwald E, Kasper DL, et al., eds. *Harrison's Textbook of Medicine.* 17th ed. New York, NY: McGraw-Hill; 2008.

Horton CH. Disorders of the eye. In: Fauci AS, Braunwald E, Kasper DL, et al., eds. *Harrison's Textbook of Medicine.* 17th ed. New York, NY: McGraw-Hill; 2008.

Langford CA, Fauci AS. The Vasculitis syndromes. In: Fauci AS, Braunwald E, Kasper DL, et al., eds. *Harrison's Textbook of Medicine.* 17th ed. New York, NY: McGraw-Hill; 2008.

Lowenstein DH. Seizures and epilepsy. In: Fauci AS, Braunwald E, Kasper DL, et al., eds. *Harrison's Textbook of Medicine.* 17th ed. New York, NY: McGraw-Hill; 2008.

Sudarsky L. Gait and balance disorders. In: Fauci AS, Braunwald E, Kasper DL, et al., eds. *Harrison's Textbook of Medicine.* 17th ed. New York, NY: McGraw-Hill; 2008.

Wells BG, DiPiro JT, Schwinghammer TL, et al. *Pharmacotherapy Handbook.* 7th ed. New York, NY: McGraw-Hill; 2009.

CHAPTER 11

Internal Medicine: Pulmonology

Jill Reichman, MPH, PA-C

Matthew A. McQuillan, MS, PA-C

DIRECTIONS: Each of the numbered items or incomplete statements in this section is followed by answers or completion of the statement. Select the ONE-lettered answer or completion that is BEST in each case.

1. A 19-year-old male college student presents with a 4-day history of fever, headache, sore throat, myalgia, malaise, and a nonproductive cough. On examination, you note an erythematous pharynx without exudate. The lung examination is unimpressive. A chest X-ray reveals a right-sided lower lobe patchy infiltrate. Which of the following is the most likely cause?

   (A) *Mycoplasma pneumoniae*
   (B) *Klebsiella pneumoniae*
   (C) *Streptococcus pneumoniae*
   (D) *Staphylococcus aureus*

2. A 40-year-old woman presents with the sudden onset of cough productive of blood-speckled sputum, chest pain with cough, shaking chills, high fever, and myalgias for the last 12 hours. On examination, she appears acutely ill, is tachypneic, and is coughing. Auscultation of the chest reveals rales and chest X-ray reveals unilateral lobar consolidation consistent with pneumonia. Which of the following is the most likely cause?

   (A) *Mycoplasma pneumoniae*
   (B) *Streptococcus pneumoniae*

   (C) *Chlamydia pneumoniae*
   (D) aspiration pneumonia

3. A 3-year-old patient presents with sudden onset of coughing and wheezing, which began at the dinner table this evening. Vital signs are pulse 120, respirations 26, and temperature 98.6°F. The most likely diagnosis is a partial obstruction secondary to tracheal foreign body. What is the next step in the management of this patient?

   (A) chest physiotherapy
   (B) intubation
   (C) tracheostomy
   (D) bronchoscopy

4. An otherwise healthy 30-year-old patient presents with a 3-week history of cough and malaise. The history reveals that prior to this episode he had an upper respiratory tract infection that was treated with acetaminophen, bedrest, and fluids. The physical examination reveals a normal lung examination result and no fever. The patient is coughing while in the office. The chest X-ray is normal. What is the most effective treatment for this patient?

   (A) clarithromycin
   (B) albuterol HFA
   (C) Flumadine
   (D) fluticasone

5. A 32-year-old patient with a 3-week history of fever, malaise, weight loss, joint pain, and dry cough presents to your office. The chest X-ray reveals bilateral hilar adenopathy with no parenchymal abnormalities. You suspect and would like to rule out sarcoidosis. How can the definitive diagnosis be made?

(A) biopsy of the mediastinal nodes
(B) perform a bronchoalveolar lavage
(C) administer an intradermal purified protein derivative
(D) measure serum angiotensin-converting enzyme

6. What is the most common mode of transmission of the *Mycobacterium tuberculosis* bacteria?

(A) aerosolized droplets
(B) blood borne
(C) transplacental
(D) transdermal

7. A 65-year-old alcoholic male patient presents with the acute onset of fever, cough productive of purulent sputum, hemoptysis, chest pain, and shortness of breath. On examination, he is noted to be confused and hypotensive. Chest X-ray shows bilateral infiltrates and cavitations. Sputum smear reveals gram-negative rods. Which of the following is the most likely cause of this pneumonia?

(A) *Pneumocystis jiroveci*
(B) *Mycoplasma pneumoniae*
(C) *Chlamydia pneumoniae*
(D) *Klebsiella pneumoniae*

8. What is the drug treatment of choice for *Mycoplasma pneumoniae*?

(A) penicillins
(B) cephalosporins
(C) aminoglycosides
(D) macrolides

9. What is the empirical drug treatment of choice for a known case of community-acquired?

(A) gentamycin
(B) penicillin

(C) clarithromycin
(D) vancomycin

10. A 50-year-old man presents with a history of persistent cough, hemoptysis, and weight loss over the past 6 months. He has smoked 2 packs per day for 30 years and also complains of shoulder and chest pain. On examination, he is noted to be pale, febrile, and dyspneic upon exertion. The chest X-ray shows hilar adenopathy. What is the most likely diagnosis?

(A) asthma
(B) bronchiectasis
(C) bronchogenic carcinoma
(D) chronic obstructive pulmonary disease (COPD)

11. A 43-year-old woman with a history of COPD presents to the office with worsening dyspnea, especially at rest. She also complains of dull, retrosternal chest pain. On examination, she has narrow splitting of S1. Radiographic findings demonstrate peripheral "pruning" of the large pulmonary arteries. What is the most likely diagnosis?

(A) congestive heart failure
(B) pericarditis
(C) pulmonary embolus
(D) pulmonary hypertension

12. What radiologic finding(s) is/are most suggestive of chronic silicosis?

(A) eggshell calcification of enlarged hilar lymph nodes
(B) pneumothorax and atelectasis
(C) large nodules that appear primarily in the lower lobes
(D) pleural thickening and plaques

13. A 50-year-old patient presents with a fever of 102°F, productive cough, mild chest pain on deep breathing and coughing, and general malaise for the last 2 days. Prior to the onset of these symptoms, the patient had a "bad cold" for 5 days. What physical finding would be most consistent with this history?

(A) vesicular breath sounds

(B) decreased transmitted voice sounds

(C) inspiratory crackles

(D) diffuse hyperresonance

14. Which histological type of lung cancer has the lowest 5-year survival rate?

(A) bronchioalveolar

(B) large cell

(C) small cell

(D) squamous cell

(E) adenocarcinoma

15. A 43-year-old female patient who is HIV negative is recently diagnosed with pulmonary tuberculosis via a positive purified protein derivative (PPD) and culture. She receives annual PPD testing and prior to this test has been negative. What is the current recommended treatment?

(A) 3 months of isoniazid (INH), rifampin (RIF), and pyrazinamide (PZA) and ethambutol (EMB)

(B) 2 months of INH, RIF, PZA, and streptomycin (SM) followed by 1 month of INH and RIF

(C) 6 months of INH and RIF

(D) 2 months of INH, RIF, PZA, and EMB followed by 4 months of INH and RIF

16. A 35-year-old man who is HIV positive presents to the emergency department (ED) complaining of high fever, pleuritic chest pain, and grossly purulent sputum. History also reveals that he was recently at a local conference and spent most of the time indoors. The ED has seen three other patients this week with the same complaints. On examination, he is toxic appearing with a temperature of 103°F. The chest film demonstrates focal patchy infiltrates. What is the treatment of choice?

(A) doxycycline

(B) erythromycin

(C) levofloxacin

(D) penicillin

17. A 19-year-old woman, post motor vehicle accident, is hospitalized with a femur fracture. She develops sudden onset of dyspnea, cough, and anxiety with retrosternal chest pain. On examination, her pulse is 120, respirations 32, and blood pressure 120/80 mm Hg. Chest X-ray shows mild bilateral atelectasis. Electrocardiogram (ECG) is normal. What is the most likely diagnosis?

(A) pulmonary thromboembolus

(B) aortic dissection

(C) pneumonia

(D) pneumothorax

18. What imaging study is the "gold standard" used to confirm the diagnosis of deep vein thrombosis?

(A) arteriography

(B) contrast venography

(C) Doppler ultrasound

(D) ventilation-perfusion scan

19. A 70-year-old patient with a long history of COPD presents to the office for a regular office visit. The patient's history is unchanged and the physical examination is consistent with a long-term history of COPD. One of the findings is distal phalanges that are rounded and bulbous. Upon palpation, the proximal nail folds feel spongy. This finding is consistent with what condition?

(A) acute dyspnea

(B) chronic hypoxia

(C) transient hypercapnia

(D) chronic hyponatremia

20. What is the mainstay bronchodilator treatment for mild intermittent asthma?

(A) beta-adrenergic agents

(B) theophylline

(C) aminophylline

(D) antileukotrienes

21. A 29-year-old patient with a history of HIV presents to the emergency department with signs and symptoms consistent with *Pneumocystis jiroveci* pneumonia. What chest X-ray findings are considered the "classic" pattern associated with this diagnosis?

    (A) diffuse interstitial infiltrates
    (B) focal consolidation
    (C) multiple pulmonary nodules
    (D) upper lobe cavitation

22. What is considered the primary therapy for patients with pulmonary thromboembolism (PTE) who are hemodynamically unstable?

    (A) anticoagulation with heparin
    (B) anti-embolization stockings
    (C) insertion of an inferior vena caval filter
    (D) thrombolysis with tissue plasminogen activator (t-Pa)

23. A 79-year-old woman who is 7 days post a total hip replacement complains of sudden onset of dyspnea, cough, and retrosternal chest pain. On examination, she appears anxious with vital signs as follows: pulse 120, respirations 32, and blood pressure 138/92 mm Hg. A chest X-ray demonstrates mild bilateral atelectasis and other than tachycardia a normal ECG. What imaging modality will best confirm the diagnosis?

    (A) arteriography
    (B) contrast venography
    (C) helical CT scan
    (D) ventilation-perfusion scan

24. A 17-year-old girl presents complaining of a nonproductive cough, postnasal drip, and nasal congestion. Examination reveals inflamed nasal turbinates, cobblestoning of the posterior pharynx, and diffuse bilateral end expiratory wheezes. Which laboratory test will provide the best information to assist in making the diagnosis?

    (A) arterial blood gas
    (B) chest X-ray
    (C) peak flow measurements
    (D) spirometry

25. A 7-year-old boy with a history of asthma presents with nocturnal cough occurring every night along with daily exacerbations of wheezing and shortness of breath. How would his asthma be classified?

    (A) intermittent
    (B) mild persistent
    (C) moderate persistent
    (D) severe persistent

26. A 13-year-old girl presents complaining of intermittent episodes of wheezing, which occur only when she is exercising. Which of the following medications is most appropriate to prevent her symptoms?

    (A) ipratropium
    (B) fluticasone
    (C) salmeterol
    (D) terbutaline

27. A 35-year-old woman with a history of severe persistent asthma has been treated with inhaled corticosteroids, a long-acting bronchodilator, and prednisone tablets for several years. In order to decrease the severity of side effects of this treatment regimen, which of the following should be prescribed?

    (A) benzodiazepines
    (B) beta-blockers
    (C) folic acid
    (D) vitamin D and calcium

28. A 17-year-old girl with a history of cystic fibrosis presents with a chronic cough productive of copious, foul smelling, purulent sputum. The patient is afebrile and the lung examination reveals crackles at the lung bases bilaterally. What is the most likely diagnosis?

    (A) asthma
    (B) bronchiectasis
    (C) bronchiolitis
    (D) pneumonitis

29. Which of the following disorders of the large bronchioles is characterized by the destruction of bronchial walls?

    (A) asthma
    (B) bronchiectasis
    (C) cystic fibrosis
    (D) pneumonia

30. A 35-year-old man is suspected of having a small right-sided pleural effusion. What imaging modality is most sensitive to detect a small amount of pleural fluid?

    (A) chest CT
    (B) lateral chest film
    (C) left lateral decubitus chest film
    (D) standard upright chest film

31. A 58-year-old man with a history of hypertension and left ventricular hypertrophy presents with shortness of breath. Examination reveals dullness to percussion bilaterally with decreased breath sounds. Pleural fluid is aspirated and analyzed. Which of the following results is consistent with his most likely diagnosis?

    (A) glucose 40 mg/dL
    (B) LDH 300 IU/L
    (C) protein 2.5 mg/dL
    (D) WBC 2,000/mm^3

32. A 75-year-old male smoker presents with hemoptysis, weight loss, and chronic cough. Chest film reveals a hilar mass greater than 5 cm and fluid in the costophrenic sulcus. An analysis of the pleural fluid is completed. Which of the following results is consistent with his most likely diagnosis?

    (A) glucose 40 mg/dL
    (B) LDH 100 IU/L
    (C) protein 2.9 g/dL
    (D) WBC 787/mm^3

33. A 14-year-old healthy boy presents to the emergency department complaining of an acute onset of unilateral chest pain and dyspnea that occurred without a precipitating event. Examination reveals unilateral chest expansion and decreased breath sounds. What is the most likely diagnosis?

    (A) atypical pneumonia
    (B) pericarditis
    (C) pulmonary embolus
    (D) spontaneous pneumothorax

34. A 25-year-old patient with a history of tobacco use presents complaining of the acute onset of right-sided chest pain and dyspnea. He has no other symptoms. Examination reveals a tall, thin man, who is mildly anxious and short of breath. An expiratory film shows a visceral pleural line. What chest examination findings are consistent with this patient's diagnosis?

    (A) decreased tactile fremitus; hyperresonant to percussion
    (B) increased tactile fremitus; dullness to percussion
    (C) decreased tactile fremitus; dullness to percussion
    (D) increased tactile fremitus; hyperresonant to percussion

35. Which of the following chest films will best demonstrate a small pneumothorax?

    (A) expiratory
    (B) lateral decubitus
    (C) lordotic
    (D) oblique

36. A 65-year-old man presents with a chronic productive cough, dyspnea, and wheezing. Examination reveals cyanosis, distended neck veins, and a prominent epigastric pulsation. What is the most likely diagnosis?

    (A) cor pulmonale
    (B) chronic bronchitis
    (C) emphysema
    (D) pneumonia

37. A 4-year-old child is brought to the emergency department with a low-grade fever, barking cough, and respiratory stridor with activity but not at rest. On examination, you note the cough and the absence of drooling. What is the most appropriate treatment for this child?

(A) dexamethasone IM
(B) endotracheal intubation and IV antibiotics
(C) inhaled budesonide
(D) nebulized racemic epinephrine
(E) supportive therapy with oral hydration

38. An otherwise healthy 2-year-old is brought to your office in late winter with a low-grade fever, wheezing, and cough. On physical examination, you note diffuse wheezing and retractions. The patient is not having any trouble feeding or swallowing. This is the fifth child you have seen this week with the same symptoms. What is the most likely diagnosis?

(A) bronchiolitis due to respiratory syncytial virus
(B) epiglottitis due to *Haemophilus influenzae* type B
(C) pharyngitis due to Group A *Streptococcus*
(D) pneumonia due to *Mycoplasma pneumoniae*
(E) tracheitis due to *Staphylococcus aureus*

39. What is a common initial presentation of cystic fibrosis?

(A) congestive heart failure
(B) failure to thrive
(C) biliary cirrhosis
(D) ulcerative colitis

40. Which viral illness is transmitted via the respiratory route by droplet nuclei?

(A) arbovirus
(B) influenza
(C) respiratory syncytial virus (RSV)
(D) rhinovirus
(E) severe acute respiratory syndrome (SARS)

41. A 4-year-old child presents with a 2-week history of cough, rhinitis, and sneezing without fever. In the last 2 days, the cough has become more severe and is now paroxysmal (10 to 20 forceful coughs at a time). The paroxysms are accompanied by a loud high-pitched inspiratory sound. The child's medical history reveals that immunizations were not completed in infancy. What is the most likely diagnosis?

(A) diphtheria
(B) *Haemophilus influenzae* type B
(C) legionella
(D) pertussis

42. A 37-year-old man who recently immigrated to the United States and is otherwise well presents to the office complaining of severe paroxysms of cough that have persisted for the past 4 weeks. He describes the cough as severe, causing him to have difficulty catching his breath and making him feel as if he will vomit. He states that before the onset of cough, he was fatigued and complained of symptoms of a head cold. What is the treatment of choice for the most likely diagnosis? ?

(A) ceftriaxone
(B) erythromycin
(C) isoniazid
(D) penicillin

43. Which laboratory/diagnostic finding is consistent with coal workers' pneumoconiosis (CWP)?

(A) CT scan showing predominance of ground-glass abnormality
(B) chest X-ray with eggshell calcifications in hilar lymph nodes
(C) decreased FEV_1
(D) positive antinuclear antibodies
(E) positive rheumatoid factor

44. What is the most commonly prescribed initial treatment of idiopathic pulmonary fibrosis (IPF)?

(A) colchicine in combination with a broad-spectrum antibiotic

(B) corticosteroids in combination with immunosuppressive agents

(C) hospitalization, intubation, and broad-spectrum antibiotics

(D) lung transplantation

(E) methotrexate in combination with low-dose corticosteroids

45. A patient diagnosed with lung cancer presents with a 4-cm tumor in the mainstem bronchus. The tumor is not within 2 cm of carina. There is no invasion of the visceral pleura or associated atelectasis. There are no distant metastases or nodal involvement. The TNM descriptor is T2N0M0. Given these findings, what is the correct stage of the patient's disease?

(A) 0

(B) IA

(C) IB

(D) IIA

(E) IIB

46. A preterm infant (33 weeks) presents at 10 days of age. The mother complains that the infant is experiencing an increasing number of apneic episodes of 20 to 30 seconds associated with cyanosis. After a careful history, physical examination, and workup, the decision is made to treat the infant. What is the appropriate treatment for this infant?

(A) corticosteroids alone

(B) corticosteroids in combination with broad-spectrum antibiotics

(C) IV glucose and careful electrolyte management

(D) methylxanthines

47. Which of the following combination of findings would provide a definitive diagnosis of cystic fibrosis (CF)?

(A) family history of CF; abnormal PFT

(B) abnormal PFT; pancreatic insufficiency

(C) abnormal sweat test; pancreatic insufficiency

(D) abnormal chest X-ray; family history of CF

48. A premature infant is born at 32 weeks and after several hours develops rapid shallow respirations at 60/min, grunting retractions, and duskiness of the skin. The chest X-ray reveals diffuse bilateral atelectasis, ground glass appearance, and air bronchograms. What is the most likely diagnosis?

(A) hyaline membrane disease

(B) meconium aspiration

(C) Tetralogy of Fallot

(D) ventral septal defect

49. A child presents to the office with respiratory symptoms consistent with influenza. What would be most helpful in supporting the diagnosis?

(A) chest X-ray with air bronchograms

(B) elevated WBC count

(C) epidemiologic and overall clinical data

(D) history of no influenza immunization

(E) presence of pneumonia

50. A 5-month-old patient is diagnosed with bronchiolitis, which occurred during an annual outbreak in the early spring. You are now concerned about the sequelae of this infection. What etiologic agent is most likely to cause persistent airway reactivity later in life?

(A) coxsackievirus

(B) influenza A

(C) parvovirus

(D) respiratory syncytial virus

51. Which of the following recommendations for annual influenza immunization is correct?

(A) Healthy children aged 0 to 6 months should be immunized.

(B) Live attenuated vaccine (nasal spray) is contraindicated in children younger than 12 years.

(C) Pregnant women in the second or third trimester should be immunized.

(D) Two doses of vaccine are recommended for children older than 9 years who are receiving vaccine for the first time.

52. What antiviral agent is indicated for the treatment of influenza A?

(A) acyclovir
(B) oseltamivir
(C) famciclovir
(D) lamivudine
(E) vidarabine

53. A 50-year-old presents to the office complaining of progressive dyspnea over the past few years. History reveals that he has worked in construction for the past 20 years demolishing and refurbishing old buildings. He rarely uses any protective breathing equipment. Physical examination demonstrates an afebrile man in mild respiratory distress with inspiratory crackles. The chest X-ray reveals a reticular linear pattern with basilar predominance, opacities, and honeycombing. What is the most likely diagnosis?

(A) asbestosis
(B) coal workers' pneumoconiosis (CWP)
(C) acute hypersensitivity pneumonitis
(D) silicosis

54. Classically, pertussis is an illness that lasts for weeks and is divided into stages. A patient who presents with 5 days of congestion, rhinorrhea, low-grade fever, and sneezing is in which stage?

(A) catarrhal
(B) convalescent
(C) paroxysmal
(D) prodromal

55. A 30-year-old patient presents to the office complaining of an acute onset of fever of 101°F, chills, productive cough, and chest pain. The pain is described as severe, knife-like, and worsened by coughing and/or deep inspiration. What is the name given to this type of chest pain?

(A) ischemic
(B) neuralgic
(C) pleuritic
(D) visceral

56. A 47-year-old man is admitted to the ICU in shock following a near-drowning 3 hours ago. While in the ICU, he suddenly develops dyspnea. Examination reveals labored breathing, tachypnea, and rales. The chest film demonstrates air bronchograms and patchy bilateral infiltrates that spare the costophrenic angles. There is no cardiomegaly or pleural effusions. What is the most likely diagnosis?

(A) ARDS
(B) congestive heart failure
(C) pneumothorax
(D) pulmonary embolism

57. A 7-year-old previously healthy patient presents with acute onset of respiratory distress following ingestion of a piece of candy. Which of the following signs or symptoms is most ominous?

(A) aphonia
(B) cough
(C) drooling
(D) stridor

58. A 55-year-old smoker with lung cancer presents with ptosis and miosis. What is the third clinical finding that comprises this syndrome found in patients with lung cancer?

(A) anhidrosis
(B) pericarditis
(C) pneumonitis
(D) systemic acidosis

59. A 32-year-old African American woman with a history of erythema nodosum presents with nonspecific complaints such as fatigue and malaise. Based on the fact that she is a smoker with these symptoms, a chest X-ray is ordered that demonstrates bilateral hilar adenopathy. A transbronchial lung biopsy reveals noncaseating granulomas. What is the most likely diagnosis?

(A) bronchogenic carcinoma
(B) mesothelioma
(C) sarcoidosis
(D) tuberculosis

60. A 25-year-old man presents for preadmission testing (PAT) to correct a ventral hernia. The PAT includes a chest X-ray, which reveals a single, smooth, well-defined node with dense central calcification of approximately 2 cm in diameter. What is the most appropriate next step in the management of this patient?

    (A) obtain a CT scan
    (B) obtain old films for comparison
    (C) proceed directly to biopsy
    (D) watchful waiting

61. A 47-year-old patient with a history of HIV presents with fever, tachypnea, shortness of breath, and a nonproductive cough. Bronchoalveolar lavage reveals *Pneumocystic jiroveci*. What is the treatment of choice?

    (A) amoxicillin/clavulanate
    (B) azithromycin
    (C) doxycycline
    (D) trimethoprim-sulfamethoxazole

62. A 61-year-old woman who was recently diagnosed with COPD presents with an acute exacerbation of chronic bronchitis. She is allergic (anaphylaxis) to penicillin and develops a rash when she takes Bactrim. What is the most appropriate antibiotic to prescribe?

    (A) Augmentin
    (B) azithromycin
    (C) ceftriaxone
    (D) cefuroxime

63. A 3-year-old child presents to the emergency department with a sudden onset of fever, difficulty swallowing, drooling, and dyspnea. Examination reveals a febrile child who is sitting, leaning forward with his neck extended. Chest examination reveals soft stridor with inspiratory retractions. What is the next step in the management of this patient?

    (A) inspection and intubation under controlled conditions
    (B) IV cephalosporin therapy
    (C) treatment with nebulized albuterol
    (D) treatment with nebulized epinephrine

64. In which gender and age group is a spontaneous pneumothorax most likely to occur?

    (A) male between 2 and 10 years of age
    (B) female between 2 and 10 years of age
    (C) male between 20 and 40 years of age
    (D) female between 20 and 40 years of age

65. A 32-year-old patient with a history of Wilson disease is 14 months status post liver transplant. The result of a routine pre-employment PPD is induration of 7 mm. What is the recommended management?

    (A) no treatment
    (B) isoniazid
    (C) isoniazid and rifampin
    (D) isoniazid, rifampin, pyrazinamide, and ethambutol

66. A 59-year-old patient presents complaining of a daily productive cough for the last 3 years, which is worse in the winter months. He has also noted some shortness of breath with moderate to heavy exertion. He has no other symptoms. The patient admits to smoking a pack of cigarettes per day for 38 years but quitting 9 months ago. Physical examination is normal. What is the most likely diagnosis?

    (A) asthma
    (B) bronchiectasis
    (C) chronic bronchitis
    (D) tuberculosis

67. A 60-year-old patient presents with the insidious onset of dyspnea with exertion and a non-productive cough and fatigue. The physical examination reveals bi-basilar inspiratory crackles and clubbing of the fingers. The chest X-ray shows a reticular pattern of densities in the lower lung fields. What is the most definitive method of establishing a diagnosis in this patient?

    (A) CT scan
    (B) pulmonary function tests
    (C) surgical lung biopsy
    (D) ventilation-perfusion scan

68. Which disease entity is defined as a condition of the lung characterized by abnormal permanent enlargement of the air spaces distal to the terminal bronchioles accompanied by destruction of their walls and without obvious fibrosis.

    (A) emphysema
    (B) hyaline membrane disease
    (C) sarcoidosis
    (D) silicosis

Answers and Explanations

1. **(A)** Mycoplasma pneumonia often presents after days of constitutional symptoms and a nonproductive cough. Generally, the examination reveals little more than a reddened throat and rarely, bullous myringitis. Diagnosis is made on clinical grounds. Cold agglutinins are a common confirmatory test. *(Baum, 2008, pp. 2272-2274)*

2. **(B)** Pneumococcal pneumonia is the most common cause of pneumonia. Classically it presents with the abrupt onset of fever, cough (productive of rusty sputum), and pleuritic chest pain. Chest X-ray usually reveals a lobar consolidation. *(Mandell, 2008, pp. 2173-2174)*

3. **(D)** Patients with obstruction of the trachea typically present with cough, wheezing, dyspnea, and/or cyanosis. In most cases, the definitive diagnosis is made by endoscopy, and treatment can be accomplished at the same time by removal of the object. *(Hollinger, 2007)*

4. **(B)** In patients with acute bronchitis, bronchodilators may give symptomatic relief. Studies show that bronchodilator therapy may lead to quicker resolution of cough and return to normal functioning. Antibiotics have not been shown to be effective in patients with acute bronchitis. Corticosteroid therapy and antiviral therapy are not appropriate for acute bronchitis. *(Hueston, 2008, pp. 278-279)*

5. **(A)** Diagnosis is confirmed by finding well-formed noncaseating granulomas in affected tissues. Because the lung is involved so commonly, the routine chest X-ray is almost always abnormal but cannot be used as the sole criteria. *(Weinberger, 2008, pp. 667-671)*

6. **(A)** *Mycobacterium tuberculosis* is most commonly transmitted from a patient with infectious pulmonary tuberculosis to other persons by droplet nuclei, which are aerosolized by coughing, sneezing, or speaking. Crowding in poorly ventilated rooms is one of the most important factors in the transmission of tubercle bacilli, since it increases the intensity of a contact with a case. *(Iseman, 2008, pp. 2298-2306)*

7. **(D)** *Klebsiella pneumoniae* is the most likely cause. It is common, along with other gram-negative bacilli, in alcoholic and in debilitated patients. It typically causes the acute onset of cough, chest pain, and shortness of breath. Cavitations are likely to be seen in pneumonias caused by *Klebsiella*. *(Chesnutt et al., 2009, pp. 237-241)*

8. **(D)** Macrolides such as erythromycin or tetracyclines are the drugs of choice in treating *Mycoplasma pneumoniae*. Gastrointestinal intolerance is common with erythromycin. Doxycycline, azithromycin, or clarithromycin may be used as alternatives. *(Baum, 2008, p. 2274)*

9. **(C)** The pneumococcus is the most common cause of community-acquired pyogenic bacterial pneumonia. The prevalence of penicillin-resistant pneumococci is increasing in the United States; therefore, macrolides are the class of choice (Level I evidence) and may be

used in penicillin-allergic patients. *(Limper, 2008, p. 679)*

10. **(C)** The clinical manifestations of bronchogenic carcinoma can vary and is largely based on the location of the tumor and extent of disease. Anorexia, weight loss, asthenia, and cough are some of the more common clinical manifestations. Chest X-ray may demonstrate hilar adenopathy, infiltrates, or single or multiple nodules. Asthma and chronic obstructive pulmonary disease usually reveal hyperinflation of the lungs and flattened diaphragms. The medical history is not consistent with bronchiectasis where the chest film may demonstrate dilated, thickened bronchi, scattered opacities, and atelectasis. *(Chesnutt et al., 2009, pp. 210-234; Rugo, 2009, pp. 1429-1435)*

11. **(D)** Peripheral "pruning" of the large pulmonary arteries is characteristic of pulmonary hypertension in severe emphysema. *(Chesnutt et al., 2009, pp. 266-268)*

12. **(A)** Eggshell calcification of hilar or mediastinal lymph nodes is characteristic of silicosis. The disease may also be recognized by the presence of small nodules, which appear predominately in the upper lobes. Pneumothorax, atelectasis, and pleural thickening and plaques are not radiologic features of silicosis. *(Samet, 2008, p. 657)*

13. **(C)** In a patient with pneumonia, inspiratory crackles along with bronchial breath sounds, increased tactile fremitus and transmitted voice sounds (the presence of egophony, bronchophony, and/or whispered pectoriloquy), and dullness to percussion over the involved area would be consistent findings on physical examination. *(Bickley and Szilagyi, 2007, p. 276)*

14. **(C)** The prognosis for each type of lung cancer varies according to the pathologic stage. However, in general, small cell lung carcinoma has the worst prognosis, with the median survival period of 12 to 16 months with only 5% to 25% surviving 2 years, whereas patients with extensive disease have a median survival period of only 7 to 11 months, with only 1% to 3% surviving 2 years. *(Theodore and Jablons, 2006, p. 385)*

15. **(D)** The Centers for Disease Control and Prevention currently recommends a minimum of 6 months of INH and RIF with initial 2 months of PZA and SM or EMB for immunocompetent persons. *(Iseman, 2008, pp. 2302-2306)*

16. **(C)** The treatment of choice for immunocompromised patients with legionella infection is either azithromycin or clarithromycin, or a fluoroquinolone such as levofloxacin. Erythromycin and doxycycline are acceptable treatments for immunocompetent patients with legionella. Penicillin is ineffective against legionella *(Schwartz B and Chambers, 2009, p. 1278)*

17. **(A)** Pulmonary thromboembolism is most often caused by the embolization of thrombus from the deep veins of the lower extremities. People at risk for pulmonary embolus are those with hypercoagulable states, which may arise from the use of birth control pills, local stasis, immobilization that may be the result of an accident or illness, fractures, obesity, and congestive heart failure. Signs and symptoms often begin abruptly and include dyspnea, cough, and chest pain (frequently pleuritic in nature). Hemoptysis may occur; tachypnea and tachycardia are common in this illness. A low-grade fever, wheezing, rales, or pleural rub are also signs of pulmonary embolism. *(Tapson, 2008, pp. 688-689)*

18. **(B)** Contrast venography is the imaging study of choice to diagnose a deep vein thrombosis. Doppler ultrasound can be used for screening. Arteriography and V/Q scans would not be appropriate studies to diagnose deep vein thrombosis. *(Ginsberg, 2008, pp. 575-576)*

19. **(B)** This description is consistent with digital clubbing. It accompanies chronic hypoxia associated with conditions such as COPD, lung cancer, heart disease, and cirrhosis. *(Bickley and Szilagyi, 2007, p. 150)*

20. **(A)** Beta-adrenergic agents are the mainstay bronchodilator treatment for mild asthma. Theophylline and aminophylline are bronchodilators of moderate potency and are usually reserved for patients with moderate to severe asthma. Antileukotrienes are controller medications, not bronchodilators. *(Drezen, 2008, pp. 615-618)*

21. **(A)** The classic X-ray finding of pneumonia caused by *Pneumocystis jiroveci* is diffuse interstitial infiltrates. Cavitations, consolidations, and nodules may also appear but not as commonly. *(Feinberg, 2008, p. 2361)*

22. **(D)** Primary therapy consists of clot dissolution with thrombolysis or removal of PTE by embolectomy and is reserved for patients at high risk of death from right heart failure and for those patients at risk of recurrent PTE despite adequate anticoagulation. Anticoagulation with heparin is useful to prevent further clot development, but it does not directly dissolve thrombi or emboli. The use of filters is considered a preventative measure, as is the recommended use of antiembolism stockings. *(Chesnutt et al., 2009, pp. 264-266)*

23. **(A)** Pulmonary arteriography is the "gold standard" for the diagnosis of PTE. An intraluminal defect in more than one projection establishes a definitive diagnosis. Contrast venography is the reference standard for the diagnosis for deep vein thrombosis. Helical CT is replacing V/Q scans as the initial diagnostic study for suspected PTE but is less sensitive than pulmonary arteriography. V/Q scans are helpful for screening especially if they are either normal or indicate high probability of PTE. *(Tapson, 2008, pp. 690-692)*

24. **(D)** Evaluation for asthma should include spirometry before and after the administration of a short-acting bronchodilator to determine whether airflow obstruction is immediately reversible. Peak expiratory flow meters are designed for home use to assess severity and provide objective data to guide treatment. Arterial blood gas measurement may be normal in mild exacerbations, but respiratory alkalosis is also common in severe cases. Chest films may show only hyperinflation and are indicated only if pneumonia or pneumothorax is expected. *(Chesnutt et al., 2009, pp. 211-217)*

25. **(D)** In this case, the nighttime symptoms and daily exacerbations would classify his asthma as severe persistent. The National Asthma Education and Prevention Program has outlined the classification of severity of chronic asthma, which is useful in directing asthma therapy. The classification is based on the frequency of symptoms, nighttime severity, and peak flow measurements. *(Chesnutt et al., 2009, p. 211)*

26. **(C)** Long-acting bronchodilators, such as salmeterol, are indicated for long-term prevention of asthma symptoms and nocturnal symptoms, and for the prevention of exercise-induced bronchospasm. It is critical to educate the patient that this should not be used as a treatment for acute bronchoconstriction. Fluticasone is an inhaled corticosteroid that can be used as part of the treatment strategy for mild persistent, moderate persistent, and severe persistent asthma. Ipratropium is an anticholinergic agent used to reverse vagally mediated bronchospasm but not allergen or exercise-induced bronchospasm. Theophylline is a phosphodiesterase inhibitor that is not recommended for therapy of asthma exacerbations. *(Chesnutt et al., 2009, p. 221)*

27. **(D)** Concurrent treatment with calcium supplements, vitamin D, and bisphosphonates can be prescribed to prevent steroid-induced bone mineral loss that occurs with long-term use of steroids. Benzodiazepines, folic acid, and bile acid sequestrants are not indicated for patients on long-term steroids. *(Chesnutt et al., 2009, p. 217)*

28. **(B)** Symptoms of bronchiectasis include chronic cough, purulent sputum, hemoptysis, and recurrent pneumonia. In addition, weight loss, anemia, and other systemic manifestations are common. Cystic fibrosis causes about half of all cases. Asthma can cause cough but is generally characterized as nonproductive and presents

with expiratory wheezes. Bronchiolitis is common in infants and children and is most commonly caused by respiratory syncytial virus or adenovirus. Pneumonitis is a general term for inflammation of the lung (alveolitis) and may be the result of an infectious or environmental insult. *(Chesnutt et al., 2009, pp. 235-236)*

29. **(B)** Bronchiectasis is characterized by permanent, abnormal dilation and destruction of bronchial walls. Asthma is a chronic inflammatory disorder of the airways. Cystic fibrosis causes altered chloride transport and water flux across the apical surface of epithelial cells. Pneumonia is caused by the infiltration of the lower respiratory tract by microorganisms. *(Chesnutt et al., 2009, pp. 233-234)*

30. **(A)** A chest CT can identify as little as 10 mL of fluid. On the lateral view, at least 75 to 100 mL of pleural fluid must accumulate in the posterior sulcus to be visible. To make fluid in the right side become visible, the patient must be in the right lateral decubitus position. The frontal view requires that at least 175 to 200 mL must be present. *(Chesnutt et al., 2009, pp. 275-278)*

31. **(C)** The patient is most likely in congestive heart failure, which would result in a transudative effusion. Pleural findings consistent with a transudate include glucose greater than 60 mg/dL; protein less than 3.0 g/dL; WBCs less than 1,000 McL; LDH less than 200 IU/L. *(Celli, 2008, p. 699)*

32. **(A)** The patient most likely has carcinoma, which would result in an exudative effusion. Pleural findings consistent with an exudate include glucose less than 60 mg/dL; protein greater than 3.0 g/dL; WBCs less than 1,000 McL; LDH greater than 200 IU/L. *(Celli, 2008, pp. 699-700)*

33. **(D)** These findings are most consistent with a spontaneous pneumothorax, which is primarily found in tall, thin mens between the ages of

10 and 30. Pericarditis is an acute inflammatory process of the pericardium due to either an infectious process or systemic disease, neoplasm, radiation, drug toxicity, or other processes. The clinical presentation includes chest pain, which is relieved by leaning forward. Pulmonary embolus presents as acute onset of chest pain with tachycardia. Breath sounds are usually normal and fremitus is symmetrical. *(Chesnutt et al., 2009, pp. 278-279; Bickley and Szilagyi, 2007, pp. 276-277)*

34. **(A)** This patient has a pneumothorax. Because of the accumulation of air in the pleural space, fremitus on the affected side will be decreased and percussion will be hyperresonant. *(Chesnutt et al., 2009, pp. 278-279; Bickley and Szilagyi, 2007, pp. 276-277)*

35. **(A)** Small pneumothoraces may only be seen on an expiratory film. Other findings include a visceral pleural line on a chest film and a "deep sulcus sign" on a supine film. *(Chesnutt et al., 2009, pp. 278-279)*

36. **(A)** Cor pulmonale is right ventricular hypertrophy and failure resulting from pulmonary disease. It is most commonly caused by chronic obstructive pulmonary disease, which is this patient's underlying disorder precipitating the failure. While the other three diagnoses may have similar symptoms, none of them would present with distended neck veins and prominent epigastric pulsations. *(Chesnutt et al., 2009, pp. 228-230)*

37. **(E)** Viral croup is the most likely diagnosis in the patient. It is most often caused by the parainfluenza virus. This patient displays mild symptoms: low-grade fever, cough, and stridor only with activity. In this case, the most appropriate treatment is supportive. If this patient was more seriously ill and had stridor at rest, other treatment including inhaled, oral, or intramuscular (IM) steroids and/or epinephrine would be appropriate. Intubation is reserved for the most severe patients with impending respiratory failure. The use of intravenous (IV) antibiotics is

inappropriate in a viral illness. *(Kerby et al., 2009, pp. 478-479)*

38. **(A)** Bronchiolitis due to respiratory syncytial virus is the best answer. Respiratory syncytial virus peaks in late winter and is common in young children. It is often a diagnosis made on the basis of symptoms, particularly during an outbreak. Epiglottitis presents more acutely with sudden onset of fever, dysphagia, drooling, and cyanosis. Tracheitis is also more severe; patients develop high fever, toxicity, and upper airway obstruction. Pneumonia due to mycoplasma is not usually seen in this age group; generally, patients with mycoplasma are older than 5 years. Pharyngitis generally presents with sore throat and fever; cough and wheezing are not part of the clinical presentation. *(Kerby et al., 2009, pp. 478-479, 484-485)*

39. **(B)** More than 40% of patients with cystic fibrosis present in infancy with failure to thrive, and respiratory compromise. The age of presentation may be variable from infancy into adulthood. Biliary cirrhosis becomes symptomatic in only 2% to 3% of patients. Congestive heart failure is not usually part of the initial presentation. Gastrointestinal disease is equally common and most commonly caused by distal intestinal obstruction syndrome, not by ulcerative colitis. *(Boat and Acton, 2007)*

40. **(B)** Influenza is transmitted via droplet nuclei. RSV, rhinovirus, and SARS are transmitted via fomites or large particle aerosols. Arbovirus is transmitted by arthropods or ticks and produces a variety of encephalitides including West Nile fever, St. Louis encephalitis, and California encephalitis. *(Shandera and Coroles-Medina, 2009, pp. 1226, 1237-1242)*

41. **(D)** The most likely diagnosis is pertussis, which is typically preceded by 2 to 3 weeks of cough and coryza without fever: the characteristic "whooping" cough is a high-pitched inspiratory sound. Diphtheria typically presents with sore throat, fever, and malaise and produces a pseudomembrane, most often in the pharynx. *Haemophilus influenzae* type B causes a severe febrile illness that presents with meningitis, epiglottitis, septic arthritis, and cellulitis. Legionella causes abrupt onset with fever, chills, and headache, which progress rapidly to pneumonia. *(Ogle and Anderson, 2009, pp. 1147-1149, 1162-1165, 1172)*

42. **(B)** This is a classic presentation of pertussis. Although the classic post-tussive "whoop" is described in the literature, it is a more common symptom in children and found less frequently in adults. Because of the waning of immunity to pertussis in adults who are not receiving booster vaccinations, the incidence of pertussis is increasing. Treatment of pertussis is erythromycin, clarithromycin, or azithromycin. Household contacts should also be treated. The other drugs listed would not be appropriate for the treatment of pertussis. *(Schwartz and Chambers, 2009, p. 1275)*

43. **(C)** A decreased FEV_1 is typically found in patients with CWP. Chest X-ray with eggshell calcifications is found in a small percentage of patients with silicosis. A CT scan showing a ground-glass abnormality may be found in nonspecific interstitial pneumonia. A positive antinuclear antibody may be found in silicosis but is nonspecific. A positive rheumatoid factor may be found in rheumatoid arthritis with pulmonary involvement. *(Samet, 2008, pp. 656-657)*

44. **(B)** No treatment to date has demonstrated improvement in survival; however, oral corticosteroids with an immunosuppressive agent is the most commonly prescribed treatment. Lung transplantation is considered only if medical therapy fails. Colchicine, methotrexate, and broad-spectrum antibiotics are not used in the treatment of IPF. Initial treatment does not generally require hospitalization or intubation. *(Raghu, 2008, p. 647)*

45. **(C)** This is stage IB. Stage IA is T1N0M0; stage IIA is T1N1M0; and stage IIB is T2N1M0 or T3N0M0. *(Ettinger, 2008, pp. 1460-1462)*

46. (D) Methylxanthines in the form of caffeine citrate (20 mg/kg as loading dose and 5 to 10 mg/kg/day) is the drug of choice. The other treatments offered play no role in treating apnea in the preterm infant. *(Thilo and Rosenberg, 2009, p. 33)*

47. (C) An elevated quantitative pilocarpine iontophoresis sweat test is one of the most consistent findings in CF. Only 2% of CF patients have a normal result. Genetic testing may also be performed. *(Welsh, 2008, p. 629)*

48. (A) Hyaline membrane disease is the most common cause of respiratory distress in the preterm infant. It is caused by a deficiency in surfactant that results in poor lung compliance and atelectasis. Meconium aspiration causes a chest X-ray characterized by patchy infiltrates and coarse streaking, with flattening of the diaphragms. In an infant with ventral septal defect (VSD), the chest X-ray would be normal or show cardiomegaly depending on the size of the VSD. Tetralogy of Fallot does not usually cause symptoms at birth. *(Thilo and Rosenberg, 2009, p. 34)*

49. (C) Epidemiologic and clinical data are most helpful. Influenza is otherwise indistinguishable from any number of acute respiratory illnesses. Leukocytosis may be present but does not assist in making the diagnosis. Chest X-ray findings are nonspecific and may reveal atelectasis and/or an infiltrate in about 10% of children. Lack of vaccination may contribute to the diagnosis but would not by itself be diagnostic. Pneumonia is a common complication of influenza but is not diagnostic. *(Wright, 2007; Levin and Weinberg 2009, pp.1078-1079)*

50. (D) Respiratory syncytial virus is a common cause of bronchiolitis and is most often associated with reactive airway disease later in life. Coxsackievirus usually occurs in the summer months. Influenza A is usually transmitted in the fall or winter and would not cause concern for airway reactivity later in life. Parvovirus rather than bronchiolitis is the cause of erythema infectiosum in children. *(Chesnutt et al., 2009, pp. 236-237;*

Shandera and Coroles-Medina, 2009, pp. 1236-1239, 1243, 1245-1246)

51. (C) Pregnant women in the second and third trimester are among the groups targeted for influenza vaccine. The vaccine should not be given to children younger than 6 months. The live virus vaccine should not be given to children younger than 5 years. Two doses of vaccine are recommended for children younger than 9 years who are vaccinated for the first time. *(Daley et al., 2009, pp. 253-254; Jacobs et al., 2009, p. 1167)*

52. (B) Influenza A may be treated with inhaled zanamivir or oral oseltamivir. Acyclovir, famciclovir, lamivudine, and vidarabine are all antiviral agents used to treat other viral illnesses but are not recommended to treat influenza. *(Shandera and Coroles-Medina, 2009, pp. 1237-1239)*

53. (A) The clinical presentation described best fits asbestosis. CWP and silicosis cause a nodular pattern with upper lobe predominance. Acute hypersensitivity pneumonitis would not be a likely diagnosis in this patient who presents with a chronic condition and not an acute process. *(Chesnutt et al., 2009, pp. 272-273)*

54. (A) Catarrhal: the first stage of illness. The second stage—paroxysmal—is marked by the onset of coughing. The third and final stage is the convalescent stage where the number, severity, and duration of coughing episodes diminish. There is no formal prodromal phase in pertussis. *(Long, 2007; Ogle and Anderson, 2009, pp. 1164-1166)*

55. (C) The description best fits pleuritic chest pain. Visceral pain is poorly localized and usually described as aching or heaviness. Ischemic pain and neurologic pain can be very variable in presentation. Neither would fit the description above. *(Bickley and Szilagyi, 2007, pp. 268-269)*

56. (A) This is a classic presentation of acute respiratory distress syndrome (ARDS). Common risk factors for ARDS include sepsis, shock, and trauma. Air bronchogram on chest X-ray is found in 80% of patients with noncardiogenic acute respiratory distress syndrome. There may also be peripheral distribution of infiltrates that typically spare the costophrenic angles. Kerley B lines and flattened diaphragms are not part of the picture. The heart is usually of normal size. *(Chesnutt et al., 2009, pp. 284-286; Hudson and Slutsky, 2008, pp. 723-729)*

57. **(A)** Aphonia, the inability to vocalize, is a sign of a complete obstruction of the airway as is an inability to cough. Signs and symptoms of a partial obstruction include cough, stridor, and drooling. *(Kerby et al., 2009, pp. 482-484)*

58. **(A)** Horner syndrome (ipsilateral ptosis, miosis, and anhidrosis) is due to involvement of the inferior cervical ganglion and the paravertebral sympathetic chain. Pericarditis, pneumonitis, and systemic acidosis are not components of Horner syndrome. *(Rugo, 2009, p. 1430)*

59. **(C)** Sarcoidosis is a systemic disease of unknown etiology, which is generally characterized by granulomatous inflammation of the lung. In the United States, the incidence is highest in blacks. Symptoms may include malaise, fatigue, and dyspnea but can also include others. Erythema nodosum is not an uncommon finding. Bronchogenic carcinoma may also present with bilateral hilar adenopathy and a biopsy would also confirm such a diagnosis. Mesothelioma and tuberculosis do not present with these signs or symptoms. *(Weinberger, 2008, pp. 667-672)*

60. **(B)** The findings mentioned are highly suggestive of a benign lesion and evaluation of old radiographs would be warranted to determine stability. A CT should be ordered if it is determined that there is an increase in size. Rapid progression (doubling times less than 30 days) suggests infection; long-term stability (doubling time over 465 days) suggests benignity. *(Chesnutt et al., 2009, pp. 253-255)*

61. **(D)**. The treatment of choice for *Pneumocystic jiroveci* is trimethoprim-sulfamethoxazole. It is a pneumonia-causing fungus found in mammals and humans worldwide. Patients with HIV and other immunosuppressive disorders are at high risk for developing this infection. Amoxicillin/clavulanate, azithromycin, and doxycycline are not appropriate for the treatment of *P jiroveci*. *(Feinberg, 2008, p. 2363)*

62. **(B)** First-line agents for the treatment of acute exacerbations of chronic bronchitis include macrolides, fluoroquinolones, and Augmentin. Considering that this patient is allergic to penicillin, the best choice would be azithromycin. Because both cefuroxime and ceftriaxone are cephalosporins, these would be contraindicated given the patient's severe allergy (anaphylaxis) to penicillin. *(Chesnutt et al., 2009, pp. 230-233)*

63. **(A)** In a patient with suspected epiglottitis, the definitive diagnosis is made by direct inspection of the epiglottis by an experienced specialist under controlled conditions (such as an OR). The most common finding is a red and swollen epiglottis. After intubation, IV antibiotics can be started. Treatment with albuterol and epinephrine is not appropriate. *(Kerby et al., 2009, p. 479)*

64. **(C)** Spontaneous pneumothorax may occur in any age group but is most common in previously healthy males 20 to 40 years of age. *(Celli, 2008, p. 703)*

65. **(D)** The combination of isoniazid, rifampin, pyrazinamide, and ethambutol is the appropriate treatment for a recently converted and previously untreated patient. Although the PPD induration is only 7 mm, in this patient with recent organ transplantation, induration of greater than or equal to 5 mm is considered positive. *(Chesnutt et al., 2009, p. 247)*

66. **(C)** This clinical picture best fits a diagnosis of chronic bronchitis, which characteristically presents in the 50s and 60s with chronic cough. Asthma is more likely to present with episodic wheezing and chest tightness along with

episodic cough. Bronchiectasis would be more likely to present with recurrent pneumonia, hemoptysis, and digital clubbing on physical examination. Tuberculosis is more likely to present with weight loss, fever, night sweats, and cough. *(Chesnutt et al., 2009, pp. 228-229)*

67. (C) The most likely diagnosis in this patient is interstitial pulmonary fibrosis (IPF). The definitive diagnostic test for IPF is a surgical lung biopsy. CT scan may show marked peripheral and subpleural distribution of the interstitial densities but this does not make a definitive diagnosis. Pulmonary function tests may show decreased lung volume and flow rates but these findings are nonspecific. Ventilation-perfusion lung scans are not recommended as a routine part of the evaluation of IPF. *(Chesnutt et al., 2009, p. 256)*

68. (A) This definition best fits the description of emphysema. Permanent enlargement of distal air spaces are not seen in hyaline membrane disease, sarcoidosis, or silicosis. *(Chesnutt et al., 2009, p. 228)*

REFERENCES

Baum S. Mycoplasma infections. In: Goldman L, Ausiello D, eds. *Cecil, Textbook of Medicine.* 23rd ed. Philadelphia, PA: Saunders; 2008.

Bickley LS, Szilagyi PG. *Bates' Guide to Physical Examination and History Taking.* 9th ed. Philadelphia, PA: Lippincott Williams & Wilkins; 2007.

Boat T and Acton J. In: Kliegman RM, ed. *Nelson Textbook of Pediatrics.* 18th ed. Philadelphia, PA: Saunders; 2007.

Celli B. Diseases of the diaphragm, chest wall, pleura, and mediastinum. In: Goldman L, Ausiello D, eds. *Cecil, Textbook of Medicine.* 23rd ed. Philadelphia, PA: Saunders; 2008.

Chesnutt M et al. Pulmonary disorders. In: McPhee S, Papadakis M, eds. *Current Medical Diagnosis and Treatment.* New York, NY: McGraw-Hill; 2009.

Daley M et al. Immunization. In: Hay WW, et al., eds. *Current Pediatric Diagnosis and Treatment,* 19th ed. New York, NY: McGraw-Hill; 2009.

Drezen J. Asthma. In: Goldman L, Ausiello D, eds. *Cecil, Textbook of Medicine.* 23rd ed. Philadelphia, PA: Saunders; 2008.

Ettinger D. Lung cancer and other pulmonary neoplasms. In: Goldman L, Ausiello D, eds. *Cecil, Textbook of Medicine.* 23rd ed. Philadelphia, PA: Saunders; 2008.

Feinberg J. Pneumocystis pneumonia. In: Goldman L, Ausiello D, eds. *Cecil, Textbook of Medicine.* 23rd ed. Philadelphia, PA: Saunders; 2008.

Ginsberg J. Peripheral venous disease. In: Goldman L, Ausiello D, eds. *Cecil, Textbook of Medicine.* 23rd ed. Philadelphia, PA: Saunders; 2008.

Hollinger L. Foreign bodies of the airway. In: Kliegman RM, ed. *Nelson Textbook of Pediatrics.* 18th ed. Philadelphia, PA: Saunders; 2007.

Hudson L and Slutsky A. Acute respiratory failure. In: Goldman L, Ausiello D, eds. *Cecil, Textbook of Medicine.* 23rd ed. Philadelphia, PA: Saunders; 2008.

Hueston W. Respiratory problems. In: South-Paul, ed. *Current Diagnosis and Treatment in Family Medicine.* 2nd ed. McGraw-Hill; 2008.

Iseman M. Tuberculosis. In: Goldman L, Ausiello D, eds. *Cecil, Textbook of Medicine.* 23rd ed. Philadelphia, PA: Saunders; 2008.

Jacobs R et al. Common problems in infectious disease. In: McPhee S, Papadakis M, eds. *Current Medical Diagnosis and Treatment.* New York, NY: McGraw-Hill; 2009.

Kerby G et al. Respiratory tract and mediastinum. In: Hay WW, et al., eds. *Current Pediatric Diagnosis and Treatment,* 19th ed. New York, NY: McGraw-Hill; 2009.

Levin M and Weinberg A. Infections: viral and rickettsial. In: Hay WW, et al., eds. *Current Pediatric Diagnosis and Treatment,* 19th ed. New York, NY: McGraw-Hill; 2009.

Limper A. Overview of pneumonia. In: Goldman L, Ausiello D, eds. *Cecil, Textbook of Medicine.* 23rd ed. Philadelphia, PA: Saunders; 2008.

Long S. Pertussis. In: Kliegman RM, ed. *Nelson Textbook of Pediatrics.* 18th ed. Philadelphia, PA: Saunders; 2007.

Mandell L. Pneumococcal pneumonia. In: Goldman L, Ausiello D, eds. *Cecil, Textbook of Medicine.* 23rd ed. Philadelphia, PA: Saunders; 2008.

Ogle J and Anderson M. Bacterial and spirochetal infections. In: Hay WW, et al., eds. *Current Pediatric Diagnosis and Treatment*, 19th ed. New York, NY: McGraw-Hill; 2009.

Raghu G. Interstitial lung disease. In: Goldman L, Ausiello D, eds. *Cecil, Textbook of Medicine.* 23rd ed. Philadelphia, PA: Saunders; 2008.

Rugo H. Cancer. In: McPhee S, Papadakis M, eds. *Current Medical Diagnosis and Treatment.* New York, NY: McGraw-Hill; 2009.

Samet J. Occupational pulmonary disorders. In: Goldman L, Ausiello D, eds. *Cecil, Textbook of Medicine.* 23rd ed. Philadelphia, PA: Saunders; 2008.

Schwartz B and Chambers H. Bacterial and chlamydial infections. In: McPhee S, Papadakis M, eds. *Current Medical Diagnosis and Treatment.* New York, NY: McGraw-Hill; 2009.

Shandera W and Coroles-Medina V. Viral and rickettsial infections. In: McPhee S, Papadakis M, eds. *Current Medical Diagnosis and Treatment.* New York, NY: McGraw-Hill; 2009.

Tapson V. Pulmonary embolism. In: Goldman L, Ausiello D, eds. *Cecil, Textbook of Medicine.* 23rd ed. Philadelphia, PA: Saunders; 2008.

Theodore P and Jablons D. Thoracic wall, pleura, mediastinum, and lung. In: Way LW, Doherty GM, eds. *Current Surgical Diagnosis and Treatment.* 12th ed. New York, NY: McGraw-Hill; 2006.

Thilo E and Rosenberg A. The newborn infant. In: Hay WW, et al., eds. *Current Pediatric Diagnosis and Treatment*, 19th ed. New York, NY: McGraw-Hill; 2009.

Weinberger S. Sarcoidosis. In: Goldman L, Ausiello D, eds. *Cecil, Textbook of Medicine.* 23rd ed. Philadelphia, PA: Saunders; 2008.

Welsh M. Cystic fibrosis. In: Goldman L, Ausiello D, eds. *Cecil, Textbook of Medicine.* 23rd ed. Philadelphia, PA: Saunders; 2008.

Wright P. Influenza. In: Kliegman RM, ed. *Nelson Textbook of Pediatrics.* 18th ed. Philadelphia, PA: Saunders; 2007.

CHAPTER 12

Rheumatology

Donna L. Yeisley, MEd, PA-C

DIRECTIONS: Each of the numbered items or incomplete statements in this section is followed by answers or by completion of the statement. Select the ONE-lettered answer or completion that is BEST in each case.

1. Which of the following clinical manifestations is most characteristic of polymyalgia rheumatica (PMR)?

    (A) subcutaneous inflammatory lesions
    (B) pain and stiffness of proximal muscle groups
    (C) insidious onset of symmetrical joint involvement
    (D) widespread musculoskeletal pain and tender points
    (E) symmetrical weakness initially in the legs that progresses caudally

2. A 53-year-old obese man presents with a third attack of gout within 1 year. Following the treatment of this acute attack, further laboratory testing is performed and the patient is found to have an elevated serum uric acid level and a 24-hour uric acid secretion of 950 mg. Which of the following medications would be most appropriate to initiate for prevention of further gouty attacks?

    (A) colchicine
    (B) probenecid
    (C) prednisone
    (D) allopurinol
    (E) indomethacin

3. A 32-year-old woman with history of anxiety presents with worsening fatigue and sleep disturbance associated with unbearable "pain all over the body" for the past several months. The physical examination is essentially unremarkable except for localized painful tenderness to palpation over the trapezius, upper back, and buttocks. Which of the following is the most likely diagnosis?

    (A) fibromyalgia
    (B) polymyositis
    (C) Paget disease
    (D) polymyalgia rheumatica
    (E) systemic lupus erythematosus

4. The diagnosis of systemic lupus erythematosus (SLE) is supported by a positive initial antibody screen; however, this test is not specific. Which of the following tests is most specific in the diagnostic evaluation of SLE?

    (A) gliadin antibody
    (B) antibody to double-stranded DNA (anti-dsDNA)
    (C) antinuclear antibody (ANA)
    (D) anticentromere antibody
    (E) antiribosomal P antibody

5. Tumor necrosis factor (TNF) inhibitors are most often considered for use in patients with rheumatoid arthritis (RA) that does not respond to initial therapy. Which of the following screenings should occur before a patient is placed on this class of medication?

   (A) chest x-ray
   (B) allergy testing
   (C) liver function tests
   (D) purified protein derivative (PPD) test
   (E) serum BUN (blood urea nitrogen) and creatinine test

6. Skin thickening that begins as swelling of the fingers and hands associated with telangiectasia, dysphagia, and hypomotility of the gastrointestinal tract is most likely seen with which of the following?

   (A) sarcoidosis
   (B) scleroderma
   (C) dermatomyositis
   (D) eosinophilic fasciitis
   (E) eosinophilia–myalgia syndrome

7. A 6-year-old girl is diagnosed with juvenile rheumatoid arthritis (JRA). Which of the following referrals is indicated, especially if the patient also has a positive antinuclear antibody test?

   (A) ophthalmologist for a screening eye examination
   (B) otolaryngologist for a screening hearing examination
   (C) dermatologist for evaluation of skin expression of the disease
   (D) endocrinologist for evaluation of potential growth restriction
   (E) gastroenterologist for evaluation of potential peptic ulcer disease

8. Which of the following conditions is strongly associated with systemic sclerosis (scleroderma)?

   (A) polymyositis
   (B) reactive arthritis
   (C) dermatomyositis
   (D) Sjögren disease
   (E) Raynaud phenomenon

9. A 65-year-old man presents with complaints of acute onset of pain and swelling of the right great toe. He denies recent alcohol ingestion or trauma to the area. On physical examination, the patient is afebrile, and the first metatarsophalangeal joint is erythematous, swollen, and warm to the touch. Laboratory evaluation reveals a WBC (white blood cells) count of $12,000/\mu L$ and a normal differential. Serum uric acid level is found to be 5 mg/dL. Synovial fluid analysis reveals the presence of rhomboid-shaped crystals. Which of the following is the most likely diagnosis?

   (A) acute gout
   (B) pseudogout
   (C) psoriatic arthritis
   (D) infectious arthritis
   (E) rheumatoid arthritis

10. Which of the following treatment options for osteoporosis has the added benefit of reducing the risk of breast cancer?

   (A) calcitonin
   (B) raloxifene
   (C) alendronate
   (D) teriparatide
   (E) conjugated estrogen

11. Which of the following patterns of stiffness is most characteristic of patients with rheumatoid arthritis?

   (A) morning stiffness lasting at least 1 hour
   (B) exacerbation of joint stiffness with walking
   (C) frequent, brief episodes of stiffness after inactivity
   (D) stiffness reflected by a major delay in muscle relaxation
   (E) stiffness evidenced by increased resistance to passive movement

12. Related infections that have been identified as triggers of reactive arthritis include sexually transmitted infections and which of the following other types of infections?

    (A) ear infections
    (B) eye infections
    (C) enteric infections
    (D) musculoskeletal infections
    (E) central nervous system infections

13. A 59-year-old woman with a known history of rheumatoid arthritis presents with relatively severe complaints of pain, notable bony deformity of the hands with extra-articular findings of cutaneous nodules, scleritis, and pleurisy. On physical examination, the patient is found to have splenomegaly. Which of the following is the most appropriate laboratory evaluation to order to further evaluate the suspected diagnosis?

    (A) complete blood count (CBC)
    (B) uric acid
    (C) C-reactive protein
    (D) antinuclear antibodies
    (E) erythrocyte sedimentation rate

14. A 45-year-old woman with recent diagnosis of rheumatoid arthritis has begun treatment with celecoxib. She has been on this medication for 3 months and notes that her pain continues. Early signs of joint involvement are present in the patient's hands. Which of the following medications is the most appropriate to add to her treatment?

    (A) aspirin
    (B) rituximab
    (C) etanercept
    (D) leflunomide
    (E) methotrexate

15. A 12-year-old girl presents with complaints of intermittent pain and stiffness involving her hands. This pain has been progressively worsening over the past 3 years. She relates that for the past 2 months she has been feeling increasingly tired and has experienced swelling and stiffness of her hands, which appears worse in the morning and is relieved as the day progresses. The physical examination shows she has a low-grade fever. There are multiple symmetrical joint swelling of the proximal interphalangeal and metacarpophalangeal joints with associated warmth, tenderness, and effusion. Initial laboratory findings include a CBC that reveals mild anemia, an elevated erythrocyte sedimentation rate, a positive rheumatoid factor, and a negative antinuclear antibody (ANA) test. X-rays of the hands and wrists show soft tissue swelling and periarticular osteopenia. Which of the following is the most likely diagnosis?

    (A) reactive arthritis
    (B) infectious arthritis
    (C) systemic juvenile rheumatoid arthritis
    (D) polyarticular juvenile rheumatoid arthritis
    (E) pauciarticular juvenile rheumatoid arthritis

16. A 48-year-old woman presents with a chief complaint of gradually progressing difficulty in climbing stairs over the past 3 months. The physical examination shows there is notable proximal muscle weakness of the upper and lower extremities. The remainder of the examination is unremarkable. The laboratory evaluation shows an elevated serum creatinine phosphokinase level, and a muscle biopsy reveals lymphoid inflammatory infiltrates. Which of the following is the appropriate initial treatment of choice in this patient?

    (A) prednisone
    (B) azathioprine
    (C) methotrexate
    (D) immunoglobulin
    (E) hydrochloroquine

17. Which of the following is the correct term to describe the abrupt onset of swelling and extreme tenderness to palpation involving the metatarsophalangeal joint of the great toe?

    (A) crepitus
    (B) podagra
    (C) xerostomia
    (D) trigger point
    (E) chondrocalcinosis

18. Which of the following is an established risk factor for osteoporosis and is also an indication for measuring bone density?

    (A) obesity
    (B) alcoholism
    (C) hypercalcemia
    (D) history of scoliosis
    (E) short-term corticosteroid therapy

19. A 22-year-old man presents with an insidious onset of low back pain over the last 6 months. He describes the pain as dull and has difficulty localizing the pain. The pain often radiates to his thighs. The pain is worse in the morning and associated with stiffening that lessens during the day. The patient notes that there is no history of trauma. The initial laboratory evaluation shows an elevated erythrocyte sedimentation rate, positive HLA-B27, and a negative rheumatoid factor. Plain films of the lumbar spine reveal bilateral blurring of the sacroiliac joints. Which of the following is the most likely diagnosis?

    (A) systemic lupus
    (B) lumbar disc disease
    (C) rheumatoid arthritis
    (D) ankylosing spondylitis
    (E) polymyalgia rheumatica

20. A 65-year-old woman with long-standing rheumatoid arthritis presents for a preoperative evaluation appointment. She is scheduled for a total joint arthroplasty in 2 weeks. Which of the following is the most appropriate intervention to detect an associated condition that may lead to complications during anesthesia?

    (A) HLA (human leukocyte antigen) typing
    (B) slit-lamp examination
    (C) thorascopic lung biopsy
    (D) repeat rheumatoid factor
    (E) flexion and extension x-rays of cervical spine

21. Which of the following clinical manifestations is associated with systemic disorders that are HLA-B27 related, including ankylosing spondylitis, reactive arthritis, psoriasis, and Behçet syndrome?

    (A) uveitis
    (B) dysentery
    (C) vasculitis
    (D) hyperuricemia
    (E) thoracic involvement

22. A 67-year-old man presents with pain and stiffness in his shoulders and hips lasting for several weeks with no history of trauma. He also has complaints of headache, throat pain, and jaw claudication. It is imperative to diagnose this patient promptly in order to prevent which of the following complications?

    (A) anemia
    (B) cerebral aneurysms
    (C) mononeuritis multiplex
    (D) ischemic optic neuropathy
    (E) respiratory tract complications

23. Which of the following is a cause of inflammatory polyarthritis?

    (A) gout
    (B) osteoarthritis
    (C) reactive arthritis
    (D) psoriatic arthritis
    (E) systemic lupus erythematosus

24. A 65-year-old woman presents with severe mid-back pain of 2 weeks duration. She has no history of trauma. Radiographic evaluation reveals compression fractures of T11 and T12. A complete blood count, erythrocyte sedimentation rate, serum protein, serum calcium, phosphate, and parathyroid hormone levels are all within normal ranges. In addition to ordering a dual-energy x-ray absorptiometry (DEXA) scan, which of the following laboratory evaluations is most helpful in evaluating this patient for secondary causes of this presentation?

    (A) bone biopsy
    (B) rheumatoid factor
    (C) serum magnesium

(D) 25-hydroxyvitamin D

(E) antinuclear antibodies test

25. Which of the following HLA haplotypes is strongly associated with rheumatoid arthritis?

(A) HLA-B8

(B) HLA-B27

(C) HLA-B51

(D) HLA-DR4

(E) HLA-DRB3

26. Reactive arthritis most commonly presents with a tetrad of urethritis, conjunctivitis, mucocutaneous lesions, and oligoarthritis. Which of the following joints are most commonly involved with this condition?

(A) sacroiliac joints

(B) metatarsophalangeal joints

(C) large weight-bearing joints

(D) metacarpophalangeal joints

(E) distal interphalangeal joints

27. A 58-year-old postmenopausal woman presents for a routine annual examination. She is concerned about osteoporosis and is currently taking no medications. While counseling the patient about calcium intake along with the appropriate amount of vitamin D, what amount of calcium per day should be recommended for this patient?

(A) 700 mg

(B) 1,000 mg

(C) 1,200 mg

(D) 1,500 mg

(E) 2,000 mg

28. Which of the following medications has been shown to have a definite association with the potential development of systemic lupus erythematosus?

(A) isoniazid

(B) penicillin

(C) gold salts

(D) allopurinol

(E) griseofulvin

29. A 52-year-old man with hypertension associated with recent unexplained weight loss presents with fever, malaise, and gradual onset of pain and weakness of his leg muscles for the past month. Physical examination reveals a mottled reticular pattern overlying portions of both calves and an area of ulceration with surrounding induration on the left lateral malleolus. Initial laboratory results reveal mild normochromic anemia, leukocytosis, and elevation of C-reactive protein, BUN, and creatinine. Which of the following is the most appropriate diagnostic evaluation to confirm the suspected diagnosis?

(A) HLA-B27 typing

(B) rheumatoid factor

(C) MRI of sacroiliac joints

(D) antinuclear antibodies test

(E) tissue biopsy of area of induration

30. Patients diagnosed with Sjögren syndrome should be counseled to avoid which of the following class of medications?

(A) penicillins

(B) decongestants

(C) antihistamines

(D) corticosteroids

(E) fluoroquinolones

Answers and Explanations

1. **(B)** An abrupt onset of proximal muscle pain and stiffness in the shoulder and pelvic girdle areas, usually associated with fever, malaise, and weight loss, is characteristic of polymyalgia rheumatica. Subcutaneous inflammatory lesions denote erythema nodosum. These lesions are associated with pregnancy and several systemic disorders, such as sarcoidosis, tuberculosis (TB), and streptococcal infections. Insidious onset of symmetrical joint involvement is most commonly associated with rheumatoid arthritis. Widespread musculoskeletal pain and tender points, referred to as "trigger points," are seen with fibromyalgia syndrome. Trigger points may be found anywhere on the body but are most common in the neck, shoulders, hands, low back, and knees. Symmetrical weakness initially in the legs that progresses caudally is characteristic of Guillain–Barré syndrome. *(Hellmann and Imboden, 2008, p. 739)*

2. **(D)** Medications used to prevent gout exacerbations include allopurinol and uricosuric drugs, such as probenecid. Allopurinol inhibits the production of uric acid and is indicated for patients who overproduce uric acid, and uricosuric drugs are used in patients who undersecrete uric acid. Criterion to classify a patient as an overproducer of uric acid is a 24-hour uric acid excretion test. The result showing uric acid excretion of 800 mg or greater indicates that the patient is an overproducer. In this patient scenario, there is an overproduction of uric acid, making the case for the use of allopurinol. If this patient's 24-hour uric acid excretion was less than 800 mg, the use of a uricosuric drug would then be appropriate. Prednisone, colchicine, and indomethacin are alternative treatments for acute attacks of gout and are not used for preventive measures. *(Furst et al. 2009, pp. 637-639; Hellmann and Imboden, 2008, pp. 706-709)*

3. **(A)** Fibromyalgia is the most likely diagnosis in this patient. It is most frequently seen in woman between the ages of 20 and 50. Patients complain of chronic musculoskeletal pain commonly associated with fatigue and sleep disturbances as well as headaches and numbness. Physical examination is normal except for the presence of multiple "trigger points." Polymyositis most commonly presents with weakness rather than pain, and although it may present at any age, it is most common in the fifth and sixth decades of life. Paget disease is most commonly diagnosed after the age of 40 and is usually asymptomatic and mild, but if symptomatic, presents with bone pain. Polymyalgia rheumatica is commonly seen in patients older than 50 years and presents with shoulder and pelvic pain. Systemic lupus erythematosus does affect mainly young female patients but involves multiple organ systems that include skin lesions, joint symptoms, ocular manifestations as well as lung, heart, and neurological symptoms. *(Hellmann and Imboden, 2008, p. 715)*

4. **(B)** Autoantibody production is the primary immunological abnormality seen in patients with systemic lupus erythematosus (SLE); the antinuclear antibody (ANA) is most characteristic of SLE and seen in 95% of patients with SLE but is not specific for the diagnosis of SLE. A positive ANA can also be found in patients with lupoid hepatitis, scleroderma, rheumatoid arthritis, Sjögren disease, dermatomyositis,

and polyarteritis. ANA testing should be employed as the initial screening test in a patient suspected of having SLE. A negative total ANA test is strong evidence against the diagnosis of SLE, whereas a positive test is not confirmatory of the diagnosis. The most specific antibody tests for SLE are antibodies to double-stranded DNA (anti-dsDNAs) and anti-Smith (anti-SM). Although these tests are more specific for SLE, they are less sensitive than the ANA test. Anti-dsDNA is positive in 60% of patients with SLE and anti-SM is positive in 30% of patients. Anti-dsDNA is more likely to reflect disease activity. Gliadin antibody assay is utilized to assess patients with suspected celiac disease. Anticentromere antibody is associated with CREST (calcinosis, Raynaud phenomenon, esophageal dysmotility, sclerodactyly, and telangiectasia) syndrome in scleroderma. Antibodies to ribonucleoprotein are present in patients with a mixture of overlapping rheumatological symptoms known as "mixed connective tissue disease." *(Hellmann and Imboden, 2008, pp. 725-729)*

5. **(D)** Patients being treated for rheumatoid arthritis with tumor necrosis factor (TNF) inhibitors are at increased risk for developing an opportunistic infection, such as tuberculosis (TB). It is recommended that screening for the presence of latent TB occur before TNF inhibitors are started. There is no specific indication to order a chest x-ray, allergy testing, liver function tests, or serum BUN and creatinine prior to initiation of TNF inhibitors. *(Furst et al, 2009, pp. 633-635; Hellmann and Imboden, 2008, p. 734)*

6. **(B)** Scleroderma is characterized by diffuse thickening of the skin and is associated with areas of telangiectasia and changes in skin pigmentation. Most patients with scleroderma also have an associated polyarthralgia, Raynaud phenomena, and gastrointestinal involvement. Sarcoidosis more commonly presents with pulmonary symptoms and erythema nodosum. Dermatomyositis presents with scaly patches over the dorsum of the hands (Gottron sign) and lilac discoloration of the eyelids (heliotrope rash). Eosinophilic fasciitis is a rare disorder associated with skin changes similar to those seen in scleroderma; however, there is no association with Raynaud phenomena. Eosinophilia–myalgia syndrome is associated with chronic ingestion of tryptophan, which is an amino acid previously found in over-the-counter preparations for insomnia and premenstrual syndrome, now banned by the Food and Drug Administration. Cutaneous findings in eosinophilia–myalgia syndrome present with a range of expression from hives to swelling of the extremities. *(Hellmann and Imboden, 2008, pp. 731-732)*

7. **(A)** The most common type of juvenile rheumatoid arthritis (JRA) is the pauciarticular form that is oligoarticular, involving four or less joints. A risk with this form of JRA is the development of insidious, asymptomatic uveitis, which may lead to blindness if not detected and treated. Routine ophthalmologic screening with slit-lamp examination is recommended every 3 months if the patient has a positive antinuclear antibody (ANA) and every 6 months if the patient has a negative ANA. Patients with JRA are not at increased risk of hearing impairment; thus a referral to the otolaryngologist is unnecessary. Patients with JRA who have a systemic presentation do have a characteristic rash, but a dermatology consultation is usually not warranted. Growth restriction may occur with any form of JRA, more commonly found in systemic onset and polyarticular onset JRA. There is no current method to predict which patients will have growth restriction, and a routine referral is not often indicated. Even though the use of nonsteroidal anti-inflammatory drugs (NSAIDs) is the first line of treatment in JRA, they are usually well tolerated in children as long as the medication is taken with food. Referral to a gastroenterologist is not indicated. *(Soep and Hollister, 2009, pp. 796-797)*

8. **(E)** Most patients with systemic sclerosis (scleroderma) will also have vascular dysfunction, most commonly Raynaud phenomenon. There is no increased association of scleroderma with polymyositis, reactive arthritis, dermatomyositis, or Sjögren disease. *(Hellmann and Imboden, 2008, pp. 731-732)*

9. **(B)** Pseudogout presents similarly to acute gout and is best diagnosed by the finding of the rhomboid-shaped crystals of calcium pyrophosphate in joint aspirates. Joints commonly involved in pseudogout are the knees and wrists and other joints such as the metacarpophalangeals, hips, shoulders, ankles, and elbows. The diagnosis of pseudogout is further supported by the finding of a normal serum uric acid level. Acute gout would more likely be associated with an elevated serum uric acid level. Psoriatic arthritis commonly presents with asymmetrical oligoarticular involvement of two to four joints, and in a higher percentage of patients, there is known presence of the dermatological expression of psoriasis. Infectious arthritis is ruled out with the findings of an afebrile patient and WBC count of 12,000/μL. In acute infectious arthritis, the WBCs would be expected to be elevated in the range of 50,000 to 200,000/μL. Rheumatoid arthritis usually presents with symmetrical polyarticular involvement of three or more joints. *(Hellmann and Imboden, 2008, p. 709)*

10. **(B)** Raloxifene, a selective estrogen receptor modulator, has the added benefit of reducing the risk of breast cancer while increasing bone density and reducing the risk of vertebral fractures in patients with osteoporosis. Calcitonin, bisphosphonates (alendronate), and teriparatide, although utilized in the treatment of osteoporosis, do not have an added benefit of reducing the risk of breast cancer. Conjugated estrogens, such as Premarin (Wyeth Pharmaceuticals, Philadelphia, PA), may actually increase the risk of breast cancer in patients. *(Bikle, 2009, p. 766; Fitzgerald, 2008, pp. 996-997)*

11. **(A)** Morning stiffness lasting at least 1 hour is characteristic of rheumatoid arthritis (RA). Exacerbation of joint stiffness with weight bearing (such as walking) and frequent, brief episodes of stiffness (lasting <30 minutes) after inactivity are both more characteristic of degenerative joint disease, not RA. Stiffness reflected by a major delay in relaxation after muscle contraction is seen in myotonic dystrophy. Stiffness evidenced by increased resistance to passive movement describes the "rigidity" associated with parkinsonism. *(Hellmann and Imboden, 2008, pp. 720-721)*

12. **(C)** Reactive arthritis, previously known as Reiter syndrome, typically presents with the clinical triad of urethritis, conjunctivitis, and arthritis. Most cases of reactive arthritis are associated with either a sexually transmitted infection (STI) or an enteric infection. Common STI etiological triggers are *Chlamydia trachomatis* or *Ureaplasma urealyticum*. Enterically *Shigella*, *Salmonella*, *Yersinia*, or *Campylobacter* are organisms associated with reactive arthritis. Common ear, eye, musculoskeletal, and central nervous system infections are usually not associated with reactive arthritis. *(Hellmann and Imboden, 2008, p. 749)*

13. **(A)** This patient presentation of known rheumatoid arthritis with severe deformities, extra-articular findings, and splenomegaly is most likely Felty syndrome. Felty syndrome is characterized by the triad of deforming rheumatoid arthritis, splenomegaly, and neutropenia. The appropriate laboratory test to order would be a CBC to evaluate for neutropenia. Uric acid testing is helpful in evaluating gout but is not relevant to this patient presentation. Ordering an erythrocyte sedimentation rate or C-reactive protein is not necessarily helpful in diagnosing Felty syndrome; in an acute inflammatory flare, both would most likely be elevated. Antinuclear antibodies could be present in 20% to 40% of patients but are not diagnostic of Felty syndrome. *(Hellmann and Imboden, 2008, p. 721; Linker, 2008, p. 438)*

14. **(E)** The treatment of rheumatoid arthritis (RA) is aimed at reduction of pain, preservation of function, and prevention of deformity. Although non-steroidal anti-inflammatory drugs (NSAIDs) provide symptomatic relief, they do not alter progression or prevent erosion of the joint. Consequently, in addition to NSAID therapy, disease-modifying antirheumatological drugs (DMARDs) should also be initiated as soon as the diagnosis is confirmed. The most common initial DMARD used as treatment of choice in RA is methotrexate. Aspirin should not be added because of the increased risk of gastrointestinal side effects as well as having no effect on altering RA disease progression. Rituximab is a biological

DMARD and is indicated to be added in patients with RA refractory to treatment with combination therapy of methotrexate and a tumor necrosis factor inhibitor (TNF). Etanercept is a TNF inhibitor. This class of medication is often added in patients with RA who are not responding to methotrexate therapy alone. Leflunomide is a pyrimidine synthesis inhibitor that is approved for the treatment of RA; however, it is contraindicated for use in premenopausal women secondary to its carcinogenic and teratogenic potential. *(Hellmann and Imboden, 2008, pp. 722-725)*

15. **(D)** The most likely diagnosis in this patient is polyarticular juvenile rheumatoid arthritis (JRA). This form of JRA is seen in approximately 35% of patients with JRA. It is characterized by symmetrical involvement of five or more joints. Two subsets of the disease exist that are distinguished by the presence or absence of rheumatoid factor. A positive rheumatoid factor is most commonly seen in girls with later disease onset (at least 8 years old). An antinuclear antibody (ANA) test may be positive but is more likely to be positive with the pauciarticular form. In the early stage of the disease, the x-ray may be normal or show soft tissue swelling and periarticular osteopenia. In addition to the positive ANA of pauciarticular JRA patients, the arthritis must be present in four or fewer joints. Early onset disease is commonly seen in girls aged 1 to 5 years and has a positive ANA; up to 30% of patients will also have eye involvement. Late onset disease is more common in male patients, with involvement of the large joints. Systemic JRA, also known as "Still disease," is seen in about 10% to 15% of children with JRA. It is characterized by daily intermittent fever spikes and a transient, nonpruritic, pale pink, blanching macular, or maculopapular rash found on the trunk. A positive rheumatoid factor is rare in this form of JRA. Reactive arthritis is usually associated with a recent viral or bacterial infection. Infectious arthritis more commonly presents as monarticular and is usually acute in onset. *(Soep and Hollister, 2009, pp. 796-797)*

16. **(A)** The most likely diagnosis in this patient is polymyositis. This is supported by the finding of a gradual progressive proximal muscle weakness and elevation of creatinine phosphokinase level. The finding of lymphoid inflammatory infiltrates on muscle biopsy confirms the diagnosis. Initial treatment of choice in this condition is the use of a corticosteroid (prednisone). Patients who do not respond to prednisone may then benefit from the use of methotrexate or azathioprine. Both intravenous immune globulin and hydroxychloroquine are effective for the treatment of patients with dermatomyositis that is resistant to prednisone therapy. *(Hellmann and Imboden, 2008, pp. 733-735)*

17. **(B)** Podagra is the term utilized to denote the involvement of the great toe in cases of gout. *Crepitus* refers to a sound or feeling associated with the movement of joints due to joint irregularities. *Xerostomia* is the term applied to symptoms of dryness of the mouth, which may be seen in Sjögren syndrome. Trigger points typically describe areas of pain revealed by palpation of involved muscle areas in patients with fibromyalgia. *Chondrocalcinosis* refers to the presence of calcium-containing salts in articular cartilage associated with metabolic diseases, such as pseudogout. *(Hellmann and Imboden, 2008, pp. 706-707)*

18. **(B)** Risk factors for osteoporosis and indications for measuring bone density include alcoholism. Low body mass index (BMI <19 kg/m^2), not obesity; hypocalcemia, not hypercalcemia; loss of height or thoracic kyphosis, not scoliosis and long-term corticosteroid therapy (more than 6 mg of prednisone for more than 1 month), not short-term corticosteroid therapy are also indications for measuring bone density. *(Fitzgerald, 2008, pp. 995)*

19. **(D)** Ankylosing spondylosis is the most likely diagnosis in this patient. This condition is a chronic inflammatory disorder of the joints of the axial skeleton and commonly presents in the late teens or twenties. Male patients have a higher incidence than do female patients. A common presentation is pain in the lower back with radiation to the thighs and associated limitation of movement that may lessen during the day. Laboratory findings include an elevated

erythrocyte sedimentation rate and positive HLA-B27. The HLA-B27 is not a specific test for ankylosing spondylitis; a small percentage of the normal population has a positive finding of this antigen. The earliest radiographic findings occur in the sacroiliac joints, with the detection of erosion and blurring of the joint space. Systemic lupus commonly affects women of childbearing years and presents with exacerbations and remissions of arthritis, rash, fatigue, and the potential for organ system involvement. Lumbar disc disease is usually seen in the age group of 35 to 45 years and is more likely to be associated with trauma. Rheumatoid arthritis does have the potential to affect this age group, but it would more likely be associated with smaller joints of the hands, along with a positive rheumatoid factor. Polymyalgia rheumatica more commonly affects patients older than 50 years and is associated with fatigue, malaise, chronic pain, and stiffness of the proximal muscles, shoulders, neck, and pelvic girdle. *(Hellmann and Imboden, 2008, pp. 746-747)*

20. **(E)** Cervical spine disease in long-standing rheumatoid arthritis (RA) may lead to C1–C2 subluxation and spinal cord compression. Flexion and extension x-rays of the cervical spine will detect the possibility of subluxation to avoid potential complications with neck movement during anesthesia. Although HLA-DR4 is associated with RA, it has no prognostic value in detecting potential complications with anesthesia. Slit-lamp examination will diagnose scleritis or episcleritis, which is a nonarticular manifestation of RA, but the presence of either of these conditions is also not associated with increased risk from anesthesia. Although lung disease may develop in patients with RA, thorascopic lung biopsy is not indicated prior to anesthesia. Patients with RA who are seropositive are more likely to have severe erosive disease, rheumatoid nodules, and extra-articular manifestations but are not at increased risk, per se, during anesthesia. *(Hellmann and Imboden, 2008, p. 722; Merkel and Simms, 2007, p. 806)*

21. **(A)** Uveitis is an associated finding in patients with ankylosing spondylitis, reactive arthritis, psoriasis, and Behçet disease. These disorders can cause a nongranulomatous anterior uveitis that usually presents unilaterally with pain, redness, photophobia, and visual loss. Uveitis associated with Behçet disease can be aggressive and result in blindness. Dysentery is more likely to be associated with reactive arthritis. Vasculitis is seen with Behçet disease. Hyperuricemia may be found with psoriasis. Thoracic involvement is often found in ankylosing spondylitis. *(Riordan-Eva, 2008, pp. 149-150)*

22. **(D)** The most urgent need for diagnosis of a patient with symptoms of polymyalgia rheumatica (PMR) and giant cell arteritis is to prevent blindness caused by ischemic optic neuropathy as a result of occlusive arteritis of the ophthalmic artery. Early diagnosis is imperative as the neurological damage to the optic nerve is not reversible. Most patients with this diagnosis will have a normochromic-normocytic anemia, but this does not create urgency in treatment. Cerebral aneurysms are not common findings with PMR; large vessels such as the subclavian and aorta may be involved in giant cell arthritis in 15% of patients. Mononeuritis multiplex commonly presents with painful paralysis of a shoulder, and respiratory tract complications are more nonclassic findings with the presentation of PMR. *(Hellmann and Imboden, 2008, pp. 739-740)*

23. **(E)** Inflammatory causes of polyarthritis include systemic lupus erythematosus and rheumatoid arthritis. Gout, although inflammatory, is most commonly monarticular. Osteoarthritis is a noninflammatory process that is also usually monarticular. Both reactive arthritis and psoriatic arthritis involve two to four joints and are therefore classified as oligoarticular. *(Hellmann and Imboden, 2008, p. 704)*

24. **(D)** This patient has typical findings associated with osteoporosis. Most patients with osteoporosis are asymptomatic until fractures present. Fractures occur spontaneously and are associated with back pain of varied degrees. Serum calcium, phosphate, and parathyroid hormone levels are often normal. Since vitamin D deficiency state is common in osteoporosis, a 25-hydroxyvitamin D should be

ordered. Bone biopsy is not indicated with this patient; this would be reserved for evaluating for osteomalacia. Rheumatoid factor and antinuclear antibodies would not be of importance with this patient presentation. Serum magnesium is associated more with evaluating for parathyroid or thyroid disorder and has no value with osteoporosis. *(Fitzgerald, 2008, pp. 994-995)*

25. **(D)** Rheumatoid arthritis (RA) is associated with HLA-DR4. Patients with a positive DR4 will most likely have more serious and seropositive RA disease. HLA-B8 is associated with Graves hyperthyroidism and myasthenia gravis. HLA-B27 is associated with multiple diseases that are classified as spondyloarthropathies, including ankloysing spondylitis, reactive arthritis (Reiter syndrome), and psoriatic spondylitis. HLA-B51 is associated with Behcet disease, and HLA-DRB3 is associated with type 1 diabetes mellitus. *(Merkel and Simms, 2007, p. 804)*

26. **(C)** The most common joints involved in reactive arthritis are the large weight-bearing joints of the knees and ankles. The sacroiliac joints are involved in only 20% of patients with reactive arthritis. The small joints of the feet, such as metatarsophalangeal joints, are not likely joints involved in reactive arthritis. Metacarpophalangeal joints are primarily involved in rheumatoid arthritis or systemic lupus erythematosus. Distal interphalangeal joints are commonly involved in osteoarthritis and psoriatic arthritis. *(Hellmann and Imboden, 2008, p. 749)*

27. **(D)** The recommended calcium intake for postmenopausal women not on estrogen replacement therapy is 1,500 mg. For premenopausal women and postmenopausal women on estrogen replacement therapy, the recommended adult dose is 1,000 mg. The average adult has

a daily dietary intake of 700 mg of calcium, which falls below the standard recommendation. Calcium is found in dairy products, green leafy vegetables, and fish with bones. There is no current recommendation for 2,000 mg of calcium intake. *(Baron, 2008, p. 1097)*

28. **(A)** Drugs that have a definite association with systemic lupus erythemaosus include isoniazid. Penicillin, gold salts, allopurinol, and griseofulvin are all classified as having an unlikely association. *(Hellmann and Imboden, 2008, p. 726)*

29. **(E)** This patient most likely has polyarteritis nodosa (PN). A major obstacle in making the diagnosis is the absence of a disease-specific serological test. The diagnosis requires confirmation with either a tissue biopsy or angiogram. HLA-B27 antigens are not associated with the suspected diagnosis. While classic PN will have low titers of rheumatoid factor and antinuclear antibodies, both are nonspecific findings and will not confirm the diagnosis. An MRI of the sacroiliac joints is indicated in evaluation of the early stages of suspected ankylosing spondylitis and plays no role in the evaluation of PN. *(Hellmann and Imboden, 2008, pp. 738-739)*

30. **(B)** Sjögren syndrome is an autoimmune disorder that commonly presents with dryness of the eyes, mouth, and other areas of the body covered by mucous membrane. Because of the chronic dysfunction of the exocrine glands and chronicity of dryness of the eyes and the mouth, patients should be counseled to avoid decongestants and atropinic drugs. The use of these medications can further exacerbate their symptoms. Penicillins, antihistamines, corticosteroids, and fluoroquinolones are not directly associated with encouraging exocrine dysfunction. *(Hellmann and Imboden, 2008, pp. 735-736)*

REFERENCES

Baron RB. Nutritional disorders. In: Tierney LM, McPhee SJ, Papadakis MA, eds. *2008 Current Medical Diagnosis and Treatment.* New York, NY: McGraw-Hill Companies, Inc; 2008:1085-1102.

Bikle DD. Agents that affect bone mineral homeostasis. In: Katzung BG, Masters SB, Trevor AJ, eds. *Basic and Clinical Pharmacology.* New York, NY: McGraw-Hill; 2009:753-772.

Fitzgerald PA. Endocrine disorders. In: Tierney LM, McPhee SJ, Papadakis MA, eds. *2008 Current Medical Diagnosis and Treatment.* New York, NY: McGraw-Hill; 2008:949-1031.

Furst DE, Ulrich RW, Varkey-Altamirano C. Nonsteroidal anti-inflammatory drugs, disease-modifying antirheumatic drugs, nonopioid analgesics, and drugs used in gout. In: Katzung BG, Masters SB, Trevor AJ, eds. *Basic and Clinical Pharmacology.* New York, NY: McGraw-Hill; 2009:621-642.

Hellmann DB, Imboden JB. Arthritis and musculoskeletal disorders. In: Tierney LM, McPhee SJ, Papadakis MA, eds. *2008 Current Medical Diagnosis and Treatment.* New York, NY: McGraw-Hill; 2008:703-756.

Linker CA. Blood disorders. In: Tierney LM, McPhee SJ, Papadakis MA, eds. *2008 Current Medical Diagnosis and Treatment.* New York, NY: McGraw-Hill; 2008:422-472.

Merkel PA, Simms RW. Rheumatoid arthritis. In: Andreoli TE, Carpenter CCJ, Griggs RC, Benjamin IJ, eds. *Andreoli and Carpenter's Cecil Essentials of Medicine.* Philadelphia, PA: Saunders Elsevier; 2007:804-808.

Riordan-Eva P. Disorders of the eyes and lids. In: Tierney LM, McPhee SJ, Papadakis MA, eds. *2008 Current Medical Diagnosis and Treatment.* New York, NY: McGraw-Hill; 2008:141-167.

Soep JB, Hollister JR. Rheumatic diseases. In: Hay WW, Levin MJ, Sondheimer JM, Deterding RR, eds. *Current Diagnosis and Treatment Pediatrics.* New York, NY: McGraw-Hill; 2009:796-803.

SECTION II
Obstetrics and Gynecology

17. A 25-year-old G1, P1 presents with 2 days of right-sided pelvic pain and a history of menstrual irregularities for 2 months. She denies fever, chills, or nausea. She has a negative pregnancy test. Her pelvic examination reveals an approximately 5-cm mobile adnexal mass. Which element of the history or physical examination is MOST specific for the diagnosis of ovarian cysts and not for the diagnoses of appendicitis, viral gastroenteritis, endometriotic cysts, carcinoma, or tubo-ovarian abscess?

    (A) right-sided pelvic pain
    (B) denial of fever, chills, or nausea
    (C) menstrual irregularities
    (D) adnexal mass

18. A very firm ovarian mass estimated at 8 cm is found in a 33-year-old woman at her annual examination. Which of the following interventions should be considered first?

    (A) combination chemotherapy
    (B) radiation therapy
    (C) surgical consult
    (D) exploratory laparoscopy

19. In women with a *BRCA1* gene mutation, which of the following types of cancer are they MOST at increased risk for developing?

    (A) cervical cancer
    (B) ovarian cancer
    (C) endometrial cancer
    (D) vaginal cancer

20. A Papanicolaou (Pap) smear is performed on a 40-year-old patient who has not had a Pap smear since the birth of her last baby (15 years ago). Today's Pap smear result indicates squamous cell carcinoma. The reason she sought medical care was for postcoital bleeding. At the time of the Pap smear, there was a friable lesion present. At this point, the MOST appropriate step in this patient's management is

    (A) repeat Pap smear in 4 to 6 months
    (B) biopsy visualized lesion and refer patient for gynecologic consult
    (C) colposcopy with endocervical curettage and directed biopsy

    (D) loop electrosurgical excision procedure (LEEP) or cervical conization
    (E) radical hysterectomy and radiation therapy

21. On physical examination of a 24-year-old nulligravida, an erythematous cervix with a yellow discharge is visualized. The patient has had one new partner in the past 60 days. She uses oral contraceptives for birth control and rarely uses condoms. She has not noticed any pruritis, discharge, or vaginal pain. The wet prep reveals no hyphae or clue cells. Which of the following etiologic organisms BEST fits the clinical information given?

    (A) *Staphylococcus aureus*
    (B) *Chlamydia trachomatis*
    (C) *Gardnerella vaginalis*
    (D) *Candida albicans*
    (E) Human papillomavirus (HPV)

22. Cervical cysts are noted while performing a Papanicolaou test. The MOST likely diagnosis is

    (A) Bartholin cysts
    (B) Nabothian cysts
    (C) cervicitis
    (D) HPV
    (E) cervical carcinoma

23. A 25-year-old G1, P1 presents to the clinic for her annual examination. She has no history of abnormal Pap smears, but the results from today's test show low-grade squamous intraepithelial lesions (LSIL). Which of the following is the BEST option for what should be done next?

    (A) recheck Pap in 1 year
    (B) repeat Pap smear in 4 to 6 months, using traditional method
    (C) repeat Pap smear in 4 to 6 months, using liquid-based cytology
    (D) HPV testing
    (E) colposcopy

24. A 58-year-old woman who is postmenopausal since 8 years complains of urinary urgency, frequency, and occasional incontinence. On pelvic examination, her vaginal mucosa appears shiny,

pale pink with white patches, and bleeds slightly to touch. Her urinalysis and urine cultures are negative. Which of the following is the BEST treatment for this patient?

(A) antibiotic by mouth

(B) testosterone cream to be applied to affected areas

(C) vaginal suppositories containing sulfa antibiotics

(D) estrogen-containing vaginal cream or vaginal ring

(E) surgical procedure

25. Human papillomavirus (HPV) is a nonenveloped DNA virus that causes essentially all cervical neoplasia. More than 100 HPV subtypes have been identified. HPV testing is becoming more and more common after the finding of an abnormal Pap smear, but not all HPV subtypes cause cancer. Which of the following subtype profiles account for 95% of cervical cancer cases?

(A) 6, 8, 9, 10, 9, 10, 11, and 12

(B) 11, 12, 13, 21, 34, 66, and 73

(C) 16, 18, 31, 33, 35, 45, and 58

(D) 22, 24, 27, 31, 44, 46, 51, and 78

(E) 39, 51, 52, 56, 59, 68, 73, and 82

26. A 26-year-old mother who is nursing presents to clinic complaining of right breast tenderness and fever. Upon physical examination, she has a 2-cm fluctuant mass at the site of erythema and tenderness. The patient had been seen 4 days ago and was placed on oxacillin, which she has been taking. At this point, the BEST treatment is

(A) changing antibiotic to vancomycin and discontinuing nursing

(B) surgical drainage and continuation of nursing

(C) discontinuation of nursing and hot soaks

(D) incision and drainage, hot soaks, antibiotics, and breast emptying

(E) hot packs and manual emptying of breasts

27. A 48-year-old woman comes in for her annual physical examination and biannual screening mammogram. Her family history is negative for breast cancer. Her breast physical examination reveals no palpable masses; however, a screening and diagnostic mammogram demonstrates several coarse calcifications that are suspicious for breast cancer. Which of the following statements is MOST accurate?

(A) fine needle aspiration would be the best diagnostic method for this finding

(B) because there is no palpable mass on physical examination, the patient may be observed with additional mammography in 3 months

(C) an image-guided, local excisional biopsy provides the most definitive diagnosis

(D) a reasonable option for this patient is a core tissue biopsy done with stereotaxis

(E) ultrasound imaging is the diagnostic method of choice for ductal carcinoma in situ (DCIS)

28. A 30-year-old woman who is 6 months postpartum (G2, P2) presents to clinic because of a sense of "heaviness and pressure" low in her pelvis. Onset was 2 days ago after a 3-mile run. She was pushing a stroller uphill as she ran. She has dribbling of urine when she coughs or exercises, but denies any other problems with urination. She takes no medications and uses an intrauterine device (IUD) for contraception. She is lactating. On physical examination, it is noted that when the patient is asked to strain, there is a bulging in the upper one-third of her vagina, just posterior to her urethra. There is no protrusion noted when the patient is not straining, but with straining the bulge comes to about 0.5 cm, just inside of the introitus. Also noted is a lack of pelvic muscle tone and vaginal dryness. At this point, what is the MOST likely diagnosis?

(A) urethrocele

(B) enterocele

(C) cystocele

(D) rectocele

(E) uterine prolapse

29. For the treatment of pelvic organ prolapse in a 32-year-old postpartum and breastfeeding woman, what would be the MOST appropriate first-line therapy?

(A) systemic estrogen therapy
(B) anticholinergics
(C) Kegel exercises
(D) surgery
(E) pessary

30. Which of the following is the MOST common symptom of a cystocele?

(A) difficulty defecating
(B) straining to urinate
(C) low back pain
(D) dribbling urine when coughing

31. A 30-year-old, G2, P0 presents to an outpatient clinic at 32 weeks' gestation. Her prenatal care up until this point has been routine for twin gestations and without any problems. Today, she is complaining of low pelvic "cramping." While in the office she has had four cramping episodes in the last 20 minutes and she is at least 1 cm dilated. Which of the following conditions is this patient at greatest risk?

(A) fetal anomalies
(B) preeclampsia
(C) intrauterine growth retardation
(D) gestational diabetes
(E) preterm labor

32. At 8 weeks' gestation, a 24-year-old primipara was seen a week prior complaining of vaginal bleeding and lower abdominal cramping. Her β-hCG level was 1,000 mIU/mL at that time. Today, she has no abdominal pain or evidence of tissue passed per vagina. Transvaginal ultrasound (TVUS) shows no adnexal masses as well as no clear pregnancy. Her repeat β-hCG level is 1,100 mIU/mL. What can be concluded from this information?

(A) The patient has a pregnancy that is nonviable but its location is unknown.
(B) She has had a spontaneous abortion and must have a dilation & curettage.

(C) The hCG level needs to be repeated in 48 hours for more information on viability.
(D) This is definitely an ectopic pregnancy.
(E) This is a molar pregnancy.

33. A 24-year-old Hispanic woman (G3, P2) presents for routine prenatal care at 20 weeks' gestation. Her urine is positive for glucosuria (2+). This finding would likely indicate

(A) gestational diabetes
(B) need to follow-up with a 3-hour glucose tolerance test
(C) need for a 50-g, 1-hour glucose challenge test
(D) need for instituting dietary control
(E) normal increase in renal threshold for glucose

34. A 39-year-old woman G2, P2 (SAb 1, living 1) presents to the ED with lower abdominal pain, vaginal bleeding, and a 6-week history of amenorrhea. Her history is significant for oral contraceptive use in the past and a spontaneous miscarriage. In addition, she has had an episode of pelvic inflammatory disease (PID). On presentation, she was orthostatic, and a culdocentesis performed in the ED was positive for blood. Exploratory laparotomy revealed an ectopic pregnancy. What risk factor did this patient have that has the highest association with developing an ectopic pregnancy?

(A) history of spontaneous abortion
(B) history of oral contraceptive use
(C) advanced maternal age
(D) history of PID

35. A 65-year-old G4, P4 presents to the clinic complaining of a vulvar mass. She says she does not know how long it has been there but her husband noticed it two nights ago. She denies any pain, itching, or discharge. She had a complete hysterectomy 10 years ago for fibroid tumors. Her history is otherwise unremarkable. On physical examination, the mass appears to be approximately 1 cm in size and is hard. There is no induration or tenderness. It is located on the right lower labia majora at

approximately 4 o'clock. Of the following neoplasms, which is the MOST likely diagnosis?

(A) adenocarcinoma of Bartholin gland

(B) carcinoma in situ of the vagina

(C) sarcoma botryoides

(D) invasive vaginal cancer

(E) Paget disease

36. A 35-year-old primipara at 39 weeks' gestation is in the labor and delivery suite for a nonstress test. She has had an uneventful pregnancy but has not felt the fetus moving much in the past 24 hours. A subsequent external fetal monitor tracing demonstrates a repetitive late heart rate deceleration. The first step in managing this patient is

(A) evaluation of maternal hypotension

(B) evaluation of fetal acid–base status

(C) administration of a tocolytic agent

(D) repositioning the patient

(E) checking maternal oxygen saturation

37. A 30-year-old woman who is nursing presents to the clinic complaining of breast tenderness. Physical examination reveals a warm, erythematous tender area with induration of the right breast. The next step in management would be to

(A) prescribe a penicillinase-resistant penicillin, eg, dicloxacillin

(B) prescribe topical mupirocin and continue breastfeeding

(C) discontinue nursing, empty breasts, and apply hot soaks to affected breast

(D) observe for fever and rest while continuing breastfeeding without medication

(E) breast drainage should be cultured to determine causative organism

38. Fibroadenoma of the breast is a common benign neoplasm. Which of the following clinical descriptions is MOST consistent with the diagnosis of fibroadenoma?

(A) 25-year-old patient with a nontender, round, freely movable breast mass approximately 1 cm in diameter

(B) 55-year-old patient with a 6-cm fixed, hard, breast mass, and palpable lymph nodes on the same side

(C) 30-year-old patient with a unilateral, bloody nipple discharge

(D) 40-year-old patient with tender, bilateral breast masses that seem to fluctuate in size monthly

(E) 60-year-old with an erythematous rash on her right breast and nipple

39. A 30-year-old woman presents with bilateral breast pain and nodularity. The tenderness and size of the nodules increase premenstrually. She has no family history of breast cancer. On physical examination, multiple tender "rope-like" nodules are palpated. There is no dominant mass and the lymph nodes are not palpable. After reassuring the patient regarding cancer probability, you recommend which of the following for INITIAL management?

(A) 200-mg danazol daily during luteal phase of menses

(B) decreasing use of caffeine and tobacco

(C) galactography to determine if lesions are focal

(D) fine-needle aspiration to determine atypia

(E) ultrasound for definitive diagnosis

40. A 32-year-old woman (G2, P1) with gestational diabetes is delivering at 39 weeks' gestation. The fetus appears to be about 4,100 g. The woman has experienced 5 hours of stage 1 labor, and currently in her second hour of stage 2 labor. The head is delivering but the shoulders are not. Which of the following descriptions include the BEST option for delivering this infant:

(A) flexing of the mother's thighs, pitocin augmentation, and suprapubic pressure

(B) flexing of the mother's thighs, suprapubic pressure, and cutting an episiotomy

(C) elevation of the mother's legs, suprapubic pressure, and oxygen for the mother

(D) no elevation of the mother's legs, pitocin, and fundal pressure

(E) no elevation of the mother's legs, suprapubic pressure, and cutting an episiotomy

41. A 32-year-old woman (G1, P1) at 35 weeks' gestation presents with a complaint of intermittent bleeding over the past week; however, she has had no evident pain or cramping. Upon physical examination, fetal heart rate is noted to be normal. These clinical characteristics are MOST consistent with

    (A) placental abruption
    (B) premature labor with bloody mucous discharge
    (C) placenta previa
    (D) vasa previa
    (E) premature rupture of membranes

42. At 33 weeks, a 28-year-old patient (G1, P1) calls the office with a complaint of a fluid gush from her vagina. She is not having contractions or evidence of bleeding. You advise her to go to labor and delivery to be examined. Which of the following procedures should be performed first?

    (A) induction of labor
    (B) sterile speculum examination or Nitrazine testing
    (C) ultrasound to estimate amniotic fluid volume
    (D) digital cervical examination to determine whether patient is in labor
    (E) administration of antibiotics to prevent infection

43. At 16 weeks' gestation, a 19-year-old G1, P0 Asian patient presents with a complaint of vaginal bleeding. She also has been experiencing severe nausea and vomiting. Her quantitative β-hCG is much higher than expected for 16 weeks' gestation, and her fundal height is approximately at 18- to 20-week size. Although she denies a past history of hypertension, her blood pressure is 140/90 mm Hg. No fetal heart sounds can be heard on Doppler, and there is no sign of a fetus on ultrasound. What is the MOST likely diagnosis?

    (A) threatened abortion
    (B) incomplete abortion
    (C) hydatidiform mole

    (D) fetal demise at 16 weeks
    (E) twin gestation

44. A 66-year-old woman who has had a hysterectomy presents with the complaints of chronic constipation and pelvic fullness. She says that at times it feels as if her insides are falling out. Pelvic organ prolapse is found on physical examination. On the basis of her history and physical examination findings, which of the following types of pelvic relaxation would MOST likely account for her prolapse?

    (A) urethrocele
    (B) enterocele
    (C) cystocele
    (D) rectocele
    (E) uterine prolapse

45. A 28-year-old woman presents to clinic complaining of vaginal pain and dyspareunia. The pain started 2 years ago after the birth of her second child. She sustained a fourth-degree laceration. She was raped 10 years ago. She denies dysuria. The pain can be provoked by the insertion of the speculum on examination, but otherwise the physical examination is unremarkable. There is no discharge, erythema, or masses. Wet prep and vaginal cultures are negative. What is the most likely diagnosis?

    (A) vaginitis
    (B) vulvodynia
    (C) cervicitis
    (D) pelvic inflammatory disease

46. Which of the following BEST describes the clinical characteristics of abruptio placenta?

    (A) variable amount of blood loss, no pain, and normal fetal heart rate, with no significant maternal history
    (B) scant blood loss, soft and nontender uterus, grand multiparity
    (C) moderate amount of blood loss, uterine hypertonus, history of maternal hypertension
    (D) bloody mucous plug, regular contractions

(E)   variable amount of blood loss, abdominal pain, and history of cesarean delivery

47.   A 20-year-old sexually active woman complains of a profuse, whitish gray vaginal discharge with a fishy odor that becomes stronger after intercourse and during menses. She denies any irritation and states that her sexual partner has no symptoms. Microscopic evaluation of the discharge reveals granular-appearing epithelial cells ("clue cells"). Which of the following is the BEST therapy?

(A)   metronidazole
(B)   ciprofloxacin
(C)   miconazole cream
(D)   fluconazole
(E)   doxycycline

48.   In a pregnant woman with the diagnosis of vaginal candidiasis, which of the following treatments would be preferred?

(A)   metronidazole
(B)   ciprofloxacin
(C)   miconazole cream
(D)   fluconazole
(E)   doxycycline

49.   A 17-year-old complains of severe dysmenorrhea since her first menses at age 13. The dysmenorrhea is often accompanied by nausea and vomiting the first 2 days of her menstrual period; analgesics or heating pads do not relieve the pain. She is sexually active and does not want to get pregnant. Her pelvic examination is normal. Which of the following medications is MOST appropriate for this patient?

(A)   narcotic analgesics
(B)   prostaglandin inhibitors
(C)   oxytocin
(D)   oral contraceptives
(E)   luteal progesterone

50.   A lactating woman, diagnosed with mastitis is treated appropriately with dicloxacillin 250 mg every 6 hours. She continues her antibiotic therapy and also continues to breastfeed, but her infection does not resolve and after 48 hours is getting worse. At this point, what is the appropriate course of action?

(A)   increase the dose of doxacillin to 500 mg every 6 hours
(B)   discontinue the breastfeeding
(C)   refer to a lactation specialist
(D)   refer for surgical consult
(E)   apply hot compresses

51.   Which of the following tests is essential to good routine prenatal care for the multipara with a normal medical history?

(A)   plasma blood glucose 1 hour after a 50-g oral glucose load
(B)   trichomonas vaginalis screening
(C)   X-ray pelvimetry
(D)   protein-bound iodine
(E)   erythrocyte sedimentation rate (ESR)

52.   A 25-year-old G1, P0 presents to labor and delivery with increasingly severe and frequent contractions over the previous 5 hours and spontaneous rupture of membranes 1 hour ago. Cervical examination shows dilation to 4 cm. The stage of labor for this patient would be assessed as

(A)   Phase 1
(B)   Phase 2, first stage, latent phase
(C)   Phase 2, first stage, active phase
(D)   Phase 2, second stage
(E)   Phase 2, third stage

53.   Which of the following nonstress tests results is most reassuring?

(A)   no change in the fetal heart rate with fetal movements over a 30-minute period
(B)   two decelerations with fetal movements over a 40-minute period
(C)   one acceleration with fetal movements over a 1-hour period
(D)   five decelerations with fetal movements over a 20-minute period
(E)   two accelerations with fetal movements over a 20-minute period

54. A 28-year-old primigravid woman at 42 weeks' gestation delivers a 4,000-g (8 lb 13 oz) newborn. Labor stages are as follows: first stage, 17 hours; second stage, 4 hours; third stage, 35 minutes. After a midline episiotomy was performed, the baby was delivered with low forceps. The placenta appeared to be intact. Ten minutes after delivery, she experiences vaginal bleeding estimated to be 500 mL over a 5-minute period. Upon examination, her uterus feels soft and boggy. Which of the following is the MOST likely cause of the hemorrhage?

(A) retained placental tissue

(B) uterine atony

(C) genital tract laceration

(D) disseminated intravascular coagulation

(E) uterine inversion

55. A 22-year-old woman (G1, P0) presents at 38 weeks' gestation complaining of dizziness, headache, and fatigue. Pertinent findings include BP of 148/90 mm Hg, 1+ bilateral ankle edema, normal electrolyte levels, normal deep tendon reflexes, and 1+ albuminuria. The MOST appropriate treatment at this time is

(A) immediate delivery

(B) administration of a mild diuretic once daily and prenatal visits every 2 to 5 days

(C) bed rest and prenatal visits every 2 to 5 days

(D) hospitalization with administration of magnesium sulfate via intravenous (IV) pump, 1 to 2 mg/h

(E) hospitalization with constant fetal monitoring

56. A previously unsensitized Rh-negative woman in her second pregnancy is seen in her 26th week. She complains of edema in her legs and some tingling in her left hand. What is the next step in managing this patient?

(A) analysis of the husband's blood type

(B) intramuscular Rho (anti-D) immune globulin

(C) ultrasonic evaluation of amniotic fluid volume

(D) Rh antibody titer

(E) amniocentesis

57. A 26-year-old G1, P0 at 28 weeks' gestation presents to labor and delivery complaining of low abdominal pain. Her contractions are regular and occur every 15 minutes. The fetal heart rate is 139 bpm and the nonstress test is reassuring. Cervical dilation is 1 cm with no effacement. Patient denies any fluid loss via the vagina—no blood or fluid. Which of the following medications should be administered to promote fetal lung development?

(A) ritodrine

(B) betamethasone

(C) nifedipine

(D) terbutaline

(E) magnesium sulfate

58. A patient had her last menstrual period on October 10, 2009. Her estimated date of delivery will be

(A) July 17, 2010

(B) July 4, 2010

(C) August 10, 2010

(D) June 30, 2010

(E) July 10, 2010

59. A woman at 22 weeks' gestation presents for her regular check-up. Her hemoglobin level is 10.8 g/dL. Which of the following statements regarding this patient's hemoglobin level is TRUE?

(A) This patient has iron deficiency anemia.

(B) The reason for this hemoglobin level in this trimester is physiologic: because of the expansion of red cell volume relative to the red blood cell mass.

(C) This patient should receive ferrous sulfate, 300 mg, not more often than twice daily.

(D) Screening for anemia should take place later in pregnancy when hemoglobin levels reach their nadir.

(E) A complete evaluation of the anemia, including serum ferritin, needs to be done.

60. There is good evidence that screening women at risk for chlamydial infection reduces the incidence of PID. The U.S. Preventive Services Task Force strongly recommends which of the following statements with regard to routine screening for *Chlamydia trachomatis*?

(A) Sexually active women with risk factors should be screened annually.

(B) Sexually active women aged 30 or younger should be screened.

(C) All pregnant women should be screened at first and third trimesters.

(D) Asymptomatic men should be routinely screened for chlamydial infection as it reduces the incidence of new infections in women.

(E) Age is the MOST important risk factor in determining whether to screen.

61. A thin, white 53-year-old woman who had her last menstrual period 2 years ago presents to the office complaining of hot flashes, vaginal dryness, and sleep loss from night sweats. She inquires about the benefits and risks of hormone replacement therapy (HRT) (combination estrogen–progesterone therapy), especially after hearing so much confusing information from the news media. When counseling the patient regarding the risks and benefits of a shorter course (<5 years) of HRT, which of the following is a documented risk of HRT that should be discussed?

(A) increased risk of endometrial cancer

(B) increased risk of breast cancer

(C) decreased bone mineral density

(D) increased risk of thromboembolism

(E) increased risk of colon cancer

62. A 30-year-old G1, P0 woman whose last menses was 8 weeks ago presents with heavy vaginal bleeding and left lower quadrant (LLQ) pain. She noted passage of something that "looked like liver" the previous day. Pelvic examination reveals a 2-cm cervical dilation. Which of the following is the MOST likely diagnosis?

(A) incomplete abortion

(B) complete abortion

(C) threatened abortion

(D) incompetent cervix

(E) missed abortion

63. A 44-year-old G2, P2 woman who had two normal pregnancies (13 and 11 years ago) presents with the complaint of amenorrhea for 8 months. She has remarried and would like to become pregnant again. A pregnancy test is negative. Her physical examination is normal. Which of the following tests is next indicated in the evaluation of this patient's amenorrhea?

(A) endometrial biopsy

(B) luteinizing hormone (LH), follicle-stimulating hormone (FSH), and estradiol levels

(C) ovarian antibody assay

(D) testosterone and dehydroepiandrosterone (DHEAS) levels

(E) hysterosalpingogram

64. A 27-year-old G1, P0 woman has received regular prenatal care throughout her pregnancy. She presents to the ED at 34 weeks with facial edema, severe headache, and epigastric pain. On physical examination, she has a blood pressure of 160/110 mm Hg, elevated liver function tests, and a platelet count of 60,000/uL. The baby is noted to be alive. Urinalysis indicates 4+ proteinuria. Which therapeutic measure should be taken next in managing this patient?

(A) oral antihypertensive therapy

(B) intravenous immunoglobulin therapy

(C) magnesium sulfate therapy and induction of labor

(D) platelet transfusion

(E) a colloid solution for plasma volume expansion

65. A 28-year-old primigravida presents for routine prenatal care at 32 weeks' gestation. Her pregnancy has been uneventful and she has been receiving regular prenatal care. At her visit today, the fundal height measurement is 36 cm. Of the possibilities below, which of the following is the LEAST likely cause for the increased fundal height?

    (A) fetal macrosomia
    (B) multiple gestation
    (C) oligohydramnios
    (D) fetal position
    (E) fibroid uterus

66. A 39-year-old G1, P0 at 39 weeks' gestational age is seen for a routine obstetric (OB) visit and has a blood pressure reading of 150/100 mm Hg. During her pregnancy thus far, baseline blood pressures have been 100–120/60–70 mm Hg. She is sent to labor and delivery. She denies any headache, visual changes, nausea, vomiting, or abdominal pain. The cervix is 50% effaced and 2- to 3-cm dilated. A repeat BP shows 160/90 mm Hg. Her hematocrit is 34, platelets are 160,000, AST is 22, ALT is 15, and urinalysis is negative for protein. Which of the following is the MOST likely diagnosis?

    (A) pregnancy-induced hypertension (gestational hypertension)
    (B) chronic hypertension
    (C) preeclampsia
    (D) eclampsia
    (E) HELLP syndrome

67. Which of the following statements regarding management of labor in a low-risk pregnancy is TRUE?

    (A) food and oral fluids are acceptable if labor is progressing normally
    (B) electronic fetal monitoring (EFM) improves perinatal outcomes
    (C) walking during labor decreases duration of labor

    (D) bed rest is associated with shorter duration of labor and less need for analgesia

68. Treating preterm labor with β-adrenergic agonists has been shown to decrease the rate of which one of the following?

    (A) delivery within 48 hours of treatment
    (B) low birth weight infants
    (C) preterm delivery
    (D) perinatal deaths
    (E) perinatal infection

69. The MOST common cause of spontaneous abortion in the first 12 weeks of pregnancy is

    (A) the presence of maternal lupus anticoagulant
    (B) chromosomal anomalies
    (C) an incompetent cervix
    (D) maternal drug abuse
    (E) inadequate progesterone

70. In the surgical repair of a marked uterine prolapse, which of the following structures MOST likely needs to be repaired in a 45-year-old G4, P4?

    (A) transverse and uterosacral ligaments
    (B) sacral nerve
    (C) detrusor muscles
    (D) pelvic floor muscle

71. Which of the following represents the primary effect of oral contraceptives?

    (A) changes in tubal mobility and ovum transport
    (B) sperm penetration
    (C) disruption of implantation
    (D) suppression of FSH and LH
    (E) change in fertile mucus

72. A healthy 20-year-old woman is using a low-dose triphasic contraceptive pill for birth

control. She experiences breakthrough bleeding during the third week of each cycle for the past few months. Her pregnancy test is negative. The physical examination is normal. There is no infection or thyroid problem. The patient desires to stay on oral contraceptives. What is the BEST way to manage her therapy?

(A) continue current oral contraceptive pill (OCP), but add extra estrogen during the third week

(B) prescribe a progestin-only pill

(C) change to a pill with a higher progestin component

(D) switch to a pill with a higher estrogenic component

(E) reassure her and have her return in 1 month

73. Which of the following is the recommended time frame for emergency contraception's greatest effectiveness in preventing pregnancies?

(A) 0 to 20 hours

(B) 21 to 40 hours

(C) 40 to 60 hours

(D) 60 to 80 hours

(E) less than 72 hours

74. In a pregnant woman with an incompetent cervix, which of the following is the BEST way to avoid a miscarriage or a premature birth?

(A) pessary

(B) bed rest

(C) cerclage

(D) magnesium sulfate

(E) terbutaline

75. Which of the following lists of patient problems BEST typifies the classical presentation of endometriosis?

(A) dysmenorrhea, deep thrust dyspareunia, infertility, abnormal bleeding, pelvic pain, and headache

(B) dysmenorrhea, headache, insomnia, infertility, abnormal bleeding, and pelvic pain

(C) infertility, abnormal bleeding, polycystic ovarian syndrome, insomnia, pelvic pain

(D) dysmenorrhea, deep thrust dyspareunia, infertility, abnormal bleeding, and pelvic pain

76. When microscopically examining a lesion taken from a fallopian tube, what does the presence of endometrial glands, stroma, and hemosiderin-laden macrophages indicate?

(A) chronic pelvic inflammatory disease

(B) cervical cancer

(C) polycystic ovarian syndrome

(D) endometriosis

77. A 32-year-old nulliparous woman is seeking contraceptive advice. She is in a monogamous relationship and is a nonsmoker and has a history of one ectopic pregnancy 5 years ago. She wishes to consider childbearing in the future. Her history includes mild, well-controlled hypertension, and frequent urinary tract infections. Which one of the following contraceptive options would be contraindicated?

(A) condoms and spermicide

(B) intrauterine device

(C) low-dose combined oral contraceptive

(D) diaphragm

(E) progesterone-only oral contraceptive

78. Genital warts are caused by low-risk human papillomavirus (HPV) types. Low-risk HPV are rarely associated with cancer. Which of the following HPV types cause genital warts?

(A) 6 and 11

(B) 11, 12, and 73

(C) 31 and 58

(D) 22 and 78

(E) 39 and 82

79. A 16-year-old female patient comes into the office for a prescription of oral contraceptives. She has been sexually active for 3 months and uses condoms for prevention of pregnancy and prevention of STDs. Her β-hCG test is negative and a combined oral contraceptive (COC) pill is prescribed. She is also interested in receiving the "HPV vaccine." The first dose is administered today in the office. When does the patient need to return for her follow-up vaccine, and how many total injections for HPV prophylaxis are needed?

(A) She should return at 1 month and 3 months, for a total of three vaccine doses.

(B) She should return at 2 months and 6 months, for a total of three vaccine doses.

(C) She should return at 3 months, for a total of two vaccine doses.

(D) She should return at 4 months and 6 months, for a total of three vaccine doses.

80. A 72-year-old G2, P2 presents to the clinic for her annual examination. She has been getting yearly wellness examinations that include a Pap smear and mammogram, but today she is wondering how much longer she needs to continue having Pap smears and mammograms. Given a healthy woman, with no history of abnormal Paps and no history of abnormal mammograms, what is the minimum age she can stop getting Pap smears and mammograms?

(A) age 66 years

(B) age 68 years

(C) age 70 years

(D) age 72 years

81. A 27-year-old G3, P3 presents to an outpatient clinic for her wellness examination. Last year her Pap smear was normal. This year, however, her Pap results indicate Atypical squamous cells of undetermined significance (ASCUS) and the reflex HPV testing results show high-risk (HR) HPV. What is the most appropriate next step in her evaluation?

(A) repeat cytology at 6 and 12 months

(B) repeat reflex HPV testing

(C) endometrial biopsy

(D) colposcopy

82. A 16-year-old nulligravida patient's Pap smear results are "LSIL," or low-grade squamous intraepithelial lesion. What is the most appropriate next step in her evaluation?

(A) repeat cytology at 12 months

(B) repeat reflex HPV testing

(C) endometrial biopsy

(D) colposcopy

83. A 42-year-old woman presents for her annual examination. Her only complaint is chronic vaginal itching, associated with dyspareunia and postcoital bleeding. She is concerned that she has recurrent yeast infections and wants something to treat the problem. On physical examination, flat topped, white papules are noted on the vulva and no vaginal discharge or internal erythema is seen. Which of the following vaginal diagnoses is most likely?

(A) candidiasis

(B) bacterial vaginosis

(C) lichen planus

(D) herpes virus

(E) Bartholin gland cyst

84. A 20-year-old female college student presents complaining of recent onset vaginal pruritis, discharge, and odor. On physical examination, a thin yellow discharge is observed along with "strawberry spots" on the cervix. The wet prep reveals a pH of 6.0, positive whiff test, and mobile protozoan. What is the best treatment?

(A) oral Diflucan 150 mg, one dose

(B) metronidazole 500 mg, twice daily, for 7 days

(C) metronidazole 1,000 mg, one dose

(D) Acyclovir 400 mg, 3 times daily, for 7 days

(E) miconazole 2% cream, 5 g intravaginally, for 7 days

85. Hormone therapy is currently indicated for which of the following conditions?

    (A) irritability, vasomotor symptoms, memory disturbance
    (B) night sweats, depression, osteoporosis prevention
    (C) hot flushes, mood swings, and vaginal dryness
    (D) vasomotor symptoms, vaginal atrophy, and osteoporosis prevention

86. A 24-year-old G2, P1 woman presents during the second trimester complaining of constipation and difficulty passing her bowel movements. Her last delivery was uncomplicated. On physical examination of her introitus and vagina, you notice a bulging of the pelvic floor when she bears down. Your assessment is that the common problem of constipation during pregnancy is being made worse because of the presence of a(n)

    (A) incompetent cervix
    (B) prolapsed uterus
    (C) cystocele
    (D) rectocele
    (E) vaginal mass

Answers and Explanations

1. **(C)** The high-dose regimen of metronidazole is for the treatment of Trichomoniasis. *Trichomonas vaginalis* causes this common sexually transmitted disease. The clinical characteristics include a profuse yellow, frothy, malodorous, pruritic discharge. Sometimes a strawberry cervix (subepithelial redness) is seen. The pH is between 4.5 and 6. The treatment for chlamydia is azithromycin or doxycycline. Candidiasis would be treated with an imidazole. *Staphylococcus* infection could be treated by many different antibiotics other than metronidazole. *(MacKay, 2009, pp. 658-659)*

2. **(C)** Although exercise-induced secondary amenorrhea may seem apparent in this case, it is imperative that pregnancy is ruled out as a cause of the amenorrhea. All amenorrheic women of reproductive age should be assumed to be pregnant until proven otherwise. Therefore, an hCG test is indicated as a first step in the evaluation of this patient. Sudden weight loss and increased physical activity can cause secondary amenorrhea, as can hypothyroidism and hyperprolactinemia. If ordering serum estradiol concentrations, an FSH level should also be ordered. Serum estradiol levels alone are less useful than FSH in deciphering cause of amenorrhea. Decreased estradiol occurs with either hypothalamic–pituitary axis failure or ovarian failure. Decreased FSH indicates hypothalamic–pituitary axis failure whereas elevated FSH indicates ovarian failure. Ordering serum testosterone levels should only be considered if the patient has symptoms of PCOS or androgen excess. *(Halvorson, 2008a, pp. 375-380)*

3. **(D)** Anovulatory bleeding is seen in 10% to 15% of all gynecologic patients and is the most common cause of abnormal vaginal bleeding in adolescents. In perimenarchal adolescents, it is caused by an immature hypothalamic–pituitary–ovarian axis. The top five causes of vaginal bleeding in the adolescent are listed by frequency: anovulation, pregnancy, exogenous hormone use, and coagulopathy. The top six causes of vaginal bleeding in the reproductive-aged woman listed by frequency are pregnancy, anovulation, exogenous hormone use, uterine leiomyomas, cervical and endometrial polyps, and thyroid dysfunction. The top four causes of vaginal bleeding in perimenopausal women listed by frequency are anovulation, uterine leiomyomas, cervical and endometrial polyps, and thyroid dysfunction. The top four causes of vaginal bleeding in postmenopausal women listed by frequency are endometrial lesions, exogenous hormone use, atrophic vaginitis, and other tumors. *(Tintinalli, 2004, pp. 647-653)*

4. **(C)** Polycystic ovarian syndrome (PCOS) is suggested by her being moderately overweight and having hirsutism and acne. As has been claimed in many clinical medicine lectures over the years, 80% to 90% of the diagnosis can be made from the medical history. The essential parts of the history when investigating the causes of dysfunctional uterine bleeding are age of menarche, menstrual history, date of the first day of the last normal menstrual period, contraceptive use, signs and symptoms of coagulopathy (nosebleeds, petechiae, and ecchymoses), endocrine symptoms, menopause symptoms, weight changes, and stress. *(Tintinalli, 2004, pp. 647-653)*

5. **(A)** Generally, infertility is defined as the inability for a couple to conceive after reasonably frequent unprotected intercourse for 1 year. In approaching the diagnostic work-up for infertility, with a thorough physical examination and history of both partners, the clinician should establish the following points: (1) does the woman ovulate? (if not, why not); (2) does the semen have normal characteristics? (3) is there a female reproductive tract abnormality? Noninvasive tests should be done first line. For the male partner, semen analysis is noninvasive and helpful, though not diagnostic. In the initial evaluation of the female partner, noninvasive procedures, such as the measurement of LH and mid-luteal phase progesterone (to determine ovulatory function) and TVUS (to rule out the possibility of fibroids or polycystic ovaries), are first-line investigations. Pelvic ultrasound should also be part of the routine gynecologic evaluation because it allows a more precise evaluation of the position of the uterus within the pelvis and provides more information about its size and irregularities. Hysterosalpingography is an invasive procedure and therefore not first line in the evaluation. Endometrial biopsy and postcoital testing are no longer recommended for the routine infertility evaluation because they have poor predictive value. *(Halvorson, 2008b, pp. 426, 431, 435, 439, 444)*

6. **(B)** It is important to evaluate why this patient has an enlarged and tender uterus; therefore, the next step in evaluation would be ultrasound. Common causes of secondary dysmenorrhea in this age group are endometriosis, adenomyosis, and the presence of an intrauterine device. For this patient, it would be important also to rule out leiomyomas, endometrial polyps, and tumors. Given the most common causes, endometriosis and adenomyosis, noninvasive studies with transvaginal and abdominal ultrasound would be a reasonable (and economical) first choice. The imaging diagnosis of adenomyosis is usually made by using TVUS or, more expensively, by MRI. Abdominal ultrasound alone can be highly sensitive for detecting masses, but often lacks specificity for the diagnosis of adenomyosis or endometrio-

sis. Hysterosalpingography is more invasive and is used to exclude endometrial polyps, leiomyomas, and congenital abnormalities of the uterus. The inability to resolve subtle differences in soft tissue attenuation limits the usefulness of computed tomography (CT). Laparoscopy is often needed as a last resort to make the diagnosis of endometriosis where surgical correction can occur simultaneously. *(Hoffman, 2008e & Hoffman, 2008f, pp. 197, 209, 257)*

7. **(B)** More than 90% of patients with endometrial cancer present with postmenopausal bleeding, thus making it the hallmark history component. In the United States, endometrial cancer is the most common gynecologic cancer. There are approximately 39,000 cases of endometrial cancer diagnosed each year and about 7,400 patients die from the disease. Of all endometrial cancer cases, 75% are type I and 25% are type II. There are several risk factors for developing type I endometrial cancer, but in general excessive estrogen is the cause. Therefore, women who are taking postmenopausal unopposed estrogen replacement or tamoxifen and women who are 50 lb above their ideal body weight, are at risk for endometrial hyperplasia and endometrial cancer. Type II endometrial cancers tend to occur in older, thinner women without exogenous estrogen exposure. *(Miller, 2008, pp. 687-692)*

8. **(B)** Oral contraceptives are the best treatment for this patient. Treatment for premenopausal abnormal uterine bleeding is varied. Once infection, fibroid tumors, pregnancy, neoplasm, and iatrogenic causes (eg, medication related) are ruled out, a woman may be treated hormonally to control bleeding. In this patient, the most likely cause of the bleeding is anovulatory cycles caused by estrogen excess due to her obesity; in addition, the iron deficiency anemia also can cause menometrorrhagia. In patients with irregular cycles, secondary to chronic anovulation, or oligo-ovulation, combined oral contraceptive (COC) pills help to prevent the risks associated with prolonged unopposed estrogen stimulation of the endometrium. Treatment with cyclic progestins for days 16 through 25 following the first day of the most

recent menstrual flow is preferred when OCP use is contraindicated, such as in smokers older than age 35 and women at risk for thromboembolism. *(Hoffman, 2008a, pp. 186-188)*

9. **(D)** Although approximately 40% of menstruating women experience one or more of the cluster of physical, emotional, or behavioral symptoms associated with the luteal phase of the menstrual cycle (premenstrual syndrome or premenstrual tension), a small percentage have symptoms so severe that they meet the DMS-IV diagnosis of premenstrual dysphoric disorder (PMDD). For the treatment of mild to moderate symptoms, lifestyle and dietary changes may be effective. Therefore, a trial of regular aerobic exercise, decrease in caffeine and alcohol intake, 1,200 mg of dietary calcium with 800 IU of Vitamin D per day, and eating complex carbohydrates as opposed to simple sugars could be initiated. For patients whose symptoms affect jobs and relationships, it is warranted to prescribe serotonin reuptake inhibitor such as fluoxetine. Fluoxetine 20 mg can be taken daily or only premenstrually. *(MacKay, 2009, pp. 657-658)*

10. **(C)** The combination of dysmenorrhea, deep dyspareunia, low back pain, and chronic pelvic pain are most suggestive of endometriosis. The other conditions could all present with a pelvic pain component, but would have a different combination of other symptoms. Adenomyosis is commonly associated with menorrhagia and dysmenorrhea. Ovarian cancer would present with nonspecific findings such as ascites, abdominal discomfort, vague gastrointestinal symptoms, pelvic or abdominal mass, and pain. Interstitial cystitis typically presents with urinary frequency and urgency, as well as suprapubic, perineal, vulvar, or vaginal pain before, during, or after urination. *(Hoffman, 2008b, Hoffman, 2008c, & Hoffman, 2008i, pp. 229-231, 257-260, 719-720)*

11. **(D)** Diagnostic laparoscopy is the only definitive way to diagnose endometriosis. Ultrasound and MRI may be helpful in the diagnostic workup, but laparoscopy is the most certain method of diagnosing endometriosis. *(Sarajari et al., 2007, p. 715)*

12. **(E)** This patient has a leiomyoma of the uterus (or fibroid tumors), which is the most common benign neoplasm, but she is also significantly anemic. The labs suggest iron deficiency anemia. It is important to control her bleeding and treat her anemia prior to surgery. The heavy bleeding that typically accompanies fibroid tumors can be minimized by using intermittent progestin supplementation (depot methodroxyprogesterone acetate 150 mg IM every 28 days) and/or prostaglandin synthetase inhibitors. In general, the size of the mass can be decreased and the bleeding can be lessened, but the only curative treatment is a myomectomy or hysterectomy. *(MacKay, 2009, pp. 664-665)*

13. **(A)** Gestational trophoblastic neoplasia (GTN) consists of benign GTN, most often a hydatidiform mole and malignant GTN, which includes nonmetastatic and metastatic GTN. Approximately, 15% to 20% of women who have a complete hydatidiform mole and 2% to 4% of partial moles, will go on to develop some form of malignant GTN. Complete and partial molar pregnancies differ clinically, genetically, and histologically. Because of the risk for progression to malignancy, these patients must be monitored. After molar evacuation, serum radioimmunoassay β-hCG levels should be monitored weekly until they have become undetectable. Historically, monitoring has continued monthly after the undetectable levels for at least 6 additional months. However, studies have shown that it is safe to cease monitoring after a single blood sample demonstrates undetectable levels of β-hCG. Urine pregnancy tests are inadequate, and a sensitive radioimmunoassay is mandatory. Prophylactic chemotherapy is controversial because of significant drug toxicity and possible lack of efficacy; it is usually reserved for highest risk cases or for patients who are unable to return for regular follow-up. Routine chest X-ray at every visit is not warranted unless hCG values rise. *(Schorge, 2008, pp. 755-761)*

14. **(C)** Leiomyomata are benign growths of the myometrium and the majority of patients do not require surgical or medical treatments. Only if myomas cause significant pressure on the

uterus, bladder, or bowel, or if the uterine bleeding causes anemia or a significant alteration in lifestyle or hygiene, medical or surgical therapy is needed. Medical treatment to reduce the size of the tumors may be all the therapy that is necessary. Their growth is stimulated by estrogen; therefore, a 2- to 3-month course of leuprolide acetate (Lupron Depot), a Gn-RH analog, would be the best choice. Gn-RH analogs produce a sustained and continuous release of Gn-RH on the pituitary that eventually results in a decrease in the release of pituitary gonadotropins and subsequent decreased production of estrogen from the ovaries. Because the risk of surgical complications increases with the size of the myoma, it is best to reduce the size of the tumor preoperatively and also to treat anemia preoperatively. *(MacKay, 2009, pp. 664-665)*

15. **(B)** The patient's diagnosis is PID. For her age group, the most likely pathogens are the sexually transmitted ones, *C. trachomatis* and *N. gonorrhoeae*. Of these two sexually transmitted diseases (STDs), *C. trachomatis* is more prevalent. Because the causes are often polymicrobial, treatment should be broad-based and for a long duration. As long as the patient is medically stable and can tolerate oral medication, she can be treated as an outpatient. One recommended outpatient treatment is Ofloxacin 400 mg once daily for 14 days; with or without metronidazole 500 mg twice daily for 14 days. *(Hemsell, 2008, pp. 66, 73-76)*

16. **(B)** A functional ovarian cyst is a much more likely diagnosis than any of the others listed. A follicular cyst develops when an ovarian follicle fails to rupture. The granulosa cells lining the cyst continue to enlarge and fluid continues to accumulate. Symptoms associated with a functional ovarian cyst include mild to moderate unilateral pain and alteration in the menstrual cycle. On occasion, rupture of the follicular cyst causes acute pelvic pain and may need laparoscopic surgery for complete evaluation. In most cases, pain control for 4 to 5 days is what is indicated as well as the consideration of contraception to suppress future ovarian cyst formation. *(Hoffman, 2008, pp. 210-212)*

17. **(C)** Menstrual irregularities are most specific for the functional ovarian cysts. Right-sided pain could be associated with many items on the differential for abdominal pain. The presence of fever and chills would be more likely seen in appendicitis infections. The negative pregnancy test makes ectopic pregnancy much less likely. The adnexal mass could be a tubo-ovarian abscess or an ovarian cyst. *(Hoffman, 2008, pp. 210-212)*

18. **(C)** The size and firmness of the ovarian mass suggests endometrioid carcinoma, a tumor in which the potential for malignancy is 100%. Referral to a gynecologic oncologist should be considered first whenever an ovarian malignancy is suspected. Standard of care is complete surgical staging, excision of all visible masses, and abdominal hysterectomy and bilateral salpingo-oophorectomy followed by chemotherapy. Radiation oncology could also be considered. *(MacKay, 2009, pp. 670-671)*

19. **(B)** *BRCA1* and *BRCA2* gene mutations are known genetic markers for breast and ovarian cancers. There is a syndrome of inherited breast–ovarian cancer. Of all breast cancer cases in the United States, 5% to 7% cases have the syndrome. About 45% of the syndrome cases carry the *BRCA1* gene and 35% carry the *BRCA2* mutation. *(Euhus, 2008, pp. 282-283)*

20. **(B)** There is no generalized clinical picture of cervical carcinoma, but there are two symptoms often associated with it. They are postcoital bleeding and abnormal uterine bleeding. The average age at diagnosis is 50. Lesions on the cervix that should be considered for immediate biopsy include new exophytic, friable, or bleeding lesions. In this patient, the lesion should have been biopsied at initial examination and this would have helped to make the diagnosis. When lesions are visualized and the biopsy confirms carcinoma, no colposcopic assessment is needed. This patient should definitely not wait 4 to 6 months for a repeat Pap smear. The gynecologic oncologist should stage the cancer and decide on appropriate therapy. *(Beckmann et al., 2005, pp. 268-272, 277)*

21. **(B)** Chlamydia should be suspected when there is eversion of the cervix and a mucopurulent cervicitis. Because of this patient's use of hormonal birth control, her cervix would likely appear to have erosion, but she has a mucopurulent cervicitis. Bacterial vaginosis (BV) typically presents with a white discharge, amine (or "fishy") odor, and possible itching. Candidiasis often presents with a history of pruritis and a thick white discharge. On wet prep, BV is diagnosed by the presence of clue cells and a positive KOH (potassium hydroxide) "whiff test" (amine odor) and vaginal candidiasis is diagnosed by the presence of yeast hyphae. *(Beckmann et al., 2006, pp. 265-267; MacKay, 2009, pp. 658-659)*

22. **(B)** Nabothian follicles, or epithelial inclusion cysts, present a characteristic appearance: they contain a dense, yellow, mucoid material. They warrant no further treatment. A Bartholin duct cyst is the most common cystic growth in the vulva. When infected, it would be visualized as a fluctuant swelling of the inferior portion of the labia minora, presenting with periodic pain and dyspareunia. Cervicitis will present with a mucopurulent drainage from the cervical os; occasionally, with columnar evasion in chronic cases. Cervical polyps are benign, pedunculated growths of various sizes that extend from the ectocervix or endocervical canal. *(Gala, 2008a, pp. 65-67, 96, 101)*

23. **(E)** On the basis of the 2006 Consensus Guidelines for the Management of Women with Cervical Cytological Abnormalities (www.asccp.org), it is recommended that colposcopy be done following LSIL on Pap smears. Viewing the cervix and its transformation zone with 10–20× magnification of colposcopy allows for visual assessment. Two solutions are used to further enhance visualization and determination of normal from abnormal tissue. When a dilute solution of acetic acid is applied to the cervix, abnormal areas will look white. After painting the cervix with Lugol solution (a strong iodine solution), the normal squamous epithelial will take on the stain whereas the abnormal tissue will not. All abnormal-appearing tissue is biopsied. *(Griffith, 2008, pp. 628-635)*

24. **(D)** The patient's symptoms describe postmenopausal atrophic changes affecting the vagina, bladder, and urethra. In women with more severe changes, vaginal irritation, dyspareunia, and fragility may become problems. Atrophy is diagnosed by the presence of a thin, clear, or bloody discharge; a vaginal pH of 5 to 7; loss of vaginal rugae; and the finding of parabasal epithelial cells on microscopic examination of a wet-mount preparation. These symptoms are all due to estrogen depletion. Treatment with topical estrogen preparations (cream, tablet, or ring) appears equally effective. Complete relief of symptoms usually occurs within weeks; in the interim, patients may obtain relief through use of vaginal lubricants and moisturizers (eg, Astroglide, Replens). Rarely, endometrial hyperplasia can be a side effect of vaginal estrogen treatment. *(Land, 2007, pp. 969-672)*

25. **(C)** Greater than 95% of cervical cancers are associated with High-risk (HR) HPV types 16, 18, 31, 33, 35, 45, and 58. There are more than 100 strains of HPV, some of them low risk for causing cancer and some high risk. The other HR HPV types that are less often associated with cancer are types 39, 51, 52, 56, 68, 73, and 82. HPV 18 is associated with cancers that develop rapidly, often 1 to 3 years from the time of documented negative Pap smears. *(Griffith, 2008, pp. 619-623)*

26. **(D)** A true abscess will require surgical drainage and therapy with antibiotics, rest, warm soaks, and complete emptying of the breasts every 2 hours. The abscess drainage should be cultured and sensitivities determined. There have been no formal studies of treatment of lactation mastitis associated abscesses. However, incision and draining is recommended along with parenteral antibiotics administered with added coverage for anaerobic bacteria. As soon as the pain of the wound permits, breastfeeding or pumping should be resumed in order to drain the affected breast. *(Euhus, 2008, p. 277)*

27. **(C)** For mammographic abnormalities that are nonpalpable and that require biopsy, image-guided tissue sampling is necessary. Tissue for

diagnosis can be obtained by open surgical biopsy with needle localization. Although it has less morbidity, core-needle biopsy for small foci of highly suspicious microcalcifications with no associated mass is less beneficial because sampling errors are more common and local excision provides definitive treatment. With nonpalpable lesions, core needle or excisional biopsy is preferred over fine needle aspiration biopsy (FNAB), because the sample provides adequate tissue for histologic diagnosis and is more accurate. Ultrasonography is helpful if the radiologist thinks that the lesion has the appearance of a cyst (not this case), but DCIS cannot be diagnosed until tissue samples and pathology are done. *(Euhus, 2008, pp. 270-274)*

28. **(C)** Pelvic pressure and stress incontinence in a multiparous woman are common symptoms of pelvic relaxation. The bulging in the anterior portion of the vagina, which was seen on physical examination, confirms the diagnosis of a cystocele. The structures that support the pelvic organs can be weakened by birth trauma, chronic elevation of intra-abdominal pressure (as seen in chronic cough and obesity), intrinsic weaknesses, or atrophic changes from estrogen loss. In the case outlined in the question, the following factors contributed to her cystocele: birth trauma, decreased estrogen because of lactation, and increased intra-abdominal pressure from pushing a stroller uphill while running. *(Schaffer, 2008, pp. 532-547)*

29. **(C)** The patient may benefit from all of the options to some degree, but the most conservative approach would be to start with Kegel exercises. By strengthening the pelvic floor muscles, this problem may become much less bothersome and once natural estrogen levels are restored after the cessation of breastfeeding, the problem may completely be resolved. Systemic estrogens are contraindicated in breastfeeding because they decrease breast milk production. A pessary may be considered after failure of Kegel exercises. Pessaries could be especially helpful if the patient's symptoms significantly interfere with her lifestyle. Surgery should be reserved for a patient whose

symptoms do not improve with conservative therapy or who have significant prolapse. *(Schaffer, 2008, pp. 532-547)*

30. **(D)** The most common symptom of general pelvic relaxation in general is a feeling of pressure or as if something is protruding from the vagina. With a rectocele, patients may have difficulty defecating. Straining to urinate may be a symptom of a cystocele, but the most common symptom of a cystocele is stress incontinence, which is often described by patients as dribbling when they cough, sneeze, or jump. Pelvic relaxation may be improved with Kegel exercises, although once the exercises are discontinued the symptoms often return. Pessaries can also be used to prevent stress incontinence. Ultimately, a surgical referral may be needed to correct the problem. *(Beckmann et al., 2006, pp. 289-298)*

31. **(E)** Of the answer choices, preterm labor is the greatest risk because multiple gestations are at risk for preterm labor to begin with and also because the patient has signs and symptoms of preterm labor. The American College of Obstetricians and Gynecologists (ACOG) suggests the following criteria to diagnose preterm labor: (1) four contractions in 20 minutes or 8 contractions in 60 minutes; (2) cervical dilation greater than 1 cm; (3) cervical effacement of greater than 80%. Multiple gestations include various complications for the mother and fetus. For the mother, twin pregnancies are associated with higher risk of pregnancy-induced hypertension, anemia, hyperemesis, abruption, placenta previa, postpartum hemorrhage (PPH), and increased risk of operative delivery. For the fetus, twin pregnancy increases risk of intrauterine death, spontaneous abortion, congenital anomalies, cerebral palsy, and intrauterine growth retardation. Twin pregnancies have a similar risk of gestational diabetes compared to singleton pregnancies, and so this is not a risk for this patient at all. *(Cunningham, 2005k, pp. 867, 912, 921-938)*

32. **(A)** This is a nonviable pregnancy, but whether or not the pregnancy was located intrauterine

or ectopic is not something which can be concluded with the data presented. Because there is a plateau in the hCG level after 1 week (48 hours is usually sufficient), the pregnancy is nonviable. The hCG level need not be repeated at this point. TVUS appears to demonstrate no visualized products of conception. It should be noted, however, that this could represent an incomplete abortion. An ectopic pregnancy cannot be ruled in or out yet. If β-hCG levels are 1,500 mIU/mL and the uterus is empty, a live uterine pregnancy is very unlikely. When hCG is less than 1,500 IU/L and an ectopic pregnancy is not seen, progesterone level needs to be determined. If the progesterone level is greater than 25 ng/mL then an ectopic pregnancy is unlikely. At this point, a D&C should be considered. The low hCG levels and lack of findings on ultrasound (eg, "snowstorm" appearance) would help rule out a molar pregnancy. (*Cunningham, 2005c, pp. 260-261*)

33. **(C)** Although glycosuria is more common during pregnancy because of the lowering of the renal threshold for glucose excretion, this patient may be at an increased risk for gestational diabetes (GDM) because of her ethnicity. Normal screening for GDM occurs at 24 weeks' gestation. Because glycosuria has been detected, screening with a 50-g, 1-hour glucose challenge test would be indicated at this time. Patients do not have to fast for this test. To be considered normal, serum or plasma glucose values should be less than 130 mg/dL (7.2 mmol/L) or less than 140 mg/dL (7.8 mmol/L). Using a value of 130 mg/dL or higher will increase the sensitivity of the test from 80% to 90% and decrease its specificity, compared with using the 140 mg/dL cutoff. An abnormal 1-hour screening test should be followed by a 100-g, 3-hour venous serum or plasma glucose tolerance test. Normal blood sugars at 0, 1, 2, and 3 hours, respectively, are:

- fasting blood sugar 95 mg/dL or less
- 1-hour blood sugar 180 mg/dL or less
- 2-hour blood sugar 155 mg/dL or less
- 3-hour blood sugar 140 or less

A diagnosis of GDM is made if two or more samples are increased or if any is greater than

200 mg/dL and the patient should be advised regarding dietary control, regardless. (*Cunningham, 2005d, pp. 1170-1173*)

34. **(D)** Of the options listed, PID would be the most likely risk factor for this patient as women with a prior history of PID are at 7 to 10 times increased risk in having an ectopic pregnancy. In decreasing order, the next most common risk factors include tubal surgery, intrauterine contraceptive devices, previous ectopic pregnancy, in vitro fertilization, smoking, previous abdominal surgery, and induced abortions. (*Gala, 2008b, pp. 157-161; Beckmann et al., 2010, pp. 141-142*)

35. **(A)** Adenocarcinoma of Bartholin gland is rare (1% of vulvar cancer), but if at anytime a new asymptomatic mass in the area of Bartholin gland is discovered in a postmenopausal woman, it should be investigated aggressively. Its incidence peaks in the mid-sixties and typically presents as an asymptomatic mass. (*Jayanthi, 2008, pp. 665-675*)

36. **(D)** Fetal heart rates by EFM are described by rate and pattern of variability. Baseline is defined as 120 to 160 bpm. Late decelerations are a symmetrical fall in FHR beginning at or after the peak of the uterine contraction and returning to baseline only after the contraction has ended. They indicate possible uteroplacental insufficiency and imply some degree of fetal hypoxia. Remedial techniques are empirically designed to overcome uteroplacental insufficiency or to decrease cord compromise and improve placental and fetal oxygenation. Changing maternal position to right/left side lying recumbent or knee–chest position is a reasonable and quick first step. Late fetal heart rate (FHR) decelerations, however, are an ominous sign and should be evaluated quickly and seriously. Persistent nonreassuring tracings indicate the need for emergent delivery. Other remedial techniques include the following: IV infusion, mask oxygen, stopping oxytocics, subcutaneous terbutaline, and amnioinfusion. (*Cunningham, 2005g, pp. 452-462*)

37. **(A)** Mastitis is an inflammation of the breast that is common in breastfeeding women. In

order to make a diagnosis of mastitis, there must be an area of hardness, pain, redness, and swelling in the breast. It can be caused by engorgement, a blocked milk duct, or a cracked nipple that allows bacteria to enter. The most common pathogen in infective mastitis is penicillin-resistant *Staphylococcus aureus.* Less common pathogens are *Streptococcus* or *Escherichia coli.* The preferred antibiotics are usually penicillinase-resistant penicillins such as dicloxacillin, with patients usually responding within 24 to 26 hours. In addition to antibiotic treatment, regular emptying of the breast by breastfeeding and/or pumping is necessary to prevent more bacteria from collecting in the breast. There is no evidence of risk to the healthy, term infant from continuing breastfeeding. Symptomatic treatment such as application of heat (eg, a shower or a hot pack) to the breast prior to feeding may help with the milk flow. *(Cunningham, 2005l, p. 703)*

38. **(A)** Fibroadenomas are the second most common type of benign breast disease. The most common type is fibrocystic breast changes. A firm, nontender, rubbery, freely movable nodule, 1 to 4 cm, in a premenopausal woman is a classic description. Fibroadenoma, unlike fibrocystic changes, do not change with the menstrual cycle. Fine needle aspiration would be acceptable in the diagnostic workup of a possible fibroadenoma, with confirmation by histology. A triple test is the combination of clinical examination, imaging, and needle biopsy. The test is considered to be "concordant" when all three tests suggest a benign lesion, or when all three tests suggest a cancerous lesion. When a concordant triple test is benign, it is 99% accurate and the lesion can be followed by clinical observation at 6-month intervals. A physical examination that contains features worrisome for breast cancer includes any mass that is fixed, nipple retraction or bloody nipple discharge, accompanied by lymphadenopathy. An erythematous or eczematous-appearing rash on the breast or nipples brings Paget disease of the breast to mind; ductal carcinoma of the nipple needs to be diagnosed by biopsy and usually requires mastectomy. *(Euhus, 2008, p. 273)*

39. **(B)** Cyclic mastalgia in usually managed symptomatically and requires no evaluation. Fibrocystic breast changes are the most common type of benign breast mass. Clinically they are often described as "rope-like," meaning they have the characteristic on palpation of feeling like a coiled rope. There is often diffuse nodularity, although solitary cysts may range in size. Also, the size of an individual cyst may fluctuate throughout the menstrual cycle. Pain is the most common presenting symptom of fibrocystic breast change. Often, women will respond to dietary changes, such as decreased caffeine and/or tobacco. Danazol as well as bromocriptine, tamoxifen, and GnRH agonists are usually reserved for women with the most severe symptoms. *(Euhus, 2008, pp. 277-278)*

40. **(B)** Shoulder dystocia is a complication associated with macrosomia. Although there is no evidence that any one maneuver is superior to another in releasing an impacted shoulder or reducing the chance of injury, American College of Obstetricians and Gynecologists guidelines recommend performance of the McRoberts maneuver (B) as a reasonable initial approach. Fundal pressure (D) should never be attempted. *(Cunningham, 2005l, p. 703)*

41. **(C)** Placenta previa can be distinguished from abruptio placenta by many factors. Placenta previa is most commonly characterized by painless hemorrhage, which usually does not present until the end of the second trimester or later. No abdominal discomfort, a normal FHR, and no significant maternal history are usually associated with the problem. Abruptio placenta, on the other hand, is associated with severe pain, abnormal FHR, usually continuous bleeding, and associated with a history in the mother such as cocaine use, abdominal trauma, maternal hypertension, multiple gestations, and polyhydramnios. In this case, one will need to rule out early labor (accompanying contractions, bloody mucus discharge), coagulopathy, hemorrhoids, vasa previa, cervical or vaginal lesion, or trauma. Vasa previa also occurs late in pregnancy, with vaginal bleeding occurring concomitantly with rupture of membranes. Vasa previa occurs when umbilical cord

blood vessels transverse the membranes and cross the cervical os below the fetus. Fetal distress will also accompany vasa previa because the blood loss will be fetal; it requires immediate delivery and is accompanied by a high rate of fetal death. *(Cunningham, 2005h, pp. 819-823)*

42. **(B)** The accurate diagnosis of spontaneous rupture of membranes is important in order to ascertain whether the patient has begun labor or if the patient has premature rupture of membranes (this patient is 33 weeks). To evaluate for spontaneous rupture of membranes, a sterile speculum examination is performed with the patient in the dorsal lithotomy position. Evidence of rupture of membranes would be clear when blood-tinged fluid in the posterior fornix of the vagina, or pooling, and escape of clear fluid from the cervical os occurs when the patient coughs. Nitrazine testing can distinguish amniotic fluid from urine or vaginal secretion samples from speculum examination. If the pH is 7.1 to 7.3, it will show positive on Nitrazine paper (dark blue). False positives can occur, however, with cervical mucus, blood, or semen in the sample. Until rupture of membranes has been ascertained, this patient should not be induced because of risk of prematurity in the fetus. Ultrasound determination of amniotic fluid volume is an important means of evaluating premature and preterm rupture of membranes, but it is not a means of diagnosing rupture of membranes. Digital cervical examination should not be performed because this would increase the risk of ascending infection. *(Cunningham, 2005k, pp. 864-865)*

43. **(C)** Hydatidiform mole is one component of gestational trophoblastic neoplasm (GTN). Moles occur in a gestation in which there is a proliferation of trophoblastic tissue. It can be a complete mole, in which there is no sign of a fetus, or a partial mole, in which the fetus may be viable, or there are findings consistent with a nonviable fetus. Young pregnant women (<20) and older (>40) reproductive ages have increased incidence as do patients with Asian, Latino, or Filipino ethnicity. The most common symptom of hydatidiform mole is several episodes of vaginal bleeding. A size-to-dates

discrepancy also is common. Severe nausea and vomiting may occur as well. When signs and symptoms of preeclampsia present earlier than 24 weeks' gestation, molar pregnancy should be high on the differential. The trophoblast is responsible for production of human chorionic gonadotropin (hCG); therefore, the levels of β-hCG in the serum are greater than expected for the weeks of gestation. Ultrasound demonstrates a characteristic "snowstorm" appearance and is the best means of diagnosing a mole. An incomplete abortion usually occurs prior to 12 to 14 weeks and is often characterized by a decreasing β-hCG level. A fetal demise at 16 weeks would also have decreasing β-hCG levels and would not be associated with hypertension. In twin gestation, there would be a higher level of β-hCG and a larger fundal height, but at 16 weeks, fetal heart tones should be heard. *(Schorge, 2008, pp. 755-757)*

44. **(B)** Pelvic organ prolapse (POP) is a health concern affecting women, and in the United States it is the third leading indication for a hysterectomy. In diagnosing POP, the patient is placed in the lithotomy position and is asked to perform a Valsalva maneuver while the introitus is observed. The names cystocele, uterine prolapse, rectocele, and enterocele refer to the location of the prolapse and which organ is bulging into the vagina. A cystocele is due to an anterior wall defect and on physical examination the bladder is protruding. Uterine prolapse is present when the cervix moves toward the introitus with Valsalva. A rectocele is due to a defect in the posterior vaginal wall and on physical examination one sees the vaginal floor protrude. An enterocele is a true hernia of the peritoneal cavity. It may be noticed as a separate bulge above the rectocele, and if it is large enough it may prolapse through the vagina. An enterocele can only be diagnosed if small-bowel peristalsis is observed. *(Schaffer, 2008, pp. 532-546)*

45. **(B)** The most likely diagnosis is vulvodynia. It is defined as vulvar discomfort occurring in the absence of relevant visible findings or a specific neurologic disorder. It is a diagnosis of

exclusion. The other answer options all have diagnostic criteria that include specific signs and symptoms. One effective treatment for vulvodynia is not present, but often a multi-disciplinary approach to treatment is required. Treatment options include psychologic, biofeedback, tricyclic antidepressants, topical anesthetics, and surgical therapy. *(Gala, 2008, pp. 97-100)*

46. (C) Abruptio placentae (ie, placental abruption) refers to separation of the normally located placenta after the 20th week of gestation and prior to birth. Patients usually present with the following symptoms: vaginal bleeding—78%, back pain or uterine tenderness—66%, fetal distress—60%, high frequency contractions—17%, premature labor—22%, and fetal death—15%. Maternal and fetal death may occur because of hemorrhage and coagulopathy. The fetal perinatal mortality rate is approximately 15%. Likely risk factors for abruptio placentae are maternal hypertension, abdominal trauma, smoking, cocaine use, and advanced maternal age among others. *(Cunningham, 2005h, pp. 809-819)*

47. (A) The most likely diagnosis of this vaginitis is bacterial vaginosis (BV) and the treatment is metronidazole 500 mg twice daily for 7 days. Other treatments include vaginal preparations of metronidazole and also vaginal preparations of clindamycin. The other treatments would be inappropriate for the treatment of BV. Ciprofloxacin is a treatment for a urinary tract infection. Miconazole cream and fluconazole are treatments for yeast vaginitis. Doxycycline is the treatment for *Chlamydia trachomatis*. *(MacKay, 2009, pp. 664-665)*

48. (C) The only acceptable treatment option presented is miconazole cream or any vaginal preparation of an imidazole compound because they are poorly absorbed vaginally. Fluconazole is a category C and therefore should not be used. Metronidazole is a category B, but effectively treats BV and yeast candidiasis. Ciprofloxacin is a category C, but it is ineffective in the treatment of yeast infections. Doxycycline is the treatment for *Chlamydia trachomatis* and is a category C. It can cause permanent discoloration of the

tooth enamel and, therefore, doxycycline should not be used during the latter half of pregnancy, during lactation, and during infancy through age 8. *(MacKay, 2009, pp. 664-665)*

49. (D) Conservative measures for treating dysmenorrhea include heating pads, mild analgesics, and outdoor exercise. Evidence suggests that primary dysmenorrhea is due to prostaglandin F2 alpha (PGF2 alpha), a potent myometrial stimulant and vasoconstrictor, in the secretory endometrium. Prostaglandin synthase inhibitors such as naproxen, ibuprofen, indomethacin, and mefenamic acid can be very effective. However, for patients with dysmenorrhea who are sexually active, oral contraceptives will provide needed protection from unwanted pregnancy and generally alleviate the dysmenorrhea. The OCPs minimize endometrial prostaglandin production during the concurrent administration of estrogen and progestin. *(Hoffman, 2008d; p. 208 Hoffman, 2008f, p. 258)*

50. (D) The woman was treated appropriately with the doxacillin, and it is best if she continues to breastfeed during the mastitis in order that she does not become engorged. Hot compresses may help, but what might be happening now is an abscess that may need surgical drainage. So, it is best that she be referred to someone who can perform that procedure. *(Giuliano, 2009, pp. 630-633)*

51. (A) Initial screening for gestational diabetes is accomplished by performing a 50-g, 1-hour glucose challenge test at 24 to 28 weeks of gestation. Chest X-ray (and all nonessential radiography) would be contraindicated as part of any antepartum screening. X-ray pelvimetry would not be indicated in a multipara who has previous successful vaginal deliveries. Screening and treatment for trichomoniasis is not recommended because it has not been shown to prevent preterm delivery. Protein-bound iodine and ESR would not be considered a routine test for any normal pregnancy, but may be indicated in specific cases. *(Cunningham, 2005j, pp. 207-226)*

52. (C) The first stage of labor is divided into two stages: latent and active. The latent stage refers to cervical effacement and early dilation. The active phase occurs when dilation has reached 3 to 4 cm or greater. The second stage of labor begins when cervical dilation is complete and ends with delivery of the infant. The third stage of labor begins after the infant is delivered and ends with placental expulsion. The percentage of effacement varies with first and subsequent births, and does not necessarily correlate with the stage of labor. By the time the woman is in the first stage active labor (4 cm), 100% effacement has occurred. Phase 1 of parturition is the preparation for labor. Phase 2 of parturition is the process of labor and is divided into the 3 stages above. Phase 3 of parturition is the puerperium. (*Cunningham, 2005i, pp. 152-161*)

53. **(E)** A reactive stress test (normal) is defined as two or more fetal heart rate increases in 20 minutes. The accelerations increase by 15 beats for 15 seconds and are related to fetal movement. A nonreactive stress test (abnormal) requires monitoring for two 20-minute periods where neither period yields adequate accelerations. (*Cunningham, 2005k, pp. 374-385*)

54. **(B)** Uterine atony is responsible for ~50% of postpartum hemorrhage (PPH). Several factors may predispose to uterine atony including conditions that enlarge the uterus (eg, multiple gestations, multiparity, microsomy, hydramnios), abnormal labor (eg, precipitous or prolonged delivery, general anesthesia, prolonged labor, use of forceps), and conditions that interfere with uterine contraction (eg, uterine leiomyomas, magnesium sulfate use). Vaginal and cervical lacerations are less common than uterine atony, but are serious and require prompt surgical attention. Retained placenta, secondary to lack of complete separation from the uterus and abnormally adherent placenta, such as placenta accreta, are less common causes of postpartum hemorrhage. Although coagulation studies should be part of the workup, in the immediate postpartum period, disorders of the coagulation system and platelets do not usually result in excessive bleeding. Fibrin deposition over the placental site and clots within supplying vessels play a significant role in the hours and days following delivery,

and abnormalities in these areas can lead to late PPH or exacerbate bleeding from other causes, most notably, trauma. Uterine inversion is a rare condition. (*Poggi, 2007, pp. 477-483*)

55. **(A)** In this case, the elevated BP, ankle edema, and 1 + albuminuria are indicative of moderate preeclampsia. In addition, complaints of headache and dizziness would indicate a CNS component. Therapy for mild to moderate preeclampsia consists of bed rest and close monitoring, which increases central blood flow to the kidneys, heart, brain, and placenta and may improve the condition. However, at 38 weeks' gestation, a diagnosis of moderate and certainly severe preeclampsia would likely be managed by induction of labor and delivery, once precise knowledge of the age and maturity of the fetus has been established. (*Miller, 2007, pp. 318-325*)

56. **(D)** An Rh-negative woman must be tested for the presence of antibodies at the beginning of the third trimester (usually at 28 weeks) so that the rare Rh sensitization of that pregnancy can be detected. If she is negative she is given Rho (anti-D) immune globulin. If she is positive for Rh sensitization, she may require intrauterine blood transfusion to prevent erythroblastosis fetalis. In mothers who receive Rh immunoglobin, the risk of isoimmunization is reduced from 16% to 0.2%. (*Roman, 2007, pp. 283-286*)

57. **(B)** Corticosteroids accelerate lung maturation and are given to expectant mothers who are less than 34 weeks' gestation and are in preterm labor. Some clinicians believe it is appropriate to use tocolytics to stop preterm contractions, but this is controversial. Tocolytics may temporarily stop contractions, but they do not consistently prevent preterm labor and they carry a significant risk. Examples of tocolytics are terbutaline, magnesium sulfate, ritodrine, and nifedipine. In general, if tocolytics are given they should be given with corticosteroids and generally not after 34 weeks. (*Cunningham, 2005b, pp. 374-385*)

58. **(A)** The estimated date of confinement (EDC) or due date is calculated after obtaining a

thorough menstrual history. The date of the last onset of normal menses is crucial and a light bleeding episode should not be mistaken for a normal period. A "normal" pregnancy lasts 40 ± 2 weeks. Calculated from the first day of the last normal menses, one adds 7 days to the first day of the last normal menstrual flow and subtracts 3 months. *(Cunningham, 2005j, p. 208)*

59. **(B)** In healthy pregnant women who are not deficient in iron or folate, a modest fall in hemoglobin levels at this point of gestation is usually due to the relative greater expansion of plasma volume compared with the increase in hemoglobin mass and red blood cell volume that accompanies normal pregnancy. In healthy nonpregnant women, anemia is defined as a hemoglobin of less than 12 g/dL. During pregnancy, a patient is not considered anemic until the hemoglobin falls below 10 g/dL. In the first trimester and at term, the hemoglobin level for most healthy women is 11 g/dL or greater. During the second trimester, women experience a nadir in their hemoglobin between 22 and 24 weeks. *(Cunningham, 2005e, p. 1144)*

60. **(E)** Age is the most important risk marker. The Centers for Disease Control and Prevention (CDC) recommends that all sexually active women younger than 25 be screened for chlamydia. The optimal interval for screening is open to clinical judgment. For example, in women with a previous negative screening test, timing for rescreening should take into account changes in sexual partners. For those at low risk for infection (eg, in a mutually monogamous relationship with no history of chlamydial infection), it may not be necessary to screen frequently. For previously infected patients, rescreening at 6 to 12 months may be appropriate because of high rates of reinfection. Screening in pregnancy should be done for all women less than age 25. The timing for the screening, however, is also uncertain. Screening early in pregnancy provides a chance to improve pregnancy outcomes associated with chlamydial infection (eg, low birth weight and premature delivery). Screening in the third trimester could be more effective in preventing transmis-

sion to the infant during birth. Until the advent of urine-based screening tests, routine screening of men was rarely performed because so many men were not interested in urethral swabs. *(Hoffman, 2008, p. 8; Hemsell, 2008, p. 66)*

61. **(D)** Currently, hormone replacement therapy (HRT) is indicated only for the treatment of vasomotor symptoms of menopause, vaginal atrophy, and for the treatment and prevention of osteoporosis. HRT increases an older woman's risk of CHD, and in all women it increases their risk of breast cancer, stroke, and thromboembolism. Increased risks of breast cancer are seen in women who use HRT for longer than 5 years. Estrogen-only therapy given to women with an intact uterus increases the risk of endometrial hyperplasia (thickening of the lining of the uterus) and eventually endometrial cancer. Daily estrogen combined with progesterone given for 10 to 14 days per month (sequential HRT) reduces this risk but does not eliminate it. *(Euhus, 2008, pp. 494-495)*

62. **(A)** In the classification of spontaneous abortions, an incomplete abortion is characterized by the passage of tissue and an open cervical os. A complete abortion would have a similar history of passing tissue; however, pain or cramping would have subsided and the cervix would be closed. In a threatened abortion, there will be bleeding but no passage of tissue, and the cervical os would be closed. A missed abortion is defined by no symptoms and a closed os. With an incompetent cervix, women present with painless cervical dilation. The treatment of an incomplete abortion is dilation and curettage. Serum-hCG levels are useful to follow after spontaneous abortion; hCG levels should halve every 48 to 72 hours, and a plateau could indicate residual retained tissue. *(Cunningham, 2005a, pp. 239-241)*

63. **(B)** This patient has secondary amenorrhea. The most common reason for amenorrhea in a woman of reproductive age is pregnancy, which has been ruled out. In the differential diagnosis for her secondary amenorrhea, possibilities include (among others) endometriosis, hypothyroidism, and premature ovarian failure

(if patient is aged less than 40), and ovarian failure or menopause if patient is older than 40. For a patient of this age, ovarian failure is more likely. Studies for establishing the diagnosis of ovarian failure are as follows: (1) serum FSH level, (2) serum LH, and (3) serum estradiol. Persistently elevated gonadotropin levels (especially when accompanied by low serum estradiol levels) are diagnostic of ovarian failure. Ovarian antibody assay is a test with low sensitivity and specificity for determining the diagnosis of autoimmune ovarian failure. Serum testosterone and DHEAS levels should be ordered only if the patient shows symptoms of androgen excess (acne, hirsutism, male pattern balding, clitoromegaly) or hypertension. The hysterosalpingogram is part of an infertility work-up that may demonstrate Asherman syndrome, but is more invasive and not indicated until ovarian failure has been excluded. (*Halvorson, 2008, pp. 365-366, 369; Bradshaw, 2008, pp. 468-471*)

64. **(C)** This patient has preeclampsia (BP $\geq 140/90$ mm Hg, proteinuria, platelets $< 100,000$, increased liver enzymes, headache, and epigastric pain). Because gestational hypertension also referred to commonly as pregnancy-induced hypertension has been associated with raised rates of maternal morbidity and mortality and with many increased risks to the fetus, patients with moderate to severe preeclampsia should be delivered if the disease develops after 34 weeks' gestation. Magnesium sulfate is the treatment of choice for preeclampsia as it reduces the risk of eclampsia and probably maternal death. Hypertension disease is classified into five types: gestational (also called pregnancy-induced), preeclampsia, eclampsia, preeclampsia superimposed on chronic hypertension, and chronic hypertension. Oral hypertensive drug therapy, though decreasing the risk of severe hypertension, has not been associated with decreased risk in the infant or mother. There is insufficient evidence for any effects of plasma volume expansion. Intravascular volume expansion carries a serious risk of volume overload, which could lead to pulmonary or cerebral edema. Patients with a platelet count greater than $40,000/mm^3$ are unlikely to bleed and do not require transfu-

sion unless the platelet count drops to less than $20,000/mm^3$. (*Cunningham, 2005l, pp. 762-764, 781-784*)

65. **(C)** Oligohydramnios, diminished amniotic fluid volume, may be associated with intrauterine growth retardation, and would result in a fundal height lower than expected. The fundal height directly correlates with gestational age in weeks from 20 to 32 weeks' gestation—eg, at 32 weeks it should measure 32 cm. This measurement, however, is subject to measurement problems. A full bladder can cause an increase of 3 cm and obesity can also distort the correlation. (*Cunningham, 2005j, pp. 208-212*)

66. **(A)** Pregnancy-induced hypertension (gestational hypertension) is defined as blood pressure of greater than 140/90 mm Hg. It is considered when maternal blood pressure reaches 140/90 mm Hg or greater for the first time during pregnancy, and proteinuria is not present. Preeclampsia is defined by a blood pressure increase $\geq 140/90$ mm Hg post 20 weeks' gestation with proteinuria. Other features of preeclampsia are headache, epigastric pain, and elevated liver enzymes. Eclampsia is defined by the development of seizures in a woman with preeclampsia. Chronic hypertension is defined as that occurring prior to the pregnancy or before 20 weeks' gestation (blood pressure of 140/90 mm Hg or greater). The diagnosis of HELLP syndrome requires the presence of hemolysis (H) on the basis of the examination of the peripheral smear, elevated indirect bilirubin levels or low serum haptoglobin levels in association with significant elevation in liver enzymes (ELL), and a platelet (P) count below $100,000/mm^3$ after ruling out other causes of hemolysis and thrombocytopenia. (*Cunningham, 2005f, pp. 761-764, 773*)

67. **(A)** Eating and drinking during early labor in a low-risk pregnancy is acceptable, but should be avoided during active labor. There are no randomized controlled studies that show a benefit of using electronic fetal monitoring (EFM) in low-risk women versus no monitoring. ACOG supports either intermittent auscultation or EFM. During the first stage of labor, the

pregnant woman may ambulate or sit as desired. *(Decherney, 2007, pp. 204, 257)*

68. **(A)** In women with premature labor, β-adrenergic agonists have been clearly shown to reduce the incidence of delivery within 24 and 48 hours of administration. The benefits of this delay are questionable. These tocolytic agents have not been shown to consistently reduce the rates of preterm delivery, low birth weight, severe respiratory distress, or perinatal death. It appears that more effective use of the 24 to 48 hours gained by tocolysis with β-adrenergic agonists holds promise for reducing perinatal morbidity and mortality, perhaps through more liberal use of predelivery glucocorticoid therapy. *(Cunninham, 2005, pp. 870-871)*

69. **(B)** The most common cause of spontaneous abortion in the first 12 weeks of pregnancy is chromosomal anomalies (accounting for about half of abortions). Maternal lupus anticoagulant, incompetent cervix, maternal tobacco abuse, and inadequate progesterone during the luteal phase can also be associated with early abortion. Maternal disease is more likely to be responsible in second trimester miscarriage. *(Cunningham, 2005a, pp. 232-237)*

70. **(A)** Childbirth can injure the pelvic floor muscles resulting in a prolapsed uterus. The transverse and uterosacral ligaments are particularly affected. The degree of protrusion of the uterus in relationship to the introitus determines the classification. Grade 0 is normal position of the uterus. Grade 1 or slight prolapse is when the uterus descends toward the introitus, but is still in the vagina. Grade 2 or moderate prolapse is when the uterus and cervix descend to the introitus, and grade 3 or marked prolapse is when the cervix and uterus descend past the hymen halfway. Grade 4 is when the uterus is at the maximum descent. When the prolapse interferes with daily life or quality of life, a surgical repair is indicated. *(Hughes, 2008, pp. 536-551)*

71. **(D)** Suppression of FSH and LH is the primary effect of oral contraceptives. They may also cause changes in tubal mobility and ovum transport, sperm penetration of the egg, disruption of implantation of a fertilized egg, and change in cervical mucus to make it harder for sperm to swim toward the egg. *(Cunningham, 2005a, p. 107)*

72. **(C)** During the initial 3 months of oral contraceptive use, breakthrough bleeding is a common side effect and can be best managed by encouraging the patient to continue on the contraceptives. After initiating therapy, when breakthrough bleeding occurs during the third week of the cycle, it is due to a lack of progestin and is best managed by changing to a pill with a higher progestin component. *(Beckmann et al., 2006, pp. 246-247)*

73. **(E)** Emergency contraception is most effective when taken within 72 hours of unprotected intercourse. When taken within the recommended time frame, emergency contraception is 75% effective in preventing pregnancies. It is not an abortive and therefore will not cause an already established pregnancy to be terminated. The Yuzpe method is the most common method. It utilizes four tablets of oral contraceptives containing 0.05-mg ethinyl estradiol and 0.5-mg DL-Norgestrel (Ovral). Two tablets are taken at once and then two more tablets 12 hours later. An alternate regimen is the progestin-only emergency contraceptive (Plan B). *(Beckmann et al., 2006, p. 257)*

74. **(C)** Although all the methods listed (bed rest, devices, and pharmacologic agents and surgery) work to some degree to treat an incompetent cervix, the generally accepted treatment is surgical. A cervical cerclage is a suture or bands that are placed surgically on the cervix to keep it closed prior to delivery. The sutures are removed after fetal maturity has been achieved (about 37 weeks). Labor and delivery occurs rapidly after the removal of the cerclage. The terbutaline and magnesium sulfate are pharmacologic agents used for the medical management of preterm labor with a competent cervix *(Cunningham, 2005a, pp. 237-239)*

75. **(D)** There is great variability in the symptoms with which endometriosis will present. Some women may even be asymptomatic, but endometrial lesions may be found during

laparoscopy for other gynecologic reasons. The classic symptoms of endometriosis are dysmenorrhea, deep thrust dyspareunia, infertility, abnormal bleeding, and pelvic pain. Thorough history taking greatly helps in the diagnosis, but the definitive diagnosis is made when the lesions are visualized during laparoscopic surgery or by tissue biopsy. *(Beckmann et al., 2006, pp. 310-307)*

76. **(D)** When the presence of endometrial glands, stroma, and hemosiderin-laden macrophages is noted microscopically on a tissue sample taken from the pelvic cavity, outside of the uterus, the diagnosis of endometriosis can be made. *(Beckmann et al., 2006, p. 301)*

77. **(B)** A prior tubal pregnancy contraindicates IUD use. Condoms and spermicides are free of hormonal side effects and, if used in combination, are reasonably effective. This patient's hypertension is mild and controlled and unlikely to be negatively affected by either low-dose or progesterone-only oral contraceptives. Although there can be an association between urinary tract infections and diaphragm use in susceptible women, this would not be an absolute contraindication to diaphragm use. *(Cunningham, 2008, pp. 118-121)*

78. **(A)** Low-risk human papillomavirus types 6 and 11 cause almost all genital warts. Although they are very prevalent, they are not associated with malignancy or neoplasia. The HR HPV types 16, 18, 31, 33, 35, 45, and 58 are associated with 95% of all cervical cancers worldwide. Gardasil, a recombinant quadrivalent HPV vaccine is for prophylactic protection from HPV types 6, 11, 16, and 18. *(Griffith, 2008, pp. 619-623)*

79. **(B)** Gardasil, the recombinant quadrivalent HPV vaccine should be administered in 3 doses. The schedule is, first dose 1 is administered, then dose 2 is administered 2 months after the first dose, and then dose 3 is administered 6 months after the first dose. Gardasil protects against HPV types 6, 11, 16, and 18. The CDC recommends it be given to girls at ages 11 to 12, but the minimum age is 9 and the maximum age is 26. *(Griffith, 2008, pp. 619-623; Jacobs, 2009, p. 1163)*

80. **(C)** The minimal accepted age for women to stop getting yearly Pap smears and mammograms is 70 years old. A woman must have documented three consecutive normal Pap smears and no history of pre-invasive lesions and also no risk factors that would put her at increased risk for cervical cancer. In women of any age who have undergone a hysterectomy and who have no history of invasive or pre-invasive cervical disease, Pap smears may be discontinued. Similarly, women may elect to stop having mammography at age 70 years as well. *(Hoffman, 2008, p. 5; Euhus, 2008, p. 283)*

81. **(D)** The most appropriate evaluation of this patient is for her to be referred for a colposcopy. A Pap smear is a medical consultation that interprets a laboratory test. The interpretation is not a diagnosis. The final diagnosis is made in conjunction with clinical and often histological data. In this patient, it would be inappropriate to repeat the HPV test or repeat the Pap smear. The consensus guidelines for the management of abnormal Pap smears recommend that following the results of atypical cells of undetermined significance (ASCUS), there are three evaluation possibilities: HPV DNA testing, repeat cytology at 6 and 12 months, and colposcopy. If either the HPV testing or the repeat cytology is abnormal, then immediate referral for colposcopy is recommended. ASCUS has about a 5% chance of progressing to cervical intraepithelial neoplasia (CIN) 2 or 3. *(Werner, 2008, pp. 628-629)*

82. **(A)** Abnormal Pap smears of adolescents are managed differently from those of other women. In women 20 years and younger there is a high HPV positivity, a high rate of spontaneous regression of neoplasia, and a low incidence of cervical cancer. Because of these factors, the standards recommend that abnormal Pap results such as ASCUS and LSIL be managed and a repeat cytology be performed at 12 months. *(Werner, 2008, pp. 628-629)*

83. **(C)** Lichen planus is an uncommon disease. Vaginal complaints are typically chronic discharge, itching, dyspareunia, and postcoital bleeding. When this diagnosis is suspected, a biopsy should be done. Treatment of topical

hydrocortisone applied to the affected area has been shown to improve symptoms and clinical manifestations in 75% of cases. The external lesions are not congruent with the signs of candidiasis or bacterial vaginosis, both of which would have vaginal erythema and discharge. Herpes lesions would be tender and red. A Bartholin gland infection or abscess would present with unilateral tenderness and swelling at the 4 o'clock or 8 o'clock position of the vulva. *(Gala, 2008a, pp. 91-95)*

84. **(C)** The diagnosis is trichomoniasis and the CDC-recommended treatment is metronidazole single 1-g dose orally. The metronidazole 500 mg dose listed is for the treatment of bacterial vaginosis. The Diflucan and miconazole are for the treatment of vaginal candidiasis. The Acyclovir is for the treatment of an initial herpes outbreak. *(Hemsell, 2008, pp. 62-65)*

85. **(D)** As a result of clinical research studies, hormone therapy (HT) is indicated only for the treatment of vasomotor symptoms (hot flushes and night sweats), vaginal atrophy, and for the prevention or treatment of osteoporosis. The other associated symptoms of menopause (depression, irritability, and insomnia) should be treated with other modalities. Hormones should be prescribed in the lowest effective doses and for the shortest period of time. The risks of HT include increased risk of coronary heart disease, breast cancer, stroke, venous thromboembolism, and cholecystitis. *(Bradshaw, 2008, pp. 494-495)*

86. **(D)** Pelvic organ prolapse (POP) is a health concern affecting women, and in the United States it is the third leading indication for a hysterectomy. While diagnosing POP, the patient is placed in the lithotomy position and asked to perform a Valsalva maneuver while the introitus is observed. The names cystocele, uterine prolapse, rectocele, and enterocele refer to the location of the prolapse and which organ is bulging into the vagina. A cystocele is due to an anterior wall defect and on physical examination the bladder is protruding. Uterine prolapse is present when the cervix moves toward the introitus with Valsalva. A rectocele is due to a defect in the posterior vaginal wall and on physical examination one sees the vaginal floor protrude. *(Schaffer, 2008, pp. 532-546)*

REFERENCES

Beckmann CR, Ling FW, Barzansky BM, et al. *Obstetrics and Gynecology*. 6th ed. Philadelphia, PA: Lippincott, Williams & Wilkins; 2010.

Bradshaw KD. Menopausal transition. In: Schorge JO, Schaffer JI, Halvorson LM, et al., eds. *Williams Gynecology*. New York, NY: McGraw-Hill; 2008.

Cunningham FG. Contraception and sterilization. In: Schorge JO, Schaffer JI, Halvorson LM, et al., eds. *Williams Gynecology*. New York, NY: McGraw-Hill; 2008.

Cunningham FG, Leveno KJ, Bloom SL, et al., Abortion. In: Cunningham FG, Leveno KJ, Bloom SL, et al., eds. *Williams Obstetrics*. 22nd ed. New York, NY: McGraw-Hill; 2005.

Cunningham FG, et al., Antepartum assessment. In: Cunningham FG, Leveno KJ, Bloom SL, et al., eds. *Williams Obstetrics*. 22nd ed. New York, NY: McGraw-Hill; 2005.

Cunningham FG, et al., Ectopic pregnancy. In: Cunningham FG, Leveno KJ, Bloom SL, et al., eds. *Williams Obstetrics*. 22nd ed. New York, NY: McGraw-Hill; 2005.

Cunningham FG, et al., Diabetes. In: Cunningham FG, Leveno KJ, Bloom SL, et al., eds. *Williams Obstetrics*. 22nd ed. New York, NY: McGraw-Hill; 2005.

Cunningham FG, et al., Hemotologic disorders. In: Cunningham FG, Leveno KJ, Bloom SL, et al., eds. *Williams Obstetrics*. 22nd ed. New York, NY: McGraw-Hill; 2005.

Cunningham FG, et al., Hypertension disorders in preganancy. In: Cunningham FG, Leveno KJ, Bloom SL, et al., eds. *Williams Obstetrics*. 22nd ed. New York, NY: McGraw-Hill; 2005.

Cunningham FG, et al., Intrapartum assessment. In: Cunningham FG, Leveno KJ, Bloom SL, et al., eds. *Williams Obstetrics*. 22nd ed. New York, NY: McGraw-Hill; 2005.

Cunningham FG, et al., Obstetrical hemorrhage. In: Cunningham FG, Leveno KJ, Bloom SL, et al., eds. *Williams Obstetrics*. 22nd ed. New York, NY: McGraw-Hill; 2005.

Cunningham FG, et al., Parturition. In: Cunningham FG, Leveno KJ, Bloom SL, et al., eds. *Williams Obstetrics.* 22nd ed. New York, NY: McGraw-Hill; 2005i.

Cunningham FG, et al., Prenatal care. In: Cunningham FG, Leveno KJ, Bloom SL, et al., eds. *Williams Obstetrics.* 22nd ed. New York, NY: McGraw-Hill; 2005j.

Cunningham FG, et al., Preterm birth in multifetal gestation. In: 22nd ed. Cunningham FG, Leveno KJ, Bloom SL, et al., eds. *Williams Obstetrics.* New York, NY: McGraw-Hill; 2005k.

Cunningham FG, et al. Puerperium. In: Cunningham FG, Leveno KJ, Bloom SL, et al., eds. *Williams Obstetrics.* 22nd ed. New York, NY: McGraw-Hill; 2005l.

Euhus DM. Breast disease. In: Schorge JO, Schaffer JI, Halvorson LM, et al., eds. *Williams Gynecology.* New York, NY: McGraw-Hill; 2008.

Gala RB. Benign disorders of the lower reproductive tract. In: Schorge JO, Schaffer JI, Halvorson LM, et al., eds. *Williams Gynecology.* New York, NY: McGraw-Hill; 2008a.

Gala RB. Ectopic pregnancy. In: Schorge JO, Schaffer JI, Halvorson LM, et al., eds. *Williams Gynecology.* New York, NY: McGraw-Hill; 2008b.

Griffith WF. Preinvasive lesions of the lower genital tract. In: Schorge JO, Schaffer JI, Halvorson LM, et al., eds. *Williams Gynecology.* New York, NY: McGraw-Hill; 2008.

Giuliano AE. Breast disorders. In: McPhee SJ, Papadakis MA, eds. *Lange 2009 Current Medical Diagnosis and Treatment.* 48th ed. New York, NY: McGraw-Hill; 2009.

Halvorson LM. Amenorrhea. In: Schorge JO, Schaffer JI, Halvorson LM, et al., eds. *Williams Gynecology.* New York, NY: McGraw-Hill; 2008a.

Halvorson LM. Evaluation of the infertile couple. In: Schorge JO, Schaffer JI, Halvorson LM, et al., eds. *Williams Gynecology.* New York, NY: McGraw-Hill; 2008b.

Hemsell DL. Gynecologic infections. In: Schorge JO, Schaffer JI, Halvorson LM, et al., eds. *Williams Gynecology.* New York, NY: McGraw-Hill; 2008.

Hoffman BL. Abnormal uterine bleeding. In: Schorge JO, Schaffer JI, Halvorson LM, et al., eds. *Williams Gynecology.* New York, NY: McGraw-Hill; 2008a.

Hoffman BL. Endometriosis. In: Schorge JO, Schaffer JI, Halvorson LM, et al., eds. *Williams Gynecology.* New York, NY: McGraw-Hill; 2008b.

Hoffman BL. Epithelial ovarian cancers. In: Schorge JO, Schaffer JI, Halvorson LM, et al., eds. *Williams Gynecology.* New York, NY: McGraw-Hill; 2008c.

Hoffman BL. Well woman care. In: Schorge JO, Schaffer JI, Halvorson LM, et al., eds. *Williams Gynecology.* New York, NY: McGraw-Hill; 2008d.

Hoffman, BL. Pelvic mass. In: Schorge JO, Schaffer JI, Halvorson LM, et al., eds. *Williams Gynecology.* New York, NY: McGraw-Hill; 2008e.

Hoffman BL. Pelvic pain. In: Schorge JO, Schaffer JI, Halvorson LM, et al., eds. *Williams Gynecology.* New York, NY: McGraw-Hill; 2008f.

Hughes D. Pelvic organ prolapse. In: Schorge JO, Schaffer JI, Halvorson LM, et al., eds. *Williams Gynecology.* New York, NY: McGraw-Hill; 2008.

Jacobs RA, Guglielmo BJ, Chin-Hong PV. Common problems in infectious disease. In: McPhee SJ, Papadakis MA, eds. *Lange 2009 Current Medical Diagnosis and Treatment.* 48th ed. New York, NY: McGraw-Hill; 2009.

Jayanthi SL. Invasive cancer of the vulva. In: Schorge JO, Schaffer JI, Halvorson LM, et al., eds. *Williams Gynecology.* New York, NY: McGraw-Hill; 2008.

Land N, Judd HL. Menopause & postmenopause. In: Decherney AL, Nathan L, Goodwin TM, et al., eds. *Lange Current Diagnosis & Treatment Obstetrics & Gynecology.* 10th ed. New York, NY: McGraw-Hill; 2007.

MacKay HT. Gynecologic disorders. In: McPhee SJ, Papadakis MA, eds. *Lange 2009 Current Medical Diagnosis and Treatment.* 48th ed. New York, NY: McGraw-Hill; 2009.

Miller DS. Endometrial cancer. In: Schorge JO, Schaffer JI, Halvorson LM, et al., eds. *Williams Gynecology.* New York, NY: McGraw-Hill; 2008.

Miller DA. Hypertension in pregnancy. In: Decherney AL, Nathan L, Goodwin TM, et al., eds. *Lange Current Diagnosis & Treatment Obstetrics & Gynecology.* 10th ed. New York, NY: McGraw-Hill; 2007.

Poggi SBH. Postpartum hemorrhage & the abnormal puerperium. In: Decherney AL, Nathan L, Goodwin TM, et al., eds. *Lange Current Diagnosis & Treatment Obstetrics & Gynecology.* 10th ed. New York, NY: McGraw-Hill; 2007.

Roman AS, Pernoll ML. Late pregnancy complications. In: Decherney AL, Nathan L, Goodwin TM, et al., eds. *Lange Current Diagnosis & Treatment Obstetrics & Gynecology.* 10th ed. New York, NY: McGraw-Hill; 2007.

Sarajari S, Muse KN, DeCherney AH. Endometriosis. In: Decherney AL, Nathan L, Goodwin TM, et al., eds. *Lange Current Diagnosis & Treatment Obstetrics & Gynecology.* 10th ed. New York, NY: McGraw-Hill; 2007.

Schaffer JI. Pelvic organ prolapse. In: Schorge JO, Schaffer JI, Halvorson LM, et al., eds. *Williams Gynecology.* New York, NY: McGraw-Hill; 2008.

Schorge JO. Gestational trophoblastic disease. In: Schorge JO, Schaffer JI, Halvorson LM, et al., eds. *Williams Gynecology.* New York, NY: McGraw-Hill; 2008.

Tintinalli JE, Kelen JD, Stapczynski JS, eds. *Emergency Medicine, A Comprehensive Study Guide.* 6th ed. New York, NY: McGraw-Hill; 2004.

Werner CL. Preinvasive lesions of the lower genital tract. In: Schorge JO, Schaffer JI, Halvorson LM, et al., eds. *Williams Gynecology.* New York, NY: McGraw-Hill; 2008.

Pediatrics

CHAPTER 14

Pediatrics

Rachel A. Carlson, MSBS, PA-C

DIRECTIONS: Each of the numbered items or incomplete statements in this section is followed by answers or by completion of the statement. Select the ONE lettered answer or completion that is BEST in each case.

1. Which of the following is the most likely pathogen responsible for bronchiectasis?

   (A) *Corynebacterium diphtheriae*
   (B) *Streptococcus pneumoniae*
   (C) parainfluenza virus
   (D) rhinovirus

2. A 3-month-old infant had a mild microcytic, hypochromic anemia at birth and the screen was negative for sickle cell disease/trait. She was started on iron therapy and presents today for follow up. The hemoglobin (Hgb) electrophoresis laboratory results are:

   Hemoglobin 8.8 mg/dL (normal: 10.5–14.0)

   Hematocrit 25% (normal: 33–42)

   Mean corpuscular volume (MCV) 60 fL (normal: 70–90)

   Mean corpuscularhemoglobin concentration (MCHC) 32 g/dL (normal: 33–37)

   Hgb A_2 27% (normal: 1.5%–4%); Hgb A_1 30% (normal: 76%–99%); HgF (fetal hemoglobin) 50% (normal: 0%–20%); Bart Hgb 0% (normal: 0%)

   Which of the following is the MOST likely diagnosis?

   (A) heterozygous alpha thalassemia
   (B) homozygous alpha thalassemia
   (C) beta thalassemia major
   (D) beta thalassemia minor

3. Which of the following is the most common etiologic agent for acute tonsillitis in the United States?

   (A) adenovirus
   (B) group A beta-hemolytic *Streptococcus Pyogenes*
   (C) Epstein–Barr virus
   (D) *Mycoplasma pneumoniae*

4. In a pediatric patient with suspected congestive heart failure, which of the following signs and symptoms would be least likely seen on physical examination?

   (A) bradycardia
   (B) cardiomegaly
   (C) hepatosplenomegaly
   (D) tachypnea

5. A 14-year-old girl presents to the office for a third visit over the past month complaining of fatigue and pain in her pelvic bones. Her previous evaluation included the following laboratory tests:

Heterophile antibody test: negative

Hematocrit: 34%

Since her last visit to the office, she has lost 4 lb. Her mother reports she has a poor appetite. On physical examination, she is noted to be pale, has several large ecchymotic areas on her legs, and has inguinal lymphadenopathy. Her complete blood cell count (CBC) results are given below:

White blood cell (WBC): 500	Polymorphonucleocytes (PMNs): 10%
Red blood cell (RBC): 2.4	Lymphocytes: 70% (90% blasts)
Hgb: 8.9	Monocytes: 1%
Hct: 25%	Basophils: 0%
Platelets: 90,000	Eosinophils: 0%

Which of the following is the MOST likely diagnosis?

(A) Hodgkin's lymphoma
(B) acute lymphoblastic leukemia
(C) acute myelogenous leukemia
(D) infectious mononucleosis/Epstein–Barr virus

6. Which of the following is the most common etiologic agent of bacterial meningitis in the pediatric population of the United States?

(A) *Streptococcus pneumoniae*
(B) *Haemophilus influenzae* type B
(C) *Listeria monocytogenes*
(D) *Neisseria meningitides*

7. Three weeks ago, an 8-year-old child was diagnosed with *Streptococcal* pharyngitis based upon a positive throat culture for group A beta-hemolytic streptococcus. Today, she returns to the clinic with evidence of carditis. The differential diagnosis includes rheumatic fever. What additional finding would allow you to make the diagnosis of rheumatic fever based upon the modified Jones criteria?

(A) leukocytosis
(B) polyarthritis
(C) elevated erythrocyte sedimentation rate (ESR)
(D) erythema multiforme

8. In a patient who has newly diagnosed Hemophilia B, which of the following laboratory results would be expected on a coagulation panel?

(A) Increased aPTT (activated partial thromboplastin time), normal PT (prothrombin time), factor VIII deficiency
(B) + von Willebrand factor, decreased aPTT, and increased PT
(C) Increased PT, increased bleeding time, decreased platelets, decreased fibrinogen
(D) Increased aPTT, normal PT, normal thrombin time

9. A routine physical examination of a 12-year-old girl demonstrates dark, coarse, curly pubic hair spread sparsely over the pubic symphysis, as well as elevation of the breast and areola without separation of their contours. According to Tanner stages of sexual maturation, at what stage would you assess her sexual maturity?

(A) Tanner Stage II
(B) Tanner Stage III
(C) Tanner Stage IV
(D) Tanner Stage V

10. During the first year of life, what would be the expected average growth for an infant who weighs 8 lb at birth?

(A) 7 lb at 2 weeks, 14 lb at 6 months, 21 lb at 12 months
(B) 7 lb at 2 weeks, 21 lb at 4 months, 28 lb at 12 months
(C) 8 lb at 2 weeks, 16 lb at 4 months, 24 lb at 12 months
(D) 8 lb at 2 weeks, 24 lb at 6 months, 32 lb at 12 months

11. A 3-year-old child presents to the emergency department (ED) with bruises on his body. His mother claims that her son sustained these bruises when he tumbled down the stairs 3 days ago. Which of the following colors would you expect the bruises to be if this occurred as stated?

(A) brown

(B) purple

(C) red

(D) yellow

12. An 8-month-old infant, whose parents elected not to immunize, presents with a 5-day history of a runny nose in late January. Then, over the past 3 days she has developed a temperature of 101.2°F and vomiting (three times in 24 hours). This morning she developed watery, non-bloody, nonmucous diarrhea. Which of the following is the MOST likely causative organism for her illness?

(A) *Clostridium difficile*

(B) *Giardia lamblia*

(C) Shigella species

(D) rotavirus

13. In a 4-year-old female child who presents with "toeing in," which of the following is the likely etiology?

(A) femoral anteversion

(B) genu valgum

(C) genu varum

(D) tibial torsion

14. Which of the following is the first sign of puberty in a normal male?

(A) appearance of axillary hair

(B) appearance of pubic hair

(C) deepening of the voice

(D) enlargement of the testes

15. Huntington disease has which of the following types of genetic patterns of inheritance?

(A) autosomal dominant

(B) autosomal recessive

(C) X-linked dominant

(D) X-linked recessive

16. A 9-year-old child, who was diagnosed with a viral upper respiratory infection 2 weeks ago, returns to the clinic with a complaint of a 2-day history of drooping of one side of her mouth. She is afebrile with a blood pressure of 110/60 mm Hg. Her physical examination reveals an inability to completely close her left eye, inability to wrinkle her forehead, and the drooping of her mouth on the left side. Her smile is asymmetric. The remainder of her examination is otherwise normal. Which of the following is the MOST likely diagnosis?

(A) Bell's palsy

(B) botulism

(C) brainstem glioma

(D) Guillain–Barré syndrome

17. A 5-year-old child presents to the office for a school physical examination. His medical history is unremarkable, including normal growth and development. His physical examination is normal except for a grade II/VI high-pitched, vibratory, systolic ejection murmur heard best at the left lower sternal border with radiation to the apex. When the child is in a supine position, the murmur is louder. Which of the following murmurs is the MOST likely diagnosis?

(A) physiologic peripheral pulmonic stenosis murmur

(B) pulmonary ejection murmur

(C) Still's murmur

(D) venous hum

18. Which of the following sleeping positions for a healthy infant should be recommended to parents during anticipatory guidance in order to reduce the risk for sudden infant death syndrome?

(A) prone position

(B) seated position

(C) side position

(D) supine position

19. A previously healthy 12-month-old infant has been coughing and experiencing fever on and off for 2 months. He was diagnosed and treated for pneumonia approximately 3 months ago. On physical examination, he is noted to be in no acute respiratory distress; however, he is tachypneic with bibasilar rales and scattered rhonchi. Which of the following is the MOST likely diagnosis?

    (A) bronchiectasis
    (B) chronic bronchitis
    (C) croup
    (D) bronchopulmonary dysplasia

20. The second most common etiologic agent of otitis externa is which of the following?

    (A) *Staphylococcus aureus*
    (B) *Corynebacterium*
    (C) *Anaerobes*
    (D) *Streptococcus pyogenes*

21. At 12 hours of age, a physical examination is performed on a neonate who has intrauterine growth retardation. He is noted to have microcephaly, jaundice, and hepatosplenomegaly. Which of the following is the MOST likely congenital viral infection in this neonate?

    (A) cytomegalovirus
    (B) herpes simplex virus
    (C) rubella
    (D) syphilis

22. A previously healthy, 5-month-old infant is admitted to the hospital due to lethargy progressing to semiconsciousness. The physical examination reveals a depressed mental status and bilateral retinal hemorrhages. Which of the following is the MOST likely diagnosis?

    (A) child abuse
    (B) retinitis pigmentosa
    (C) Reye syndrome
    (D) viral encephalitis

23. A 2-year-old child presents to the emergency department via ambulance due to a seizure lasting approximately 2 minutes with jerking and somnolence. En route in the ambulance her vital signs are: temperature 39°C rectal; pulse 120/min; respirations 32/min; blood pressure 110/64 mm Hg. Upon further questioning, her mother claimed she had a runny nose yesterday. On physical examination, she is sleepy but arousable with negative Kernig and Brudzinski signs. Which of the following seizures is the MOST likely diagnosis?

    (A) absence seizure
    (B) complex partial seizure
    (C) febrile seizure
    (D) simple partial seizure

24. A 6-month-old uncircumcised male infant presents with a 2-day history of a fever (39.6°C rectal today), vomiting, and poor feeding. Urinalysis of a catheterized specimen reveals 50 to 100 white blood cells per high-power field and moderate bacteria. Two days later, the urine culture results are available. Which of the following is the MOST common pathogen responsible for this infant's first urinary tract infection?

    (A) *Enterococcus*
    (B) *Escherichia coli*
    (C) *Klebsiella*
    (D) *Staphylococcus saprophyticus*

25. A 6-month-old infant presents to the emergency department with a 2-day history of vomiting and diarrhea. Upon physical examination, she appears to be intermittently irritable and restless with minimal tearing when crying and dry mucous membranes. Her capillary refill is 2 to 3 seconds. Her urine sodium is less than 20 mEq/L and mildly oliguric. On the basis of these clinical manifestations, what is the magnitude of her dehydration?

    (A) less than 3%
    (B) approaching 3% to 5% (mild)
    (C) approaching 6% to 10% (moderate)
    (D) approaching 11% to 15% (severe)

26. A previously well, 15-month-old baby boy is brought to the emergency department in the middle of the night with increased irritability

and severe paroxysmal colicky abdominal pain followed by vomiting. On physical examination, a tubular mass is palpated in the abdomen. The rectal examination reveals bloody mucus. Which of the following is the MOST likely diagnosis?

(A) appendicitis

(B) infectious enteritis

(C) intussusception

(D) pyloric stenosis

27. Which of the following daily maintenance fluid requirements is the closest approximation for a 24-kg child who is refusing to eat?

(A) 1,080 mL

(B) 1,200 mL

(C) 1,580 mL

(D) 2,000 mL

28. Which of the following is the recommended treatment for a 4-year-old child with presumed bacterial meningitis?

(A) cefotaxime or ceftriaxone plus ampicillin

(B) cefotaxime or ceftriaxone plus vancomycin

(C) gentamicin plus ampicillin

(D) ampicillin plus chloramphenicol

29. At a 2-month-old well-child checkup, a female infant is noted to have the following physical findings: widely open anterior and posterior fontanels, large protruding tongue, coarse facial features, low-set hair line, and an umbilical hernia. In the newborn period, there was a prolongation of physiologic icterus. The results of the newborn screening test are abnormal. Which of the following is the MOST likely diagnosis?

(A) congenital adrenal hyperplasia

(B) congenital hypothyroidism

(C) Crigler–Najjar syndrome

(D) galactosemia

30. Within hours of birth, a healthy infant is noted to have a superficial swelling over the right occipitoparietal region that extends across the suture line. Which of the following conditions is it MOST likely to be?

(A) caput succedaneum

(B) cephalohematoma

(C) craniotabes

(D) subgaleal hemorrhage

31. A 2-year-old male child is brought to the emergency department by his mother with a sudden onset of choking, gagging, coughing, and wheezing. Vital signs are temperature 37°C; pulse 120/min; and respirations 28/min. The physical examination reveals decreased breath sounds over the right lower lobe with inspiratory rhonchi and localized expiratory wheezing. The chest X-ray reveals normal inspiratory views but expiratory views show localized hyperinflation with mediastinal shift to the left. Which of the following is the MOST likely diagnosis?

(A) asthma

(B) epiglottitis

(C) foreign body aspiration

(D) pulmonary embolism

32. A 16-year-old girl is brought to the emergency department by ambulance after reportedly ingesting "a bottle of aspirin." Vital signs are temperature 37.8°C oral; pulse 94/min; respirations 30/min; blood pressure 100/68 mm Hg. What would you expect the blood gases to show that would confirm she had swallowed the aspirin?

(A) anion gap metabolic acidosis with respiratory acidosis

(B) nonanion gap metabolic acidosis with respiratory alkalosis

(C) anion gap metabolic acidosis with respiratory alkalosis

(D) nonanion gap metabolic acidosis with respiratory acidosis

33. A 16-year-old high school boy presents to the emergency department 4 hours after sustaining an abrasion to his knee after a fall while rollerblading on the school playground. His school immunization record reveals that his last diphtheria, tetanus, and pertussis (DTaP) booster was administered at age 4. In this situation, which of the following is the MOST appropriate plan?

    (A) administer tetanus toxoid
    (B) administer adult tetanus and diphtheria toxoid (Td)
    (C) administer diphtheria, tetanus toxoid, and acellular pertussis (Tdap) vaccine
    (D) administer tetanus immune globulin

34. Which of the following newborn reflexes should still be present at the 9-month check-up?

    (A) Galant reflex
    (B) Landau reflex
    (C) rooting reflex
    (D) parachute reflex

35. A 3-day-old infant has bilateral copious, yellow-green eye discharge and conjunctival inflammation. A Gram stain of this discharge reveals gram-negative intracellular diplococci. Which of the following antibiotics is the drug of choice for this infection?

    (A) ceftriaxone
    (B) cephalexin
    (C) erythromycin
    (D) gentamicin

36. A 10-year-old boy presents to the office, complaining of a painful, swollen area along his right jaw and neck. On physical examination, he is noted to be febrile and has diffuse tenderness over the right parotid gland. His laboratory tests include an elevated serum amylase. His parents elected not to vaccinate him. In this patient, based on the most likely diagnosis, which of the following is a complication of his disease?

    (A) hepatitis
    (B) nerve deafness

    (C) pneumonitis
    (D) testicular torsion

37. Which of the following physical examination findings in a newborn infant should cause the clinician to suspect a genetic disorder?

    (A) café au lait spots
    (B) subconjunctival hemorrhages
    (C) miliaria
    (D) vernix caseosa

38. The newborn examination at 1 minute shows a heart rate of 120 bpm, strong cry, some flexion in the upper extremities, sneezing with nasal catheter suction, and bluish hands and feet; but the remainder of the body is pink. What is the Apgar score?

    (A) 7
    (B) 8
    (C) 9
    (D) 10

39. Which of the following is the most common congenital heart malformation?

    (A) atrial septal defect
    (B) tetralogy of Fallot
    (C) ventricular septal defect
    (D) transposition of the great vessels

40. A 5-year-old male child presents to the office for his kindergarten physical examination. Assuming that the patient's immunizations have been up to date, which of the following are the immunizations that the patient should receive at the end of today's visit?

    (A) hepatitis B, inactivated poliovirus (IPV), diphtheria, tetanus, acellular pertussis (DTaP), measles, mumps, rubella (MMR), varicella
    (B) IPV, DTaP, MMR, pneumococcal (PCV)
    (C) IPV, DTaP, MMR, *Haemophilus influenzae* type B (Hib)
    (D) DTaP, IPV, MMR, varicella

41. Which of the following is an absolute contraindication to breastfeeding?

    (A) tuberculosis of the mother
    (B) methadone treatment (20 mg/d)
    (C) maternal smoking
    (D) infant with cystic fibrosis

42. A 4-month-old infant presents to the office for her "well-check." The parents state that they have no concerns and think she is doing well. She is being breastfed every 4 to 6 hours and has four wet diapers a day and two dirty diapers a day. Her birth weight was 7 lb 7 oz (50th percentile); she missed her 2-month appointment and at today's visit her weight is 11 lb 5 oz (5th percentile). The clinician, however, is very concerned and diagnoses the infant with which of the following?

    (A) dwarfism
    (B) growth deficiency
    (C) lactose intolerance
    (D) Beckwith–Wiedemann syndrome

43. During influenza season, a 15-year-old boy presents to the emergency department, unresponsive. The parents state that when they tried to wake him up in the morning he would not get up and was barely breathing. They deny any drug or alcohol use and state that he just had some cold symptoms the past few days. A spinal tap shows decreased glucose, increased pressure, and increased proteins, but there were no cells found. The rest of the blood work shows elevated liver enzymes, but normal serum bilirubin and alkaline phosphatase. A liver biopsy demonstrates microvesicular steatosis without glycogen and large mitochondria. Which of the following is the best treatment for this patient?

    (A) high-dose steroids
    (B) broad-spectrum antibiotics until the cultures come back
    (C) supportive treatment, including maintenance fluids and hyperventilation
    (D) liver transplant

44. A 5-year-old female child presents for her kindergarten physical examination and her mother mentions that she thinks she looks a bit yellow to her. The clinician notes diffuse jaundice, icterus, and Kayser–Fleischer rings. Which of the following is the treatment of choice for this patient?

    (A) alpha-interferon therapy
    (B) D-penicillamine therapy
    (C) methylprednisolone
    (D) protease inhibitor therapy

45. A 24-month-old infant presents for his routine physical examination. The parents state that he has been following all of his developmental milestones. On examination, the clinician hears a grade II/VI murmur along the left sternal border, which radiates into the left axilla and the left side of the back. The child also has decreased femoral pulses bilaterally. The clinician orders a chest X-ray. Which of the following is the expected finding on X-ray based on the presentation?

    (A) notching or scalloping of the ribs
    (B) boot-shaped heart—right ventricular hypertrophy
    (C) "egg on string"—narrowed mediastinum
    (D) absence of the main pulmonary artery

46. An 8-year-old female child presents to the emergency department with her parents. They state she has been coughing all night the past few nights, to the point she sounds like she is choking. On examination, the clinician notes mild retractions at rest. Retractions worsen with the lung examination and there is diffuse stridor on auscultation. Pulse oximetry is 92% on room air and the child is afebrile. Which of the following is the recommended treatment for this patient?

    (A) supportive care only—mist therapy
    (B) IV (intravenous) antibiotics, with gram-negative coverage
    (C) IM (intramuscular) dexamethasone
    (D) nebulized racemic epinephrine and oral dexamethasone

47. A neonate presents with meconium ileus that is successfully unobstructed. The infant returns at her 4-month appointment with signs of failure to thrive. Which of the following is the most likely diagnosis for this patient?

    (A) cystic fibrosis
    (B) Wilson disease
    (C) intussusception
    (D) volvulus

48. Which of the following is NOT a cyanotic heart lesion?

    (A) transposition of the great arteries
    (B) atrioventricular septal defect
    (C) hypoplastic left heart syndrome
    (D) tricuspid atresia

49. A 2-week-old male infant presents for a routine checkup. The mother complains that he nurses every hour, but vomits (nonbilious) after every time he eats. He has only had three bowel movements since he has been home. On examination, the infant has not gained any weight since leaving the hospital, and the clinician notes gastric peristaltic waves. Which of the following is the treatment of choice for this patient?

    (A) pyloromyotomy
    (B) metoclopramide
    (C) laparotomy
    (D) omeprazole

50. A 6-month-old infant presents for her checkup. Her father mentions that they started solid foods after her 4-month check. She has had foul-smelling diarrhea off and on for the first month of solids; it now occurs after every meal and looks greasy. They have tried different formulas and different cereals without improvement. What is the diagnostic test of choice for the most likely disorder?

    (A) sweat chloride test
    (B) RAST (radioallergosorbent assay test)
    (C) gastrin level
    (D) intestinal biopsy

51. A 9-year-old child presents to the urgent care center with her mother. The child is complaining of dark colored urine. The mother mentions that the child was complaining of sore throat and cold symptoms a few weeks ago. The urine shows gross hematuria without nitrites or leukocytes. Which of the following is the best test to help the clinician confirm the diagnosis?

    (A) monospot
    (B) antistreptolysin O titer
    (C) immunoglobulin electrophoresis
    (D) renal biopsy

52. Upon performing a newborn examination, the clinician notes a widened pulse pressure, paradoxical splitting of S_2, and a "machine"-like murmur heard best at the second intercostal space, left sternal border, and inferior to the clavicle. Which of the following is the most likely diagnosis?

    (A) tetralogy of Fallot
    (B) ventricular septal defect
    (C) atrial septal defect
    (D) patent ductus arteriosus

53. A 15-year-old boy suddenly collapses on the basketball court; his sports physical conducted at the beginning of the year did not elicit any abnormal findings. Basic life support initiated at the scene, however, is unsuccessful in resuscitation. Which of the following is the most likely etiology of his sudden death?

    (A) mitral valve prolapse
    (B) surgically corrected aortic stenosis
    (C) hypertrophic cardiomyopathy
    (D) rheumatic heart disease

54. A 7-year-old male child presents to the emergency department with complaints of severe dyspnea, dysphagia, drooling, muffled voice, and fever. The pulse oximetry is 91% on room air; lung examination shows stridor and inspiratory retractions. Which of the following is the expected chest X-ray finding for the suspected diagnosis?

(A) thumbprint sign

(B) Scottie dog sign

(C) steeple sign

(D) figure 3 sign

55. Which of the following is one of the most common lethal genetic disorders in the United States?

(A) trisomy 13

(B) trisomy 21

(C) cystic fibrosis

(D) neurofibromatosis

56. Which of the following is the initial treatment step in an adolescent who presents to the emergency department with status epilepticus?

(A) IV glucose

(B) stabilize airway

(C) arterial blood gas

(D) IV diazepam therapy

57. A 12-year-old boy presents to the urgent care center complaining of burning pain in his lower extremities with weakness. On examination, the clinician notes symmetric weakness with severely decreased active range of motion of the lower extremities. In addition, there is decreased position and vibratory sensation in the distal portions bilaterally. Upon further questioning, the patient admits to being diagnosed with mononucleosis 2 weeks ago. Which of the following is the most likely diagnosis?

(A) poliomyelitis

(B) botulism

(C) Tick-bite paralysis

(D) Guillain–Barré syndrome

58. Which thoracic curvature is an indication for treatment with bracing in an adolescent with scoliosis?

(A) less than 20°

(B) 20° to 40°

(C) 40° to 60°

(D) 40° with lumbar curvature of 30°

59. A 6-year-old female child presents with complaints of chronic hip pain so severe that she has not been able to walk to the school bus. Examination shows severe tenderness at the left hip with markedly decreased active and passive range of motion. Radiologic examination demonstrates joint effusion with widening. Which of the following is the most likely diagnosis?

(A) osteochondritis dissecans

(B) slipped capital femoral epiphysis

(C) septic hip arthritis

(D) Legg–Calvé–Perthes disease

60. A 16-year-old boy presents to the office with thumb pain. He just returned from a skiing trip. On examination, the practitioner notes a positive ulnar collateral ligament laxity test. What is the most likely diagnosis?

(A) mallet finger

(B) gamekeeper thumb

(C) boxer fracture

(D) nondisplaced scaphoid fracture

61. A 3-year-old child is brought in by her parents to the urgent care center stating that the child "will not bend her arm." They are obviously worried and distraught. The clinician notices the elbow is held in strict pronation and there is tenderness over the radial head. X-ray examination shows no findings. Which of the following is the treatment of choice for this disorder?

(A) place elbow in full supination and move from full extension to full flexion

(B) immobilization of the elbow in a splint for 2 weeks

(C) referral to the orthopedic surgeon for suspected radial head fracture

(D) call child protective services for suspected battery

62. A 7-year-old child is brought into the office by her mother who states that the child "is still wetting the bed at night." The child has already decreased liquid intake and uses the bathroom before going to bed. The mother is worried that there is something wrong with the child. Upon examination there is no abnormality. Urinalysis is negative. Which of the following is the treatment of choice for this disorder?

(A) bed-wetting alarm
(B) desmopressin acetate (DDAVP)
(C) imipramine
(D) amitriptyline

63. A 13-year-old boy presents with fever and blood in his urine. Examination shows an asymptomatic mass in the left lower quadrant. Urinalysis shows hematuria and small leukocytes. Which of the following is the most likely diagnosis?

(A) renal cell carcinoma
(B) intussusception
(C) volvulus
(D) nephroblastoma

64. A mother brings in her 20-month-old female child to the office because she noticed pubic hair growing. On examination, the clinician notices that the clitoris is enlarged; the rest is unremarkable. Which of the following is an expected laboratory finding on this patient?

(A) increased aldosterone
(B) increased estrogen
(C) increased androstenedione
(D) increased luteinizing hormone

65. A 5-year-old child presents for her kindergarten checkup. The clinician notes that over the past couple of years, her height decreased from the 50th percentile to the 5th percentile. On examination, the clinician also notes truncal adiposity. Her CBC and lead levels were normal. Which of the following is the most likely diagnosis?

(A) growth hormone deficiency
(B) Cushing disease
(C) congenital hypothyroidism
(D) congenital adrenal hyperplasia

66. An Rh-negative, 5-year-old male child presents with acute onset of petechiae and purpura after an acute viral illness. In addition, he has episodes of epistaxis. Which of the following is a treatment option if his platelet count falls below 20,000/mm^3, but he is not actively bleeding?

(A) platelet transfusions
(B) IV anti-D (WinRho SD) 50–70 mg/kg/dose
(C) prednisone 2.4 mg/kg/24 hours × 2 weeks
(D) splenectomy

67. A 9-year-old female child presents with tachycardia, tachypnea, shortness of breath, bibasilar rales, and distended jugular veins. Which of the following is the least likely cause for her signs and symptoms?

(A) rheumatic heart disease
(B) sickle cell anemia
(C) viral myocarditis
(D) patent ductus arteriosus

68. A 12 year-old girl patient was treated for a urinary tract infection 3 days ago. She presents today with severe conjunctivitis, target lesions on her trunk, and bullous eruptions in her mouth. Which of the following medications is the likely cause of her symptoms?

(A) ciprofloxacin
(B) erythromycin
(C) amoxicillin
(D) trimethoprim-sulfamethoxazole (TMP-SMX)

69. Which of the following is a complication of infection with Parvovirus B19?

(A) aplastic crisis
(B) leukopenia
(C) aseptic meningitis
(D) congenital defects (if mother contracts during pregnancy)

70. A 9-year-old male child presents with a painful rash of his upper extremity. His mom states it started 4 days ago and seems like it is spreading. Physical examination demonstrates a vesicular rash across the right upper arm and chest but does not cross the midline. Which of the following prescriptions would be most appropriate for this patient at today's visit?

(A) hydration
(B) nonsteroidal anti-inflammatory drugs (NSAIDs)
(C) Varicella-Zoster immunoglobulin (VZIG)
(D) oral acyclovir

71. Which of the following findings would suggest a specific child abuse diagnosis of Munchausen syndrome by proxy?

(A) fractures in various stages of healing
(B) retinal hemorrhages
(C) head or abdominal trauma
(D) recurrent polymicrobial sepsis

72. Which of the following is a contraindication for the meningococcal (Menomune) vaccine?

(A) history of Guillain-Barré
(B) complement deficiency
(C) college freshman in dormitories
(D) persons with functional asplenia

73. A 7-year-old Caucasian female child presents to the office with "an itchy head." The child's mother, who is with her, states that this has been bothering her daughter for about a week and she has noticed a lot of "dandruff" in the child's hair that will not come out. She also mentions that several of her daughter's friends are having the same problem. On the basis of the most likely diagnosis, what is the best treatment for this patient?

(A) permethrin 1% shampoo
(B) ketoconazole cream
(C) tar-based shampoo
(D) silver sulfadiazine 1% cream

74. A young mother brings her 4-year-old son to the clinic for evaluation of a rash on his umbilicus and hands. She has been treating it with an over-the-counter ointment for about a week, without success. She says that she has noticed that he scratches the rash periodically, and it seems to bother him the most at night. She also says that she noticed this same rash on the hands on one of the other boys at his daycare center. On examination, there are excoriated papules and nodules on his hand and umbilicus. What is the most likely diagnosis?

(A) herpes simplex
(B) scabies
(C) pediculosis
(D) tinea corporis

75. A new mother brings her 3-month-old daughter to the clinic for a rash on the infant's head. On examination, the skin affected by the rash is thickened, yellowish white in color, scaly, and looks waxy. In addition, it involves only the scalp and bilateral postauricular areas. What is the most likely diagnosis?

(A) contact dermatitis
(B) lichen planus
(C) pityriasis rosea
(D) seborrheic dermatitis

76. An 8-year-old male child presents with brown, nonpruritic, annular lesions on the back of his hands and feet. Intradermal nodules are seen on the extensor surfaces of the elbows and knees that have been present for several months. At today's visit, the lesions are essentially unchanged since his last visit about a month ago. What is the best treatment for this suspected disorder?

(A) excision and biopsy
(B) no treatment
(C) topical steroids
(D) wet to dry dressings

77. Which of the following is the recommended treatment of a 2- to 5-cm, single, nonpainful, common wart on the hand of a 7-year-old?

(A) 40% salicylic acid plaster
(B) burning laser surgery
(C) electrocautery
(D) liquid nitrogen

78. In treating uncomplicated, comedonal acne (open and closed comedones) in adolescents, which of the following treatments is best?

    (A) topical antibiotics

    (B) topical keratolytics

    (C) oral retinoids

    (D) systemic antibiotics

79. The most common fracture of newborns is a fracture of the

    (A) clavicle

    (B) humerus

    (C) radius

    (D) ulna

80. A 13-year-old boy presents to the clinic for a complaint of right knee pain that he first noticed about a year ago. It started out as mild discomfort in the area just below the kneecap, but has been getting progressively worse. Now, it hurts anytime he uses his leg, even when walking. He does not remember any injury to his knee. When you examine his knee, you notice swelling and exquisite tenderness over the tibial tubercle. X-rays are normal. What is the most likely diagnosis?

    (A) chondromalacia patellae

    (B) Osgood–Schlatter disease

    (C) patellar dislocation

    (D) patellofemoral overuse syndrome

81. The eggs of this parasite are detected by microscopic examination of clear adhesive tape that has been pressed to the child's anus in the morning, prior to bathing. What parasite is most likely to be identified by this test method?

    (A) *Ancylostoma duodenale* (hookworm)

    (B) *Ascaris lumbricoides* (ascaris)

    (C) enterobiasis (pinworm)

    (D) trichuriasis (whipworm)

82. A 13-year-old boy presents with complaints of pain in both knees and his right ankle. The pain is worse in the morning. He denies any injuries, but does notice he tires more easily when playing baseball. He says this has been going on for

about 8 weeks. His father admits to having chronic low back pain, but otherwise the family medical history is noncontributory. On the basis of this history, which of the following is the most likely diagnosis?

    (A) juvenile idiopathic arthritis

    (B) Lyme arthritis

    (C) psoriatic arthritis

    (D) enteropathic arthritis

83. An 8-year-old female child presents with complaints of a red itchy right eye with a lot of yellowish green color discharge for 3 days. She denies any injury. Her visual acuity is normal but she does have moderate tearing and mild photophobia. What is the most likely diagnosis?

    (A) allergic conjunctivitis

    (B) bacterial conjunctivitis

    (C) viral conjunctivitis

    (D) reactive arthritis/Reiter syndrome

84. While seeing a 12-week-old baby girl for her well-child checkup, it is noticed that she has tearing from her left eye. There is a small reddened area that is swollen and she cries when it is touched. The swollen area is just below the medial inferior eyelid. There is also constant tearing from this same eye. Her mother says it just started about 2 days ago and is getting worse. What is the most likely cause of this problem?

    (A) blepharitis

    (B) conjunctivitis

    (C) dacryocystitis

    (D) anterior uveitis

85. The majority of cases of halitosis in young children can be traced to which of the following causes?

    (A) dental caries

    (B) nasal foreign body

    (C) poor dietary habits

    (D) upper respiratory tract infection

86. Of the following, which is the most frequent cause of epistaxis in children?

   (A) bleeding disorders
   (B) choanal atresia
   (C) digital trauma
   (D) foreign bodies

87. A 5-year-old male child in the clinic is being evaluated for a firm, painful lump that is slightly reddened and approximately 3 cm in diameter, in his right axilla. His mother tells you the lump has been there for a couple of days. The boy does not look acutely ill. The mother informs you that they got a new kitten and puppy about a month ago but otherwise nothing else is new at home. Which of the following is the most likely etiology for his rash?

   (A) *Bartonella henselae*
   (B) parvovirus
   (C) Hodgkin disease
   (D) Osgood–Schlatter disease

88. When considering infections caused by nematodes, which of the following is most consistent with iron deficiency anemia, abdominal discomfort, weight loss, and the presence of ova in the feces?

   (A) ascariasis
   (B) hookworm
   (C) pinworms
   (D) whipworm

89. Erythema migrans, the characteristic rash of Lyme disease, occurs in what percent of patients with this disease?

   (A) 20% to 40%
   (B) 40% to 60%
   (C) 60% to 80%
   (D) 80% to 100%

90. A 2-week-old male infant is being seen in the clinic for a profuse mucoid discharge from both eyes, with some associated tearing. On examination, you notice both eyes are hyperemic and the eyelids are red and swollen. Which of the following is the most likely cause of this patient's ophthalmia neonatorum (conjunctivitis in the newborn)?

   (A) allergic
   (B) gonococcal
   (C) chlamydial
   (D) viral

91. Which of the following neurologic disorders is least likely to be associated with Lyme disease?

   (A) aseptic meningitis
   (B) Bell palsy
   (C) polyradiculitis
   (D) seizures

92. A young mother brings her 3-week-old daughter for care of a rash in her mouth. The mother indicates the baby was doing fine until 2 days ago when she noticed white spots in the infant's mouth. On examination, they do not come off easily with a tongue blade. She is bottle-feeding the infant without any problem. Which of the following is the most likely diagnosis of this problem?

   (A) leukoplakia
   (B) hand–foot–mouth disease
   (C) herpangina
   (D) oral candidiasis

93. A 14-year-old boy presents for evaluation of behavior problems that his mother reports have been present for about a year, but have been worsening in the past few months. She complains that her son has been having problems in school, is not behaving, and is getting into fights. He seems to only want to talk about science fiction movies and occasionally seems to be talking to people who are not really there. Sometimes, he seems really depressed and at other times, "full of energy and happy." On the basis of this mother's observations, which of the following is the most likely diagnosis?

   (A) attention-deficit/hyperactivity disorder (ADHD)
   (B) bipolar disorder
   (C) conduct disorder
   (D) depression

94. A 9-year-old male child presents in August with complaints of a red rash on the palms of his hands, soles of his feet, and a little on his legs. His mother states that this rash started about 2 days ago, and just before it appeared her son had been complaining of a severe headache and aching all over. She said he felt "hot to the touch" during that time, as well. The child mentions he was camping in Arkansas about 10 days ago with his dad but did not eat anything abnormal. On the basis of this history, what is the most likely diagnosis?

(A) endemic typhus
(B) human ehrlichiosis
(C) Q fever
(D) Rocky Mountain spotted fever

95. In young children, which of the following is the most common cause of lower respiratory tract infections?

(A) adenovirus
(B) human parvovirus
(C) parainfluenza virus
(D) respiratory syncytial virus

96. A 3-year-old male child presents to the clinic for a cough that occurs only after he has been running, according to his mother. She says she first noticed this about 6 months ago, after he had had one of his usual winter colds, and his cough persisted for about a week. On the basis of this history, what is the most likely diagnosis?

(A) airway foreign body
(B) asthma
(C) cystic fibrosis
(D) laryngomalacia

97. A 12-month-old male infant presents with his mother's concerns that he does not seem to play with other children as his brother and sister did at this age. She indicates she has noticed that he does not seem to respond when she or other children call him by name, he is indifferent to other children or adults when they are present, and he does not seem to know any and "just grunts." On the basis of this his-

tory, the most likely diagnosis for this problem is which of the following?

(A) attention-deficit/hyperactivity disorder (ADHD)
(B) autism
(C) fragile X syndrome
(D) schizophrenia

98. When evaluating a newborn, the inability to pass a small catheter through the nasal cavity is most indicative of which of the following conditions?

(A) choanal atresia
(B) meconium ileus
(C) nasal infection
(D) nasal polyps

99. Anorexia nervosa is an eating disorder commonly affecting teenage girls. Which of the following best represents the percentage of the teenage girls affected?

(A) 1% to 5%
(B) 5% to 10%
(C) 10% to 15%
(D) 15% to 20%

100. Which of the following is the most common childhood nutritional disorder in the United States?

(A) binge eating disorder
(B) folate deficiency
(C) obesity
(D) rickets

101. By which age do infants develop heart failure secondary to congenital heart lesions?

(A) birth
(B) 6 months
(C) 9 months
(D) 12 months

102. Which of the following is the antibiotic of choice for a patient who is diagnosed with *Bordetella pertussis*?

(A) erythromycin 40–50 mg/kg/24 hours in divided doses × 14 days

(B) ampicillin 100 mg/kg/34 hours in divided doses × 7 days

(C) amoxicillin 80–90 mg/kg/24 hours in divided doses × 10 days

(D) cephalexin 30 mg/kg/24 hours in divided doses × 7 days

103. Which of the following is indicated for an incarcerated inguinal hernia present for more than 12 hours?

(A) watchful waiting

(B) manual reduction

(C) surgical reduction

(D) bilateral surgical reduction

104. A 6-year-old female child presents with neck pain and fever for 2 days. Her remote history consists of 2 to 3 days of diarrhea and vomiting. She attends a local daycare where other kids had similar nausea/vomiting, but recovered. The LP was positive for gram-negative bacilli, decreased glucose, increased protein, and increased neutrophils. Which of the following is the most likely etiologic agent?

(A) rotavirus

(B) Salmonella species

(C) *Corynebacterium diphtheria*

(D) *Clostridium botulinum*

105. In an infant with highly suspected vitamin K deficiency, which laboratory finding would be expected?

(A) prolonged PT (prothrombin time)

(B) elevated fibrinogen

(C) decreased platelet count

(D) decreased aPTT (activated partial thromboplastin time)

106. In a 12-month-old male infant presenting with acute onset ear pain that is disrupting his sleep, which of the following findings on clinical examination would confirm a diagnosis of acute otitis media?

(A) erythematous tympanic membrane

(B) tenderness upon palpation of the tragus

(C) bulging tympanic membrane

(D) flat tracing on tympanometry

107. Which of the following requirements for child safety restraints is TRUE?

(A) Infants weighing less than 20 lb and longer than 20 inches may sit in forward-facing seats.

(B) Children weighing between 20 and 30 lb may sit in upright booster seats.

(C) Children who weigh less than 80 lb should be in a certified child safety seat/booster.

(D) Children weighing more than 40 lb may sit in the front seat in four-door vehicles.

108. Which of the following is the most common cause for childhood gynecomastia?

(A) neoplasms

(B) medications

(C) illicit drug use

(D) idiopathic

109. In the evaluation of a child with newly diagnosed hypertension, which of the following evaluations will help rule in the most common etiology?

(A) urinalysis

(B) serum uric acid

(C) electrocardiogram

(D) chest radiography

110. The Centers for Disease Control and Prevention recommend the first lead screening for children living in high risk areas in the United States at which age?

(A) 6 months

(B) 9 months

(C) 15 months

(D) 24 months

Answers and Explanations

1. **(B)** Bronchiectasis has numerous etiologies. Most commonly, cultures reveal normal oral flora from the lower respiratory tract: *Streptococcus pneumoniae, Staphylococcus aureus, Haemophilus influenzae, Pseudomonas aeruginosa.* Parainfluenza viruses typically are responsible for croup. *Corynebacterium diphtheriae* is the causative organism for diphtheria. Rhinovirus is the most common pathogen isolated with acute viral rhinitis or the common cold. *(Kerby et al., 2009, pp. 478-480, 487-488)*

2. **(D)** The typical hemoglobin electrophoresis for beta thalassemia minor has an elevated level of hemoglobin A_2. In a normal infant there is mainly HgF and HgA_1 with minimal amounts of A_2. Bart hemoglobin is diagnostic for the alpha thalassemias after the neonatal period is over. Beta thalassemia major will only have fetal hemoglobin on electrophoresis. Because of the high incidence of false-negatives in hemoglobin screenings in the neonatal period, it is important for the provider to do a full work-up of microcytic, hypochromic anemias to ensure proper diagnosis. *(Scott, 2006, pp. 704-707; Ambruso et al., 2009, pp. 815-817)*

3. **(B)** In children who present with symptoms of sore throat and fever, approximately 50% to 70% of these cases are due to a viral infection. Adenovirus is one of the most common etiologic viral agents. Epstein–Barr virus is the etiologic agent for mononucleosis and while very common in the United States it is still less than rhinoviruses and coronaviruses. The two remaining choices are bacterial pathogens of which group A beta-hemolytic streptococcus (GAS) is the most common followed by the less common pathogens (group C *Streptococcus, Arcanobacterium haemolyticus,* and *Streptococcus pneumoniae*). As a single agent, GAS is the most common etiology of acute tonsillitis and pharyngitis *(Jenson and Baltimore, 2006, pp. 488-490; Kelley et al., 2009, pp. 460-463)*

4. **(A)** In left-sided congestive heart failure, the signs of tachycardia, tachypnea, intercostal retractions, rales, and rhonchi are found. Hepatosplenomegaly is a sign of right-sided congestive heart failure. Bradycardia is not associated with either left- or right-sided congestive heart failure in the pediatric patient. *(Schneider, 2006, pp. 680-683)*

5. **(B)** Leukemia is the most common form of childhood cancer. Acute lymphoblastic leukemia is the most common form of leukemia in childhood, accounting for approximately 4 out of 100,000 children younger than the age of 15. The clinical presentation is variable, ranging from severe with a life-threatening infection to asymptomatic at a routine well-child visit. Often, there is a 3- to 4-week history of an illness prior to the diagnosis, with signs and symptoms including malaise, anorexia, intermittent fever, bone tenderness, pallor, petechiae, purpura, and abdominal pain. Findings noted on the physical examination include pallor, petechiae, purpura, retinal hemorrhages, lymphadenopathy (either localized or generalized to cervical, axillary, or inguinal areas), bone and joint tenderness (especially in the pelvis, lower vertebral bodies, and femur), hepatosplenomegaly, and nephromegaly. Initially, the most useful test is a complete blood count with differential, revealing multiple cytopenias and leukemic blasts.

The bone marrow examination is diagnostic, revealing a homogeneous infiltration of leukemic blasts replacing normal marrow. Acute myelogenous leukemia typically presents with hyperleukocytosis (WBC > 100,000) or with myeloblasts on peripheral smears and bone marrow biopsies. It accounts for 25% of leukemias in childhood. Patients with chronic Epstein–Barr virus infections present with sore throat, fever, posterior cervical lymphadenopathy, and malaise associated with atypical lymphocytosis and a positive heterophile antibody test. Hodgkin's lymphoma typically presents with painless cervical adenopathy and a normal CBC. However, typically the C-reactive protein and erythrocyte sedimentation rates are elevated. *(Maloney et al., 2009, pp. 853-865; McLean and Wofford, 2006, pp. 737-742)*

6. **(A)** Despite the increase in vaccination of infants in the United States, *Streptococcus pneumoniae* remains the most common etiologic agent for bacterial meningitis in the pediatric population. *Haemophilus influenzae* type B is the second most common, but has gone down significantly due to the widespread vaccination of children. *Neisseria meningitides* has approximately 2,400 to 3,000 cases a year. Meningitis due to *Listeria monocytogenes* is typically seen in the neonatal period due to transmission from the mother. It is present in normal fecal matter in around 10% of the population. Its rates have gone down due to strict guidelines for the food industry, resulting in less than 1,000 cases per year. *(Ogle and Anderson, 2009, pp. 1131-1132, 1138-1139, 1162-1164, 1166-1167; Jenson and Baltimore, 2006, pp. 481-483)*

7. **(B)** The diagnosis of rheumatic fever is based on clinical grounds using the modified Jones criteria. Two major manifestations or one major and two minor manifestations in addition to supporting evidence of a preceding streptococcal infection are needed to make the diagnosis of rheumatic fever. The major manifestations are polyarthritis, carditis, erythema marginatum, subcutaneous nodules, and Sydenham chorea. The minor manifestations are fever, arthralgia, previous rheumatic fever or rheumatic heart disease, an elevated sedimentation rate or C-reactive protein, and a prolonged P–R interval.

The supporting evidence of a preceding streptococcal infection includes elevated titers of antistreptolysin O or other streptococcal antibodies and positive throat culture for group A beta-hemolytic streptococcus. *(Schneider, 2006, pp. 683-684; Sondheimer et al., 2009, p. 554t)*

8. **(D)** Hemophilia B, also known as Christmas disease and factor IX deficiency. Factor IX is activated on the intrinsic side of the coagulation cascade right before the common pathway and the result is an increased aPTT, with a normal prothrombin time, thrombin time, and INR. It does not affect platelets nor bleeding time. *(Ambruso et al., 2009, pp. 837-838; Scott, 2006, pp. 717-719)*

9. **(B)** Tanner stages of sexual maturation categorize the progression of pubertal development in girls according to pubic hair and breast development. Menarche usually occurs 18 to 24 months following the onset of breast development. In female breast development, Tanner Stage I is an absence of breast development; Stage II is a small, raised breast bud; Stage III shows further enlargement/elevation of breast and alveolar tissue; Stage IV is the areola and papilla forming a secondary mound on breast contour; and Stage V is the mature breast with alveolar area as part of the breast contour. For the stages of pubic hair development, Stage I is prepubertal, an absence of hair; Stage II shows sparse, fine hair, primarily on the border of labia; Stage III is pigmented and curly and increases in quantity on the mons pubis; Stage IV is increased quantity of coarser texture with labia and mons pubis well covered; and Stage V is mature adult distribution with spreading to medial thighs. *(Kaplan and Love-Osborne, 2009, p. 110; Blake and Davis, 2006, pp. 343)*

10. **(C)** During the first year of life, the average, expected increase in weight of a full-term infant is to regain the birth weight by 2 weeks of age, double the birth weight by 4 months of age, and triple the birth weight by 1 year of age. *(Goldson and Reynolds, 2009, pp. 63-80)*

11. **(B)** When evaluating children with physical injuries, the major difficulty is distinguishing

intentional injuries from unintentional injuries. Inconsistencies between the stated story and the injury are suspect. Discoloration caused by healing bruises tends to follow a distinctive pattern. On the first day, there is swelling without discoloration. From day 1 through day 5, the bruise is purple in color. For days 5 through 7, the bruise is green. Then, from day 7 through day 10, the bruise is yellow, followed by a brownish color from day 10 to day 14. *(Sirotnak et al., 2009, pp. 209-215; Christian and Blum, 2006, pp. 109-116)*

12. **(D)** Rotavirus is one of the most important causes of acute gastroenteritis in infants and young children primarily 6 to 24 months of age. In the United States, there are 65,000 to 70,000 hospitalizations and 200 deaths per annum. Peak incidences occur in the fall and winter. Most initial infections are characterized by diarrhea (watery, nonbloody, nonmucous), fever, and vomiting. Nasal congestion and coryza often precede the gastrointestinal symptoms. *Clostridium difficile* produces a toxin that causes a self-limited diarrhea in which symptoms characteristically begin following the administration of antibiotics that reduce normal bowel flora. *Giardia lamblia*, a flagellated protozoa, characteristically causes a mild diarrhea, with or without a low-grade fever, anorexia, flatulence, and abdominal cramps. It is not associated with vomiting nor upper respiratory tract symptoms. Shigella gastroenteritis in young children classically presents acutely with a high fever or seizures along with vomiting followed by bloody, mucoid, diarrheal stools. *(Sondheimer and Sundaram, 2009, p. 594; Dominguez et al., 2009, pp. 1199-1200; Ogle and Anderson, 2009, p. 1156; Jenson and Baltimore, 2006, pp. 512-517)*

13. **(A)** "Toeing in" in children before the age of 2 is typically due to tibial torsion; however, any "toeing in" after the age of 2 to 3, is usually due to femoral anteversion. The femur has more internal rotation that results in the presentation. Genu varum is known as bowleg and genu valgum is known as knock-kneed. *(Polousky and Eilert, 2009, pp. 755-756; Thompson, 2006, pp. 914-917)*

14. **(D)** The first sign of pubertal development in boys is the enlargement of testicular size and occurs at the mean age of 11.6 years. Genital stages accelerate before pubic hair development, which occurs, on average, at 13.4 years of age. The deepening of the voice and the development of chest and axillary hair usually occurs in midpuberty or 2 years after the growth of pubic hair. *(Kaplan and Love-Osborne, 2009, p. 109; Blake and Davis, 2006, pp. 345-348)*

15. **(A)** Huntington disease is an autosomal dominant hereditary disease. Its occurrence is between 1:5,000 and 1:20,000. It is caused by a defect on chromosome 4p16.3 that results in a repeat of "CAG" in the "Huntington" protein gene. *(Levy and Marion, 2006, p. 218)*

16. **(A)** Bell's palsy is the acquired peripheral facial weakness (cranial nerve VII) of sudden onset and unknown etiology. It often follows a viral illness with notable improvement within 2 weeks and near complete recovery within 2 months. Prednisone therapy may promote recovery of facial strength. Guillain–Barré syndrome (acute idiopathic polyneuritis) generally presents with symmetrical weakness of the lower extremities, which may ascend rapidly to the arms, trunk, and face. Nonspecific respiratory or gastrointestinal symptoms may occur 5 to 14 days preceding the infection. Physical examination will yield symmetric flaccid weakness, which is usually proximal in distribution. Rarely, there is cranial nerve (III–VI, IX–XI) involvement. Botulism is most often caused by the ingestion of food containing the *Clostridium botulinum* toxin or rarely from an infected wound. Children will present with blurred or double vision, ptosis, or choking. Physical findings include a weak swallow paralysis of accommodation and eye movements. In this case, there was not a history of food ingestion or wound infection to support this diagnosis. Children with a brain stem tumor may present with facial and extraocular muscle palsies, hemiparesis, gait disturbances, and hydrocephalus (25%). Changes in personality such as lethargy, irritability, and aggressive behavior are particularly common findings. Speech and swallowing difficulties are not unusual. Later in the illness, patients will develop vomiting and headaches. *(Lewis, 2006, pp. 843-844; 2006,*

p. 186; Ogle and Anderson, 2009, p. 1182; Maloney et al., 2009, p. 860)

17. **(C)** Still's murmur is the most common innocent murmur of early childhood and is usually appreciated in children from 3 to 6 years of age. It is a grade I–III/VI early systolic ejection murmur of musical or vibratory quality heard best between the apex and the left lower sternal border. It is loudest when the patient is in a supine position. The murmur may diminish or disappear with inspiration, during the Valsalva maneuver, or when the patient is standing or seated. A physiologic peripheral pulmonic stenosis murmur is a soft, short, high-pitched, grade I–II/VI systolic ejection murmur. Typically, it is auscultated with equal intensity at the left upper sternal border, along the back, and in both axillae. It is usually found in newborns and generally disappears by 3 to 6 months of age. A pulmonary ejection murmur is the most common innocent murmur of later childhood and is usually seen in children 8 to 14 years of age. It is a soft, early to midsystolic ejection, grade I–III/VI murmur heard best along the left upper sternal border. It is louder when the patient is supine or with increased cardiac output. It diminishes with standing or during the Valsalva maneuver. A venous hum is a continuous musical, grade I–II/VI murmur heard at the right or left superior infraclavicular area. The murmur is obliterated when the patient is in a supine position, with head rotation, and with compression of the jugular vein. It is usually auscultated in children from 3 to 6 years of age. *(Sondheimer et al., 2009, p. 538; Bickley and Szilagyi, 2009, pp. 822-823)*

18. **(D)** Sudden infant death syndrome (SIDS) is defined as the sudden, unexplained death of an apparently healthy infant that is unexpected and not adequately explained by a comprehensive medical history, a postmortem physical, and investigation of the death scene. SIDS is a leading cause of death in infants between the ages of 1 month and 1 year, second only to congenital anomalies. The exact etiology of SIDS is unclear. Prevention of SIDS has become a focus of public health measures. In 1994, The American Academy of Pediatrics initiated a campaign called "Back to Sleep," which rec-ommended placing infants in the supine position for sleep. Following the institution of this campaign in the United States, the annual death rate decreased from 1.3 per 1,000 to 0.7 per 1,000. *(Marshall and Debley, 2006, pp. 634-636; Kerby et al., 2009, pp. 516-517)*

19. **(A)** Bronchiectasis, meaning "dilation of the bronchi," results from destruction of the airway and poor drainage, often associated with cystic fibrosis, foreign body aspiration, or an infection. It is uncommon in the general population. The presentation may vary from a chronic productive cough to recurrent pneumonia with or without hemoptysis. Persistent rhonchi, rales, and decreased breath sounds are noted over the affected atelectatic area. Croup is an inflammatory disease of the larynx most frequently affecting young children during the fall and early winter months. Typically, there is an upper respiratory tract prodrome followed by stridor and a "barky cough" in the absence of drooling. Subglottic narrowing with a normal epiglottis is diagnostic on a lateral neck X-ray. The most common pathogen is parainfluenza virus. Bronchopulmonary dysplasia is most commonly seen in infants in the neonatal intensive care unit. It is a chronic condition seen in patients whose clinical course included hyaline membrane disease. These infants typically need oxygen for a few months as they grow and some need permanent tracheostomy and ventilation for up to 2 years. Chronic bronchitis falls into the chronic obstructive pulmonary disease category typically seen in older adults and does not typically present with acute symptoms. *(Kerby et al., 2009, pp. 478-480, 487-491)*

20. **(A)** Otitis externa is an infection of the auditory canal. The most common etiologic agent is pseudomonas. However, *Staphylococcus aureus* is a very close second and therefore antibiotic treatment should provide coverage for both organisms. *Corynebacterium* is part of the normal flora of the auditory canal and does not typically cause infections. *Streptococcus pyogenes* is the most common cause of acute bacterial pharyngitis. *(Jenson and Baltimore, 2006, pp. 495-496; Kelley et al., 2009, p. 437)*

21. **(A)** Cytomegalovirus (CMV) is one of the congenital neonatal TORCH infections (*t*oxoplasmosis, *o*ther [syphilis, varicella-zoster, and parvovirus in this list], *r*ubella, *c*ytomegalovirus, and *h*erpes simplex/*h*epatitis/ *H*IV). CMV is the most common congenital infection. The disease-specific manifestations for CMV include microcephaly with periventricular calcifications, neonatal jaundice with direct hyperbilirubinemia, and hepatosplenomegaly. Other associated manifestations include intrauterine growth retardation, thrombocytopenia, and purpura. Disease-specific manifestations for herpes simplex virus include skin/eye/mouth vesicles, encephalitis, respiratory distress, and sepsis. Disease-specific manifestations of rubella include congenital heart lesions (patent ductus arteriosus, pulmonary artery stenosis, aortic stenosis, ventricular defects), thrombocytopenic purpura characterized by purple macular lesions ("blueberry muffin" appearance), cataracts, retinopathy, and sensorineural deafness. Disease-specific manifestations of syphilis include mucocutaneous lesions (snuffles), periostitis, osteochondritis, and hemolytic anemia. Often, these babies are stillborn. Syphilis is caused by a spirochete, *Treponema pallidum*, not a virus. (*Levin and Weinberg, 2009, 1086-1088, 1091-1094, 1103-1104; Ogle and Anderson, 2009, pp. 1175-1178*)

22. **(A)** Approximately 40% of children who have been physically abused showed evidence of ocular trauma. Retinal hemorrhages are the most frequent ocular finding that result from violent shaking. This form of child abuse is termed shaken baby syndrome. The finding of retinal hemorrhages in an infant without an appropriate medical condition (eg, clotting disorder, leukemia) should raise concerns about nonaccidental trauma. Some of the most common presenting complaints of infants with shaken baby syndrome are lethargy, coma, seizures, vomiting, and respiratory distress. Retinal hemorrhages are not associated with retinitis pigmentosa, retinoblastoma, Reye syndrome, or viral encephalitis. With Reye syndrome, an antecedent viral illness is followed by vomiting and progressive lethargy. On examination, there is usually fever, tachypnea, and stupor. Laboratory hallmarks include elevated serum hepatocellular enzyme assays and elevated serum ammonia. Retinitis pigmentosa is a progressive retinal degeneration and is characterized by pigmentary changes, optic atrophy, and progressive impairment of visual function. The presenting clinical manifestation is usually an impairment of dark adaptation or night vision. Clinical manifestations of viral encephalitis vary in severity depending upon the etiologic organism (eg, cytomegalovirus, mumps, echovirus). Some children will have mild symptoms lapsing into a coma leading to death, whereas others are febrile, with convulsions and hallucinations followed by full recovery. (*Sirotnak et al., 2009, pp. 209-215; Levin and Weinberg, 2009, pp. 1096-1098; Levine, 2006, p.52; Jenson and Baltimore, 2006, pp. 484-486*)

23. **(C)** A febrile seizure is a brief (less than 15 minutes), generalized, symmetric, tonic–clonic seizure associated with a febrile illness (temperature greater than 38.8°C) without any central nervous system infection or neurologic cause. An absence (petit mal) seizure is a brief (2 to 25 seconds) loss of consciousness that can occur multiple times per day. There is no loss of tone, and frequently the only observable behaviors are staring or minor movements such as lip smacking and semipurposeful movements of the hands. There is no postictal period. Complex partial seizures (psychomotor) have varied symptoms including alterations in consciousness, unresponsiveness, and repetitive complex motor activities that are purposeless. Often, at the beginning of the attack, there is a psychoillusory phenomenon such as hallucinations, visual distortions, visceral sensations, or feelings of intense emotions. Simple partial seizures include focal motor, adversive, and somatosensory seizures. Manifestations of these seizures are varied including hallucinatory, psychoillusory, or complex emotional phenomena. Children will interact normally with their environment, with the exception of those limitations imposed by the seizure. Following the seizure (minutes to hours), there may be transient paralysis of the affected body part. (*Moe et al., 2009, pp. 683-700; Lewis, 2006, pp. 833-840*)

24. **(B)** Urinary tract infections (UTIs) are one of the most common infections in children. Clinical

features of a UTI vary depending upon the age and sex of the child. In newborns, the most common symptom is failure to thrive associated with poor feeding, diarrhea, and vomiting. In infants, the symptoms may be relatively nonspecific, such as poor feeding, failure to gain weight, vomiting, fever, strong-smelling urine, and irritability. As children grow older, the initial signs and symptoms become more specific to the urinary tract. In early infancy, males are two times more likely than girls to have a UTI. Also, uncircumcised males are 10 times more likely to be affected than circumcised males. *Escherichia coli* is the most common pathogen for the first UTI (80%) and of recurrent infections (75%). Other organisms that cause infections include *Pseudomonas aeruginosa*, *Proteus*, *Enterobacter*, *Klebsiella*, and *Enterococcus*. An infection with *Staphylococcus saprophyticus*, a coagulase-negative staphylococcus, is primarily seen in adolescents with a UTI. *(Lum, 2009, pp. 670-672; Jenson and Baltimore, 2006, pp. 522-524)*

25. **(B)** Dehydration is a common pathophysiologic alteration in fluid and electrolyte balance in children. Children are at an increased risk for dehydration because of their decreased oral intake, especially when ill, and their higher ratio of surface area to body weight, promoting significant evaporative losses. Important clinical features to estimate the degree of dehydration include postural blood pressure, changes in heart rate, capillary refill time, skin turgor and color, lack of tears, lack of external jugular venous filling when supine, sunken fontanel (if present), and altered mental status. This infant was estimated to have mild dehydration (3% to 5% decrease in body weight) with decreased tears, slightly longer capillary refill time (2 to 3 seconds), and intermittent irritability and restlessness. Severe dehydration (11% to 15% decrease in body weight) manifests as markedly decreased skin turgor with parched or mottled mucous membranes, absence of tears, tachycardia, capillary refill greater than 4 seconds, hypotension, circulatory collapse, and anuria. Moderate dehydration (6% to 10% decrease in body weight) manifests as decreased skin turgor; dry mucous membranes; decreased tearing; oliguria; and

normal pulse, blood pressure, and perfusion. *(Ford, 2009, pp. 1247-1249)*

26. **(C)** Intussusception is the most common cause of intestinal obstruction between 3 months and 6 years of age. It is twice as common in males than females. It is caused by intestinal invagination, usually around the ileocecal valve. The classic presentation is intermittent severe colicky abdominal pain with legs drawn up, followed by periods of comfort or falling asleep. Vomiting usually occurs in the early phase, which later becomes bilious. A passage of blood and mucus in the stool ("currant jelly stools") occurs in 60% of the cases. Palpation of the abdomen usually reveals a sausage-shaped mass in the right upper quadrant. The classic presentation of pyloric stenosis is in first-born males of 3 to 6 weeks of age, presenting with nonbilious projectile vomiting leading to dehydration with hypochloremia, hypokalemia, and metabolic alkalosis. A firm, movable, 2-cm olive-shaped mass ("olive") is palpable superior and to the right of the umbilicus in the midepigastrium. In addition, peristaltic waves may be visible on the physical examination. The classic presentation of appendicitis presents with a period of anorexia followed by steady periumbilical pain shifting to the right lower quadrant; nausea and vomiting is followed by a low-grade fever. Diarrhea (nonbloody and nonmucous), if it occurs, is infrequent. Peritoneal signs are present. The incidence increases with age and peaks during adolescence. Infective enteritis usually begins with emesis followed by crampy abdominal pain of hyperperistalsis. This sequence of symptoms with emesis preceding pain is an important factor in distinguishing it from intussusception. Masses are not palpated with infective enteritis. *(Jenson and Baltimore, 2006, pp. 512-518; Bishop, 2006, pp. 599-600, 609-610; Sondheimer and Sundaram, 2009, pp. 580-581, 584-584, 594, 596)*

27. **(C)** Dehydration is a common pathophysiologic alteration in fluid balance in children. The body has a maintenance fluid requirement to replace daily normal losses that occur through the skin, kidney, intestines, and respiratory tract. The following formula can be used to

calculate the usual amount of fluid a healthy child requires by mouth to maintain hydration:

100 mL/kg for the first 10 kg of body weight

50 mL/kg for the next 10 kg of body weight

20 mL/kg for the weights above 20 kg

For this question, a 24-kg child would require:

100 mL/kg × 10 kg = 1,000 mL for the first 10 kg

50 mL/kg × 10 kg = 500 mL for the next 10 kg

20 mL/kg × 4 kg = 80 mL for the next 4 kg

Total = 1,580 mL 24 kg

(Ford, 2009, pp. 1247-1250)

28. **(B)** The most common etiologic organisms for bacterial meningitis in children are *S pneumoniae*, *N Meningitidis*, *and H influenzae*. Because of an increase in resistant *S pneumoniae*, coverage with vancomycin and a third-generation cephalosporin such as cefotaxime or ceftriaxone is needed for best coverage. Gentamicin can be used but, as with all aminoglycosides, caution is needed regarding toxicity. Ampicillin, rifampin, and chloramphenicol are alternative treatments if necessary. *(Jenson and Baltimore, 2006, pp. 483-484)*

29. **(B)** Congenital hypothyroidism is one of the most common disorders tested for in newborn screening tests, revealing an elevated TSH (thyroid stimulating hormone) and a decreased T_4 (thyroxine). Symptoms suggestive of congenital hypothyroidism in the neonate include hypotonia, coarse facial features, hirsute forehead, large fontanels (anterior and posterior), widely open sutures, umbilical hernia, protruding/large tongue, hoarse cry, distended abdomen, and prolonged jaundice. Signs of congenital hypothyroidism include lethargy or hypoactivity, poor feeding, constipation, mottling, and hypothermia. Congenital adrenal hyperplasia (CAH) is not universally screened for in the newborn screening test, as it is included in only 14 of the 50 states. In females with CAH, there may be virilization with abnormalities of the external genitalia varying from mild enlargement of the clitoris to complete fusion of the labioscrotal folds. Signs of adrenal insufficiency (salt loss) may present in the first few days of life. Crigler–Najjar syndrome is not one of the disorders tested for in the standard newborn screening tests. It is an inherited disease producing congenital nonobstructive, nonhemolytic, unconjugated severe hyperbilirubinemia. The physical findings in this infant do not correlate with Crigler–Najjar syndrome. Galactosemia is tested for in the newborn screening test in nearly all 50 states. The infant may have symptoms of cataract, hepatomegaly, and prolonged jaundice. Often, these neonates have *Escherichia coli* sepsis, leading to death in the first 2 weeks of life if not treated promptly. *(Zeitler et al., 2009, pp. 922-923, 942-945, 962-963; Sokol and Narkewicz, 2009, 620-621)*

30. **(A)** Caput succedaneum is a result of fluid and blood accumulation in the occipitoparietal region of the newborn's scalp due to the vacuum effect of membrane rupture. A cephalohematoma is a firm, tense external swelling of the cranium that does *not* extend across suture lines because it is limited to the surface of one cranial bone. It occurs most often in the parietal area. This subperiosteal hemorrhage usually is not present at birth, but develops within the first 24 hours of life. Craniotabes is a condition caused by the osteoporosis of the outer table of the involved membranous bone, generally over the temporoparietal or parietooccipital areas, creating a "ping-pong ball" sensation when gentle pressure is applied. A subgaleal hemorrhage is a firm, fluctuant external swelling of the cranium that does extend across suture lines and increases in size over time. *(Bickley and Szilagyi, 2009, pp. 765-766)*

31. **(C)** Foreign body aspiration into the respiratory tract is associated with an acute choking or coughing episode with expiratory wheezing (indicative of a lower airway obstruction) in children aged 6 months to 4 years of age. Often, there is a history of the child playing with small toys that are commonly aspirated. Asymmetrical physical findings of decreased breath sounds and localized wheezing are present with foreign body aspiration. A positive forced expiratory chest X-ray shows a mediastinal shift away from the affected side. Radiolucent foreign bodies such as plastic toys may not appear on an

X-ray, but there will be evidence of this mediastinal shift. Asthma is generally characterized by wheezing, but it is not unilateral nor is it of sudden onset. A chest X-ray reveals bilateral hyperinflation with flattening of the diaphragm. Epiglottitis is a life-threatening upper airway obstructive condition that presents with a sudden onset of fever, dysphagia, drooling, and inspiratory retractions with stridor. A lateral neck X-ray reveals an enlarged, indistinct epiglottis ("thumb sign"); however, the chest X-ray is normal. Pulmonary embolism, rare in children, presents clinically with acute dyspnea, tachypnea, and tachycardia. There may be mild hypoxemia, rales, and focal wheezing. Chest X-rays may be normal, or there may be a peripheral infiltrate, small pleural effusion, or elevated hemidiaphragm. *(Elias et al., 2009, pp. 1018-1034; Ogle and Anderson, 2009, p. 1162; Kerby et al., 2009, pp. 482, 508; Marshall and Debley, 2006, p. 639t)*

32. **(C)** An acute salicylate overdose (greater than 150 mg/kg) will produce symptoms of salicylate intoxication. Chronic salicylate intoxication occurs with ingestion of greater than 100 mg/kg/day for at least 2 days. Salicylates affect most organ systems, leading to various metabolic abnormalities. Because salicylates are a gastric irritant, symptoms of vomiting and diarrhea occur soon after the overdose, which may contribute to the development of dehydration. Salicylates stimulate the respiratory center leading to hyperventilation and hyperpnea resulting in respiratory alkalosis and compensatory alkaluria. A characteristic feature of salicylate intoxication is the coexistence of a respiratory alkalosis with a widened anion gap metabolic acidosis. *(Rumack and Dart, 2009, pp. 334-335; Marcdante, 2006a, pp. 206-213)*

33. **(C)** Generalized tetanus (lockjaw) is a neurologic disease caused by *Clostridium tetani*. Although any open wound is a potential source for contamination with *C tetani*, those with dirt, soil, feces, or saliva are at increased risk. Tetanus-prone wounds contain devitalized tissue, especially those caused by punctures, frostbite, crush injury, or burns. Recommendations for tetanus prophylaxis in a child with a laceration or abrasion depend upon the number of previous vaccinations, occurrence of last booster, type of wound (clean or tetanus-prone), and age of child. In this case, the patient is older than 7 years and had all of his previous immunizations; however, his most recent booster was greater than 10 years ago. Thus, he should receive an adult-type diphtheria and tetanus toxoid with acellular pertussis. In most cases, when tetanus toxoid is required for wound prophylaxis in a child older than 7 years, the Td instead of tetanus toxoid alone is recommended so that diphtheria immunity is maintained. If tetanus immunization is not up to date at the time of wound treatment, then the immunization series should be completed according to the primary immunization schedule. If a child is younger than 7 years, then the diphtheria, tetanus, acellular pertussis (DTaP) booster is indicated, unless there is a contraindication for pertussis, in which case the diphtheria and tetanus (DT) booster should be administered. Tetanus immune globulin (TIG) is recommended for treatment of tetanus. Under special circumstances, a patient infected with the human immunodeficiency virus (HIV) with a tetanus-prone wound should also receive TIG in addition to the prophylactic vaccine. *(Ogle and Anderson, 2009, pp. 1144-1147; Centers for Disease Control and Prevention, 2009a)*

34. **(D)** Normally, primitive reflexes are present at birth and should not persist beyond the age of 6 months. However, the parachute reflex is a postural response that normally appears around 7 months of age to coincide with volitional movement and persists for life. It occurs when an infant is held prone by the waist over a surface and lowered with the head downward and extends the arms and legs as a form of protection. The rooting reflex occurs when the cheek is stroked on the infant and they turn his/her head to feed. Galant and Landau reflex disappear by the age of 2 months (trunk incurvation upon stroking the back) and 6 months (the baby lifts head and straightens spine upon being held prone), respectively *(Bickley and Szilagyi, 2009, pp. 794-795t)*

35. **(A)** Gonococcal ophthalmia neonatorum presents as a unilateral or bilateral serosanguineous discharge and then within 24 hours the discharge

becomes mucopurulent, followed by conjunctival injection and edema of the eyelids. The usual incubation period for *Neiserria gonorrhea* is 2 to 5 days; however, the infection may be present at birth or delayed greater than 5 days if there has been instillation of silver nitrate prophylaxis. A presumptive diagnosis is made by the demonstration of gram-negative intracellular diplococci on Gram stain. Definitive diagnosis is made by culture. Following a positive Gram stain and pending culture results, treatment should be promptly initiated with ceftriaxone (50 mg/kg/24 hours IV or IM for one dose not to exceed 125 mg), a third-generation cephalosporin with good coverage for gram-negative bacteria. An alternate drug is cefotaxime (100 mg/kg/24 hours IV or IM every 12 hours for 7 days or 100 mg/kg as a single dose), which is also a third-generation cephalosporin. Although erythromycin drops (0.5%) are used prophylactically for *N gonorrhea*, this is not an effective treatment. Gentamicin would be used for Pseudomonas, and Chlamydia is treated with erythromycin. Cephalexin as a first-generation cephalosporin does not have coverage for gram-negative bacteria. *(Braverman, 2009, pp. 408-409; Jenson and Baltimore, 2006, pp. 539-543)*

36. **(B)** The most likely diagnosis in this patient is mumps. It is endemic in most unvaccinated populations. The onset is characterized by pain and swelling in one or both parotid glands. The pain can be exacerbated by tasting sour liquids such as lemon juice. An elevated serum amylase level is common and coincides with the parotid swelling. Unilateral, rarely bilateral, nerve deafness is a complication of mumps that may be transient or permanent. Other complications include meningoencephalomyelitis, orchitis, epididymitis, pancreatitis, arthritis, and rarely thyroiditis and myocarditis. *(Daley et al., 2009, pp. 254-257; Levin and Weinberg, 2009, pp. 1105-1106)*

37. **(A)** Café au lait spots are brown macules that may be found on any part of the body. The presentation of six or more spots greater than 1.5 cm is a sign of neurofibromatosis, a genetic disorder that results in neurofibromas that can develop in any organ/tissue system. Miliaria are blocked sweat gland ducts that are commonly

found on the face, scalp, or intertriginous areas. Vernix caseosa is a normal finding in newborns and is a whitish, greasy layering on the body—it decreases as an infant comes to full term. Subconjunctival hemorrhages are a common finding in infants secondary to birth trauma. *(Morelli and Burch, 2009, p. 378; Levy and Marion, 2006, p. 222; Lembo, 2006, p. 885)*

38. **(B)** The Apgar score assesses the newborn at 1-minute and 5-minute intervals to determine the need for resuscitative care. The infant is evaluated by heart rate, respiratory effort, muscle tone, response to catheter in nostril, and color, and each is rated on a scale of 0, 1, or 2 for a total score of 10. The heart rate is scaled 0–2 for absent, less than 100 bpm (slow), and greater than 100 bpm; respiratory effort of absent, slow/irregular, and good crying. Muscle tone scale (0–2) consists of limp, some flexion, and active motion; response to catheter stimulation (0–2) is scaled no response, grimace, and cough/sneeze. Finally, color is scored 0–2 for blue/pale, body pink with blue extremities, and completely pink. *(Thilo and Rosenberg, 2009, p. 4t; Gowen, 2006, p. 285)*

39. **(C)** Ventricular septal defect, a hole between the two ventricles, can be cyanotic or acyanotic based on the size of the defect, and accounts for 30% of cases of congenital heart disease. Atrial septal defect occurs in approximately 10% of congenital heart disease cases. Transposition of great vessels is an embryonic malformation resulting in the aorta arising from the right ventricle and the pulmonary artery arising from the left ventricle. It is responsible for about 10% of all congenital malformations. Tetralogy of Fallot, consisting of a ventricular septal defect, overriding aorta, pulmonic/subpulmonic stenosis, and right ventricular hypertrophy, accounts for 10% of congenital heart disease. *(Sondheimer et al., 2009, pp. 531-551; Schneider, 2006, p. 669-670, 674-676)*

40. **(D)** The immunization schedule is developed biannually by the Centers for Disease Control and Prevention. Assuming that the child has had the appropriate immunizations at the regularly scheduled examinations, the recommended immunizations at the 4- to 6-year-old

range are the DTaP (diphtheria, tetanus, acellular pertussis), IPV (inactivated polio), and the MMR (measles, mumps, and rubella). The hepatitis series should have been completed by the age of 6 months and the *Haemophilus influenzae* type B (Hib) should be completed by the age of 12 to 15 months. Varicella is given from 12 to 18 months and again from 4 to 6 years; the PCV (pneumo-coccal) should be finished by 12 to 15 months. *(Centers for Disease Control and Prevention, 2009b)*

41. **(A)** There are only two known absolute con-traindications to breastfeeding: tuberculosis of the mother and galactosemia of the infant. The highly contagious nature of tuberculosis makes the risk greater than the benefit, and infants with galactosemia are unable to digest any lactose due to an enzyme deficiency. Infants of mothers in a methadone program may be breastfed as long as the mother's dose is less than 40 mg. While nicotine is transmitted in breast milk and is therefore strongly discouraged, it is not an absolute contraindication. As long as a breastfed infant with cystic fibrosis is maintaining normal growth with supplemented pancreatic enzymes, breastfeeding is encouraged. *(Krebs and Primak, 2009, pp. 275-282; Ogle and Anderson, 2009, pp. 1167-1170; Krebs and Primak, 2006, pp. 133-134)*

42. **(B)** Failure to thrive is diagnosed in infants younger than the age of 6 months with a decrease in growth velocity that results in a decrease in two major percentile lines on the growth chart. In the case of this patient, she was initially in the 50th percentile and crossed the 25th and 10th percentile and fell into the 5th percentile. Failure to thrive is also known as growth deficiency and may also be diagnosed if the child is younger than 6 months and has not grown for two consecutive months or if a child is older than 6 months and has not grown for 3 consecutive months. Growth hormone defi-ciency/dwarfism may present with decreased growth velocity later in childhood; the drop in percentiles is grossly below the 5th percentile mark. Lactose intolerance presents with varying gastrointestinal symptoms without the marked decrease in weight. Beckwith–Wiedemann syn-drome consists of macrosomia, macroglossia, and omphalocele and they are at increased risk

for malignancies, hypoglycemia, and dysmor-phism (usually of the ears). *(Brayden, 2009, pp. 234-235; Sondheimer and Sundaram, 2009, p. 603; Zeitler et al., 2009, pp. 913-917; Elias et al., 2009, pp. 1008-1009; Christian and Blum, 2006, pp. 105-108; Bishop, 2006, p. 584t; Jospe, 2006, pp. 792-796)*

43. **(C)** This patient has presented with classical findings of Reye syndrome—upper respiratory infection followed by unresponsiveness. Reye syndrome is usually preceded by an upper res-piratory tract illness, which progresses into vomiting, strange behavior, stupor, and coma. Liver function tests (LFTs) will be markedly ele-vated (without jaundice); however, the serum bilirubin and alkaline phosphatase are normal. Unresponsive patients who have a spinal tap will show no cells in the CSF and glucose may be low with increased CSF pressure. If arterial blood gases are ordered, they will show a mild respiratory alkalosis and metabolic acidosis. A liver biopsy will show little inflammatory changes with diffuse microvesicular steatosis and absent glycogen from the hepatocytes. The mitochondria of the hepatocytes are large and polymorphic with decreased matriceal density. Treatment for patients with Reye syndrome is largely supportive—specifically decreasing cerebral edema. There is no place for antibiotics or steroids. The liver will fully recover if the cerebral edema is decreased. *(Seashore, 2006, p. 245, Jenson and Baltimore, 2006, pp. 471, 487)*

44. **(B)** Wilson disease is a result in a genetic muta-tion on chromosome 13 that causes decreased bile excretion of copper and results in accumu-lation of copper by the liver, specifically the ceru-loplasmin. The build-up of copper causes damage to the liver, basal ganglia, and other tis-sues. Physical examination shows jaundice, hepatosplenomegaly, Kayser–Fleischer rings (a brown band at the junction of the iris and cornea under slit-lamp), and neurologic manifestations later in the disease process. Laboratory tests show marked decrease in ceruloplasmin of the liver, anemia, hemolysis, and severely elevated bilirubin with decrease alkaline phosphatase. Urinalysis shows severe elevation in copper excretion, glycosuria, and aminoaciduria. Liver biopsy is conclusive with evidence of copper greater than 250 μg/g of dry tissue. Treatment requires copper chelation with D-penicillamine or trientine hydrochloride. Liver transplant may be required with noncompliance and in acute fulminant disease. Copper chelation is continued for life with the addition of zinc (decrease copper absorption) and vitamin B_6 (decrease optic neuritis). Genetic screening of siblings and future children should be strongly encouraged. Alpha-interferon therapy is mainly used to treat hepatitis patients. There is no place for steroids in therapy and protease inhibitors are antiviral medications that are typically used in HIV patients. *(Sokol and Narkewicz, 2009, pp. 631-633; Bishop, 2006, pp. 619-620)*

45. **(A)** The patient's presentation is consistent with findings of coarctation of the aorta. The pathognomonic finding in coarctation is decreased or absent femoral pulses. However, the majority of children show no signs of coarctation in infancy and develop signs and symptoms during childhood, most notably unequal pulses and blood pressure between arms and legs (arms lower than legs). In addition, a grade II/VI ejection murmur is heard at the aortic area and left sternal border that radiates into the left axilla and left back. Chest X-ray shows a normal-sized heart, a prominent aorta, indents at the level of the coarctation, and a dilated poststenotic segment resulting in the "figure 3" sign. Scalloping or notching of the ribs is due to enlargement of the intercostal arteries. Echocardiography is used to directly visualize the coarctation and estimate the obstruction. Asymptomatic infants and children are encouraged to have corrective surgery prior to age 5, after which they are at increased risk for myocardial dysfunction and hypertension, and require exercise testing prior to participation in aerobic activities. The boot-shaped heart is seen in patients with tetralogy of Fallot secondary to right ventricular hypertrophy; the narrowed mediastinum finding with "egg on a string" is typically seen in patients with transposition of the great vessels. *(Sondheimer et al., 2009, pp. 539-540, 545-546, 550-551; Schneider, 2006, pp. 673-676)*

46. **(D)** Viral croup usually presents with cough that may sound like a dog or a seal barking. The patients are usually afebrile and also present with stridor either at rest, in severe cases, or when agitated, in mild cases. In addition, the patient may be cyanotic and have retractions and acute shortness of breath. Radiologic examination of the neck shows subglottic narrowing with a normal epiglottis, "steeple sign." However, X-rays are usually not indicated in patients with the common presenting symptoms. Treatment for viral croup is mainly symptomatic, especially in mild cases consisting of oral hydration and mist therapy. Severe cases (stridor at rest) call for oxygen in patients who have desaturated, and nebulized racemic epinephrine and glucocorticoids. Dexamethasone as an intramuscular injection or oral as a one time dose is effective in alleviating symptoms, decreasing the need for intubation, and decreasing hospital stays. Inhaled budesonide is also effective in decreasing hospital stays and improving symptoms, but dexamethasone is more cost-effective. Patients who are unable to be stabilized need airway maintenance either by intubation with endotracheal tube or by tracheostomy if intubation fails. Because it is a self-limiting disorder, unless there is a secondary infection most children recover in a few days. *(Kerby et al., 2009, pp. 478-479; Jenson and Baltimore, 2006, pp. 496-499)*

47. **(A)** Cystic fibrosis (CF) is a major cause of gastrointestinal and pulmonary morbidity in children due to mutations in the CF genes. The mutations lead to a deficiency in cystic fibrosis transmembrane conductance regulator protein that controls movement of salt and water into and out of epithelial cells and results in production of abnormally thick mucus. About 15% of patients with CF present with meconium ileus at birth. This is typically treated with enema for disimpaction and rarely surgery. Approximately half of the infants with CF will present with failure to thrive, which is diagnosed by lack of growth for 2 consecutive months in patients younger than 6 months of age. They may also present with respiratory compromise. However, not all patients present in childhood. Diagnosis of CF is confirmed by a sweat chloride level above 60 meq/L or with genetic testing. Treatment for patients with CF is mainly symptomatic therapy for obstructions of

the digestive and respiratory tract. In addition, there is pancreatic enzyme supplementation to aid in digestion and vitamin and calorie supplementation for deficiencies in the diet. Gene therapy is now being looked at for future treatment. Intussusception (telescoping of the small intestine) typically presents in an infant with paroxysmal abdominal pain, vomiting, and diarrhea that may progress into bloody stools. Volvulus is normally the result of intestinal malrotation that causes occlusion of the superior mesenteric artery and eventual bowel necrosis. Infants typically present within 3 weeks of life with bile-stained vomiting and bowel obstruction. Wilson's disease is the defect in the ability to excrete copper in the bile that results in accumulation of copper in the liver. *(Kerby et al., 2009, pp. 485-486; Sondheimer and Sundaram, 2009, pp. 584-585; Sokol and Narkewicz, 2009, pp. 631-633; Bishop, 2006, pp. 602-603, 609, 619-620; Marshall and Debley, 2006, pp. 648-651)*

48. **(B)** Cyanotic heart lesions are a result of a right-to-left shunt. These include tetralogy of Fallot, pulmonary atresia with and without ventricular septal defect, tricuspid atresia, hypoplastic left heart syndrome, and transposition of the great arteries. The right-to-left shunt results in deoxygenated blood reaching the left ventricle, aorta, and systemic arteries. The decreased oxygen in the blood results in decreased oxygen to the tissue and subsequently causes cyanosis. Atrial septal defect, ventricular septal defect, atrioventricular septal defect, and patent ductus arteriosus most commonly present with a left-to-right shunt. *(Sondheimer et al., 2009, pp. 534-551; Schneider, 2006, pp. 673-680)*

49. **(A)** This infant is presenting with signs and symptoms of pyloric stenosis. Infants typically have vomiting (projectile at times) after every feeding and it normally starts between the age of 2 and 4 weeks. The infant nurses fervently and is hungry. In addition, there may be dehydration, constipation, weight loss, and apathy. Abdomen may be distended with gastric peristaltic waves. Occasionally, an olive-sized mass can be felt in the right upper quadrant with deep palpation after the child has vomited. Vomitus is typically nonbilious. Diagnosis is confirmed by an upper gastrointestinal series with delayed gastric emptying, enlarged pyloric muscle, and characteristic semilunar impressions on the gastric antrum. In addition, an ultrasound is needed to verify the hypertrophic muscle. The treatment of choice for these patients is pyloromyotomy, which can be done laparoscopically. These patients make full recoveries and have an excellent prognosis. *(Sondheimer and Sundaram, 2009, pp. 580-581; Bishop, 2006, pp. 599-600)*

50. **(D)** Celiac disease or gluten enteropathy typically presents with diarrhea episodes in the first 6 to 12 months of life—when whole grains are first fed. Therefore, in strictly breastfed babies, symptoms may not be noticed until solid foods are begun. The diarrhea is usually intermittent at first and then typically progresses into pale, greasy, foul-smelling, frothy stools. Additional symptoms may be constipation, vomiting, and abdominal pain, which may lead the clinician to think of intestinal obstruction. Other findings may be failure to thrive, anemia, and vitamin deficiencies. Stool sample demonstrates excessive fecal fat excretion. Blood tests show hypoproteinemia and impaired carbohydrate absorption. Intestinal biopsy is the diagnostic test of choice for celiac disease. Results show shortened celiac mucosa, absent villi, lengthened crypts of Lieberkühn, plasma cell infiltration of the lamina propria, and intraepithelial lymphocytes. Treatment consists of dietary restriction of gluten—wheat, rye, and barley. Steroids are given on an as needed basis. Sweat chloride testing is utilized in patients suspected of cystic fibrosis. Gastrin level is taken in patients suspected of Zollinger–Ellison syndrome, and RAST (radioallergosorbent assay test) is used in patients to determine different environmental-type allergens. *(Sondheimer and Sundaram, 2009, pp. 602-603; Lasley, 2006, p. 420; Bishop, 2006, pp. 607-608, 649-650)*

51. **(B)** The most likely diagnosis for this patient is poststreptococcal glomerulonephritis. The diagnosis is supported by a documented culture of group A beta-hemolytic streptococcus infection. If a culture is not available, like of the patient in this scenario, the clinician can order an antistreptolysin O titer. Antistreptolysin is an

enzyme released by group A streptococcus and is elevated for up to 1 month after strep infection. Glomerulonephritis presents with gross hematuria with or without edema. Hypertension, proteinuria, ascites, and headache may also be present. Treatment with antibiotics is useful if infection is still present, and, if necessary, symptomatic treatment for renal failure is done with hemodialysis. Symptoms typically resolve within a few weeks. The monospot is used to diagnose infectious mononucleosis. Renal biopsy could be performed on extreme cases of glomerulonephritis but is not typically necessary. Immunoglobulin electrophoresis would be utilized in patients suspected of having immunoglobulinopathies or IgA-mediated glomerulonephritis. *(Lum, 2009, pp. 656-657; Marcdante, 2006, pp. 757-759)*

52. **(D)** Patent ductus arteriosus (PDA) is an isolated abnormality that occurs in infants. The ductus arteriosus is a normal fetal vessel that joins the aorta and the pulmonary artery and spontaneously closes after 3 to 5 days. Lack of closure results in the audible murmur that is "machine-like" and maximal at the second intercostal space (ICS), at the left sternal border (LSB), and inferior to the clavicle. It is typically a pansystolic murmur with bounding pulses and a widened pulse pressure. There is also a paradoxical splitting of S_1 and S_2. Echocardiography confirms the PDA, the direction and degree of shunting, and the presence of lesions for which the PDA is needed to keep. If there are no other cardiac malformations requiring the PDA, then if the PDA is large, surgery should be completed before 1 year of age. Symptomatic PDAs that are relatively small may be closed with indomethacin in preterm infants. The murmur heard in atrial septal defect (ASD) usually is an ejection type, systolic murmur heard best at the LSB, second ICS with a wide, fixed S_2 and normal pulses. Ventricular septal defect (VSD) presents with a harsh, pansystolic murmur heard best at the third and fourth ICS. With increasing size of the VSD, heaves, thrills, and lifts are present along with radiation throughout the chest. Tetralogy of Fallot presents with a rough ejection, systolic murmur heard best at the LSB and the third ICS with radi-

ation to the back. *(Sondheimer et al., 2009, pp. 531-536, 545-546; Schneider, 2006, pp. 669-671, 674-675)*

53. **(C)** Hypertrophic cardiomyopathy in adolescence is typically due to familial hypertrophic cardiomyopathy with an incidence of 1:500. Many patients are asymptomatic until a sporting event, which may cause symptoms, specifically sudden cardiac death. Examination may demonstrate a palpable or audible S_4, an LV (left ventricular) heave, systolic ejection murmur (may need to stimulate cardiac activity), and/or a left precordial bulge. Echocardiography is the gold standard for diagnosis but family history should be assessed. Stress testing is indicated to assess for ischemia and arrhythmias. Strenuous activities are prohibited for these patients. The other cardiomyopathies (dilated and restrictive) are next but are not as common. Congenital structural abnormalities of the coronary arteries are the next most common cause. Valvular disorders, including surgically repaired aortic stenosis, are typically not causes of sudden death, but these patients should be screened for symptoms and stress tested as necessary. *(Sondheimer et al., 2009, pp. 540-542, 554-555, 558-559; Schneider, 2006, pp. 672-673, 683-685, 688)*

54. **(A)** This patient presentation describes epiglottitis. Although there is a decreased incidence of epiglottitis secondary to the introduction of the vaccine for *Haemophilus influenzae* type B (Hib), patients still present with sudden onset of fever, dysphagia, muffled voice, drooling, cyanosis, inspiratory retractions, and soft stridor. The patients are usually sitting in a tripod position to aid their breathing. Recognition of the classic symptoms needs to be immediate to stabilize the patient's airway, as these patients will decompensate into respiratory failure quickly. In the event that there is time, a lateral neck X-ray will show the "thumb sign," which is an enlarged, undistinguished epiglottis. Treatment for the patient requires intubation for airway stabilization, blood cultures and throat/epiglottis cultures, and antibiotic coverage for *H. influenzae*. The steeple sign is seen in patients with croup and is due to a subglottic narrowing. The "figure 3" sign is seen in patients with coarctation of the aorta. The "Scottie dog" sign

is seen in oblique lumbar films and is a normal finding representing the pars interarticularis. Its absence signifies spondylolysis. *(Kerby et al., 2009, p. 479; Jenson and Baltimore, 2006, pp. 497-499)*

55. **(C)** With an incidence of 1:3,000 to 1:4,000 Caucasians, cystic fibrosis is the most common lethal genetic disorder in the United States. While trisomy 21 (Down syndrome) is one of the most common genetic disorders with 1:500 newborns, it is typically not a fatal disease. It is characterized with mental retardation and physical malformations. Trisomy 13 is a fatal trisomy, with most deaths occurring in early infancy or by the age of 2, but its incidence is approximately 1:12,000 live births. Neurofibromatosis, a genetic disorder of typical autosomal dominant inheritance, occurs in approximately 1:3,000 live births. Most affected children have the skin lesions (café au lait macules or neurofibromas) and other minor problems. *(Kerby et al., 2009, pp. 485-486; Elias et al., 2009, pp. 999-1000; Levy and Marion, 2006, pp. 218-219, 232-233)*

56. **(B)** Status epilepticus is a medical emergency and is defined as seizure activity that lasts a minimum of 30 minutes. This results in hypoxia, acidosis, cerebral edema, and structural damage. In addition, fever, respiratory depression, hypotension, and death may occur. There are both convulsive and nonconvulsive types of status epilepticus. Because of its emergency status and potential complications, the clinician needs to initiate the ABCs (airway, breathing, circulation). Therefore, the first line of treatment is to establish and maintain an airway, oxygen is next, and then circulation, which encompasses pulse, blood pressure, and IV access. Once the IV is established, the orders should be for administering glucose-containing fluids and IV drug therapy with diazepam, lorazepam, or midazolam as well as administer phenytoin and phenobarbital. Arterial blood gases should be ordered and any abnormalities should be corrected appropriately. Finally, the clinician should determine the underlying cause: trauma, structural disorder, infection, lactic acidosis, toxins, and uremia. Maintenance drug therapy is necessary until the underlying cause is determined and rectified. *(Moe et al., 2009, pp. 696-697; Lewis, 2006, p. 838)*

57. **(D)** Guillain–Barré syndrome is most likely due to a delayed hypersensitivity with T-cell–mediated antibodies to mycoplasma and viral infections (CMV, EBV, hepatitis B, *campylobacter jejuni*). The patients may mention a nonspecific respiratory or gastrointestinal infection 1 to 2 weeks prior to symptoms. Complaints may be paresthesias, weakness in bilateral lower extremities with occasional ascension into the arms, trunk, and face, and rarely ataxia and ophthalmoplegia in the Miller–Fisher variant. Examination findings demonstrate symmetric flaccid weakness, with impairment of position, vibration, and touch in the distal portions of the extremities. If a spinal tap is performed, it may show few polymorphonuclear neutrophils with high protein and normal glucose. EMG is positive for decreased nerve conduction. Laboratory tests may show high titers of suspected infections or active infection of hepatitis/bacterial pathogens. Guillain-Barré is normally a self-limiting disorder within a few weeks, unless there are issues with respiratory depression. Poliomyelitis is secondary to polioviruses and presents with fever, paralysis, meningeal signs, and asymmetrical weakness. Botulism secondary to infection with *Clostridium botulinum* in older children presents with blurred vision, diplopia, ptosis, choking, and weakness. In infants, botulism presents as constipation, poor suck and cry, apnea, lethargy, and choking. Tick-bite paralysis presents with rapid onset with ascending flaccid paralysis reaching upper extremities in a couple of days of onset and patients often present with paresthesia and pain. Finding of a tick is usually confirmatory for these patients. *(Moe et al., 2009, pp. 734-735t; Levin and Weinberg, 2009, pp. 1083-1084, 1094-1098; Lewis, 2006, pp. 843-844; Marcdante, 2006, p. 186)*

58. **(B)** Scoliosis is defined by lateral curvature of the spine with rotation of vertebrae and is typically located in the thoracic or lumbar spine in the right or left directions. Idiopathic scoliosis most commonly presents as a right thoracic curve in females from 8 to 10 years of age. Scoliosis is typically asymptomatic unless curvatures are so

severe that there is pulmonary dysfunction or there is an underlying disorder (bone or spinal tumor) that is causing the scoliosis. X-rays need to be taken of the entire spine to help determine the degree of curvature. Treatment modalities are based on the degree of curvature: 20° or less does not normally require treatment; 20° to 40° is an indication for bracing in an immature child; and 40° and greater is resistant to bracing and requires surgical fixation with spinal fusion, which is best done at special centers. *(Polousky and Eilert, 2009, pp. 754-755; Thompson, 2006, pp. 926-930)*

59. **(D)** Legg–Calvé–Perthes disease is also known as avascular necrosis of the proximal femur. It typically occurs in children between 4 and 8 years old and persistent hip pain is the main symptom. On examination, the clinician notices a limp and/or limitation of motion of the affected hip. Radiologic examination demonstrates the necrosis with effusion and joint space widening with a negative aspirate. Treatment involves surgical hip replacement. Slipped capital femoral epiphysis (SCFE) is due to the displacement of the proximal femoral epiphysis owing to disruption of the growth plate. The head is normally displaced medially and posteriorly relative to the femoral neck. It typically occurs in adolescence, specifically obese males, and can also be associated with hypothyroidism. SCFE usually occurs after direct trauma to the hip or a fall. Patients complain of vague symptoms at first that progress into pain of the hip or of the knee. On examination, there is decreased internal rotation of the hip that can be confirmed by lateral X-ray of the hip. Septic hip arthritis is not common in children between the age of 5 and 12 years. The legs are held in external rotation to minimize pain and will have a positive aspirate. Osteochondritis dissecans typically presents in the knee, elbow, and talus and is characterized by a wedge-shaped necrosis of bone. *(Polousky and Eilert, 2009, pp. 755, 763-764; Thompson, 2006, pp. 910-912, 919)*

60. **(B)** Gamekeeper thumb is a result of damage to the ulnar collateral ligament during forced abduction of the metacarpophalangeal joint, an injury that is most commonly seen in skiers.

An avulsed fragment may or may not be seen on radiologic examination. If it is smaller than 2 mm, there is no fragment, a thumb spica cast can be used as seen in patients with no fragment. If the fragment is larger than 2 mm, surgery is required. Mallet finger is an avulsion of the extensor tendon and occurs in ball-handling sports. Boxer fracture is a distal neck fracture of the 5th metacarpal. Scaphoid fractures are due to hyperextension of the wrist injuries and present with pain in the anatomic snuffbox and swelling. *(Wilson and Pengel, 2009, p. 781)*

61. **(A)** Nursemaid elbow is the subluxation of the radial head due to a child or infant being lifted or pulled by the hand. The patient will present with the elbow pronated and painful and he or she will not bend the elbow. During the radiologic examination, the dislocation is usually reduced by placing the elbow in full supination and moving it slowly from full extension to full flexion. This typically provides immediate relief of pain and a sling may be given for comfort for a couple of days. Otherwise, X-rays are normal. Child protective services should be considered if this is a recurrent problem or if there are other associated signs and symptoms of battery. There is no need for orthopedic referral unless reduction is not commonly done in your setting. Immobilization of the elbow is not recommended, because the patient then may have to recover from frozen shoulder. *(Polousky and Eilert, 2009, p. 758; Thompson, 2006, p. 913)*

62. **(A)** This patient is presenting with signs and symptoms of primary nocturnal enuresis, which is the wetting only at night during sleep without any sustained period of dryness. It is mainly considered a parasomnia occurring in deep sleep. The incidence of enuresis is higher in boys, is typically related to a developmental delay, and most children become continent by adolescence. Patients need to be tested for structural abnormalities and infections, in addition to neurologic diseases, diabetes mellitus and insipidus, and seizure disorders. Treatment includes limiting liquids at bedtime and routine bathroom training during the day. If these are unsuccessful, the next option is a bed-wetting alarm. This device is attached to the child's

undergarment and vibrates when the child is wet to arouse the child to be aware of their need to urinate. If the alarm is unsuccessful, then the next step is medication—DDAVP (desmopressin acetate) or imipramine. *(Stafford et al., 2009, pp. 195-196; Gahagan, 2006, pp. 68-70)*

63. **(D)** Nephroblastoma also known as Wilms tumor typically presents with an asymptomatic abdominal mass noticed by the parent or an increasing size of the abdomen. On examination, the mass feels smooth and firm, is well defined, and usually does not cross the midline. Gross hematuria may be present, but rare, and some patients have microscopic hematuria when tested. Wilms tumor accounts for approximately 5% of cancers in children younger than 15 years. Wilms tumor arises from the kidney and the average age at diagnosis is 4 years. Ultrasound and CT of the abdomen can be used to confirm the presence of an intra-abdominal mass. Treatment includes exploratory abdominal surgery for removal and staging with a mixture of chemotherapy. Intussusception (telescoping of the small intestine) typically presents in an infant with paroxysmal abdominal pain, vomiting, and diarrhea that may progress into bloody stools. Volvulus is normally the result of intestinal malrotation that causes occlusion of the superior mesenteric artery and eventual bowel necrosis. Infants typically present within 3 weeks of life with bile-stained vomiting and bowel obstruction. *(Sondheimer and Sundaram, 2009, pp. 584-585; Maloney et al., 2009, pp. 870-871; Bishop, 2006, pp. 584, 602-603, 609; McLean and Wofford, 2006, pp. 725-726, 747-748)*

64. **(C)** Infant girls presenting with signs of precocious puberty need to be screened for congenital adrenal hyperplasia (CAH). CAH most commonly presents with pseudohermaphroditism in females—urogenital sinus, enlarged clitoris, or other signs of virilization. In males, there tends to be isosexual precocity in older males and salt-losing crisis in infant males. Both children show increased linear growth and skeletal maturation. The most common type of CAH is a deficiency in the enzyme 21-hydroxylase and laboratory tests demonstrate increased urinary and plasma androgens (DHEA, androstenedione). There may be elevated progesterone, but typically there is no effect on estrogen. There is also decreased aldosterone and elevated urinary ketosteroids. There is also no effect on the levels of leuteinizing hormone or follicle-stimulating hormone. Treatment usually involves glucocorticoids, mineralocorticoids, and reconstructive surgery, if needed. *(Zeitler et al., 2009, pp. 942-945; Levy and Marion, 2006, pp. 219, 240; Jospe, 2006, pp. 816-817)*

65. **(A)** Growth hormone (GH) deficiency is defined as a decreased growth velocity, delay in skeletal maturation, absence of other explanations for poor growth (lack of intake), and laboratory tests demonstrating decreased GH secretion. Etiology of GH deficiency can be congenital, genetic, acquired, or idiopathic, which is the most common. Infants usually have a normal birth weight and may have a slightly decreased length. In addition, most infants present with other endocrine deficiencies like hypoglycemia, hypothyroidism, and/or adrenal insufficiency. Children may present with truncal adiposity because growth hormone promotes lipolysis. Serum GH or intrinsic growth factor levels may or may not be decreased. In patients who do not have a demonstrated decrease in these hormones, a trial period with GH is indicated. These patients and positive GH-deficient patients receive a once-daily subcutaneous injection of recombinant human GH. Congenital hypothyroidism typically presents with short stature (typically noted after the 4-month newborn visit), delayed epiphyseal development, delayed closure of fontanelles, and retarded dental eruption in addition to other signs of hypothyroidism. Cushing disease typically presents with truncal adiposity with thin extremities, muscle wasting, decreased growth rate, and moon facies. Laboratory results show elevated adrenocorticosteroids both in urine and serum, hypokalemia, eosinopenia, and lymphocytopenia. Typically, in patients younger than the age of 12, Cushing disease is secondary to administration of ACTH or glucocorticoids. Congenital adrenal hyperplasia typically presents with pseudohermaphroditism in females or salt-losing crisis in males with or without isosexual

precocity. There is an increased linear growth and advanced skeletal maturation. *(Zeitler et al., 2009, pp. 913-917, 922-923, 942-946; Levy and Marion, 2006, pp. 219, 240; Jospe, 2006, pp. 792-796, 806-808, 823)*

66. **(C)** In patients with idiopathic thrombocytopenic purpura, treatment options should be initiated when platelet counts fall below 20,000, regardless of whether there is active bleeding or not. Without active bleeding the treatment options include prednisone 2–4 mg/kg/ 24 hours for 2 weeks; IV immunoglobulin 1 g/kg/24 hours for 1 to 2 days, or IV anti-D 50–75 μg/kg/dose for Rh-positive patients. Splenectomy is indicated for life-threatening bleeding. There is currently no indication for platelet transfusion and none of the above treatments are considered optimal, because in the majority of children, it will resolve on its own within 6 months. *(Scott, 2006, pp. 715-717)*

67. **(D)** This patient is presenting with signs of congestive heart failure. The most common causes of heart failure in children/adolescents are due to acquired heart disease. Congenital heart diseases, such as malformations of the heart— patent ductus arteriosus and ventricular septal defects, are the most common causes of heart failure in infants–toddlers, and are second to fluid overload in neonates. *(Schneider, 2006, pp. 680-682)*

68. **(D)** This patient has the classic presentation of erythema multiforme major or Stevens– Johnson syndrome. The most common causes in children of erythema multiforme are medications and *Mycoplasma pneumoniae*. Of the antibiotics listed, the one most commonly causing Stevens–Johnson syndrome is sulfonamide followed by penicillin and tetracycline. The most common medications causing SJS in children are nonsteroidal anti-inflammatory drugs. *(Lembo, 2006, pp. 895-896; Morelli and Burch, 2009, p. 393)*

69. **(A)** Infection with Human parvovirus B19 (also known as fifth disease) resulting in the slapped cheek appearance, can also cause aplastic anemia. This is because the virus infects the precursors of erythrocytes and halts erythro-

poiesis. Recovery is typically spontaneous with an occasional transfusion for severe anemias. *(Scott, 2006, pp. 701-702; Levin and Weinberg 2009, pp. 1100-1101)*

70. **(D)** As this patient is presenting with signs and symptoms of herpes zoster within the appropriate time frame for antiviral treatment, the treatment for this patient would be oral acyclovir. NSAIDs may help with the pain associated from zoster but will not hasten the length of the course of the virus as acyclovir will. Varicella-Zoster immunoglobulin (VZIG) is indicated for prophylaxis in exposed individuals who are immunocompromised. *(Jenson and Baltimore, 2006, pp. 470-472; Levin and Weinberg, 2009, pp. 1088-1090)*

71. **(D)** Munchausen syndrome by proxy is when the parent/caregiver is causing or complaining of signs and symptoms of illnesses in his/her children. While it is a form of child abuse and should be treated as such, it is also considered a psychiatric disorder where the parent/caregiver is desiring to be in the sick role. The most common signs or symptoms that should raise the level of suspicion for Munchausen syndrome by proxy are: recurrent polymicrobial sepsis, recurrent apnea, chronic dehydration, or other unexplained symptoms like vomiting, diarrhea, seizures, failure to thrive, and hypoglycemia. The remaining signs are seen in classical physical child abuse. *(Scheffer, 2006, pp. 86-87; Sirotnak et al., 2009, pp. 211-214)*

72. **(A)** Menomune is a tetravalent vaccine that is indicated for prevention of meningococcemia caused by the bacterium *Neisseria meningitides*. Menomune is indicated for patients between 11 and 12 years of age and at 15 years of age. It is also indicated for college freshmen in dormitories, military recruits, microbiologists working with the bacterium, persons with complement deficiency and functional or anatomic asplenia, and for those traveling to countries with endemic disease. Guillain–Barré is a rare complication of the Menomune vaccine, and if a patient has a history of developing it, is the only relative contraindication other than a known reaction to a previous administration of

the vaccine, rubber latex, and diphtheria toxoid severe allergic reaction. *(Daley at al., 2009, pp. 260-261; Centers for Disease Control and Prevention, 2007)*

73. **(A)** The most likely diagnosis is pediculosis. This parasitic infestation is most commonly seen in the young school-aged child, and more often in female and Caucasian children. The pediculosis louse lives in the hair and on the scalp and intermittently "bites" into the skin to feed. Discrete urticarial papules or erosions may arise at the bite site. By visualizing the live louse on the scalp, or in the hair, one can easily make the diagnosis. However, the louse may be difficult to see, as it is only 1 to 3 mm in size. Otherwise, nits, or the casings of the eggs laid by the louse, can often be seen on the proximal portion of the hair shaft. The nit adheres to the hair shaft and is often difficult to remove. Brown nits are representative of current infestations and white nits past infestations. Treatment of head lice can be difficult due to the increasing resistance to some of the current treatment options. First-line treatment includes permethrin (5%) and permethrin-based products. Secondary treatment options for resistant infestations may include Malathion (0.5%). Regardless of treatment, viable ova should be removed by combing the patient's wetted hair with a finely toothed comb until all are removed. Ketoconazole cream and tar-based shampoos are utilized in fungal and seborrheic dermatitis infections. Silver sulfadiazine cream is a topical antibiotic. *(Lembo, 2006, pp. 897-898; Morelli and Burch, 2009, p. 387)*

74. **(B)** Scabies, *Sarcoptes scabiei*, is the most common arthropod infestation of children, and it is highly contagious. However, its presentation varies widely and is dependent on the child's age, duration of the infestation, and immune status. Most often, the presenting complaint is severe intermittent itching. The linear papule or burrow commonly associated with scabies is often difficult to identify. Instead, most children will present with eczematous eruptions of red, excoriated papules and nodules. Usually, the distribution of the papules are the most diagnostic finding, and may include the web spaces of the fingers and toes, axillae, umbilicus, groin,

penis, and the instep of the feet. Usually, in older children and adults, the face and scalp are spared. The treatment for scabies is a 12-hour application of permethrin 5% lotion. In addition, the parents and all caregivers should be treated at the same time. Clothing and bedding should be washed and dried (heat kills scabies). The family should also be educated in the treatment and prevention of future infestations. Moreover, they should be advised that the itching associated with scabies could persist for 7 to 14 days after successful treatment. Pediculosis is an infestation of louse in the hair. Tinea corporis is a fungal infection of the torso or "ring worm" and presents with annual scaly plaques with central clearing and pustules. Herpes simplex typically presents with grouped vesicles on erythematous base and is painful. It typically is located in the lips, eyes, cheeks, or hands of children. *(Lasley, 2006, p. 410; Jenson and Baltimore, 2006, pp. 474-476; Lembo, 2006, pp. 896-898; Morelli and Burch, 2009, pp. 384-385, 387)*

75. **(D)** Seborrheic dermatitis is common in all age groups. In infants, this inflammatory skin disease is often manifested as thickened, yellowish white, scaly, waxy appearing skin of the scalp and commonly involves the postauricular areas and the forehead. The more common name is "cradle cap." Cradle cap is a self-limiting disease of infants and resolves by the child's first birthday. In all ages, the scalp scale can be treated by shampooing with zinc pyrithione (Head and Shoulders), selenium sulfide 1% to 2.5%, salicylic acid (Tsal), or ketoconazole (Nizoral). The primary lesion in lichen planus presents on the flexor surfaces and is characterized by pruritic papules that are polygonal and flat-topped. Pityriasis rosea typically presents with the "herald patch" that is a solitary pink, round patch with some central clearing typically found on the torso. The rest of the eruption is described as papulovesicular and develops a Christmas tree pattern. Contact dermatitis usually presents with red patches and plaques with scales and is localized to the area exposed to the irritant. *(Lembo, 2006, pp. 886, 890; Morelli and Burch, 2009, pp. 389-391)*

76. (B) This presentation is typical for granuloma annulare, which is a benign skin disorder, and treatment is not warranted. It is most commonly seen in children aged 6 to 10. The red to brown lesions are annular or circinate. These asymptomatic lesions are often confused with tinea corporis. The lesions will disappear on their own over a couple of years. *(Morelli and Burch, 2009, p. 391)*

77. (D) Liquid nitrogen is the treatment of choice for a single isolated wart. Forty percent salicylic acid in a plaster application is the most effective treatment of large and painful warts. Electrosurgery, burning laser surgery, and other destructive treatments should be avoided because of the potential for scarring and subsequent problems often associated with scars, as well as the possible recurrence of the wart after destructive treatment. *(Morelli and Burch, 2009, pp. 386-387; Jenson and Baltimore, 2006, pp. 476-477)*

78. (B) Topical keratolytic agents applied to the skin either as a single, once a day agent or in combination regime (retinoic acid cream, azelaic acid, and adapalene) once a day in the evening and benzoyl peroxide gel in the morning, will control approximately 80% to 85% of cases of adolescent acne. When treating inflammatory acne, papular or pustular, a daily topical antibiotic such as tetracycline, minocycline, or erythromycin can be used in addition to a daily keratolytic. The oral retinoid, 13-cis-retinoic acid (isotretinoin), Accutane is reserved for treating nodulocystic acne (severe cystic acne). This medication is not effective for the milder forms of acne such as comedonal. Isotretinoin is teratogenic in women of childbearing age and has other side effects. Therefore, strict adherence to FDA guidelines is required *(Morelli and Burch, 2009, pp. 381-383; Gowen, 2006, pp. 284-285)*

79. (A) Clavicular factures are the most common fractures in infants and children. In newborns, this fracture is usually unilateral and often occurs after a difficult delivery. Many times no treatment is required or a figure-of-eight bandage can be used. For infants and children, a sling can be used. The bump that can be seen after fracture consolidation will usually resolve in a few months to a year. The next most common fractures are of the extremities, humerus being the most common and then the femur, but still much less common than the clavicle. *(Polousky and Eilert, 2009, p. 759; Thompson, 2006, pp. 903-906)*

80. (B) Osgood–Schlatter disease is caused by microfractures of the patellar ligament where it inserts into the tibial tubercle. This condition usually occurs in the preteen and adolescent years, and is more common in males than females. The history of injury can be vague and the patient may not remember a specific injury that precipitated the pain. Often, the pain progresses to the point of interference of even routine physical activities. X-rays may or may not show any abnormalities. Upon X-ray, Type I disease appears normal, but Type II will reveal fragmentation of the tibial tubercle. Often, after healing there will be enlargement of the tibial tubercle. Generally, treatment consists of rest, limitation of activities, and isometric exercises. Chondromalacia patellae can only be diagnosed under an arthroscopic examination, not on the basis of clinical features. Patellofemoral overuse syndrome presents with medial knee pain and subpatellar pain. Additional signs are swelling and crepitus in the knee and it is more common in females than males. It is diagnosed by increased Q-angles (anterosuperior iliac spine through center of patella to tibial tubercle). Subluxation of the patella or dislocation is more common in adolescent girls and the patient presents with acute knee pain. The knee is in flexion with a mass lateral to the knee and with absence of the bony prominence of the patella (flat). X-ray confirms the dislocation. *(Polousky and Eilert, 2009, pp. 758-759,783-784; Thompson, 2006, pp. 919-920)*

81. (C) Enterobiasis or pinworms is a worldwide infection that affects people of all ages and socioeconomic levels. It especially affects children. The classic manifestation of this problem is nocturnal anal pruritis and sleeplessness. The sleeplessness may be secondary to the migration of female worms to the perianal area to lay eggs, during which the tape may pick up the larvae. Transmission of the worms occurs when children ingest the eggs that are present on their hands (from scratching), in the bedclothes, or in house dust. After hatching in the stomach, the larvae migrate to the cecum where they mature into adults. The treatment of choice for pinworms is pyrantel pamoate or mebendazole. Albendazole may also be used. For eradication of this parasite, often the entire family must be treated at once. Ascaris is a helminthiasis infection that is ingested and excreted in the stool. Diagnosis is made by stool examination for the characteristic eggs. Hookworms are found in warm, damp soil and penetrate the skin. From there the infection can spread to the lungs where they ascend into the trachea to be swallowed and live in the intestine. Diagnosis is made by stool examination for the eggs. Whipworm is ingested from the soil and lives in the intestine; detection is also made by egg in the feces. *(Dominguez et al., 2009, pp. 1202-1204; Jenson and Baltimore, 2006, pp. 562-563)*

82. **(A)** Juvenile idiopathic arthritis (JIA) presents as three distinct types. The types are based upon clinical manifestations during the first 6 months of the illness. The most common type is pauciarticular as presented by this 13-year-old boy in the scenario mentioned. Second is polyarticular disease with five or more joints being affected, and the third is systemic onset of disease that begins with high spiking fevers that are often associated with a rash that comes and goes with the fever elevations. It is recommended that patients with pauciarticular JIA have an ophthalmologic evaluation and slit lamp examination every 3 months, if the antinuclear antibody test (ANA) is positive and every 6 months, if the ANA is negative, for 4 years after the JIA is identified to catch iridocyclitis (untreated results in blindness). Lyme arthritis usually presents with a monoarticular rash that typically affects the larger joints, without morning stiffness. Enteropathic arthritis is associated with gastrointestinal symptoms occurring simultaneously as lower extremity arthritis. It encompasses Reiter syndrome, reactive arthritis (eg, post-salmonella, shigella), and arthritis associated with celiac disease and inflammatory bowel disease. Psoriatic arthritis is the arthritis accompanying the dermatological disorder of psoriasis. The build-up of epidermal cells over the joints causes inflammation and thickening

that results in arthralgia. *(Soep and Hollister, 2009, pp. 796-799; Haftel, 2006, pp. 425-428, 432-436)*

83. **(B)** Bacterial conjunctivitis is often unilateral and presents with a mucopurulent discharge. Common bacterial causes of this problem include nontypable *Haemophilus, Streptococcus pneumoniae, Moraxella catarrhalis,* and *Staphylococcus aureus*. These infections usually respond to topical antibiotics such as sulfacetamide and erythromycin. Systemic treatment is indicated for conjunctivitis caused by *chlamydia trachomatis, Neisseria gonorrhea,* or *Neisseria meningitides*. Allergic conjunctivitis is usually associated with moderate to severe itching of the eyes and clear mucoid drainage. Viral conjunctivitis is usually associated with minimal itching, profuse tearing, and minimal clear mucoid drainage. While reactive arthritis typically presents with a conjunctivitis, it is also concomitantly present with arthritis and urethritis. *(Braverman, 2009, pp. 408-410; Jenson and Baltimore, 2006, pp. 540-543)*

84. **(C)** Dacryocystitis, whether acute or chronic, is usually secondary to bacterial infections. It presents as an acutely inflamed swelling and tender area over the lacrimal sac just medial and inferior to the inner canthus of the eye. Because the lacrimal sac is inflamed and blocked there is tearing and usually purulent discharge from the eye. There may also be an orbital cellulitis. Treatment consists of oral and topical antibiotics and warm compresses, and surgical drainage may also be indicated. After the acute episode and for chronic cases, surgical correction of the nasolacrimal obstruction is required. Anterior uveitis typically presents with pain, photophobia, blurred vision, and injection without exudates. Blepharitis is an inflammation of the lid margin that presents with crusty debris along the lashes. Unless there is a concomitant conjunctival infection, there is typically no injection noted. *(Braverman, 2009, pp. 404-414; Jenson and Baltimore, 2006, pp. 540-543)*

85. **(B)** While halitosis can be caused by pharyngitis, sinusitis, and poor hygiene, the most common cause of halitosis in children is a nasal foreign body. Seeds and beads are the leading objects inserted into the nose. If not promptly removed,

they can cause nasal obstruction, infection, rhinorrhea, bleeding, halitosis, or a foul smell. They are usually easy to remove, but if there is difficulty in removing the foreign body, the child should be referred to an otolaryngologist for definitive care. Tobacco use in adolescents is a common cause of halitosis. Dental disease is the most common cause of halitosis in adults. *(Kelley et al., 2009, pp. 459, 468-469; Lasley, 2006, p. 407)*

86. **(C)** Most cases of epistaxis in the anterior portion of the nose are caused by digital trauma (nose picking) or some other mechanical cause such as nose blowing or repeated nose rubbing. Other causes may include incorrect use of steroid nasal sprays. Examination of the anterior nose will usually reveal irritation of the Kiesselbach area. Less than 5% of recurrent nosebleeds are caused by bleeding disorders. Choanal atresia, unilateral, usually appears as a chronic nasal discharge that may be mistaken for chronic sinusitis. Foreign bodies typically present with purulent discharge instead of bleeding. *(Kelley et al., 2009, pp. 458-459)*

87. **(A)** Cat scratch disease (CSD) is caused by the gram-negative bacillus, *Bartonella henselae*. The disease is more common in the fall and winter months and more males than females are affected. Typically (approximately 90%), patients report handling a cat or kitten and up to 70% will report a scratch by a cat. The most common complication of CSD is encephalitis. About half of the patients with CSD will develop a primary cutaneous papule at the site of inoculation, most often (approximately 50%) on the hands or upper extremities, 3 to 10 days after the exposure. Regional lymphadenopathy will usually develop in about 1 to 7 weeks after the cutaneous lesions and will affect the nodes draining the site of the scratch or bite. The affected lymph nodes may be inflamed and are usually tender. Occasionally, the involved nodes may suppurate. The lymphadenopathy resolves in about 2 months, but may last as long as 4 to 8 months. Treatment is usually not indicated for this self-resolving disease. However, suppurative lesions may need to be aspirated for pain relief. It has been shown that 5 days of treatment with azithromycin has helped to speed recovery for some patients.

Because Hodgkin disease involves the lymph nodes, it should be considered as a differential diagnosis when evaluating a child for CSD. However, it typically presents as a cervical lymphadenopathy. Fifth disease (erythema infectiosum) is a childhood disease caused by the human parvovirus. This common community-acquired disease does not usually require treatment, but respiratory isolation is recommended for 7 days following the onset of symptoms. The initial stage of the disease presents as red cheeks that appear to be "slapped" or "slapped cheeks" with circumoral pallor. Osgood–Schlatter disease is an orthopedic problem in children. It is the result of repetitive microtraumas to the patellar ligament at its point of insertion into the tibial tubercle. Usually, rest and anti-inflammatory medications are helpful in alleviating the pain associated with this condition. *(Jenson and Baltimore, 2006, pp. 469-447, 478-479; Scott, 2006, pp. 740-741; Thompson, 2006, p. 919; Wilson and Pengel, 2009, p. 784; Maloney et al., 2009, pp. 864-865; Levin and Weinberg, 2009, pp. 1100-1101; Ogle and Anderson, 2009, pp. 1174-1175)*

88. **(B)** Hookworm (*Ancylostoma duodenale* and *Necator americanus*) infections, if severe, can cause iron deficiency anemia. Abdominal discomfort, weight loss, and ova in the stool are more commonly associated with these nematodes. Both types of human hookworms are found in tropic and subtropical climates, which include the southeastern United States, primarily the coastal areas. The larva of this parasite is passed in the feces and incubates in warm, damp soil when they hatch into larvae. The larvae penetrate directly into the skin of humans, enter the bloodstream, and migrate to the lungs. From the lungs they move up to the trachea and are swallowed. Once swallowed, they mature in the intestines. The worms attach their mouth to the mucosal lining of the intestine where they suck blood and shed new ova. Mild infections are usually asymptomatic, but severe infestations can cause anemia. Treatment for the infestation is achieved with albendazole. In severe cases of anemia, parenteral iron or transfusion may be indicated. Pinworms are associated only with localized pruritus, specifically the anus. Treatment may help recurrent urinary tract infections in some young girls when the pinworm has infected the urethra. Ascariasis

is usually asymptomatic; however, in severe cases it may be associated with anorexia, diarrhea, vomiting, weight loss, and abdominal pain. Whipworm is also asymptomatic until the infection is severe, with general gastrointestinal symptoms—pain, diarrhea, and mild abdominal distention. Eosinophilia may also be present, although slight. *(Dominguez et al., 2009, pp. 1202-1204; Jenson and Baltimore, 2006, pp. 562-563)*

89. **(C)** Appearing in 60% to 80% of cases, the characteristic rash may not be present in all cases of acute Lyme disease. Following the bite of a deer tick (*Ixodes* species), infected with the spirochete *Borrelia burgdorferi*, an erythematous ring forms around the bite site and spreads outward. The ring may have a raised border and usually a clear center. The ring can attain a diameter of up to 20 cm. Multiple rings may form and they can form at sites distal to the original bite site. If left untreated, the rash will usually resolve within 3 weeks. Erythema migrans is a minimally tender to nontender, nonscaly rash that persists longer than many of the other erythematous rashes of childhood. *(Ogle and Anderson, 2009, pp. 1180-1182; Jenson and Baltimore, 2006, pp. 551-556)*

90. **(C)** Chlamydial infections are the most common cause of conjunctivitis in newborns in developed countries. Other causes of ophthalmia neonatorum include reactions to silver nitrate prophylaxis, other bacterial infections such as gonococcal or staphylococcal, or viral organisms such as adenovirus or echovirus. *Chlamydia trachomatis* causes conjunctivitis and pneumonia in neonates. Treatment for chlamydial conjunctivitis should be with systemic erythromycin to treat the conjunctivitis and as prophylaxis against pneumonia. *(Braverman, 2009, pp. 408-410; Jenson and Baltimore, 2006, pp. 539-543)*

91. **(D)** Seizures have not been associated with Lyme disease. Neurologic manifestations occur in up to approximately 20% of patients with Lyme disease. Primarily, these are Bell palsy, lymphocytic, aseptic meningitis, and polyradiculitis. Cranial neuropathies, such as Guillain–Barré syndrome and ataxias are less common. Additional neurologic manifestations include peripheral neuropathy, pseudotumor cerebri, and encephalitis. If untreated, most neurological symptoms are self-limited, but some will persist or become permanent. *(Ogle and Anderson, 2009, pp. 1180-1182; Jenson and Baltimore, 2006, pp. 551-555)*

92. **(D)** Oral candidiasis (thrush) is very common in the first few weeks of infancy. The diagnosis is usually done by visual inspection and does not usually require further laboratory testing. On visual examination, white, creamy plaques are found on the buccal mucosa and occasionally the gingival and lingual mucosa. For this age group, direct topical application of nystatin in oral suspension to the lesions should suffice. If the lesions are resistant to treatment or if they occur in older children, consideration should be given to the possibility of the patient being immunocompromised. All sources of candida, such as toys and bottle nipples, should be sterilized daily. Herpangina and hand–foot–mouth disease are ulcerating lesions of the oral cavity due to viruses and are self-limiting, but can be very painful. Leukoplakia is a precursor lesion to oral cancer, seen most commonly in oral tobacco users. *(Kelley et al., 2009, p. 460; Levin and Weinberg, 2009, pp. 1082-1083; Dominguez et al., 2009, pp. 1212-1214; Jenson and Baltimore, 2006, p. 489; Bishop, 2006, pp. 595-596)*

93. **(B)** Bipolar affective disorder is the most likely diagnosis for this patient. Although ADHD, bipolar disorder, and conduct disorder share many similarities in behavior disorders, such as varying degrees of school and behavior problems, defiant attitude, and distractibility, the obsession with ideas (in this case, science fiction movies) is not present in ADHD and conduct disorder. The mood swings described here, as depression and elation are consistent with bipolar disorder, which is confirmed by the presence of hallucinations. Hallucinations, when considering a differential diagnosis in a behavior disorder, are diagnostic for bipolar disorder. In up to 70% of patients with bipolar disorder, their first symptom of the disorder may be depression. However, hallucinations are not typically a manifestation of depression. *(Stafford et al., 2009, pp. 180-188; Goldson and Reynolds, 2009, pp. 65-68, 93-97)*

94. (D) Rocky Mountain spotted fever (RMSF) is the most common rickettsial infection in the United States, especially in the eastern, southeastern, and western states, and it is very common in 5- to 9-year-old children. A known tick exposure may or may not be documented. Most exposures to ticks carrying *Rickettsia rickettsii*, the causative organism of this disease, occur in the warmer months of April to September when victims are most likely to participate in outdoor activities in wooded areas. The incubation period of RMSF is 3 to 12 days (mean 7) after a tick exposure. The tick must be attached for 6 hours or greater in order to transmit the disease. Clinical presentation includes fever, often 40°C, myalgias, headache, and less characteristic, red-rose macular or maculopapular rash. The rash usually appears within 2 to 6 days, after the fever. The rash is especially prevalent on the palms, soles, and extremities. After several days, the rash, which starts peripherally and spreads centrally, becomes petechial. Conjunctivitis, edema, splenomegaly, meningismus, and confusion may occur. Up to 5% to 7% of patients with RSMF will die, and therefore, delays in treatment should be avoided. Treatment for children is doxycycline, regardless of age and the possible side effect of stained teeth. In endemic areas, treatment should be started early and is often based on suspicion alone, and prior to the appearance of the rash. Endemic typhus (murine typhus) is not transmitted by ticks but instead by the fleas from infected rodents. The rash of endemic typhus differs from that of RMSF in that it does *not* involve the palms and soles. Q fever is spread by inhalation instead of ticks. The cause of this rickettsial disease is *Coxiella burnetii* hosted by domestic animals including dogs, cats, cattle, and sheep. Unpasteurized milk from infected animals may also be a source of this infection. One form of human monocytic ehrlichiosis is carried by ticks that have fed on infected hosts that may include deer, wild rodents, and sheep, most commonly in the southeast, north, and south central United States. The presentation is usually a viral syndrome without any rash. Although this is usually a self-limiting disease, deaths do occur in children; therefore, treatment should be carried out with the antibiotic of choice, doxycycline, regardless of side effects. (*Levin and Weinberg, 2009, pp. 1107-1110; Jenson and Baltimore, 2006, pp. 553-557*)

95. (D) In young children, respiratory syncytial virus (RSV) accounts for more than 70% of bronchiolitis, approximately 40% of the cases of pneumonia, and about 10% of cases of croup. This seasonal disease occurs in the winter and early spring months of the year. More than 50% of children have been infected with RSV by age 1, and by the age of 2, almost all children have been infected. Reinfection commonly occurs but is mild. Adenovirus infections, though common in early childhood, only account for approximately up to 10% of all respiratory diseases. The peak incidence of adenovirus respiratory infections occurs in the spring, summer, and early winter. Human parvovirus infection is typically seen in school-aged children. This disease is characterized by the "slapped-cheek" appearing rash on the face that appears about 10 to 17 days following the infection. About 2 days after the appearance of this facial rash, a similar rash appears on the extremities, trunk, neck, and buttocks. The rash often persists for a few days to a few weeks (average of 10 days) and often will recur with exposure to bathing in warm water, exercise, sunlight, and stress. Parainfluenza viruses fall into four categories and are responsible for the majority of cases of croup (65%), laryngitis (50%), and tracheobronchitis (25%). Types 1 to 3 occur as seasonal outbreaks with types 1 and 2 in the fall and type 3 in the spring and summer. Type 4 is an endemic virus. Clinical symptoms of these viruses include laryngotracheitis (croup), laryngitis, bronchiolitis, and less commonly pneumonia (especially in immunocompromised children). (*Levin and Weinberg, 2009, pp. 1074-1081, 1100-1101; Jenson and Baltimore, 2006, pp. 501-502*)

96. (B) Asthma, in this case exercise-induced, is the most likely cause of this problem. The symptoms commonly associated with acute exacerbations of asthma include wheezing, cough, dyspnea, and chest pain. Some symptoms that might be suggestive of asthma include exercise-induced cough, nighttime cough, cough after cold air exposure, and cough after laughing. Airway foreign bodies, though not common, are an acute problem that may present as sudden cough, choking, and wheezing. Cystic fibrosis (CF) is the most common, lethal, genetic disease affecting the Caucasian population. Up to 50% of patients with CF are diagnosed in infancy, but others may not be diagnosed until adolescence or adulthood. Chronic or recurrent cough should be an indicator for consideration of CF as a differential diagnosis. Laryngomalacia is the most common cause of stridor in infants. It is the incomplete development of the cartilaginous support of the laryngoglottic structures. This congenital condition is usually self-limiting and occurs most commonly in infants at or just after birth. The inspiratory collapse of the epiglottis or arytenoid cartilages is heard as stridor. *(Kerby et al., 2009, pp. 477, 485-486; Boguniewicz et al., 2009, pp. 1018-1034; Lasley, 2006, pp. 396-405; Jenson and Baltimore, 2006, p. 502; Marshall and Debley, 2006, pp. 637, 641, 648-651)*

97. **(B)** Autism is the most likely diagnosis for this child. The signs of autism often present before the second year of life such as the child's failure to respond to their name, failed speech development, and appearing self-absorbed and withdrawn in the presence of other children or adults. Often in childhood, autistic children may develop ritualistic behaviors and intense interests that if interrupted may cause tantrums and rages. When speech does begin to develop, it may be nonsensical: reversal of speech patterns, echolocation, and other abnormal patterns. Goals of treatment include early intervention to address behavior and communication skills. ADHD is characterized by easy distractibility, inattention, and overactivity. Estimates for the presence of ADHD in school-aged children range from 2% to 20%. Fragile X syndrome is the most common cause of functional mental retardation. This syndrome, affecting approximately 1 in 1,250 males, is caused by a trinucleotide expansion (CGG repeated sequence) in the Fragile X Mental Retardation I (*FMR1*) gene. Fragile X syndrome is characterized by a wide range of symptoms, which may include language delay, hyperactivity, autistic behavior,

and variable levels of mental retardation. Schizophrenia is usually detected in adolescence, with prepubertal onset occurring rarely. Patients may initially present with somatic or social behavior problems. Schizophrenic children and adolescents often have the same symptoms as adults, such as hallucinations, bizarre thought processes, and rambling speech. *(Goldson and Reynolds, 2009, pp. 97-98; Stafford et al., 2009, pp. 177-186; Gahagan, 2006, pp.65-68; Scheffer, 2006, pp. 98-103; Levy and Marion, 2006, p. 227)*

98. **(A)** Choanal atresia, whether unilateral or bilateral, is a nasal obstruction that occurs relatively rarely in newborns. If bilateral choanal atresia occurs at birth, it causes a respiratory distress that requires immediate treatment (due to infants being obligate nose breathers) by placing an oral airway and subsequent surgical correction. Unilateral choanal atresia can present as a chronic, single-sided, nasal discharge that may not appear until later in childhood. Meconium ileus, intestinal obstruction secondary to inspissated meconium, occurs in approximately 10% of newborns with cystic fibrosis. Cystic fibrosis affects approximately 1 in 2,500 live Caucasian births, and is a leading cause of death in young adults. Nasal infections may occur secondary to a furuncle (infected hair follicle) in the anterior nares or as a nasal septal abscess following spread of a furuncle. Common causes of nasal infections include picking at the nose and pulling out nose hair. Nasal polyps are uncommon in children younger than age 10, and when they do occur it is usually in older children and adults with allergic rhinitis. *(Thilo and Rosenberg, 2009, p. 44; Kelley et al., 2009, pp. 457-458; Lasley, 2006, p. 407; Bishop, 2006, p. 604; Marshall and Debley, 2006, pp. 640, 649-651)*

99. **(A)** It is estimated that 1% to 5% of adolescents are affected by anorexia nervosa. There are two types of anorexia nervosa. The first is the nonpurging type when patients restrict their total caloric intake and the second involves binge eating and purging in association with the restrictive dietary habits. Otherwise, intensive exercise regimes may be used as a means to control weight. Anorexia nervosa occurs in boys but is more prevalent in girls (2:1). The

specific etiology of this familial problem is unknown; there are genetic and environmental factors. DSM-IV criteria also include refusal to keep weight at 85% of ideal weight, intense fear of gaining weight even though underweight, amenorrhea, and disturbance in the way one's body shape is experienced. *(Sigel, 2009, pp. 152-155; Blake and Davis, 2006, pp. 356-357)*

100. **(C)** Obesity is the number one nutritional disorder in children in the United States. In 2004, 17% of American children aged between 9 and 19 were considered obese. Risk factors for obesity include other obese family members and infants born to diabetic mothers. Associated environmental factors include sedentary lifestyle, total caloric intake, television watching, and computer games. All are considered contributory factors in childhood obesity. Binge eating disorder is a relatively new eating disorder category. It is most frequent in overweight or obese individuals. This disorder includes recurrent episodes of binge eating (eating more than most individuals would in a 2-hour period) and a sense of lack of control over the impulse to eat, marked distress over the episode at least 2 days a week, and is not associated with regular compensatory activity such as purging or fasting. Folate deficiency anemia (megaloblastic) can occur in infants within a few weeks after birth. This deficiency may be a result of malabsorption, low dietary intake such as with goat's milk or home-prepared formulas that have been sterilized by heating, or formulas based on pasteurized milk. Infants who are breastfed or given supplemented cows' milk formulas do not have a problem with folate deficiency. In children, rickets is most commonly a result of poor dietary intake of vitamin D and inadequate exposure to direct sunlight. Vitamin D sources include milk, cheese, and baby formula. Vitamin D in humans is produced by activation of its inactive precursors in the skin after exposure to ultraviolet light. *(Sigel, 2009, pp. 161-162; Krebs and Primak, 2009, pp. 277-278, 284-286; Ambruso et al., 2009, pp. 811-812; Krebs and Primak, 2006, pp. 140-142, 149, 151-152)*

101. **(B)** The symptoms for congestive heart failure in infants are typically failure to thrive, tachy-cardia, and poor feeding. These will typically not present at birth and will be identified by the 6-month well visit. *(Schneider, 2006, pp. 680-683; Sondheimer et al., 2009, pp. 529-553)*

102. **(A)** *Bordetella pertussis* is a gram-negative bacillus and, therefore, of all the choices, the antibiotic with good gram-negative coverage is erythromycin. The other macrolides, azithromycin and clarithromycin may also be given for shorter durations, however they are more expensive. Ampicillin, amoxicillin, and cephalexin provide mainly gram-positive coverage. *(Jenson and Baltimore, 2006, pp. 499-501; Ogle and Anderson, 2009, pp. 1164-1166)*

103. **(C)** Surgical reduction is the treatment of choice for incarcerated hernias over 12 hours. At that point the likelihood that the hernia will manually reduce is very small and the bowel is becoming necrotic and needs to be removed as soon as possible. Bilateral surgical reduction is required only in the event of two hernias, and there is no place for prophylaxis surgery for inguinal hernia repairs. *(Sondheimer and Sundaram, 2009, p. 585)*

104. **(B)** Salmonella species are gram-negative bacilli that are classified as Enterobacteriaceae, along with *E Coli*. While extremely uncommon as an etiology for meningitis, salmonella can cause lethal meningitis infections and must be watched. While there is typically no treatment for mild to moderate diarrhea from salmonella infections, these patients should be monitored for complete resolution. Viral meningitis typically does not have a positive Gram stain, unless there is contamination. Corynebacterium and clostridium are gram-positive bacilli. *(Thilo and Rosenberg, 2009, p. 52; Sondheimer and Sundaram, 2009, p. 594; Ogle and Anderson, 2009, pp. 1145-1147)*

105. **(A)** Vitamin K deficiency causes hemorrhagic disease of the newborn. Vitamin K is one of the compounds required for conversion of prothrombin, factors VII, IX, and X of the coagulation cascade. In addition, proteins C & S are also Vitamin K dependent. Therefore, the result is an increased prothrombin time and this would result in an increased aPTT. There is no

effect on platelets or fibrinogen. *(Krebs and Primak, 2006, pp. 152-153; Ambruso et al., 2009, pp. 840-841)*

106. **(C)** The diagnosis of otitis media requires the presence of middle ear effusion, acute onset of symptoms, and signs and symptoms of middle ear inflammation. Presence of the middle ear effusion can be determined by the bulging of the tympanic membrane, air-fluid levels, absent mobility of the tympanic membrane by pneumatic otoscopy, or otorrhea from perforation. Office tympanometry can be performed to confirm a diagnosis of effusion. Tenderness on palpation of the tragus typically is a sign of otitis externa. *(Jenson and Baltimore, 2006, pp 493-495; Kelley et al., 2009, pp. 437-441)*

107. **(C)** While different states have different requirements for child safety restraints, the most common guidelines state that infants must be 20 lb and 1 year of age before switching to forward-facing seats. Children between 20 lb and 40 lb should be in front-facing safety seats, typically with a 5-point harness; children between 40 and 80 lb may be in booster seats in which the back is typically required based on the height of the child. Lastly, children should be older than 12 years of age and typically at least 80 lb as the front air bags are dangerous. *(Levine, 2006, p. 39)*

108. **(D)** The most common etiology of gynecomastia is idiopathic. Occurring in 50 % to 60% of adolescent males, idiopathic gynecomastia typically is self-limited. Additional uncommon etiologies of gynecomastia include liver disease, hyperthyroidism, illicit drugs (marijuana, heroin), neoplasms (adrenal, testicular), and medications (eg, antacids, chemotherapy). *(Blake and Davis, 2006, p. 348)*

109. **(A)** A urinalysis should be performed because renal disease is the most common etiology of hypertension in children. Electrocardiograms and chest radiography should be considered as part of the evaluation for end-organ disease as well as an initial basic metabolic panel to include serum and creatinine. Although rare, elevated uric acid has also been shown to cause essential hypertension in children. *(Marcdante, 2006, pp. 763-764)*

110. **(B)** The CDC recommends that there are two age ranges for testing lead in children in the United States: 9 to 12 months and again at 24 months. These high-risk areas include poverty-stricken areas, use of lead paint pottery, lead painted homes (peeling or cracking), industrial exposures, and use of diarrhea remedies in Mexico. The CDC recommends using questions to screen all children between 6 months and 6 years of age. *(Levine, 2006, p. 35)*

REFERENCES

Ambruso DR, Hays T, Goldenberg NA. Hematologic disorders. In: Hays WW, Levin MJ, Sondheimer JM, et al., eds. *Current Diagnosis & Treatment: Pediatrics.* 19th ed. New York: McGraw-Hill; 2009.

Bickley LS, Szilagyi PG. *Bates' Guide to Physical Examination and History Taking.* 10th ed. New York: Lippincott Williams & Wilkins; 2009.

Bishop WP. The digestive system. In: Kliegman RM, Marcdante KJ, Jenson HB, et al., eds. *Nelson Essentials of Pediatrics.* 5th ed. Philadelphia: Elsevier Saunders; 2006.

Blake K, Davis V. Adolescent medicine. In: Kliegman RM, Marcdante KJ, Jenson HB, et al., eds. *Nelson Essentials of Pediatrics.* 5th ed. Philadelphia: Elsevier Saunders; 2006.

Boguniewicz M, Covar RA, Fleischer DM. Allergic disorders. In: Hays WW, Levin MJ, Sondheimer JM, et al.,

eds. *Current Diagnosis & Treatment: Pediatrics.* 19th ed. New York: McGraw-Hill; 2009.

Braverman RS. Eye. In: Hays WW, Levin MJ, Sondheimer JM, et al., eds. *Current Diagnosis & Treatment: Pediatrics.* 19th ed. New York: McGraw-Hill; 2009.

Brayden RM, Bunik M, Brown JM, et al. Ambulatory and community pediatrics. In: Hays WW, Levin MJ, Sondheimer HM, et al., eds. *Current Diagnosis & Treatment: Pediatrics.* 19th ed. New York: McGraw-Hill; 2009.

Centers for Disease Control and Prevention (2007). Prevention and control of meningococcal disease. http://www.cdc. gov/mmwr/preview/mmwrhtml/ mm5631a3.htm. August 2007. Accessed July 2, 2009.

Centers for Disease Control and Prevention (2009a). Summary of recommendations for tetanus toxoid, reduced diphtheria toxoid and acellular pertussis vaccine (Tdap) and tetanus and diphtheria toxoids (Td) use among adolescents aged 11–18 years. http://www.cdc.gov/mmwr/preview/mmwrhtml/rr55e223a4.htm. Accessed July 2, 2009.

Centers for Disease Control and Prevention (2009b). Childhood & Adolescent Immunization Schedule; 2009. http://www.cdc.gov/nip/recs/child-schedule.htm. Accessed July 2, 2009.

Christian CW, Blum NJ. Psychosocial issues. In: Kliegman RM, Marcdante KJ, Jenson HB, et al., eds. *Nelson Essentials of Pediatrics*. 5th ed. Philadelphia: Elsevier Saunders; 2006.

Daley MF, Simoes EF, Nyquist AC. Immunization. In: Hays WW, Levin MJ, Sondheimer JM, et al., eds. *Current Diagnosis & Treatment: Pediatrics*. 19th ed. New York: McGraw-Hill; 2009.

Dominguez AR, Weinberg A, Levin MJ. Infections: Parasitic & mycotic. In: Hays WW, Levin MJ, Sondheimer JM, et al., eds. *Current Diagnosis & Treatment: Pediatrics*. 19th ed. New York: McGraw-Hill; 2009.

Elias ER, Tsai ACH, Manchester DK. Genetics & dysmophology. In: Hays WW, Levin MJ, Sondheimer JM, et al., eds. *Current Diagnosis & Treatment: Pediatrics*. 19th ed. New York: McGraw-Hill; 2009.

Ford DM. Fluid, electrolyte & acid-base disorders & therapy. In: Hays WW, Levin MJ, Sondheimer JM, et al., eds. *Current Diagnosis & Treatment: Pediatrics*. 19th ed. New York: McGraw-Hill; 2009.

Gahagan S. Behavioral disorders. In: Kliegman RM, Marcdante KJ, Jenson HB, et al., eds. *Nelson Essentials of Pediatrics*. 5 ed. Philadelphia: Elsevier Saunders; 2006.

Goldson E, Reynolds A. Child development & behavior. In: Hays WW, Levin MJ, Sondheimer JM, et al., eds. *Current Diagnosis & Treatment: Pediatrics*. 19th ed. New York: McGraw-Hill; 2009.

Gowen CW. Fetal and neonatal medicine. In: Kliegman RM, Marcdante KJ, Jenson HB, et al., eds. *Nelson Essentials of Pediatrics*. 5th ed. Philadelphia: Elsevier Saunders; 2006.

Haftel HM. Rheumatic diseases of childhood. In: Kliegman RM, Marcdante KJ, Jenson HB, et al., eds. *Nelson Essentials of Pediatrics*. 5th ed. Philadelphia: Elsevier Saunders; 2006.

Jenson HB, Baltimore RS. Infectious disease. In: Kliegman RM, Marcdante KJ, Jenson HB, et al., eds. *Nelson Essentials of Pediatrics*. 5th ed. Philadelphia: Elsevier Saunders; 2006.

Jospe N. Endocrinology. In: Kliegman RM, Marcdante KJ, Jenson HB, et al., eds. *Nelson Essentials of Pediatrics*. 5th ed. Philadelphia: Elsevier Saunders; 2006.

Kaplan DW, Love-Osborne KA. Adolescence. In: Hays WW, Levin MJ, Sondheimer JM, et al., eds. *Current Diagnosis & Treatment: Pediatrics*. 19th ed. New York: McGraw-Hill; 2009.

Kelley PE, Friedman NR, Yoon PJ. Ear, nose, & throat. In: Hays WW, Levin MJ, Sondheimer, et al., eds. *Current Diagnosis & Treatment: Pediatrics*. 19th ed. New York: McGraw-Hill; 2009.

Kerby GS, Deterding RR, Balasubramaniam V, et al. Respiratory tract & mediastinum. In: Hays WW, Levin MJ, Sondheimer JM, et al., eds. *Current Diagnosis & Treatment: Pediatrics*. 19th ed. New York: McGraw-Hill; 2009.

Krebs NF, Primak LE. Normal childhood nutrition & its disorders. In: Hays WW, Levin MJ, Sondheimer JM, et al., eds. *Current Diagnosis & Treatment: Pediatrics*. 19th ed. New York: McGraw-Hill; 2009.

Krebs N, Primak L. Pediatric nutrition and nutritional disorders. In: Kliegman RM, Marcdante KJ, Jenson HB, et al., eds. *Nelson Essentials of Pediatrics*. 5th ed. Philadelphia: Elsevier Saunders; 2006.

Lasley MV. Allergy. In: Kliegman RM, Marcdante KJ, Jenson HB, et al., eds. *Nelson Essentials of Pediatrics*. 5th ed. Philadelphia: Elsevier Saunders; 2006.

Lembo R. Dermatology. In: Kliegman RM, Marcdante KJ, Jenson HB, et al., eds. *Nelson Essentials of Pediatrics*. 5th ed. Philadelphia: Elsevier Saunders; 2006.

Levine DA. Growth and development. In: Kliegman RM, Marcdante KJ, Jenson HB, et al., eds. *Nelson Essentials of Pediatrics*. 5th ed. Philadelphia: Elsevier Saunders; 2006.

Levin MJ, Weinberg A. Infections: viral & rickettsial. In: Hays WW, Levin MJ, Sondheimer JM, et al., eds. *Current Diagnosis & Treatment: Pediatrics*. 19th ed. New York: McGraw-Hill; 2009.

Levy PA, Marion RW. Human genetics and dysmorphology. In: Kliegman RM, Marcdante KJ, Jenson HB, et al., eds. *Nelson Essentials of Pediatrics*. 5th ed. Philadelphia: Elsevier Saunders; 2006.

Lewis D. Neurology. In: Kliegman RM, Marcdante KJ, Jenson HB, et al., eds. *Nelson Essentials of Pediatrics*. 5th ed. Philadelphia: Elsevier Saunders; 2006.

Lum GM. Kidney & urinary tract. In: Hays WW, Levin MJ, Sondheimer JM, et al., eds. *Current Diagnosis & Treatment: Pediatrics*. 19th ed. New York: McGraw-Hill; 2009.

Maloney K, Greffe BS, Foreman NK, et al. Neoplastic disease. In: Hays WW, Levin MJ, Sondheimer JM, et al., eds. *Current Diagnosis & Treatment: Pediatrics*. 19th ed. New York: McGraw-Hill; 2009.

Marcdante KJ. The acutely ill or injured child. In: Kliegman RM, Marcdante KJ, Jenson HB, et al., eds. *Nelson Essentials of Pediatrics*. 5th ed. Philadelphia: Elsevier Saunders; 2006.

Marcdante KJ. Nephrology and urology. In: Kliegman RM, Marcdante KJ, Jenson HB, and Behrman RE, eds. *Nelson Essentials of Pediatrics*, 5th ed. Philadelphia: Elsevier Saunders; 2006.

Marshall SG, Debley JS. The respiratory system. In: Kliegman RM, Marcdante KJ, Jenson HB, et al., eds.

Nelson Essentials of Pediatrics. 5th ed. Philadelphia: Elsevier Saunders; 2006.

McLean TW, Wofford MM. Oncology. In: Kliegman RM, Marcdante KJ, Jenson HB, et al., eds. *Nelson Essentials of Pediatrics.* 5th ed. Philadelphia: Elsevier Saunders; 2006.

Moe PG, Benke TA, Bernard TJ, et al. Neurologic & muscular disorders. In: Hays WW, Levin MJ, Sondheimer JM, et al., eds. *Current Diagnosis & Treatment: Pediatrics.* 19th ed. New York: McGraw-Hill; 2009.

Morelli JG, Burch JM. Skin. In: Hays WW, Levin MJ, Sondheimer JM, et al., eds. *Current Diagnosis & Treatment: Pediatrics.* 19th ed. New York: McGraw-Hill; 2009.

Ogle JW, Anderson MS. Infections: bacterial & spirochetal. In: Hays WW, Levin MJ, Sondheimer JM, et al., eds. *Current Diagnosis & Treatment: Pediatrics.* 19th ed. New York: McGraw-Hill; 2009.

Polousky JD, Eilert RE. Orthopedics. In: Hays WW, Levin MJ, Sondheimer JM, et al., eds. *Current Diagnosis & Treatment: Pediatrics.* 19th ed. New York: McGraw-Hill; 2009.

Scheffer R. Psychiatric disorders. In: Kliegman RM, Marcdante KJ, Jenson HB, et al., eds. *Nelson Essentials of Pediatrics.* 5th ed. Philadelphia: Elsevier Saunders; 2006.

Schneider DS. Cardiovascular. In: Kliegman RM, Marcdante KJ, Jenson HB, et al., eds. *Nelson Essentials of Pediatrics.* 5th ed. Philadelphia: Elsevier Saunders; 2006.

Scott JP. Hematology. In: Kliegman RM, Marcdante KJ, Jenson HB, et al., eds. *Nelson Essentials of Pediatrics.* 5th ed. Philadelphia: Elsevier Saunders; 2006.

Sigel EJ. Eating disorders. In: Hays WW, Levin MJ, Sondheimer JM, et al., eds. *Current Diagnosis & Treatment: Pediatrics.* 19th ed. New York: McGraw-Hill; 2009.

Sirotnak AP, Krugman RD, Chiesa A. Child abuse & neglect. In: Hays WW, Levin MJ, Sondheimer JM, et al., eds. *Current Diagnosis & Treatment: Pediatrics.* 19th ed. New York: McGraw-Hill; 2009:209–215.

Soep JB, Hollister JR. Rheumatic diseases. In: Hays WW, Levin MJ, Sondheimer JM, et al., eds. *Current Diagnosis & Treatment: Pediatrics.* 19th ed. New York: McGraw-Hill; 2009.

Sokol RJ, Narkewicz MR. Liver & pancreas. In: Hays WW, Levin MJ, Sondheimer JM, et al., eds. *Current Diagnosis & Treatment: Pediatrics.* 19th ed. New York: McGraw-Hill; 2009.

Sondheimer HM, Darst JR, Shaffer EM. et al. Cardiovascular diseases. In: Hays WW, Levin MJ, Sondheimer JM, et al., eds. *Current Diagnosis & Treatment: Pediatrics.* 19th ed. New York: McGraw-Hill; 2009.

Sondheimer JM, Sundaram S. Gastrointestinal tract. In: Hays WW, Levin MJ, Sondheimer JM, et al., eds. *Current Diagnosis & Treatment: Pediatrics.* 19th ed. New York: McGraw-Hill; 2009.

Stafford B, Hagman J, Dech B. Child & adolescent psychiatric disorders & psychosocial aspects of pediatrics. In: Hays WW, Levin MJ, Sondheimer JM, et al., eds. *Current Diagnosis & Treatment: Pediatrics.* 19th ed. New York: McGraw-Hill; 2009.

Thilo EH, Rosenberg AA. The newborn infant. In: Hays WW, Levin MJ, Sondheimer JM, et al., eds. *Current Diagnosis & Treatment: Pediatrics.* 19th ed. New York: McGraw-Hill; 2009.

Thomson GH. Orthopedics. In: Kliegman RM, Marcdante KJ, Jenson HB, et al., eds. *Nelson Essentials of Pediatrics.* 5th ed. Philadelphia: Elsevier Saunders; 2006.

Wilson PE, Pengel B. Sports medicine. In: Hays WW, Levin MJ, Sondheimer JM, et al., eds. *Current Diagnosis & Treatment: Pediatrics.* 19th ed. New York: McGraw-Hill; 2009.

Zeitler PS, Travers SH, Hoe F, et al., Endocrine disorders. In: Hays WW, Levin MJ, Sondheimer JM, et al., eds. *Current Diagnosis & Treatment: Pediatrics.* 19th ed. New York: McGraw-Hill; 2009.

SECTION IV
Pharmacology and Therapeutics

CHAPTER 15

Pharmacology and Therapeutics

Raymond J. Pavlick Jr., PhD

DIRECTIONS: Each of the numbered items or incomplete statements in this section is followed by answers or by completions of the statement. Select the ONE-lettered answer or completion that is BEST in each case.

1. A history of which of the following warrants special consideration when initially prescribing levothyroxine?

    (A) peptic ulcer disease
    (B) chronic stable angina
    (C) obesity
    (D) rheumatoid arthritis
    (E) parkinsonism

2. Which of the following medications is capable of causing agranulocytosis?

    (A) insulin
    (B) metformin
    (C) methimazole
    (D) prednisone
    (E) desmopressin

3. A 56-year-old African American woman with moderate asthma and hypertension suffers a mild, ischemic stroke. Prior to this event, her hypertension was controlled with diet and exercise, but her recent blood pressure measurements have averaged 148/90 mm Hg. Which of the following is the most appropriate antihypertensive therapy for this patient considering her history and present medical conditions?

    (A) Atenolol & lisinopril
    (B) diltiazem & hydrochlorothiazide
    (C) diltiazem & hydralazine
    (D) hydralazine & atenolol
    (E) hydrochlorothiazide & lisinopril

4. A 4-year-old child swallows several tablets of a medication that he found in his parent's bathroom cabinet underneath the sink. Approximately 2 to 3 hours after ingesting the tablets, there were no symptoms other than nausea and vomiting. Thirty hours after ingesting the tablets, elevated aminotransferase levels were detected followed by jaundice, hepatic encephalopathy, renal failure, and death. What did the child most likely swallow?

    (A) diazepam
    (B) aspirin
    (C) oxycodone
    (D) acetaminophen
    (E) phenobarbital

5. Which of the following requires drug-free periods to avoid tolerance when used as prophylaxis for chronic stable angina?

    (A) digoxin
    (B) diltiazem
    (C) metoprolol
    (D) isosorbide dinitrate
    (E) propranolol

6. Following chronic therapy for its listed indication, which of the following medications is typically tapered prior to discontinuation?

    (A) omeprazole for gastroesophageal reflux disease (GERD)
    (B) glipizide for type 2 diabetes mellitus
    (C) prednisone for systemic lupus erythematosus
    (D) metformin for type 2 diabetes mellitus
    (E) ezetimibe for hyperlipidemia

7. Which of the following medications is often prescribed in combination with digoxin for managing moderate to severe congestive heart failure, but can also be a cause of digoxin toxicity?

    (A) nitroglycerin
    (B) furosemide
    (C) triamterene
    (D) verapamil
    (E) ramipril

8. Of the following choices, which regimen is considered first-line therapy for *Helicobacter pylori*-positive individuals with peptic ulcer disease?

    (A) omeprazole & clarithromycin & amoxicillin
    (B) omeprazole & ranitidine & clarithromycin
    (C) esomeprazole & clarithromycin & ampicillin
    (D) ranitidine & amoxicillin & bismuth subsalicylate
    (E) misoprostol & clarithromycin & metronidazole

9. Following a gunshot wound to the lower abdomen, a 29-year-old man is hospitalized and treated with clindamycin for a potential anaerobic infection. After 3 days of clindamycin therapy, while recuperating in the hospital, he develops severe diarrhea, dehydration, and lower abdominal cramping. A stool culture is ordered and later discovered to contain *Clostridium difficile*. After discontinuing the clin-

damycin, which of the following would be the most appropriate treatment?

    (A) cefaclor
    (B) doxycycline
    (C) amoxicillin
    (D) metronidazole
    (E) cephalexin

10. Which of the following medications is most appropriate for the treatment of an initial case of acute uncomplicated cystitis in a 23-year-old woman?

    (A) amoxicillin
    (B) ciprofloxacin
    (C) doxycycline
    (D) azithromycin
    (E) gentamicin

11. Assuming no contraindications, which of the following class of medications is considered the preferred long-term control therapy for persistent asthma?

    (A) inhaled corticosteroids
    (B) leukotriene antagonists
    (C) long-acting B_2 agonists
    (D) methylxanthines
    (E) muscarinic antagonists

12. Which of the following type 2 diabetes mellitus medications is correctly paired with its mechanism of action?

    (A) glimepiride; enhancement of insulin secretion
    (B) metformin; reduction of postprandial glucagon secretion
    (C) miglitol; enhancement of insulin sensitivity at skeletal muscle
    (D) rosiglitazone; inhibition of intestinal sucrase and glucoamylase
    (E) sitagliptin; enhancement of hepatic insulin sensitivity

13. Along with diuretic therapy, which of the following agents is considered first-line therapy in a 52-year-old man with hypertension who develops systolic heart failure with an ejection fraction of 30% following a myocardial infarction?

    (A) diazoxide
    (B) lisinopril
    (C) prazosin
    (D) reserpine
    (E) verapamil

14. A 61-year old man arrives at the emergency department (ED) suffering an acute myocardial infarction as a result of coronary artery thrombosis. One of the agents administered to the patient is a thrombolytic agent. From the choices below, which drug is a thrombolytic agent?

    (A) abciximab
    (B) alteplase
    (C) warfarin
    (D) heparin
    (E) clopidogrel

15. A patient on a 16 mg daily dose of hydromorphone is being switched to morphine sulfate for pain control. If 7.5 mg of hydromorphone is equianalgesic with 30 mg of morphine sulfate, what dose of morphine sulfate should be prescribed if you account for 25% cross-tolerance?

    (A) 30 mg
    (B) 36 mg
    (C) 48 mg
    (D) 64 mg
    (E) 80 mg

16. A 37-year-old woman under your care is diagnosed with bipolar I disorder. As part of her drug regimen, you prescribe lithium carbonate as long-term maintenance therapy. Which of the following would be most appropriate to perform or order prior to the initiation of lithium carbonate?

    (A) electrocardiogram
    (B) fasting plasma glucose
    (C) liver function tests
    (D) serum creatinine
    (E) urine culture

17. One of the most common adverse effects with spasmolytics such as carisoprodol and cyclobenzaprine is their tendency to cause which of the following?

    (A) rash
    (B) drowsiness
    (C) hypertension
    (D) myalgia
    (E) hyperglycemia

18. A 68-year-old man is recently diagnosed with depression associated with the loss of his close sister to an automobile accident. He is currently taking oxybutynin for overactive bladder disease and lisinopril for hypertension. He has no known drug allergies. Which of the following medications would be most appropriate to prescribe for this patient?

    (A) alprazolam
    (B) amitriptyline
    (C) buspirone
    (D) desipramine
    (E) fluoxetine

19. One of the common tendencies associated with antiarrhythmic drugs is their ability to produce "proarrhythmic" effects, which means they

    _____

    (A) suppress the arrhythmia that they are being used for without any serious adverse effects
    (B) selectively block certain ion channels in the heart that are responsible for triggering the arrhythmia
    (C) create a new and often worse arrhythmia in the heart
    (D) increase the resistance of cardiac cells to premature activation by prolonging the refractory period
    (E) decrease conduction velocity through the sinoatrial (SA) and atrioventricular (AV) nodes

20. Taking aspirin or ibuprofen 30 to 45 minutes prior to taking _____ often helps to blunt intense flushing and may increase patient compliance.

    (A) atorvastatin
    (B) warfarin
    (C) niacin
    (D) ezetimibe
    (E) metformin

21. A 24-year-old man presenting to the clinic 1 week ago was diagnosed with depression and subsequently prescribed 10 mg/day of fluoxetine. He unexpectedly shows up today and states that he is not experiencing any improvement since starting the medication. What is the best treatment option at this time?

    (A) double the dose of fluoxetine to 20 mg/day
    (B) maintain the current dose of fluoxetine and comfort the patient that the medication may still take at least 1 to 2 more weeks to work
    (C) discontinue the fluoxetine and start sertraline
    (D) discontinue the fluoxetine and start amitriptyline
    (E) maintain the current dose of fluoxetine and add phenelzine to the medication regimen

22. Assuming no contraindications to their use, which of following are the antihypertensives of first choice for treating hypertension in the type 2 diabetic patient?

    (A) angiotensin converting enzyme inhibitors
    (B) Ca^{+2} channel blockers
    (C) β-blockers
    (D) thiazide diuretics
    (E) α-receptor blockers

23. Which of the following medications would be most appropriate for an otherwise healthy 57-year-old man seeking relatively quick relief from urinary obstructive symptoms with slight prostatic enlargement due to benign prostatic hyperplasia (BPH)?

    (A) finasteride
    (B) doxazosin
    (C) testosterone
    (D) desmopressin
    (E) atropine

24. Chronic therapy with which of the following medications can potentially lead to abrupt, unpredictable, and transient motor fluctuations (from mobility to immobility) often referred to as the "on–off phenomenon"?

    (A) cyclobenzaprine
    (B) diazepam
    (C) methotrexate
    (D) levodopa/carbidopa
    (E) carbamazepine

25. A 5-year-old child with no known drug allergies is diagnosed in your clinic with bilateral acute otitis media. Which of the following is the drug of choice?

    (A) levofloxacin
    (B) nitrofurantoin
    (C) amoxicillin
    (D) doxycycline
    (E) gentamicin

26. Which of the following drugs is indicated for the treatment of anemia associated with chronic renal failure?

    (A) deferoxamine
    (B) warfarin
    (C) protamine sulfate
    (D) erythropoietin
    (E) argatroban

27. A 57-year-old woman with hypertension and a recent diagnosis of chronic stable angina presents for her quarterly check-up. She is currently treated with metoprolol tartrate 100 mg bid and her blood pressure is 148/88 mm Hg with a pulse of 54 bpm. She has not experienced anginal attacks since being started on metoprolol

tartrate 4 months ago. Which of the following is the most rationale approach to managing the patient at this time?

(A) add diltiazem to the current medication regimen

(B) add ramipril to the current medication regimen

(C) discontinue the metoprolol tartrate and start diltiazem

(D) discontinue the metoprolol tartrate and start hydrochlorothiazide

(E) double the current dose of metoprolol tartrate

28. Which of the following is considered an osmotic laxative?

(A) senna

(B) polyethylene glycol

(C) docusate sodium

(D) methylcellulose

(E) loperamide

29. A 48-year-old man is brought to the emergency department by his sister after suffering from loss of consciousness, followed by muscle rigidity and rhythmic contractions, and then a return to a normal state. When asked about medication use, the patient states he is currently being treated with a drug for depression but cannot remember the name. He claims that he has never had a seizure or seizure-like activity prior to this event. Approximately 6 hours after the first episode, the patient suffers a second one while still in the ED. Which of the following medications is the patient most likely taking?

(A) bupropion

(B) duloxetine

(C) fluoxetine

(D) nortriptyline

(E) phenelzine

30. A 23-year-old man visits the clinic today for a pre-employment physical. He has a medical history of asthma that is currently being man-

aged prn with a metered-dose inhaler of albuterol. The patient tells you he has been using it daily for the past month due to increased shortness of breath and that it does not seem to be working too well. Which of the following is the most rationale approach to managing the patient at this time?

(A) add ipratropium bromide for use on a daily basis and continue albuterol prn

(B) add fluticasone for use on a daily basis and continue albuterol prn

(C) discontinue the albuterol and prescribe fluticasone for use on a daily basis

(D) add methylprednisone for use on a daily basis and continue albuterol prn

(E) increase the dose of albuterol and keep using prn

31. A progestin-only contraceptive, or "minipill," would be most appropriate for which of the following patients?

(A) a 25-year-old woman in excellent overall health

(B) a 28-year-old woman with a history of epilepsy

(C) a 32-year-old woman with a history of pelvic inflammatory disease

(D) a 37-year-old woman who smokes 2 packs per day and has a history of hypertension

(E) a 38-year-old woman with a history of asthma and bronchitis

32. Which of the following should be used cautiously in patients with chronic pulmonary disease or elevated intracranial pressure (ICP)?

(A) morphine sulfate

(B) naloxone

(C) carbamazepine

(D) methylphenidate

(E) verapamil

33. Which of the following is the drug of choice for treating herpes simplex virus (HSV) types 1 and 2?

    (A) amantadine
    (B) acyclovir
    (C) zidovudine
    (D) nystatin
    (E) zanamivir

34. Which of the following class of antihypertensives is associated with a first-dose phenomenon that is characterized by transient dizziness or faintness, palpitations, and possible syncope?

    (A) α_1-blockers
    (B) angiotensin converting enzyme inhibitors (ACEIs)
    (C) angiotensin receptor blockers (ARBs)
    (D) thiazide diuretics
    (E) potassium-sparing diuretics

35. A 35-year-old man is brought to the emergency department with unremitting, generalized convulsive status epilepticus. The initial, preferred treatment is intravenous administration of which of the following?

    (A) phenobarbital
    (B) valproate
    (C) phenytoin
    (D) lorazepam
    (E) donepezil

36. Abrupt cessation of which of the following antihypertensives can produce significant rebound hypertension, tachycardia, and excessive sweating?

    (A) angiotensin converting enzyme inhibitors (ACEIs)
    (B) angiotensin receptor blockers (ARBs)
    (C) β-blockers
    (D) thiazide diuretics
    (E) potassium-sparing diuretics

37. A 54-year-old man with chronic stable angina is being treated with daily doses of metoprolol and sublingual nitroglycerin prn to control occasional angina attacks. Approximately 45 minutes after taking sildenafil, the patient suffers a severe attack and takes several nitroglycerin tablets within a short time frame that ultimately leads to his death. Which of the following best explains what occurred?

    (A) the nitroglycerin/sildenafil combination led to a fatal arrhythmia
    (B) the nitroglycerin/sildenafil interaction triggered acute arterial thromboembolism
    (C) the nitroglycerin/sildenafil interaction led to severe hypotension
    (D) the metoprolol/sildenafil combination triggered a fatal coronary vasospasm
    (E) the metoprolol/sildenafil combination led to severe bronchospasm

38. A patient with myasthenia gravis would likely experience symptomatic benefit with which of the following?

    (A) acetylcholinesterase inhibitors
    (B) muscarinic antagonists
    (C) α_1-blockers
    (D) β-blockers
    (E) dopamine agonists

39. From the choices given below, which medication is considered the safest for use during pregnancy?

    (A) warfarin
    (B) captopril
    (C) isotretinoin
    (D) esomeprazole
    (E) misoprostol

40. The risk of extrapyramidal side effects (pseudoparkinsonism) and tardive dyskinesia is associated with which class of medications?

    (A) amphetamines
    (B) benzodiazepines
    (C) monoamine oxidase inhibitors (MAOIs)
    (D) tricyclic antidepressants (TCAs)
    (E) typical (first-generation) antipsychotics

41. Drug X is an antiepileptic medication that is labeled as a "CYP2D6 inducer." CYP2D6 enzymes do not metabolize drug X. Drug Y is an antihypertensive medication that is typically metabolized to inactive products by CYP2D6 enzymes. If drugs X and Y are taken simultaneously, a patient will:

    (A) be at greater risk for having a seizure
    (B) be at lesser risk for having a seizure
    (C) likely experience hypertension
    (D) likely experience hypotension
    (E) likely experience hypotension and be at greater risk for having a seizure

42. A 50-year-old man presents to the emergency department with an episode of paroxysmal supraventricular tachycardia (PSVT). He is hypotensive (BP 88/58 mm Hg), does not feel faint, nor is complaining of any chest pain. His electrocardiogram (ECG) shows a regular arrhythmia with no P waves, narrow QRS complexes, and a heart rate of 172 bpm. Successive Valsalva maneuvers fail to terminate the PSVT. Which of the following intravenous treatments would be most appropriate for the patient at this time?

    (A) morphine
    (B) amiodarone
    (C) atenolol
    (D) adenosine
    (E) digoxin

43. Which of the following is the primary site of action for warfarin?

    (A) kidneys
    (B) liver
    (C) blood
    (D) small intestine
    (E) red bone marrow

44. Disulfiram increases the level of which of the following to produce flushing, throbbing headache, vomiting, and palpitations during alcohol intake?

    (A) acetic acid
    (B) acetylaldehyde
    (C) alcohol dehydrogenase
    (D) creatinine
    (E) glucuronic acid

45. Which of the following exerts its action by inhibiting cell wall synthesis?

    (A) amoxicillin
    (B) ciprofloxacin
    (C) doxycycline
    (D) erythromycin
    (E) gentamicin

46. The use of triptans is contraindicated in patients with a history of which of the following?

    (A) kidney stones
    (B) gall bladder disease
    (C) cerebrovascular disease
    (D) peptic ulcer disease
    (E) schizophrenia

47. Two 0.75-mg tablets of levonorgestrel taken 12 hours apart are effective as _____

    (A) emergency contraception following unprotected intercourse
    (B) analgesia for pain associated with endometriosis
    (C) a method to increase the chances of becoming pregnant by inducing ovulation
    (D) a method for preventing hot flashes in postmenopausal women
    (E) a method of protection against HIV transmission

48. Which drug can potentially lead to oropharyngeal candidiasis, and which agent can be used to treat this type of infection?

    (A) albuterol; ketoconazole
    (B) triamcinolone; fluconazole
    (C) fluticasone; amantadine
    (D) cromolyn sodium; levofloxacin
    (E) flunisolide; metronidazole

49. A 19-year-old woman presents to the clinic with complaints of nausea, diarrhea, flatulence, stomach cramps, and bloating. A stool sample provided while at the clinic has frothy and greasy characteristics but is free of any visible blood. She explains that she just returned from a 2-week camping trip where she did a great deal of swimming in a couple of lakes. Which of the following medications would be most appropriate for this patient?

(A) metronidazole
(B) nystatin
(C) trimethoprim-sulfamethoxazole
(D) doxycycline
(E) erythromycin

50. A 34-year-old woman presents to the clinic with complaints of intermittent flushing and blushing that started 3 to 4 weeks ago. Since then, she has noticed several inflammatory papules on the cheeks, nose, and chin. Upon exam, you notice an overall rosy hue to the face and the absence of any comedones. Which of the following would be the best course of topical therapy at this time?

(A) mupirocin ointment
(B) permethrin cream
(C) tretinoin gel
(D) hydrocortisone 1% cream
(E) metronidazole gel

51. A 25-year-old woman complains of chest pain, shortness of breath, sweating and trembling. After an extensive negative work-up, the patient is diagnosed with panic disorder. Which of the following would be the most appropriate sustained treatment?

(A) buspirone
(B) clomipramine
(C) clorazepate
(D) paroxetine
(E) ramelteon

52. A 52-year-old man recently underwent surgery for a hip replacement. Upon discharge, he is prescribed oxycodone 7.5 mg and acetamino-phen 325 mg and told to take 1 to 2 tablets every 6 hours prn to help manage the pain he is expected to encounter as he recovers at home. Which of the following medications would you also recommend for the patient to help minimize potential side effects associated with his pain medication?

(A) esomeprazole
(B) diphenhydramine
(C) guaifenesin
(D) hydrocortisone 1% cream
(E) senna & docusate

53. A 64-year-old woman with a medical history of rheumatoid arthritis and deteriorating vision presents to the clinic with complaints of painful bilateral swelling of her ankles and hands, morning stiffness, loss of appetite, and fatigue. She is currently taking naproxen sodium 500 mg twice per day. Which medication(s) would be most appropriate for this patient?

(A) acetaminophen
(B) azathioprine
(C) cyclosporine
(D) hydroxychloroquine
(E) methotrexate

54. When used for advanced carcinoma of the prostate, chronic administration of leuprolide inhibits the synthesis of androgens by

_____

(A) blocking gonadotropin-releasing hormone (GnRH) receptors at the anterior pituitary
(B) blocking luteinizing hormone (LH) receptors on interstitial (Leydig) cells of the testes
(C) increasing the secretion of GnRH from the hypothalamus
(D) inhibiting pulsatile secretion of gonadotropins from the anterior pituitary
(E) upregulation of the number of GnRH receptors at the anterior pituitary

55. Mitotic inhibitors such as vinblastine and vincristine are classified as chemotherapeutic agents because they _____

    (A) block hormone receptors
    (B) cross-link or alkylate DNA
    (C) inhibit the function of microtubules
    (D) inhibit the synthesis of RNA
    (E) inhibit topoisomerase

56. A 35-year-old woman diagnosed with depression 3 weeks ago has been taking a medication prescribed by her clinician. Recently, she reports complaints of dry mouth, constipation and visual sensitivity to bright light. Which of the following medications was the patient most likely prescribed?

    (A) bupropion
    (B) nortriptyline
    (C) phenelzine
    (D) sertraline
    (E) venlafaxine

57. Which of the following is a common adverse effect associated with the use of stimulants such as methylphenidate for attention-deficit hyperactivity disorder (ADHD)?

    (A) diarrhea
    (B) hypoglycemia
    (C) hypotension
    (D) paresthesias
    (E) reduced appetite

58. A 28-year-old woman in the emergency department is administered an intravenous paralytic agent prior to endotracheal intubation. The agent produces transient muscle fasciculations, particularly over the thorax and abdomen, prior to paralysis. Which of the following was the patient most likely administered?

    (A) tubocurarine
    (B) rocuronium
    (C) carbamazepine
    (D) succinylcholine
    (E) pyridostigmine

59. A 22-year-old man with pernicious anemia can be given which of the following to correct any hematologic and neurologic defects of his condition?

    (A) vitamin K
    (B) folic acid
    (C) ferrous sulfate
    (D) vitamin B_{12}
    (E) erythropoietin

60. Which of the following are common adverse effects associated with aminoglycosides?

    (A) diarrhea and bone marrow depression
    (B) ototoxicity and nephrotoxicity
    (C) blurred vision and hyperglycemia
    (D) headache and hypoglycemia
    (E) rash and dyspepsia

61. In the treatment of asthma, long-acting β_2-agonists are _____

    (A) an effective substitute for inhaled corticosteroids as monotherapy for long-term control of any form of asthma
    (B) commonly used as an adjunct to inhaled corticosteroid therapy for providing long-term control of more severe forms of asthma
    (C) of limited use due to their low therapeutic index, risk of life-threatening toxicity, and numerous drug interactions
    (D) the drugs of choice for providing prompt relief of bronchoconstriction and its accompanying acute symptoms such as cough, chest tightness, and wheezing
    (E) the most effective at reducing inflammation of bronchial airways

62. A patient presents with signs and symptoms of moderate congestive heart failure that includes a modest degree of left ventricular dysfunction, shortness of breath, fatigue, reduced exercise tolerance, and ankle edema. Which of the following drug combinations would be the best choice for initial treatment?

    (A) digoxin and hydrochlorothiazide
    (B) metoprolol and triamterene
    (C) metoprolol and enalapril
    (D) enalapril and furosemide
    (E) isosorbide dinitrate and furosemide

63. A 24-year-old woman presents with nausea that has fluctuated in severity for the last 3 weeks. The patient states that the nausea seems to have coincided with taking a prescription for birth control pills for the first time. Substitution of her current prescription with a combined hormonal contraceptive containing a lesser amount of which compound would most likely relieve the patient's nausea?

    (A) desogestrel
    (B) ethinyl estradiol
    (C) norethindrone
    (D) luteinizing hormone
    (E) testosterone

64. Constipation, abdominal distention, bloating, and flatulence are common adverse effects associated with which class of drugs?

    (A) bile acid resins
    (B) fibrates
    (C) HMG-CoA reductase inhibitors
    (D) nonselective β-blockers
    (E) organic nitrates

65. A 25-year-old man is hospitalized with symptoms of delusion, paranoia, rambling statements coupled with disorganized thought, and flattened affect. The companion who brings him to the hospital claims this is the first time she has ever witnessed any of these symptoms and is not aware of any medication he is currently taking. Which of the fol-

lowing medications is most appropriate for this patient?

    (A) sertraline
    (B) topiramate
    (C) olanzapine
    (D) clomipramine
    (E) thioridazine

66. Which of the following is the primary mechanism by which benzodiazepines exert their sedative and anxiolytic effects?

    (A) acting as dopamine receptor agonists
    (B) acting as NMDA receptor antagonists
    (C) acting as serotonin receptor antagonists
    (D) decreasing reuptake of serotonin and norepinephrine
    (E) increasing $GABA_A$ receptor-mediated chloride conductance

67. Which of the following lists the common adverse effects caused by nitroglycerin when administered sublingually at high doses?

    (A) constipation, blurred vision, tinnitus
    (B) dyspepsia, abdominal distention, vomiting
    (C) elevated pulse, facial flushing, headache
    (D) photophobia, excessive salivation, excessive tearing
    (E) wheezing, cough, heartburn

68. Hyperkalemia is a contraindication to the use of which of the following medications?

    (A) metformin
    (B) cimetidine
    (C) triamterene
    (D) glipizide
    (E) verapamil

69. Which of the following drugs block the actions of leukotrienes and can be used for long-term control of mild persistent asthma?

    (A) cromolyn sodium
    (B) omalizumab

(C) zafirlukast

(D) nedocromil sodium

(E) ipratropium bromide

70. Which of the following has the potential for causing cyanide toxicity?

(A) clonidine

(B) diazoxide

(C) hydralazine

(D) reserpine

(E) sodium nitroprusside

71. Which of the following therapeutic regimens is most appropriate for a 17-year-old girl diagnosed with gonococcal and chlamydial urethritis?

(A) amoxicillin & clavulanate

(B) trimethoprim-sulfamethoxazole

(C) metronidazole

(D) ceftriaxone & azithromycin

(E) doxycycline & amoxicillin

72. A patient is taking an antihypertensive medication for which the prescribing information says "do not use with other cardiac depressant drugs." To which combination of antihypertensive medications would this precaution or contraindication apply?

(A) doxazosin & diltiazem

(B) hydralazine & doxazosin

(C) lisinopril & atenolol

(D) lisinopril & verapamil

(E) verapamil & atenolol

73. Which of the following is a potential adverse effect associated with unfractionated heparin (UFH)?

(A) hyperglycemia

(B) hypothyroidism

(C) thrombocytopenia

(D) excessive cough

(E) muscle cramps

74. A 31-week-pregnant woman is diagnosed with an uncomplicated urinary tract infection (UTI). Which of the following would be most appropriate in this situation?

(A) doxycycline

(B) trimethoprim-sulfamethoxazole

(C) metronidazole

(D) nitrofurantoin

(E) levofloxacin

75. A 43-year-old pilot is interested in quitting his 20-year habit of smoking. His medical history includes type 2 diabetes mellitus diagnosed 6 years ago for which he is currently taking metformin. Which of the following would be most appropriate to recommend to this patient?

(A) alprazolam

(B) clonidine

(C) nicotine replacement therapy

(D) nortriptyline

(E) varenicline

76. A 33-year-old woman treated with trifluoperazine for the past 3 months is seen in the emergency department because of recent-onset fever, stiffness and tremor, as reported by her accompanying sister. The patient also appears to be mildly confused when asked about location, day, and time. Her temperature is 104.5°F, and her serum creatine kinase (CK) level is markedly elevated. Which of the following has most likely occurred?

(A) a delayed allergic reaction has occurred with trifluoperazine

(B) tardive dyskinesia has begun to develop in the patient

(C) the patient has developed neuroleptic malignant syndrome

(D) the patient has developed serotonin syndrome

(E) the patient has overdosed on trifluoperazine

77. Which property accounts for why some β-blockers produce dizziness and drowsiness, whereas other β-blockers are not as likely to cause these problems?

    (A) selectivity for certain β-receptors
    (B) degree of lipophilicity
    (C) degree of intrinsic sympathomimetic activity (ISA)
    (D) serum half-life
    (E) margin of safety

78. Which of the following antineoplastic medications is most likely to cause cardiac toxicity and precipitate heart failure?

    (A) doxorubicin
    (B) cisplatin
    (C) cyclophosphamide
    (D) tamoxifen
    (E) 6-mercaptopurine

79. A type 1 diabetic patient who does not experience many of the normal warning signs of hypoglycemia when her blood glucose is 57 mg/dL is most likely receiving which of the following antihypertensive medications?

    (A) diltiazem
    (B) enalapril
    (C) hydrochlorothiazide
    (D) losartan
    (E) propranolol

80. Which of the following is considered first-line therapy for a nonpregnant, 24-year-old woman suffering from cervicitis believed to be due to a *Chlamydia trachomatis* infection?

    (A) 7-day course of oral doxycycline or 1 oral dose of azithromycin
    (B) 7-day course of oral erythromycin or 1 oral dose of azithromycin
    (C) 7-day course of oral penicillin or 1 oral dose of trimethoprim-sulfamethoxazole
    (D) 7-day course of oral erythromycin or 1 oral dose of trimethoprim-sulfamethoxazole
    (E) 7-day course of oral penicillin or 1 oral dose of azithromycin

81. Which of the following agents is the treatment of choice to reverse an opioid overdose?

    (A) buprenorphine
    (B) butorphanol
    (C) nalbuphine
    (D) methadone
    (E) naloxone

82. Which compound can be applied topically and acts as a keratolytic to remove corns, calluses, and common warts?

    (A) acetaminophen
    (B) salicylic acid
    (C) ibuprofen
    (D) hydroxychloroquine
    (E) colchicine

83. A 50-year-old man with asymptomatic hyperuricemia is to begin therapy for newly diagnosed hypertension. Which of the following is most likely to increase his serum uric acid levels further and possibly precipitate a gout attack?

    (A) amlodipine
    (B) candesartan
    (C) hydrochlorothiazide
    (D) metoprolol
    (E) ramipril

84. In addition to insulin and fluid replacement with 0.9% saline, which electrolyte is commonly infused in the type 2 diabetic patient who arrives in the emergency department in a hyperglycemic, hyperosmolar, nonketotic state?

    (A) bicarbonate
    (B) potassium
    (C) calcium
    (D) magnesium
    (E) sulfate

85. Both rifampin and certain antiepileptics (AEDs) such as phenytoin and carbamazepine have been shown to reduce the effectiveness of which of the following?

(A) nicotine replacement therapy

(B) combined hormonal contraceptives

(C) HMG-CoA reductase inhibitors

(D) nonsteroidal anti-inflammatory drugs

(E) proton pump inhibitors

86. Which of the following provides the greatest fracture risk reductions and greatest increases in bone mineral density in postmenopausal females with osteoporosis?

(A) alendronate

(B) calcitonin

(C) estrogen

(D) raloxifene

(E) vitamin D

87. Drugs such as donepezil and rivastigmine that are used for Alzheimer disease exert their effect by which of the following mechanisms?

(A) blocking muscarinic receptors

(B) blocking serotonin receptors

(C) inhibiting acetylcholinesterase

(D) binding to muscarinic receptors

(E) binding to serotonin receptors

88. A 46-year-old man with a 2-year history of gouty arthritis presents to the clinic with a red, swollen joint at the base of the great toe. After resolution of the acute attack with indomethacin, a drug which inhibits the synthesis of uric acid was prescribed. Which of the following was the drug most likely prescribed?

(A) allopurinol

(B) colchicine

(C) cyclosporine

(D) probenecid

(E) sulfasalazine

89. Which agent is most appropriate for the treatment of seasonal allergies in a 32-year-old male taxi driver?

(A) diphenhydramine

(B) clemastine

(C) ergotamine tartrate

(D) promethazine

(E) loratadine

90. Which class of medications now includes a boxed warning and expanded warning statements about the increased risk of suicidality in children and adolescents being treated with these drugs?

(A) benzodiazepines

(B) typical antipsychotics

(C) atypical antipsychotics

(D) opiates

(E) antidepressants

91. In general, the bioavailability of a drug will be the greatest when it is administered by which of the following routes?

(A) intramuscular

(B) intravenous

(C) oral

(D) respiratory

(E) subcutaneous

92. Which of the following is the primary emergency treatment for anaphylaxis?

(A) epinephrine

(B) antihistamines

(C) atropine

(D) aminophylline

(E) dopamine

93. A 12-year-old boy reaches under his friend's porch to retrieve a baseball and suffers a small puncture wound to his left hand as a result of a bite by the friend's cat. Within 24 hours, he becomes febrile and complains of chills, and the wound appears infected. Which drug(s) would be most appropriate to give this patient?

(A) amoxicillin & clavulanate

(B) erythromycin

(C) trimethoprim-sulfamethoxazole

(D) metronidazole

(E) gentamicin

94. A 62-year-old man with a history of parkinsonism is recently diagnosed with colorectal cancer and is to begin chemotherapy. Which of the following regimens would be most appropriate in prophylactically treating acute nausea and vomiting associated with his moderately emetogenic chemotherapeutic regimen?

    (A) metoclopramide
    (B) metoclopramide & dexamethasone
    (C) ondansetron & dexamethasone
    (D) lorazepam
    (E) prochlorperazine

95. A 52-year-old man is brought to the ED by his daughter because she recently notices that he gets extremely tired, has periodic tremors in his hands, and suffers from increasing memory lapses. Initial laboratory work shows a serum creatinine of 2.2 mg/dL. His medical history is significant for bipolar disorder, for which he has been taking the same drug for the past 32 months. Which of the following is most likely responsible for the patient's symptoms?

    (A) valproate
    (B) lithium carbonate
    (C) carbamazepine
    (D) olanzapine
    (E) risperidone

96. Angiotensin receptor blockers (ARBs) are not as likely to produce cough compared to angiotensin converting enzyme inhibitors (ACEIs) because they do not _____

    (A) cause hyperkalemia
    (B) cause hyponatremia
    (C) cross the blood-brain barrier
    (D) increase bradykinin levels
    (E) undergo a first-pass effect

97. A 56-year-old woman is currently being treated with daily warfarin for thrombophlebitis. She has contracted a serious lower respiratory tract infection and is admitted to the hospital. The patient is started on ciprofloxacin upon admission, and after 3 days of treatment, her INR increases from 2.7 to 7.4. She also reports a nosebleed on the third night in the hospital. Her lower respiratory function has improved slightly, but the infection has still not resolved. Which of the following is the most likely explanation for the increase in the patient's INR?

    (A) decreased warfarin absorption in the small intestine
    (B) decreased warfarin metabolism by the liver
    (C) increased plasma protein binding of warfarin
    (D) increased warfarin absorption in the small intestine
    (E) increased warfarin metabolism by the liver

98. Which of the following medications increases the risk of developing Reye syndrome in the pediatric patient when used to treat influenza and other viral illnesses?

    (A) acetaminophen
    (B) aspirin
    (C) ibuprofen
    (D) oseltamivir
    (E) naproxen

99. Which of the following combination of drugs can be used effectively for prophylactic treatment of variant (Prinzmetal) angina?

    (A) diltiazem & atenolol
    (B) diltiazem & isosorbide dinitrate
    (C) isosorbide dinitrate & atenolol
    (D) lisinopril & atenolol
    (E) lisinopril & diltiazem

100. A 24-year-old man is on a 2-injection regimen for his type 1 diabetes mellitus that includes NPH and regular insulin taken before breakfast and then again before dinner. One evening, he has an abnormally light dinner and in the middle of the night, he awakens in a cold sweat with his heart pounding. He obtains a glucometer reading and discovers that his blood glucose is 44 mg/dL. He eats some candy and then goes back to sleep. Immediately after awakening the next morning, his blood glucose is 277 mg/dL. What would be the most appropriate course of action at this time?

(A) take the usual morning insulin regimen after breakfast instead of before breakfast

(B) decrease the morning NPH dose and leave the morning regular insulin dose unchanged

(C) increase the morning NPH dose and leave the morning regular insulin dose unchanged

(D) leave the morning NPH dose unchanged and increase the morning regular insulin dose

(E) increase both the morning NPH and regular doses

Answers and Explanations

1. **(B)** Multiple factors influence the initial dose of levothyroxine when used for thyroid replacement therapy, including age, the duration and severity of hypothyroidism, and the presence of certain underlying conditions. Thyroid hormones are known to elevate heart rate and increase cardiac contractility, both of which demand more oxygen utilization by the heart. In hypothyroid patients with a history of chronic stable angina, initial levothyroxine doses are typically smaller and then titrated upward. This regimen prevents a more immediate increase on the heart's workload that could occur with usual doses and minimizes the chances of an exacerbation of angina. *(Sherman and Talbert, 2008, p. 1257; Barrett, 2009, p. 1051)*

2. **(C)** Methimazole is an antithyroid agent known as a thionamide or thiourea drug. It decreases the synthesis of thyroid hormone by inhibiting the oxidation of iodide and the coupling of iodotyrosines. Minor adverse reactions include skin rash, nausea, vomiting, and drowsiness. The main risk of thionamides, however, is agranulocytosis, with the incidence varying between 0.5% to 6.0%. Patients who receive methimazole should be closely supervised and cautioned to report immediately any evidence of illness, including sore throat, skin eruptions, fever, headache, or general malaise. In such cases, methimazole should be discontinued and white blood cell and differential counts should be made to determine whether agranulocytosis has developed. Because the onset is sudden, routine monitoring is not required. It is particularly important for the patient to carefully monitor for signs and symptoms during the early stages of methimazole therapy, because methimazole-induced agranulocytosis usually occurs within the first 3 months of therapy. *(Sherman and Talbert, 2008, pp. 1250-1251; Whitby and Johns, 2008, p. 1706)*

3. **(E)** There are two evidence-based antihypertensive regimens for patients with a medical history of ischemic stroke or transient ischemic attack (TIA) to reduce the risk of a recurrent stroke. The first is a combination of an ACE inhibitor with a thiazide diuretic and the second is monotherapy with an angiotensin receptor blocker (ARB). Patients with a history of ischemic stroke should have a blood pressure goal of less than 130/80 mm Hg. *(Saseen and Maclaughlin, 2008, p. 155)*

4. **(D)** Acetaminophen toxicity may result from a single toxic dose, from repeated ingestion of large doses of acetaminophen (eg, 7.5 to 10 g daily for 1 to 2 days), or from chronic ingestion of the drug. Dose-dependent hepatic necrosis is the most serious acute toxic effect associated with overdose and is potentially fatal. Acetaminophen is the second most common cause of liver failure requiring transplantation in the United States. *(Olson, 2008, pp. 1365-1366)*

5. **(D)** According to the American College of Cardiology/American Heart Association practice guidelines for chronic stable angina, β-blockers like metoprolol are generally considered among the initial antianginal drugs of choice in the long-term prophylactic management of chronic stable angina. Long-acting nitrates such as isosorbide dinitrate can be used alone or in combination as second-line therapy in patients

previously treated with a β-blocker. However, the development of tolerance is a major limiting step in their efficacy when used longterm. The degree of tolerance can be limited by utilizing a regimen that includes a minimum 8- to 10-hour period per day without nitrates no matter the route of delivery (ointment, patch, or tablets). *(Talbert, 2008, pp. 236-238; Bashore et al., 2008, pp. 307-308)*

6. **(C)** Chronic therapy with systemic corticosteroids can induce atrophy of the adrenal glands, which significantly depresses the adrenal response to adrenocorticotropic hormone (ACTH). Stopping prednisone suddenly would leave the body without a source of glucocorticoids, because the hypothalamic–pituitary–adrenal axis needs time to re-establish its normal functioning. As a result, an acute adrenal crisis (Addisonian crisis) that is marked by dehydration with severe vomiting and diarrhea, hypotension, shock, and loss of consciousness can develop and potentially lead to a fatality. *(Delafuente and Cappazzo, 2008, p. 1437; Fitzgerald, 2008, pp. 1001-1002)*

7. **(B)** Digoxin binds to Na^+/K^+ ATPases on the sarcolemmal membranes of cardiac muscle cells and inhibits them from working. This raises intracellular Na^+ levels, which facilitates Na^+/Ca^{+2} exchange. The resulting increase in intracellular Ca^{+2} enhances contractile protein cross-bridge formation and cardiac contractility, resulting in a positive inotropic effect. One of the parameters often monitored in the heart failure patient taking digoxin is serum K^+. Potassium and digoxin inhibit each others' binding to the Na^+/K^+ ATPases; therefore, hyperkalemia reduces the actions of digoxin, whereas hypokalemia increases its effect. As a result, hypokalemic patients are more susceptible to the many cardiac manifestations of digoxin toxicity, particularly ventricular arrhythmias. Rhythm disturbances are a major concern in heart failure patients, as they are already at an elevated risk for sudden cardiac death that can be linked to ventricular arrhythmias. Furosemide is a K^+-wasting, loop diuretic that is often prescribed with digoxin to provide symptomatic relief due to fluid retention,

particularly in patients with moderate to severe congestive heart failure. Hence, loop diuretics should be used cautiously as a result of their potential to cause hypokalemia and subsequently, an elevated risk of cardiac arrhythmias. *(Parker et al., 2008, pp. 198-200)*

8. **(A)** Triple-therapy regimens consisting of a proton pump inhibitor (PPI) and two antibiotics are considered first-line therapy for the eradication of *Helicobacter pylori*. PPI-based regimens that combine clarithromycin and amoxicillin or clarithromycin and metronidazole have been shown to have the most effective eradication rates. There are also 4-drug regimens that include bismuth subsalicylate that have been shown to be effective as well. Because of lower eradication rates, it is not recommended that histamine receptor antagonists like ranitidine be substituted for a PPI. Misoprostol is used for reducing the risk of nonsteroidal anti-inflammatory agent (NSAIA)-induced gastric ulcer in patients at high risk of developing complications from these ulcers and in patients at high risk of developing gastric ulceration. It has no effect on *H pylori* eradication. *(Berardi and Welage, 2008, pp. 577-578)*

9. **(D)** *Clostridium difficile* is a gram-positive, anaerobic, spore-forming bacillus that is responsible for the development of antibiotic-associated diarrhea and colitis. *C difficile* colitis results from a disturbance of the normal bacterial flora of the colon, colonization with *C difficile*, and release of toxins that cause mucosal inflammation and damage. Antibiotic therapy is the key factor that alters the colonic flora. Specific therapy aimed at eradicating *C difficile* is indicated if symptoms are persistent or severe. The drug of choice is metronidazole, 500 mg orally three times daily or 250 mg orally four times daily. Oral metronidazole and vancomycin are equally effective in treating diarrhea caused by *C difficile*. Despite the isolation of metronidazole-resistant strains of *C difficile*, metronidazole is the drug of first choice because of its lower cost and the fact that it can promote vancomycin-resistant nosocomial infections. *(Martin and Jung, 2008, p. 1863; McQuaid, 2008, pp. 543-544)*

10. **(B)** Acute uncomplicated cystitis is predominately caused by *E coli*. While trimethoprim-sulfamethoxazole has been used to treat uncomplicated cystitis in numerous cases, it is becoming more ineffective due to the emergence of resistant strains of *E coli*. As a result, fluoroquinolones such as ciprofloxacin are now considered the drugs of choice over all other antibiotics. Three-day courses of fluoroquinolones have been shown to be more effective than single-dose therapies. *(Coyle and Prince, 2008, pp. 1904-1906; Stoller et al., 2008, p. 817)*

11. **(A)** Inhaled corticosteroids (eg, beclomethasone, fluticasone, triamcinolone, etc) are the preferred long-term control therapy for persistent asthma in all patients because of their potency and consistent effectiveness. Low- to medium-dose inhaled corticosteroids offer several advantages over other medications, including the ability to reduce bronchial hyper-responsiveness, improve overall lung function, and reduce severe exacerbations that often lead to emergency department visits and hospitalizations. *(Chesnutt et al., 2008, p. 209; Kelly and Sorkness, 2008, pp. 485-486;)*

12. **(A)** Glimepiride is an example of a sulfonylurea, which, as a class of medications, enhances the secretion of insulin from pancreatic β-cells. Hence, sulfonylureas are sometimes known as insulin secretagogues. Metformin, a biguanide, enhances insulin sensitivity of both hepatocytes and skeletal muscle cells, by decreasing gluconeogenesis. Miglitol, an α-glucosidase inhibitor, inhibits intestinal enzymes that degrade carbohydrates. Thiazolidinediones (TZDs) or glitazones, such as rosiglitazone, also enhance insulin sensitivity in hepatic and skeletal muscle tissues. Sitagliptin belongs to a relatively new class of type 2 diabetes medications known as DPP-IV (dipeptidyl peptidase 4) inhibitors, which stabilize blood levels of an incretin called glucagon-like peptide-1 (GLP-1). During hyperglycemia, incretins stimulate insulin secretion and inhibit glucagon secretion. DPP-IV metabolizes incretins. Hence, DPP-IV inhibitors block this enzyme, thereby increasing the level of incretins. *(Triplitt et al., 2008, pp. 1220-1226)*

13. **(B)** The use of an ACE inhibitor with diuretic therapy is the regimen of choice in hypertensive patients with systolic heart failure and reduced cardiac output. This is based on the fact that ACE inhibitors have demonstrated reduced cardiovascular morbidity and mortality in several studies. ACE inhibitors have also been shown to slow cardiac remodeling, improve cardiac function, and reduce cardiovascular events following a myocardial infarction. *(Saseen and Maclaughlin, 2008, p. 153)*

14. **(B)** Both warfarin and heparin are anticoagulants that are indicated for the prevention of thrombi. They do not actively lyse clots, but are capable of preventing further thrombogenesis. Both abciximab and clopidogrel are considered antiplatelet agents. Abciximab inhibits the activation of glycoprotein IIb/IIIa receptors on platelets, which helps to reduce platelet aggregation. Clopidogrel blocks adenosine diphosphate (ADP) receptors on platelets. The binding of ADP to these receptors is an important cellular mechanism in stimulating platelet aggregation. Alteplase converts plasminogen to plasmin, which then actively dissolves the fibrin threads associated with a thrombus. *(Spinler and deDunus, 2008, pp. 256-262; Haines et al., 2008, pp. 335-339, 347-349)*

15. **(C)** Opioid rotation is a common practice of switching a patient from one opioid to another. This typically occurs when patients are not getting sufficient pain relief with one opioid (despite increasing its dose) or are complaining of its side effects. Opioid rotation requires the provider to determine approximate equianalgesic dosing conversions, as different opioids usually have different potencies. In this particular problem, 7.5 mg of hydromorphone is equianalgesic with 30 mg of morphine sulfate. Using this ratio of relative potencies, the first step is to determine how many milligrams of morphine sulfate is equianalgesic with 16 mg of morphine sulfate:

$$\frac{7.5 \text{ mg hydromorphone}}{30 \text{ mg morphine sulfate}} = \frac{16 \text{ mg hydromorphone}}{x \text{ mg morphine sulfate}}$$

Solving for *x*, the calculation is 64 mg.

Because of wide ranges in individual responses to the various opioids and also because of potential cross-tolerance between opioids, the calculated dose of the new opioid is typically reduced by at least 25% to ensure safety:

$$64 \text{ mg} - 16 \text{ mg} (25\% \text{ of } 64) = 48 \text{ mg}$$

(*Bauman and Strickland, 2008, pp. 994-996*)

16. **(D)** Patients on chronic lithium carbonate therapy have an approximate 10% to 20% risk of developing renal problems such as glomerulosclerosis, tubular atrophy, or interstitial nephritis. Each of these conditions can lead to filtration problems and a subsequent rise in serum creatinine. Hence, it is advised to obtain a baseline serum creatinine prior to administering lithium carbonate to follow any changes that may occur in renal function during therapy. It is also advised that lithium carbonate be avoided in patients with pre-existing renal disease. (*Drayton and Weinstein, 2008, p. 1155*)

17. **(B)** Spasmolytics like carisoprodol and cyclobenzaprine are indicated as an adjunct to rest and physical therapy for relief of muscle spasm associated with acute and painful musculoskeletal conditions. Some of the more common adverse effects include drowsiness, dizziness, and dry mouth. These effects appear to be related to the drug's antimuscarinic properties. Patients should be advised not to use these drugs with alcohol or other central nervous system (CNS) depressants, as these combinations can cause significant sedation. Operating machinery or driving a motor vehicle should be avoided while taking carisoprodol or cyclobenzaprine. (*White and Katzung, 2009, pp. 462-465*)

18. **(E)** Selective serotonin reuptake inhibitors (SSRIs) such as fluoxetine are usually considered first-line antidepressants due to their relative safeness in overdose and their minimal affinity for muscarinic, α-adrenergic, and histamine receptors, thereby causing fewer side effects. Tricyclic antidepressants such as amitriptyline and desipramine produce several adverse effects associated with their antimuscarinic properties (eg, dry mouth, constipation, blurred vision, urinary retention, etc). The

patient is already taking the antimuscarinic agent oxybutynin, so a tricyclic antidepressant could attenuate these adverse effects. Orthostatic hypotension is also common with tricyclic antidepressants, and because the patient is taking lisinopril for hypertension, the risk for a significant drop in blood pressure is high. Buspirone and alprazolam are not indicated for depression. (*Teter et al., 2008, pp. 1128-1129*)

19. **(C)** Many antiarrhythmic drugs have the potential for causing new arrhythmias or even worsening arrhythmias for which the drug is indicated. This phenomenon is referred to as a "pro-arrhythmic" effect. For example, treatment with the class 1A agent quinidine for supraventricular arrhythmias can precipitate torsade de pointes (a form of ventricular tachycardia) in 4% to 8% of patients using the drug because of its ability to prolong the QT interval. Long QT interval syndrome (LQTS) can often lead to an abrupt loss of consciousness and death. It is characterized by QT prolongation accompanied by tachycardia. In patients with LQTS who develop torsade de pointes, the symptoms can range from syncope (where the torsade de pointes stops suddenly) to cardiac arrest (when it results in ventricular fibrillation). Hence, torsade de pointes can have a particularly poor prognosis. (*Sanaski et al., 2008, pp. 304-307*)

20. **(C)** Of all the therapeutic agents currently on the market, niacin has the greatest potential to raise high-density lipoproteins (HDL-C), often by as much as 25% to 35%. The amount of niacin needed to achieve this therapeutic effect is very high compared to the recommended daily allowance (RDA) for niacin (3.0 to 4.5 g/day vs 20 mg/day). Unfortunately, compliance with niacin therapy is low because of intense (yet harmless) flushing of the skin that is quite similar to hot flashes experienced in many postmenopausal women. Aspirin and other NSAIDs can often blunt this prostaglandin-mediated response to high doses of niacin, as their mechanism of action is to decrease prostaglandin synthesis. (*Talbert, 2008, p. 397; Baron, 2008, p. 1081*)

21. **(B)** Alleviation of symptoms associated with depression is typically slow in onset following

initiation with SSRIs. Fluoxetine, for instance, can take anywhere between 2 to 6 weeks to achieve substantial benefit when used for depression. After just 1 week of therapy, there is little justification to increase the current dose or switch to another SSRI such as sertraline. Switching the patient to a TCA such as amitriptyline at this point would further delay symptom relief, as TCAs can take several weeks to produce improvement. Compared to SSRIs, TCAs are also more likely to create unwanted side effects such as weight gain, orthostatic hypotension, and constipation. Combining an SSRI with a monoamine oxidase inhibitor (MAOI) such as phenelzine can cause serotonin syndrome that can be lethal. In order to avoid interaction between SSRIs and MAOIs, it is recommended that at least 4 to 5 weeks pass after discontinuing one and starting the other. (*Eisendrath and Lichtmacher, 2008, pp. 923-924*)

22. **(A)** Aggressive treatment of hypertension in diabetic patients is essential in preventing many comorbidities, including nephropathy, myocardial infarction, and stroke. The American Diabetes Association (ADA) currently recommends the use of ACE inhibitors as first-line agents for the treatment of hypertension in diabetic patients. This recommendation is based on a number of studies that have demonstrated a clinically significant decrease in the development and progression of diabetic nephropathy, a so-called "protective renal effect." The majority of diabetic patients will actually require the use of multiple antihypertensive agents to reach their goal blood pressure, as one medication alone is often ineffective. Whatever combination regimen is selected, it should include an ACE inhibitor. Angiotensin receptor blockers (ARBs) have also recently been shown to have similar "nephroprotective" properties and could be selected in lieu of ACE inhibitor. (*Saseen and Maclaughlin, 2008, p. 154; Sutters, 2008, pp. 392-393*)

23. **(B)** α_1-adrenergic antagonists (blockers) such as doxazosin cause relaxation of the internal urethral sphincter and also decrease prostatic smooth muscle tone. As a result, urinary outflow from the bladder is enhanced and the patient is less likely to experience obstructive symptoms such as weak urine flow, straining to initiate urine flow, dribbling after urination, and the constant feeling of a full bladder. 5α-reductase inhibitors such as finasteride and dutasteride decrease the production of intraprostatic dihydrotestosterone (DHT) by inhibiting the enzyme type II 5α-reductase. Within the prostate, this enzyme converts testosterone into DHT, which causes prostatic enlargement and growth. As a result, 5α-reductase inhibitors shrink the prostate, which subsequently can provide relief of obstructive symptoms. $\alpha 1$-adrenergic antagonists are faster acting in providing symptom relief compared to the 5α-reductase inhibitors, which often take up to 6 months to maximally shrink an enlarged prostate gland. Hence, patients with troublesome symptoms seeking quick relief generally do not prefer 5α-reductase inhibitors. The use of testosterone would not be indicated as this could raise DHT levels and cause further prostatic enlargement. Desmopressin is a synthetic analog of antidiuretic hormone (ADH) and would cause urinary retention, thus exacerbating symptoms. Atropine is a muscarinic antagonist and would also worsen symptoms. (*Lee, 2008, pp. 1391-1394*)

24. **(D)** One of the drug therapies used to manage the symptoms of Parkinson disease is the combination of levodopa (L-DOPA) and carbidopa. Levodopa is the precursor to dopamine, which is the neurotransmitter whose decreased concentrations in the substantia nigra lead to symptoms of tremor, rigidity, bradykinesia, and postural instability. Levodopa is converted into dopamine by dopa decarboxylase, an enzyme found within the nervous tissue and also the peripheral circulation. Levodopa is used instead of dopamine because it can cross the blood–brain barrier. While levodopa can improve symptoms, it does not halt progression of the disease. Carbidopa inhibits peripheral dopa decarboxylase, which allows more levodopa to cross the blood–brain barrier instead of being converted into dopamine within the circulation. Carbidopa itself does not cross the blood–brain barrier. A complication that can potentially develop over time with this therapy is the "on–off

phenomenon," which is characterized by abrupt, unpredictable, and transient fluctuations in motor symptoms. The patient experiences a good response to therapy during the "on" phase, but then encounters symptoms of their underlying parkinsonism during the "off" period. Dyskinesias can occur in the "on" periods, but overall, mobility is improved. *(Aminoff, 2008, p. 869)*

25. **(C)** First choice antibiotic treatment for acute otitis media includes a 10-day course of amoxicillin (80 to 90 mg/kg/day in two divided doses) or a combination of erythromycin (50 mg/kg/day) and a sulfonamide (150 mg/kg/day). Reasons for amoxicillin therapy include spectrum of activity including both susceptible and intermediate resistant *S pneumoniae*, safety, cost, and tolerability. *(Schindler et al., 2008, p. 173)*

26. **(D)** Erythropoietin (EPO) is a naturally occurring hormone synthesized and secreted by the kidneys. Synthetic forms of EPO include Epogen and Procrit. EPO works at the red bone marrow to stimulate erythropoiesis. In patients with chronic renal failure, EPO production is usually impaired, and this EPO deficiency leads to anemia. Deferoxamine is an iron-chelating compound that can be given systemically in situations of iron overdose. Warfarin and argatroban are both anticoagulants and do not typically affect red cell count. Protamine sulfate is a heparin-chelating compound that can be given in cases of heparin overdose. *(Watnick and Morrison, 2008, p. 797)*

27. **(B)** In combination with β-blocker therapy, evidence demonstrates that ACE inhibitors further reduce cardiovascular risk in patients with coronary disease. Generally, β-blockers are not used in combination with other cardiac depressant drugs such as calcium channel blockers (eg, amlodipine). Discontinuing the patient's β-blocker therapy would be harmful, as the drug is indicated and working well for her chronic stable angina. Abrupt discontinuation of a β-blocker (without tapering) could cause problematic rebound hypertension. Doubling the metoprolol dose would pose a risk of lowering her heart rate below the current 54 bpm. *(Saseen and Maclaughlin, 2008, pp. 159, 161-162)*

28. **(B)** Polyethylene glycol (PEG) is an example of an osmotic laxative that leads to water retention in the bowel. It is often used when complete colonic cleansing is required prior to gastrointestinal endoscopic procedures or colorectal surgeries, and is not recommended for routine treatment of constipation. Senna is a plant derivative found in preparations such as Senokot and Ex-Lax. While the exact mechanism is unknown, it is believed that senna induces peristalsis by directly stimulating the enteric nervous system of the bowel. Docusate is a typical ingredient found in stool softeners, whereas methylcellulose is a plant product used in bulk-forming laxatives. Loperamide is not a laxative, but rather an antidiarrheal agent. *(Spruill and Wade, 2008, pp. 626-627)*

29. **(A)** Bupropion has been shown in some patients to cause seizures in a dose-dependent fashion, particularly in those with a history of head trauma or electrolyte abnormalities. Tricyclic antidepressants (eg, nortriptyline), selective serotonin reuptake inhibitors (eg, fluoxetine), serotonin-norepinephrine reuptake inhibitors (eg, duloxetine), and monoamine oxidase inhibitors (eg, phenelzine) have not been associated with seizures. *(Teter et al., 2008, pp. 1129-1130)*

30. **(B)** The patient is in need of long-term control therapy due to his worsening symptoms. Whenever increased use of a quick-relief medication such as a β2-agonist (albuterol) occurs, it is usually indicative of needing to add a long-term control agent to the therapeutic regimen or to increase the dose of an already prescribed long-term control medication. Inhaled corticosteroids like fluticasone are considered first-line long-term control medications for patients with persistent asthma. *(Chesnutt et al., 2008, pp. 212-213)*

31. **(D)** In the majority of cases, a combined hormonal contraceptive (ie, one that contains both an estrogen and progestin) is the preferred method of oral contraception because of its

efficacy when used perfectly (>99%). However, for women older than 35 years of age who are smokers or are obese, or who have a history of hypertension or vascular disease, progesterone-only contraceptives are recommended. Ethinyl estradiol (EE), the most common estrogen found in combined hormonal contraceptives, has been associated with an increased risk of myocardial infarction in women older than 35 years of age who are smokers. Additionally, EE has also been shown to cause increases in blood pressure in both normotensive and mildly hypertensive women. Progestin-only contraceptives, however, tend to be less effective than the combined hormonal contraceptives. (*Dickerson et al., 2008, pp. 1316-1320*)

32. **(A)** Via its interaction with mu (μ) receptors throughout the CNS, morphine and other related opioids not only produce an analgesic effect, but they also can cause respiratory depression, particularly as doses are increased. Typically, morphine will reduce the respiratory rate, which then leads to an increase in the levels of carbon dioxide (CO_2) in the blood and cerebrospinal fluid (CSF). In the patient with underlying pulmonary disease, whose ventilation and gas exchange efficiency may already be compromised, morphine has the potential to raise the CO_2 level further and also limit how much oxygen (O_2) can be breathed into the lungs. Excess CO_2 also has the effect of causing pronounced vasodilation of cerebral blood vessels, which results in an increase in ICP. Elevations in ICP can also reduce ventilation further. (*Bauman and Strickland, 2008, p. 998; Segal, 2009, p. 580*)

33. **(B)** Acyclovir is the treatment of choice for HSV disease, typically in oral doses of 200 mg five times daily or 400 mg three times daily. In situations where oral acyclovir cannot be absorbed effectively by the GI tract or tolerated by the patient, intravenous acyclovir can be administered at a rate of 15 mg/kg/day. (*Knodel, 2008, p. 1926*)

34. **(A)** α_1-blockers (eg, doxazosin, terazosin, and prazosin) can cause a potentially severe orthostatic hypotension that is associated with the

initial dose. This phenomenon can also occur with increases in dose. α_1-Blockers are peripheral vasodilators and the drop in blood pressure produces the symptoms of dizziness, faintness (as blood flow to the brain decreases due to the decrease in blood pressure), and palpitations (which is indicative of the heart trying to elevate its rate to increase blood pressure). These episodes can be better tolerated by patients if the first dose or dose increases are taken at bedtime. (*Saseen and Maclaughlin, 2008, p. 163*)

35. **(D)** In most patients suffering from generalized convulsive status epilepticus (GCSE), benzodiazepines such as lorazepam and diazepam are effective initial therapies due to their relatively high lipid solubility. As a result, they are able to cross the blood–brain barrier easily, which gives them the potential to stop seizures quickly. Lorazepam's lipid solubility is less compared to diazepam, and it also redistributes to fat more slowly. Hence, lorazepam tends to have a longer duration of action (12 to 24 hours) than diazepam (20 to 30 minutes). Phenytoin is often administered immediately after benzodiazepine administration for long-term seizure control, as it has a long half-life (20 to 36 hours) compared to diazepam. Phenytoin is not given first because its lipid solubility is less than the benzodiazepines and therefore cannot enter the brain quickly enough to terminate seizure activity. (*Phelps et al., 2008, pp. 956-958; Aminoff, 2008, pp. 847-848*)

36. **(C)** Gradual tapering of β-blockers over a period of 1 to 2 weeks is advised before discontinuation to avoid rebound hypertension, tachycardia, and sweating. Abrupt cessation of β-blockers has also been shown to cause unstable angina, myocardial infarction, and even death in the hypertensive patient with coronary artery disease. (*Saseen and Maclaughlin, 2008, p. 162*)

37. **(C)** Sildenafil and other selective phosphodiesterase (PDE) inhibitors (eg, tadalafil, vardenafil) profoundly potentiate the vasodilatory effects (eg, a greater than 25 mm Hg decrease in systolic blood pressure) of organic nitrates and

potentially life-threatening hypotension or hemodynamic collapse can result. Nitrates promote the formation of cyclic guanosine monophosphate (cGMP) by stimulating guanylate cyclase. Sildenafil acts to decrease the degradation of cGMP by inhibiting the enzyme that degrades it (PDE type 5). Together, these combined effects of the nitrate and PED-5 inhibitor result in increased accumulation of cGMP, which causes more pronounced smooth muscle relaxation and vasodilation than with either drug alone. In this scenario, the profound hypotension led to a significant decrease in coronary blood flow, thereby worsening the patient's ischemia that he was experiencing during his angina attack. Because of the serious risk of concomitant use of organic nitrates and selective PDE inhibitors, such combined use is contraindicated. *(Lee, 2008, pp. 1375-1378)*

38. **(A)** Myasthenia gravis is characterized by autoantibodies directed against nicotinic cholinergic receptors at neuromuscular junctions. By inhibiting the enzyme responsible for metabolizing acetylcholine (acetylcholinesterase), the synaptic concentration of acetylcholine increases and can bind more frequently to functional nicotinic receptors yet to be affected by the disease. This can alleviate the symptoms such as limb weakness, difficulty swallowing, and difficulty chewing associated with the disease. Examples of acetylcholinesterase inhibitors include neostigmine and pyridostigmine. *(Aminoff, 2008, pp. 892-893)*

39. **(D)** Warfarin is contraindicated in all trimesters and is listed as category X by the FDA, because it has been shown to induce fetal bleeding and cause several teratogenic effects including CNS malformations, structural deformities of the nose, and bone dysplasias. ACEIs (eg, captopril) should not be used due to their increased risk of causing fetal hypotension, fetal renal damage, and major congenital malformations. Isotretinoin is also listed as category X and is a known teratogen that causes malformations of the CNS, face, and ears. Misoprostol is a synthetic prostaglandin analog indicated for reducing the risk of NSAID-induced gastric ulcers in patients at high risk of complications

from gastric ulcer. It also has oxytocic properties, meaning that it can induce uterine contractions that may endanger pregnancy. The drug comes with a black box warning stating that administration to women who are pregnant can cause abortion, premature birth, or birth defects. Esomeprazole is category B and has not been shown to cause birth defects or threaten pregnancy. *(Saseen and Maclaughlin, 2008, p. 159; Haines et al., 2008, p. 352; Berardi and Welage, 2008, p. 582; Berger, 2008, p. 112)*

40. **(E)** Typical antipsychotics (eg, haloperidol, chlorpromazine, fluphenazine) can produce pseudoparkinsonism via blockade of dopamine (D_2) receptors in the nigrostriatum. Symptoms can include akinesia, bradykinesia, mask-like facial expression, tremor, cogwheel rigidity, and postural abnormalities. Tardive dyskinesia may also occur, as the reported incidence with first generation antipsychotics ranges from 0.5% to 62%. *(Carson et al., 2008, pp. 1111-1113)*

41. **(C)** As a CYP2D6 inducer, the antiepileptic medication will stimulate or increase the activity of the enzymes responsible for metabolizing the antihypertensive medication into harmless by-products. As a result, the patient is more susceptible to having his/her blood pressure elevate, because the dose of the antihypertensive drug is being cleared from the body more quickly. *(Bauer, 2008, p. 17)*

42. **(D)** This patient only has mild symptoms resulting from his PSVT. In these situations, nonpharmacologic measures that increase vagal activity (eg, Valsalva maneuver) to the heart can be attempted to help restore a sinus rhythm. Because this failed in our patient, drug therapy is the best option. Adenosine is often the drug of first choice in patients with PSVT, as it slows conduction and interrupts the reentry pathways through the AV node. Adenosine is capable of producing hypotension and would need to be used cautiously. However, adenosine has a short duration of action (6 to 10 seconds). Intravenous verapamil and diltiazem are equally efficacious in terminating PSVT and could also be used in this situation. *(Sanaski et al., 2008, pp. 297-298; Bashore et al., 2008, p. 326)*

43. **(B)** Warfarin interferes with the actions of vitamin K in the liver. Within hepatocytes, vitamin K is a cofactor required for the activation of clotting factors II (prothrombin), VII, IX, and X. By disrupting the actions of vitamin K, warfarin indirectly results in a slower rate of synthesis of these four clotting factors, thereby creating the anticoagulant effect. *(Haines et al., 2008, p. 347)*

44. **(B)** Disulfiram inhibits the hepatic enzyme aldehyde dehydrogenase in the biochemical pathway for alcohol degradation. This effect causes acetylaldehyde to accumulate which produces severe facial flushing, throbbing headache, nausea and vomiting, palpitations, weakness, dizziness, blurred vision, and confusion. This reaction only occurs if the patient drinks alcohol while taking disulfiram. In the absence of alcohol, disulfiram has little or no effect. *(Doering et al., 2008, p. 1088)*

45. **(A)** All β-lactam antibiotics, including the penicillins (eg, amoxicillin) and cephalosporins, prevent bacterial growth by inhibiting cell wall synthesis. Fluoroquinolones (eg, ciprofloxacin) block bacterial DNA synthesis. Erythromycin, doxycycline, and gentamicin all inhibit protein synthesis but via different mechanisms. *(Craig and Stitzel, 2004, pp. 519, 526, 538, 544)*

46. **(C)** Triptans (eg, sumitriptan, eletriptan, etc) are serotonin receptor agonists that are taken to help terminate and relieve pain associated with acute migraine attacks. During an attack, vasodilation of intracranial blood vessels occurs, leading to dural plasma extravasation, perivascular inflammation, and subsequent pain. Triptans help minimize these reactions by causing vasoconstriction of intracranial blood vessels. However, in the patient who has underlying cerebrovascular disease, vasoconstriction can further diminish blood flow, creating potentially dangerous hypoxic conditions in the brain. *(Minor and Wofford, 2008, pp. 1013-1014)*

47. **(A)** There are a few products on the market that are FDA-approved specifically for emergency contraception, including Plan B (two 0.75-mg tablets of levonorgestrel taken 12 hours apart). *(MacKay, 2008, p. 659)*

48. **(B)** If they coat the mouth and throat, inhaled corticosteroids (eg, triamcinolone, fluticasone, flunisolide) can alter the local bacteria and fungal population, thereby enhancing fungal growth. In cases of oropharyngeal candidiasis (thrush), white spots on the tongue and hard palate can be visualized, and the patient usually has pain on swallowing. In the asthma patient, the utilization of a spacer with a metered dose inhaler (MDI) can help minimize the chances of oropharyngeal candidiasis, as can routine gargling and rinsing following each inhaled treatment. Fluconazole is an antifungal agent that is effective in treating oropharyngeal candidiasis. *(Kelly and Sorkness, 2008 pp. 486-487; Schindler et al., 2008, p. 190; Chesnutt et al., 2008, p. 209)*

49. **(A)** The patient is most likely suffering from giardiasis that could have been contracted on her camping trip. While swimming, she may have inadvertently swallowed water contaminated with *Giardia lamblia*, whose incubation period is generally 1 to 3 weeks, after which symptoms develop. An effective treatment is metronidazole 250 mg taken three times daily for 5 to 7 days. *(Rosenthal and Goldsmith, 2008, pp. 1309-1310)*

50. **(E)** Metronidazole is the topical treatment of choice for rosacea, which is consistent with the clinical findings in this 34-year-old female patient. Mupirocin ointment is a treatment option for impetigo, whereas permethrin is indicated for scabies. Tretinoin is effective and is indicated for comedonal acne. Topical hydrocortisone has not been shown to be effective for rosacea. *(Berger, 2008, p. 113)*

51. **(D)** For sustained treatment of panic attacks, SSRIs are the initial drugs of choice. Sublingual benzodiazepines are often effective for urgent treatment. *(Eisendrath and Lichtmacher, 2008, p. 902)*

52. **(E)** Constipation is a common adverse effect of opioid therapy. In order to minimize or prevent constipation, the use of stool softeners (docusate) and a stimulant laxative (senna) can be initiated when opioid therapy is begun. *(Rabow and Pantilat, 2008, pp. 69, 78)*

53. **(E)** Whereas NSAIDs such as naproxen provide some symptomatic relief in rheumatoid arthritis, they do not alter disease progression like DMARDs (disease-modifying antirheumatic drugs). NSAIDs are best used in conjunction with DMARDs. Methotrexate is usually the DMARD of choice because it is well tolerated by the majority of patients and can produce beneficial effects in 2 to 6 weeks. Hydroxychloroquine is another DMARD that can be used for rheumatoid arthritis but can produce ocular toxicity. Cyclosporine and azathioprine are used less frequently today due to toxicity and lack of long-term benefits. Similar to naproxen, acetaminophen would also fail to alter disease progression. *(Schuna, 2008 pp. 1512-1513; Rabow and Pantilat, 2008, pp. 69, 78)*

54. **(D)** Leuprolide is a GnRH (LHRH) agonist that suppresses the pulsatile secretion of follicle stimulating hormone (FSH) and LH (gonadotropins) from the anterior pituitary when given chronically. Continuous administration of a GnRH agonist causes down-regulation of GnRH receptors on gonadotropes, which, in turn suppresses gonadotropin release and gonadal function. Decreased amounts of LH, in particular, lead to diminished production of androgens by the testes (especially DHT), which support prostate growth. It is believed that by interrupting the hormonal pathways that modulate prostatic growth, tumor development and metastasis is slowed. *(Kolesar, 2008, p. 2212; Jones, 2009, pp. 1151-1152)*

55. **(C)** Vinca alkaloids (eg, vincristine, vinblastine) bind to tubulin, the structural protein that forms the microtubules, which comprise the mitotic spindle. Through this binding, the microtubules are unable to assemble to form the mitotic spindle, which results in a cell's (both normal and cancerous) inability to divide. *(Medina and Fausel, 2008, p. 2098)*

56. **(B)** Tricyclic antidepressants (eg, nortriptyline) produce anticholinergic side effects not seen with other types of antidepressants such as SSRIs, SNRIs, and MAOIs. Anticholinergic side effects include dry mouth, constipation, pho-tophobia, blurred vision, urinary retention, and tachycardia. *(Teter et al., 2008, p. 1129)*

57. **(E)** Stimulants (eg, amphetamines, methylphenidate) are considered first-line therapy in the majority of cases of ADHD. Both amphetamines and methylphenidate block dopamine and norepinephrine reuptake, while amphetamines also stimulate norepinephrine release. Elevated levels of CNS norepinephrine have been associated with an anorexigenic effect, leading to reduce caloric intake. *(Dopheide et al., 2008, pp. 1030-1033)*

58. **(D)** Tubocurarine and rocuronium are classified as nondepolarizing neuromuscular blocking drugs, whereas succinylcholine is depolarizing. Nondepolarizing agents competitively block nicotinic receptors on skeletal muscle, which leads to flaccid muscle paralysis. Depolarizing agents, on the other hand, activate nicotinic receptors on skeletal muscle cells leading to membrane depolarization, initial fasciculations, and intense contractions. Succinylcholine is not metabolized efficiently at neuromuscular junctions; hence, the cells remain depolarized and are unable to repolarize or recover back to a resting state. This failure to repolarize then leads to a flaccid muscle paralysis. Pyridostigmine in an acetylcholinesterase inhibitor indicated for myasthenia gravis and causes an increase in skeletal muscle activity. *(Craig and Stitzel, 2004, pp. 341-344)*

59. **(D)** Pernicious anemia is a chronic illness caused by impaired absorption of vitamin B_{12} due to a lack of intrinsic factor (IF) production by the gastric mucosa. Replacement therapy with intramuscular injections of vitamin B_{12} is often used to treat this condition. An alternative is Nascobal, a synthetic form of vitamin B_{12} as a nasally administered gel. *(Linker, 2008, p. 429)*

60. **(B)** All aminoglycosides are ototoxic and nephrotoxic. The likelihood of experiencing these toxicities occurs when treatment lasts beyond 5 days, at higher doses, in elderly patients, and those suffering from renal insufficiency. Other agents that produce either of these toxicities should not be used concurrently. *(Craig and Stitzel, 2004, pp. 541-542)*

61. (B) Long-acting β_2-agonists are the preferred adjunctive therapy to inhaled corticosteroids in the long-term treatment of more severe forms of asthma. A combination of an inhaled corticosteroid and long-acting β_2-agonist provides greater asthma control than increasing the dose of the inhaled corticosteroid alone. Because they lack anti-inflammatory properties, long-acting β_2-agonists should not be used as monotherapy for long-term control of asthma, because alone they increase the risk of asthma-related death. *(Kelly and Sorkness, 2008, pp. 487-488)*

62. (D) A combination of a loop diuretic and an ACE inhibitor is typically the initial treatment in most symptomatic patients with congestive heart failure. ACE inhibitors have been demonstrated to not only reduce symptoms but also mortality in patients with symptomatic heart failure. Loop diuretics offer the best option to reduce the congestive symptoms in the lungs and fluid retention in the ankles. *(Bashore et al., 2008, pp. 344-345)*

63. (B) The amount of steroid in a combined hormonal contraceptive accounts for many adverse effects than occur while taking the medication. Ethinyl estradiol excess can lead to nausea and bloating, whereas low-dose ethinyl estradiol can cause early or mid-cycle breakthrough bleeding and spotting. Low-dose progestin (eg, desogestrel, norethindrone) can lead to late-cycle breakthrough bleeding and spotting, whereas high dose progestin can cause weight gain, bloating, and constipation. Combined hormonal contraceptives do not contain luteinizing hormone or testosterone. *(Dickerson et al., 2008, p. 1317)*

64. (A) Bile acid resins (eg, cholestyramine, colestipol, colesevelam) are used for lowering LDL-C. They sequester bile acids in the intestinal lumen, thereby preventing them from carrying out their normal functions of emulsification and micelle formation. Emulsification is an important process for lipid digestion, while the formation of micelles is required for lipid absorption. These actions not only inhibit lipid digestion and absorption from the intestinal lumen, but they also deplete the hepatic pool of cholesterol as a result of increased bile acid synthesis. Normally, bile acids are recirculated

(enterohepatic circulation) from the intestine and back to the liver for reincorporation into the bile. Resins cause the bile acids to be excreted with the feces, so the liver needs to continually synthesize new bile acids from endogenous cholesterol. Constipation, abdominal distention, bloating, and flatulence result from the increased lipid content of the stool, because lipids are not being absorbed across the intestinal wall. These adverse effects can often be managed by increasing fluid and fiber intake and also using stool softeners. *(Talbert, 2008, pp. 395-397)*

65. (C) The patient is showing signs and symptoms of schizophrenia for which antipsychotic agents are the treatment of choice. Olanzapine is an atypical antipsychotic (eg, second-generation) that has less risk of causing extrapyramidal side effects (EPS) compared to typical antipsychotics (eg, first-generation) such as thioridazine. Because of the risk of EPS, typical or first-generation antipsychotics are not considered first-line treatments. Even though both typical and atypical antipsychotics appear to have similar efficacy, the atypical agents also tend to be better tolerated, which enhances compliance. *(Crismon et al., 2008, pp. 1103-1105; Eisendrath and Lichtmacher, 2008, pp. 913)*

66. (E) Benzodiazepines bind to $GABA_A$ receptors, which consist of many peripheral subunits that form chloride channels at their core. GABA is one of the major inhibitory neurotransmitters in the brain; hence, benzodiazepines enhance this inhibitory influence to produce sedation and calm. *(Kirkwood and Melton, 2008, p. 1167)*

67. (C) Sublingual nitroglycerin produces venodilation and vasodilation, which causes secondary responses of flushing and headache. The elevated pulse or tachycardia is reflexive in nature, and the heart tries to compensate for the drop in blood pressure by raising its rate. *(Talbert, 2008, pp. 237-239)*

68. (C) Triamterene is a K^+-sparing diuretic based on its mechanism of action. In the kidneys, it will lead to less K^+ excretion in the urine and hence retention of plasma K^+. In patients with elevated plasma K^+, triamterene can cause further hyperkalemia, which can impact neuro-muscular and cardiac function. *(Saseen and Maclaughlin, 2008, pp. 158-159; Brophy and Gehr, 2008, p. 882)*

69. **(C)** Leukotrienes are inflammatory mediators that are generated within the lungs. When they bind to specific receptors, they induce a variety of responses, including bronchospasm and mucus production. Zafirlukast (and also montelukast) are leukotriene receptor antagonists that block these effects in the lungs and improve asthma symptoms. Zafirlukast is considered an alternative therapy for long-term control of asthma, as it has been shown to be less effective than inhaled corticosteroids. Both cromolyn and nedocromil are mast cell stabilizers and can also be used as an alternative treatment to inhaled corticosteroids. Omalizumab is an anti-IgE antibody, whereas ipratropium bromide is a muscarinic receptor antagonist. *(Kelly, 2008, pp. 478, 488-490)*

70. **(E)** Intravenous nitroprusside is a common medication used for hypertensive emergencies. It is metabolized to cyanide and then to thiocyanate, which is excreted in the urine. The level of thiocyanate should be monitored if nitroprusside infusion lasts longer than 72 hours. The risk of cyanide toxicity and thiocyanate accumulation is increased in patients with a history of impaired renal function. *(Saseen and Maclaughlin, 2008, pp. 165-166)*

71. **(D)** It is estimated that in females with gonorrhea, coexisting chlamydial infection occurs 50% of the time. For gonococcal urethritis, the treatment of choice is ceftriaxone. In cases of coexistent chlamydial infection, either doxycycline or azithromycin are recommended. *(Chambers, 2008, pp. 1257-1258)*

72. **(E)** Calcium channel blockers can cause cardiac conduction abnormalities such as bradycardia or atrioventricular block. Similarly β-blockers are associated with bradycardia and atrioventicular conduction abnormalities, particularly second- and third-degree heart block. Their effects in producing these responses can be additive, and hence, they are not rec-

ommended for concomitant use. *(Saseen and Maclaughlin, 2008, pp. 160-162)*

73. **(C)** Heparin-induced thrombocytopenia (HIT) is a potentially serious complication of unfractionated heparin therapy, usually occurring within 4 to 10 days after heparin treatment has started. Fortunately, current estimates show that it is infrequent, occurring in approximately 0.3% to 3.0% of patients receiving UFH for more than 4 days. HIT should immediately be suspected in a patient who develops deep vein thrombosis or pulmonary embolism while receiving UFH. *(Whitby and Johns, 2008, pp. 1710-1712)*

74. **(D)** Nitrofurantoin has been shown to be a safe and effective drug during pregnancy for treating UTIs. Tetracyclines, fluoroquinolones, and sulfonamides are not recommended for use in pregnancy because of the various risks they pose on the fetus. *(Crombleholme, 2008, p. 683; Watnick and Morrison, 2008, pp. 817-819)*

75. **(C)** Nicotine replacement therapy is relatively safe in the majority of patients and comes in many forms (transdermal patches, gums, sprays, and inhalers). Both clonidine and nortriptyline are considered second-line smoking cessation agents because of their many side effects. Neither has been approved by the FDA for smoking cessation. Alprazolam is also not indicated, and there is currently no evidence that it aids in smoking cessation. Varenicline is a relatively new agent for smoking cessation and is a partial agonist to α_4-β_2 nicotinic acetylcholine receptors. It has been approved by the FDA; however, varenicline is banned from use by pilots and air traffic controllers as per the Federal Aviation Administration (FAA) *(Doering et al., 2008, pp. 1090-1094)*

76. **(C)** Neuroleptic malignant syndrome is an uncommon but serious complication with therapeutic doses of antipsychotic drug therapy, particularly the first-generation (typical) class. Cardinal signs and symptoms include a body temperature above 100.4°F, altered state of consciousness, autonomic dysfunction, and rigidity. *(Crismon et al., 2008, pp. 1113-1114; Eisendrath and Lichtmacher, 2008, pp. 917-919)*

77. (B) β-Blockers are capable of crossing the blood–brain barrier and, hence, can cause CNS side effects. In general, drugs that are more lipophilic can cross the blood–brain barrier more efficiently compared to drugs that are less lipophilic. Each β-blocker has a different degree of lipophilicity based on its chemical structure. *(Saseen and Maclaughlin, 2008, p. 162)*

78. (A) Doxorubicin is a common antineoplastic drug used for a variety of cancers, including breast, bladder, ovarian, and endometrial, among many others. Unfortunately, it has a well-established, dose-dependent adverse effect on the heart that is linked to free-radical formation. *(Medina and Fausel, 2008, p. 2099)*

79. (E) Nonselective β-blockers can mask many of the signs and symptoms of hypoglycemia in patients who tightly regulate their blood glucose levels. This is due to the fact that many of the symptoms are mediated through the sympathetic nervous system and β-receptors, including tachycardia, palpitations, and tremor. Sweating is another warning sign of hypoglycemia, but should still occur with β-blocker therapy, because it is mediated via cholinergic receptors. *(Saseen and Maclaughlin, 2008, p. 154)*

80. (A) Recommended drug regimens for Chlamydial cervicitis include a single oral 1-g dose of azithromycin, 100 mg of doxycycline orally for 7 days or 500 mg of levofloxacin orally for 7 days. *(Chambers, 2008, p. 1266)*

81. (E) Naloxone is a specific opioid antagonist administered intravenously in cases of opioid overdose. It is a short-acting drug that may require repeated doses if the offending opioid has a long duration of action. *(Olson, 2008, p. 1380)*

82. (B) Salicylic acid is a commonly used keratolytic that is typically applied as a lotion or gel (2% to 10% concentration) to corn pads. It is also indicated for the treatment of common warts, but is used in higher concentrations (17%). *(Berger, 2008, pp. 122-123)*

83. (C) Thiazide diuretics can raise plasma levels of uric acid, which can be problematic in patients who already have hyperuricemia or a previous history of gout. Calcium channel blockers, ACE inhibitors, angiotensin receptor blockers, and β-blockers have not been shown to raise plasma levels of uric acid. *(Saseen and Maclaughlin, 2008, p. 158)*

84. (B) Insulin not only causes cellular uptake of glucose but also of potassium. Hypokalemia may develop when insulin is infused to correct either a hyperglycemic hyperosmolar state or a diabetic ketoacidosis. Hence, in order to avoid hypokalemia, potassium chloride can be added to a saline solution, as long as the serum potassium is not elevated. *(Masharani, 2008, pp. 1065-1067)*

85. (B) Certain medications have been implicated in decreasing the efficacy of oral contraceptives, including rifampin and some of the antiepileptics (AEDs). A back-up method of contraception is suggested for females taking rifampin and combined hormonal contraceptives concomitantly on a short-term basis. If they are taken for longer periods of time, the patient should consider an alternative method of contraception. Similarly, for those patients taking either phenytoin or carbamazepine for seizure disorder, an alternative method of contraception is highly recommended. *(Dickerson et al., 2008, p. 1322)*

86. (A) Bisphosphonates (eg, alendronate, risedronate, ibandronate) are the prescription drug of choice for osteoporosis over raloxifene, calcitonin, estrogen, and vitamin D due to their consistent ability to provide the greatest fracture risk reductions and bone mineral density increases. While some of these other medications can cause similar effects, they do so to a lesser extent. In particular, the risks of estrogen therapy outweigh the benefits on the bone as suggested by recent data from the Women's Health Initiative trials. *(O'Connell and Vondracek, 2008, pp. 1492-1497)*

87. (C) Acetylcholinesterase inhibitors for Alzheimer disease were designed around the "cholinergic hypothesis," which stated that the replenishment of acetylcholine could help restore memory and cognitive ability, both of which are lost as the disease progresses. While numerous cholinergic pathways are destroyed during Alzheimer disease, many others are also lost. Even though these acetylcholinesterase inhibitors are indicated for Alzheimer disease, they are not curative and do not restore function. *(Slattum et al., 2008, pp. 1053, 1057)*

88. **(A)** Allopurinol is an inhibitor of xanthine oxidase, a key enzyme necessary for the production of uric acid. It is the most commonly prescribed drug for the long-term management of gout and is an effective prophylactic agent. Probenecid can also be prescribed as prophylactic therapy for gout. However, it is classified as a uricosuric drug, meaning it increases the renal clearance of uric acid rather than affecting uric acid synthesis. Colchicine is an antimitotic drug that can relieve acute attacks of gout, but also does not affect uric acid synthesis. Cyclosporine and sulfasalazine are not indicated for acute management of gout or for prophylactic therapy. *(Ernst et al., 2008, pp. 1543-1544, 1546-1547)*

89. **(E)** The second-generation antihistamines such as loratadine, fexofenadine, and desloratadine are nonsedating when taken at recommended doses. Because the patient is employed as a taxi driver, remaining alert is of prime importance. First-generation antihistamines (eg, diphenhydramine, clemastine) have a much higher potential for causing sedation and should be avoided in this particular patient. *(May and Smith, 2008, pp. 1569-1571)*

90. **(E)** In March 2004, the FDA instructed manufacturers of all antidepressants to include in their labeling a boxed warning and expanded warning statements about the increased risk of suicidal thinking and behavior in children and adolescents being treated with these drugs. This directive was based on a combined analysis of several studies that concluded the risk of suicidal behavior to be twice as high (4% vs 2%) in children and adolescents receiving antidepressants versus placebo. *(Teter et al., 2008, p. 1134)*

91. **(B)** Bioavailability represents the fraction of an administered drug that reaches the systemic circulation. Because the intravenous route represents direct administration of a drug into the

circulation, the bioavailability would be 100%. All of the other routes listed as choices possess biologic barriers to a drug before it can be absorbed into the vasculature. These barriers can often impede a percentage of the drug dose from reaching the blood. Additionally, some drugs (particularly when given orally) can also be metabolized by enzymes or influenced by the first-pass effect through the liver before reaching the circulation. *(Bauer, 2008, pp. 11-12)*

92. **(A)** Intramuscular administration of epinephrine is the drug of choice to quickly reverse the considerable vasodilation (and subsequent drop in blood pressure) and bronchoconstriction that often occurs with anaphylaxis. Several adjunctive therapies (eg, intravenous fluids, antihistamines, corticosteroids) may also be necessary to help maintain blood pressure, reduce inflammation, and prevent bronchospasm. However, epinephrine should be the first drug administered. *(DiPiro, 2008, pp. 1455-1456; Kishiyama and Adelman, 2008, pp. 690-691)*

93. **(A)** *Pasteurella multocida* is the typical cause of an early infection (within 24 hours) due to a cat bite. Penicillins offer the best coverage for *P multocida*, compared to other antibiotics. *(Fish et al., 2008, pp. 1814-1816; Jacobs et al., 2008, pp. 1114-1115)*

94. **(C)** Chemotherapy-induced nausea and vomiting (CINV) is a common problem for cancer patients that can often be avoided if treated prophylactically. Patients who receive chemotherapeutic regimens that are classified as being of moderate emetic risk should receive a selective serotonin receptor inhibitor (eg, SSRI; ondansetron, granisetron, dolasetron) and dexamethasone. The efficacy of the SSRI is enhanced when used concomitantly with dexamethasone. Antiemetics known as phenothiazines (eg, prochlorperazine) and metoclopramide can cause extrapyramidal side effects, and hence would not be advised for use in patients with parkinsonism. *(DiPiro, 2008, pp. 611-612; Rugo, 2008, pp. 1445-1446)*

95. **(B)** The patient's symptoms are consistent with long-term lithium therapy, which can cause a variety of neuropsychiatric side effects (eg,

tremor, ataxia, mental confusion, fatigue, poor concentration). Lithium is also known to produce adverse effects on the kidneys that can lead to nephrogenic diabetes insipidus and increased serum creatinine concentrations. *(Drayton and Weinstein, 2008, pp. 1155-1156; Eisendrath and Lichtmacher, 2008, pp. 929-930)*

96. **(D)** ACEIs not only inhibit the conversion of angiotensin I to angiotensin II, but they also block the metabolism of bradykinin, thus elevating bradykinin levels. Cough and other side effects of ACEIs are believed to be due to increased bradykinin. ARBs do not inhibit bradykinin metabolism; instead these block angiotensin receptors. Hence, they have limited, if any, potential in causing cough. *(Saseen and Maclaughlin, 2008, pp. 159-160)*

97. **(B)** There are several clinically important warfarin drug interactions, with most of them causing an increase in the drug's anticoagulant effect (ie, increasing the INR). Warfarin metabolism occurs via hepatic cytochrome P450 enzymes that can be inhibited by a large number of drugs, including the fluoroquinolones. When this inhibition occurs, plasma levels of warfarin rise, thereby enhancing the anticoagulant effect. *(Haines et al., 2008, pp. 347-352)*

98. **(B)** The pathogenesis of Reye syndrome is unknown, but there appears to be a potential association between aspirin use and the development of the disease. Reye syndrome is marked by hepatic failure and encephalopathy and has a poor prognosis. *(Kirchain and Allen, 2008, p. 652; Koo and Shandera, 2008, p. 1210)*

99. **(B)** Both organic nitrates and calcium channel blockers are effective prophylactically for spasm of coronary arteries. The use of β-blockers is not advised because the use of these drugs can cause unopposed α_1-mediated vasoconstriction of coronary arteries, thereby worsening the ischemia. ACE inhibitors do not have a role in the treatment of variant angina. *(Talbert, 2008, p. 241; Bashore et al., 2008, p. 307)*

100. **(D)** Regular insulin is a short-acting insulin that starts working 30 to 60 minutes after administration. Increasing the dose by a few units can help quickly restore a normoglycemic state. NPH is an intermediate-acting insulin, which has an onset of action of 2 to 4 hours. Therefore, adjusting the NPH dose at breakfast time will not correct the morning hyperglycemia. If the NPH dose was increased, it could cause him to experience hypoglycemia in the middle of the day once it starts to work. *(Triplitt et al., 2008, pp. 1216-1219)*

REFERENCES

Aminoff MJ. Nervous system disorders. In: Tierney LM Jr, McPhee SJ, Papadakis MA, eds. *Current Medical Diagnosis & Treatment.* 47th ed. New York: McGraw-Hill; 2008.

Baron RB. Lipid abnormalities. In: Tierney LM Jr, McPhee SJ, Papadakis MA, eds. *Current Medical Diagnosis & Treatment.* 47th ed. New York: McGraw-Hill; 2008.

Barrett EJ. The thyroid gland. In: Boron WF, Boulpaep EL, eds. *Medical Physiology.* 2nd ed. Philadelphia, PA; Saunders Elsevier; 2009.

Bashore TM, Granger CB, Hranitzky P. Heart disease. In: Tierney LM Jr, McPhee SJ, Papadakis MA, eds. *Current Medical Diagnosis & Treatment.* 47th ed. New York: McGraw-Hill; 2008.

Bauer LA. Clinical pharmacokinetics & pharmacodynamics. In: DiPiro JT, Talbert RL, Yee GC, et al., eds. *Pharmacotherapy: A Pathophysiologic Approach.* 7th ed. New York: McGraw-Hill; 2008.

Baumann TJ, Strickland J. Pain management. In: DiPiro JT, Talbert RL, Yee GC, et al., eds. *Pharmacotherapy: A Pathophysiologic Approach.* 7th ed. New York: McGraw-Hill; 2008.

Berardi RR, Welage LS. Peptic ulcer disease. In: DiPiro JT, Talbert RL, Yee GC, et al., eds. *Pharmacotherapy: A Pathophysiologic Approach.* 7th ed. New York: McGraw-Hill; 2008.

Berger TG. Dermatologic disorders. In: Tierney LM Jr, McPhee SJ, Papadakis MA, eds. *Current Medical*

Diagnosis & Treatment. 47th ed. New York: McGraw-Hill; 2008.

Brophy DF, Gehr TWB. Disorders of potassium and magnesium homeostasis. In: DiPiro JT, Talbert RL, Yee GC, et al., eds. *Pharmacotherapy: A Pathophysiologic Approach.* 7th ed. New York: McGraw-Hill; 2008.

Carson ML, Argo TR, Buckley PF. Schizophrenia. In: DiPiro JT, Talbert RL, Yee GC, et al., eds. *Pharmacotherapy: A Pathophysiologic Approach.* 7th ed. New York: McGraw-Hill; 2008.

Chambers HF. Bacterial & chlamydial infections. In: Tierney LM Jr, McPhee SJ, Papadakis MA, eds. *Current Medical Diagnosis & Treatment.* 47th ed. New York: McGraw-Hill; 2008.

Chesnutt MS, Murray JA, Prendergast TJ. Pulmonary disorders. In: Tierney LM Jr, McPhee SJ, Papadakis MA, eds. *Current Medical Diagnosis & Treatment.* 47th ed. New York: McGraw-Hill; 2008.

Coyle EA, Prince RA. Urinary tract infections and prostatitis. In: DiPiro JT, Talbert RL, Yee GC, et al., eds. *Pharmacotherapy: A Pathophysiologic Approach.* 7th ed. New York: McGraw-Hill; 2008.

Craig CR, Stitzel RE. *Modern Pharmacology with Clinical Applications.* 6th ed. Baltimore, MD: Lippincott Williams & Wilkins; 2004.

Crismon ML, Argo TR, Buckley PF. Schizophrenia. In: DiPiro JT, Talbert RL, Yee GC, et al. eds. *Pharmacotherapy: A Pathophysiologic Approach.* 7th ed. New York: McGraw-Hill; 2008.

Crombleholme WR. Obstetrics & Obstetric Disorders. In: Tierney LM Jr, McPhee SJ, Papadakis MA, eds. *Current Medical Diagnosis & Treatment 2008.* 47th ed. New York: McGraw-Hill; 2008.

Delafuente JC, Cappazzo KA. Systemic lupus erythematosus and other collagen vascular diseases. In: DiPiro JT, Talbert RL, Yee GC, et al., eds. *Pharmacotherapy: A Pathophysiologic Approach.* 7th ed. New York: McGraw-Hill; 2008.

Dickerson LM, Shrader SP, Diaz VA. Contraception. In: DiPiro JT, Talbert RL, Yee GC, et al., eds. *Pharmacotherapy: A Pathophysiologic Approach.* 7th ed. New York: McGraw-Hill; 2008.

DiPiro CV. Nausa and vomiting. In: DiPiro JT, Talbert RL, Yee GC, et al, eds. *Pharmacotherapy: A Pathophysiologic Approach.* 7th ed. New York: McGraw-Hill; 2008a.

DiPiro JT. Allergic and pseudoallergic drug reactions. In: DiPiro JT, Talbert RL, Yee GC, et al., eds. *Pharmacotherapy: A Pathophysiologic Approach.* 7th ed. New York: McGraw-Hill; 2008b.

Doering PL, Kennedy WK, Boothby LA. Substance-related disorders: Alcohol, nicotine and caffeine. In: DiPiro JT, Talbert RL, Yee GC, et al., eds. *Pharmacotherapy: A Pathophysiologic Approach.* 7th ed. New York: McGraw-Hill; 2008.

Dopheide JA, Tesoro JT, Malkin M. Childhood disorders. In: DiPiro JT, Talbert RL, Yee GC, et al., eds. *Pharmacotherapy: A Pathophysiologic Approach.* 7th ed. New York: McGraw-Hill; 2008.

Drayton SJ, Weinstein B. Bipolar disorder. In: DiPiro JT, Talbert RL, Yee GC, et al., eds. *Pharmacotherapy: A Pathophysiologic Approach.* 7th ed. New York: McGraw-Hill; 2008.

Eisendrath SJ, Lichtmacher JE. Psychiatric disorders. In: Tierney LM Jr, McPhee SJ, Papadakis MA, eds. *Current Medical Diagnosis & Treatment.* 47th ed. New York: McGraw-Hill; 2008.

Ernst ME, Clark EC, Hawkins DW. Gout and hyperuricemia. In: DiPiro JT, Talbert RL, Yee GC, et al., eds. *Pharmacotherapy: A Pathophysiologic Approach.* 7th ed. New York: McGraw-Hill; 2008.

Fish DN, Pendland SL, Danziger LH. Skin and soft tissue infections. In: DiPiro JT, Talbert RL, Yee GC, et al., eds. *Pharmacotherapy: A Pathophysiologic Approach.* 7th ed. New York: McGraw-Hill; 2008.

Fitzgerald PA. Endocrine disorders. In: Tierney LM Jr, McPhee SJ, Papadakis MA, eds. *Current Medical Diagnosis & Treatment.* 47th ed. New York: McGraw-Hill; 2008.

Haines ST, Witt DM, Nutescu EA. Venous thromboembolism. In: DiPiro JT, Talbert RL, Yee GC, et al,. eds. *Pharmacotherapy: A Pathophysiologic Approach.* 7th ed. New York: McGraw-Hill; 2008.

Jacobs RA, Guglielmo BJ, Chin-Hong PV. Common problems in infectious diseases and antimicrobial therapy. In: Tierney LM, Jr, McPhee SJ, Papadakis MA, eds. *Current Medical Diagnosis & Treatment.* 47th ed. New York: McGraw-Hill; 2008.

Jones EE. The female reproductive system. In: Boron WF, Boulpaep EL, eds. *Medical Physiology.* 2nd. Philadelphia, PA; Saunders Elsevier; 2009.

Kelly HW, Sorkness CA. Asthma. In: DiPiro JT, Talbert RL, Yee GC, et al., eds. *Pharmacotherapy: A Pathophysiologic Approach.* 7th ed. New York: McGraw-Hill; 2008.

Kirchain WR, Allen RE. Drug-induced liver disease. In: DiPiro JT, Talbert RL, Yee GC, et al., eds. *Pharmacotherapy: A Pathophysiologic Approach.* 7th ed. New York: McGraw-Hill; 2008.

Kirkwood CK, Melton ST. Anxiety disorders I: generalized anxiety, panic and social anxiety disorders. In: DiPiro JT, Talbert RL, Yee GC, et al., eds. *Pharmacotherapy: A Pathophysiologic Approach.* 7th ed. New York: McGraw-Hill; 2008.

Kishiyama JL, Adelman DC. Allergic and immunologic disorders. In: Tierney LM Jr, McPhee SJ, Papadakis MA, eds. *Current Medical Diagnosis & Treatment.* 47th ed. New York: McGraw-Hill; 2008.

Knodel LC. Sexually transmitted diseases. In: DiPiro JT, Talbert RL, Yee GC, et al., eds. *Pharmacotherapy: A Pathophysiologic Approach.* 7th ed. New York: McGraw-Hill; 2008.

Kolesar JM. Prostate cancer. In: DiPiro JT, Talbert RL, Yee GC, et al., eds. *Pharmacotherapy: A Pathophysiologic Approach.* 7th ed. New York: McGraw-Hill; 2008.

Koo H, Shandera WX. Viral & rickettsial infections. In: Tierney LM Jr, McPhee SJ, Papadakis MA, eds. *Current Medical Diagnosis & Treatment.* 47th ed. New York: McGraw-Hill; 2008.

Lee M. Erectile dysfunction. In: DiPiro JT, Talbert RL, Yee GC, et al., eds. *Pharmacotherapy: A Pathophysiologic Approach.* 7th ed. New York: McGraw-Hill; 2008a.

Lee M. Management of benign prostatic hyperplasia. In: DiPiro JT, Talbert RL, Yee GC, et al., eds. *Pharmacotherapy: A Pathophysiologic Approach.* 7th ed. New York: McGraw-Hill; 2008b.

Linker CA. Blood disorders. In: Tierney LM Jr, McPhee SJ, Papadakis MA, eds. *Current Medical Diagnosis & Treatment.* 47th ed. New York: McGraw-Hill; 2008.

MacKay HT. Gynecology. In: Tierney LM Jr, McPhee SJ, Papadakis MA, eds. *Current Medical Diagnosis & Treatment.* 47th ed. New York: McGraw-Hill; 2008.

Martin S, Jung R. Gastrointestinal infections and enterotoxigenic poisonings. In: DiPiro JT, Talbert RL, Yee GC, et al., eds. *Pharmacotherapy: A Pathophysiologic Approach.* 7th ed. New York: McGraw-Hill; 2008.

Masharani U. Diabetes mellitus & hypoglycemia. In: Tierney LM Jr, McPhee SJ, Papadakis MA, eds. *Current Medical Diagnosis & Treatment.* 47th ed. New York: McGraw-Hill; 2008.

May JR, Smith PH. Allergic rhinitis. In: DiPiro JT, Talbert RL, Yee GC, et al., eds. *Pharmacotherapy: A Pathophysiologic Approach.* 7th ed. New York: McGraw-Hill; 2008.

McQuaid KR. Gastrointestinal disorders. In: Tierney LM Jr, McPhee SJ, Papadakis MA, eds. *Current Medical Diagnosis & Treatment.* 47th ed. New York: McGraw-Hill; 2008.

Medina PJ, Fausel C. Cancer treatment and chemotherapy. In: DiPiro JT, Talbert RL, Yee GC, et al., eds. *Pharmacotherapy: A Pathophysiologic Approach.* 7th ed. New York: McGraw-Hill; 2008.

Minor DS, Wofford MR. Headache disorders. In: DiPiro JT, Talbert RL, Yee GC, et al., eds. *Pharmacotherapy: A Pathophysiologic Approach.* 7th ed. New York: McGraw-Hill; 2008.

O'Connell MB, Vondracek SF. Osteoporosis and other metabolic bone diseases. In: DiPiro JT, Talbert RL, Yee GC, et al., eds. *Pharmacotherapy: A Pathophysiologic Approach.* 7th ed. New York: McGraw-Hill; 2008.

Olson KR. Poisoning. In: Tierney LM Jr, McPhee SJ, Papadakis MA, eds. *Current Medical Diagnosis & Treatment.* 47th ed. New York: McGraw-Hill; 2008.

Parker RB, Rodgers JE, Cavallari LH. Heart failure. In: DiPiro JT, Talbert RL, Yee GC, et al., eds. *Pharmacotherapy: A Pathophysiologic Approach.* 7th ed. New York: McGraw-Hill; 2008.

Phelps SJ, Hovinga CA, Wheless JW. Status epilepticus. In: DiPiro JT, Talbert RL, Yee GC, et al., eds. *Pharmacotherapy: A Pathophysiologic Approach.* 7th ed. New York: McGraw-Hill; 2008.

Rabow MW, Pantilat SZ. Palliative care & pain management. In: Tierney LM Jr, McPhee SJ, Papadakis MA, eds. *Current Medical Diagnosis & Treatment.* 47th ed. New York: McGraw-Hill; 2008.

Rosenthal PJ, Goldsmith RS. Protozoal and helminthic infections. In: DiPiro JT, Talbert RL, Yee GC, et al., eds. *Pharmacotherapy: A Pathophysiologic Approach.* 7th ed. New York: McGraw-Hill; 2008.

Rugo HS. Cancer. In: Tierney LM Jr, McPhee SJ, Papadakis MA, eds. *Current Medical Diagnosis & Treatment.* 47th ed. New York: McGraw-Hill; 2008.

Sanaski CA, Schoen MD, Bauman JL. The arrhythmias. In: DiPiro JT, Talbert RL, Yee GC, et al., eds. *Pharmacotherapy: A Pathophysiologic Approach.* 7th ed. New York: McGraw-Hill; 2008.

Sassen JJ, Maclaughlin EJ. Hypertension. In: DiPiro JT, Talbert RL, Yee GC, et al., eds. *Pharmacotherapy: A Pathophysiologic Approach.* 7th ed. New York: McGraw-Hill; 2008.

Schindler J, Lustig L, Jackler RK, et al. Ear, nose & throat. In: Tierney LM Jr, McPhee SJ, Papadakis MA, eds. *Current Medical Diagnosis & Treatment.* 47th ed. New York: McGraw-Hill; 2008.

Schuna AA. Rheumatoid arthritis. In: DiPiro JT, Talbert RL, Yee GC, et al., eds. *Pharmacotherapy: A Pathophysiologic Approach.* 7th ed. New York: McGraw-Hill; 2008.

Segal SS. Special circulations. In: Boron WF, Boulpaep EL, eds. *Medical Physiology.* 2nd. ed. Philadelphia, PA; Saunders Elsevier; 2009.

Sherman SI, Talbert RL. Thyroid disorders. In: DiPiro JT, Talbert RL, Yee GC, et al., eds. *Pharmacotherapy: A Pathophysiologic Approach.* 7th ed. New York: McGraw-Hill; 2008.

Slattum PW, Swerdlow RH, Hill AM. Alzheimer's disease. In: DiPiro JT, Talbert RL, Yee GC, et al., eds. *Pharmacotherapy: A Pathophysiologic Approach.* 7th ed. New York: McGraw-Hill; 2008.

Spinler SA, deDunus S. Acute coronary syndromes. In: DiPiro JT, Talbert RL, Yee GC, et al., eds. *Pharmacotherapy: A Pathophysiologic Approach.* 7th ed. New York: McGraw-Hill; 2008.

Spruill WJ, Wade WE. Diarrhea, constipation and irritable bowel syndrome. In: DiPiro JT, Talbert RL, Yee GC, et al., eds. *Pharmacotherapy: A Pathophysiologic Approach.* 7th ed. New York: McGraw-Hill; 2008.

Stoller ML, Kane CJ, Meng MV. Urologic disorders. In: Tierney LM Jr, McPhee SJ, Papadakis MA, eds. *Current Medical Diagnosis & Treatment.* 47th ed. New York: McGraw-Hill; 2008.

Sutters M. Systemic hypertension. In: Tierney LM Jr, McPhee SJ, Papadakis MA, eds. *Current Medical Diagnosis & Treatment.* 47th ed. New York: McGraw-Hill; 2008.

Talbert RL. Ischemic heart disease. In: DiPiro JT, Talbert RL, Yee GC, et al., eds. *Pharmacotherapy: A Pathophysiologic Approach.* 7th ed. New York: McGraw-Hill; 2008a.

Talbert RL. Ischemic heart disease. In: Tierney LM Jr, McPhee SJ, Papadakis MA, eds. *Current Medical Diagnosis & Treatment.* 47th ed. New York: McGraw-Hill; 2008.

Talbert RL. Hyperlipidemia. In: DiPiro JT, Talbert RL, Yee GC, et al., eds. *Pharmacotherapy: A Pathophysiologic Approach.* 7th ed. New York: McGraw-Hill; 2008b.

Teter CJ, Kando JC, Wells BG, et al., Depressive disorders. In: DiPiro JT, Talbert RL, Yee GC, et al., eds. *Pharmacotherapy: A Pathophysiologic Approach.* 7th ed. New York: McGraw-Hill; 2008.

Triplitt CL, Reasner CA, Isley WL. Diabetes mellitus. In: DiPiro JT, Talbert RL, Yee GC, et al., eds. *Pharmacotherapy: A Pathophysiologic Approach.* 7th ed. New York: McGraw-Hill; 2008.

Watnick S, Morrison G. Kidney disease. In: Tierney LM Jr, McPhee SJ, Papadakis MA, eds. *Current Medical Diagnosis & Treatment.* 47th ed. New York: McGraw-Hill; 2008.

Whitby DH, Johns TE. Drug-induced hematologic disorders. In: DiPiro JT, Talbert RL, Yee GC, et al., eds. *Pharmacotherapy: A Pathophysiologic Approach.* 7th ed. New York: McGraw-Hill; 2008.

White PF, Katzung BG. Skeletal muscle relaxants. In: Katzung BG, Masters SB, Trevor AJ, eds. *Basic and Clinical Pharmacology.* 11th ed. New York: McGraw-Hill; 2009.

Psychiatry

CHAPTER 16

Psychiatry

Michelle Heinan, EdD, DFAAPA, PA-C

Rex L. Hobbs, MPAS, PA-C

DIRECTIONS: Each of the numbered items or incomplete statements in this section is followed by answers or by completions of the statement. Select the ONE-lettered answer or completion that is BEST in each case.

1. While interviewing a 29-year-old computer programmer, you find that he denies any close friends or prior sexual relationships and has no interest in developing them. He describes little enjoyment in any activities except role play video games. He denies past emotional difficulties or stressors. His exam reveals a flat affect throughout the visit but is otherwise normal. Which is the most likely diagnosis in this scenario?

    (A) antisocial personality disorder
    (B) adjustment disorder
    (C) seasonal affective disorder
    (D) schizoid personality disorder

2. Which complication can be found in anorexia nervosa and not bulimia?

    (A) salivary gland hypertrophy
    (B) psychopathology
    (C) petechial hemorrhages
    (D) hypokalemia
    (E) osteoporosis

3. What is another name for multiple personalities?

    (A) dissociative amnesia
    (B) dissociative fugue

    (C) depersonalization
    (D) dissociative disorder not otherwise specified
    (E) dissociative identity disorder

4. Which of the following are predictive or diagnostic of anorexia nervosa?

    (A) less than 85% of normal weight than expected
    (B) homosexual orientation in females
    (C) promiscuity
    (D) menorrhagia

5. Which medication when co-administered with lithium may cause a potential fatal neurotoxicity?

    (A) calcium channel inhibitors
    (B) potassium-sparing diuretics
    (C) loop diuretics
    (D) ACE inhibitors

6. What is the most common personality disorder in prison populations?

    (A) paranoid
    (B) antisocial
    (C) borderline
    (D) avoidant

7. What diagnosis should be given to a patient who has nonbizarre delusions for at least a month and no other symptoms?

    (A) schizoaffective disorder
    (B) delusional disorder
    (C) brief psychotic disorder
    (D) schizophreniform disorder

8. A patient presented to your office with multiple somatic complaints. During the mental status exam, you notice that the patient loses the thread of conversation and discusses irrelevant topics based on an external stimulus. The patient never gets back to the main point he or she was trying to express. What is this thought process called?

    (A) tangentiality
    (B) circumstantiality
    (C) looseness of association
    (D) word salad
    (E) neologisms

9. A colleague is frustrated with one of his patients. He describes her as being extremely dramatic and overly provocative in her dress and behavior. She uses rapidly shifting emotions to maintain her position as the center of attention. He is concerned that she believes that their provider–patient relationship is much more than it actually is. Which of the following is the most likely diagnosis you might suggest to him?

    (A) narcissistic personality disorder
    (B) dependent personality disorder
    (C) histrionic personality disorder
    (D) schizotypal personality disorder

10. A person with an exaggerated sense of entitlement and uniqueness and who believes they can only be understood by people of significance is described to you by a colleague. They go on to state the person is arrogant, is lacking in empathy, and can be manipulative with relationships. What personality disorder best fits this scenario?

    (A) histrionic
    (B) narcissistic

    (C) antisocial
    (D) borderline

11. Hypochondriacal patients can mimic which disorder?

    (A) bipolar disorder
    (B) acute stress disorder
    (C) obsessive compulsive disorder
    (D) dissociative disorder

12. Mr. Smith leaves home and does not return nor does he go to work. A friend of Mr. Smith sees him in another state while on vacation. When he approaches Mr. Smith, he does not recognize him and has a total different demeanor. What type of disorder does Mr. Smith have?

    (A) amnesia
    (B) dissociative fugue
    (C) schizophrenia
    (D) dissociative identity disorder
    (E) depersonalization

13. What type of disorder develops within 3 months of an identified stressor such as finances, going to school, divorce, or illness in their life. The stressor causes impairment in their job and relationships, but the symptoms resolve within 6 months. What is the most likely diagnosis?

    (A) depression
    (B) bereavement
    (C) post-traumatic stress disorder
    (D) personality disorder
    (E) adjustment disorder

14. *DSM IV* classifies disorders into five axes. What type of information should be provided on Axis IV?

    (A) global assessment
    (B) clinical disorders
    (C) medical conditions
    (D) psychosocial stressors
    (E) personality disorders

15. What type of finding would be necessary to determine if a child has shaken baby syndrome versus a viral illness?

(A) poor feeding

(B) lethargy

(C) retinal hemorrhages

(D) irritability

(E) vomiting

16. A 9-year-old male is reported by his mother to be excessively and deliberately annoying to her and others at home and school, most always to those he knows well. She states that over the last year he frequently loses his temper, argues with adults, is easily annoyed by others and consistently blames others for his mistakes. She admits that he is not violent and really does not do anything out of the social norm. There have been no changes in his surroundings, exposures, or life events. Which of the following is the most likely diagnosis based on the information presented?

(A) Tourette disorder

(B) adjustment disorder

(C) disruptive behavior disorder

(D) oppositional defiant disorder

17. Generally, patients who are malingering:

(A) use illness to attain a goal

(B) have avoidant personalities

(C) follow prescribed treatment regimens

(D) have a history that agrees with their physical symptoms

18. What is the main communication deviance associated with autistic children?

(A) use of stereotyped phrases

(B) increased receptive language skills

(C) use of clanging speech patterns

(D) increased meaningful expressive language

19. Which of the following is a differentiating factor in diagnosing Asperger's syndrome from Autistic disorder?

(A) inflexible adherence to specific routines

(B) qualitative impairments in communication

(C) impaired peer relationship development

(D) repetitive motor mannerisms

20. Which process is *not* assessed during the mental status exam?

(A) judgment

(B) affect

(C) intelligence quotient

(D) cognition

(E) insight

21. A patient presents to your office claiming that the FBI is trying to poison him. What would these types of beliefs be called?

(A) somatic delusion

(B) delusion of persecution

(C) illusion

(D) delusion of grandeur

(E) hallucination

22. What question does the "C" represent in the alcohol abuse screening tool CAGE?

(A) Have you ever felt the need to *cut down*?

(B) Has anyone ever *cautioned* you not to drink?

(C) Have you been *caught* having an "eye opener" in the morning?

(D) Has anyone ever *criticized* you about your drinking?

(E) Do you *care* that you are feeling guilty about drinking?

23. A phobia is an excessive fear of an object or place that leads to or can be preceded by:

(A) panic attack

(B) depression

(C) hallucinations

(D) delusions

(E) confabulations

24. A 33-year-old woman presents with a 3-year history of a persistent, unfluctuating depressed mood. She also notes persistent insomnia, poor concentration, and very little appetite. She denies previous similar symptoms, substance abuse, current prescriptive drug use, and has had no change in her overall life circumstances. She remains functional at work and in most relationships. On the basis of the information presented, what is the most likely diagnosis?

    (A) dysthymic disorder
    (B) premenstrual dysphoric disorder
    (C) major depressive disorder
    (D) cyclothymic disorder

25. Of the following, which is the one criterion that differentiates a manic versus a hypomanic episode?

    (A) duration of symptoms
    (B) presence of pressured speech
    (C) involvement in high risk activities
    (D) exhibiting decreased need for sleep

26. What is the hallmark of a manic episode?

    (A) hypersomnolence
    (B) psychosis
    (C) depression
    (D) anxiety
    (E) irritability

27. Ms. Smith is diagnosed with a panic disorder. On the basis of the history gathered from the patient, you decide to treat her with an MAOI. Which side effect is considered common for this medication?

    (A) orthostatic hypotension
    (B) paresthesias
    (C) muscle pain
    (D) myoclonus
    (E) inducing mania in a bipolar patient

28. What type of pharmacological agent would be used as a first-line medication to treat obsessive compulsive disorder?

    (A) risperidone
    (B) lonazepam
    (C) fluoxetine
    (D) trazadone
    (E) venlafaxine

29. Ms. Jones wakes up from a deep sleep after having a nightmare. The nightmare caused her to re-experience the time she received third-degree burns on her arms. The next day at work, she was very jumpy and had difficulty concentrating. What diagnosis would be made in the case of Ms. Jones?

    (A) adjustment disorder
    (B) post-traumatic stress disorder
    (C) personality disorder
    (D) anxiety
    (E) schizophrenia

30. In which of the following conditions would electroconvulsive therapy (ECT) be effective?

    (A) somatization
    (B) anxiety disorders
    (C) major depressive disorders
    (D) personality disorders
    (E) geriatric patients who can take antidepressants

31. A patient who is intoxicated presents to the emergency department. On ocular exam, you notice mydriasis. Which substance could he have been using?

    (A) sedatives
    (B) PCP
    (C) opioids
    (D) cocaine

32. Which symptom is related to delirium tremens?

    (A) hypersomnolence
    (B) subnormal temperature
    (C) bradycardia
    (D) hypotension
    (E) perceptual distortions

33. A student is told that he failed a course in school and forgets that he has been given this information. Which defense mechanism is being utilized by this student?

    (A) sublimation
    (B) reaction formation
    (C) displacement
    (D) repression
    (E) denial

34. Which statement is true regarding vascular dementia?

    (A) occurs more frequently in females
    (B) patients with a stroke are at increased risk
    (C) has a chronic onset
    (D) patients have a normal funduscopic exam
    (E) cardiac chambers are normal size

35. A patient reports having repetitious impulses and images that come to the forefront of her thoughts frequently throughout the day. These cause her a great deal of anxiety even though she knows they should not. What term best fits the patient's description?

    (A) anhedonia
    (B) compulsions
    (C) abstraction
    (D) obsessions

36. A 24-year-old presents with difficulty sleeping and jumpiness since returning from his tour of duty in Iraq 1 year ago. He also notes poor concentration, fatigue, and having no emotions. He avoids leaving his home, has lost three jobs in the last few months, and has numerous speeding tickets. He remains distant from his family but finds some comfort talking to his surviving friends at the local bar. Based on the information, what is the most likely diagnosis?

    (A) bipolar I disorder
    (B) major depressive disorder
    (C) post-traumatic stress disorder
    (D) social phobia disorder

37. A misinterpretation of an external stimulus is

    (A) delusion
    (B) hallucination
    (C) illusion
    (D) neologism
    (E) tactile hallucination

38. Which of the following indicates a poor prognosis for someone diagnosed with schizophrenia?

    (A) acute onset
    (B) co-morbid mood disorder
    (C) obvious precipitating event
    (D) younger age at diagnosis

39. You are asked to see a patient who was admitted to the hospital. Upon attempts to obtain a history, you notice the patient states words that sound similar, but do not have the same meaning. He also does some rhyming of his words. What type of thought process would this be?

    (A) flight of ideas
    (B) circumstantiality
    (C) looseness of association
    (D) word salad
    (E) clanging

40. Which antidepressant has the longest half-life?

    (A) trazodone
    (B) venlafaxine
    (C) fluoxetine
    (D) paroxetine

41. A patient presents to the emergency department with alcohol withdrawal syndrome. What is the pharmacological agent of choice to be administered?

    (A) clonidine
    (B) phenobarbital
    (C) neuroleptics
    (D) benzodiazepines
    (E) methadone

42. Which pharmaceutical or group of agents can cause erectile disorders?

    (A) clomipramine
    (B) sympathomimetics
    (C) lithium
    (D) trazodone
    (E) antianxiety agents

43. A 56-year-old man presents to your office stating he has no desire to have sex. He has recently gotten back into dating after being divorced for 10 years and is being pressured by his current girlfriend. The gentleman states he has no desire to be sexually romantic with his girlfriend or any other person. What is the most likely diagnosis?

    (A) sexual aversion disorder
    (B) hypoactive sexual desire
    (C) hyperactive sexual desire
    (D) erectile disorder
    (E) sexual arousal disorder

44. A patient presents to the clinic with a family member. Upon obtaining history from the patient, he responds with excessive details of his symptoms and the reason for his visit. He is unable to answer a question directly without signification elaboration. What problem does this patient have?

    (A) circumstantiality
    (B) derailment
    (C) incoherence
    (D) tangentiality

45. Which system is *not* affected by the common side effects of lithium?

    (A) cutaneous
    (B) cardiovascular
    (C) endocrine
    (D) gastrointestinal
    (E) musculoskeletal

46. What primitive, or immature, defense mechanism is demonstrated by a patient who attributes their own, unacknowledged, feelings onto others while they search for perceived wrong-doings, no matter how small?

    (A) acting out
    (B) isolation
    (C) projection
    (D) splitting

47. A 19-year-old female college student is brought to the emergency department by emergency medical services. The paramedics were called to a frat house when the patient was found passed out on the floor. People at the party stated they had seen her take some pills, but were not sure what they were. After taking the pills, the patient became confused, depressed, and paranoid. She also became chilled, dizzy, and nauseated. Which street drug do you suspect she has taken?

    (A) ketamine (special K)
    (B) PCP
    (C) GHB (gamma hydroxybutyrate)
    (D) MDMA (ecstasy)
    (E) Rohypnol

48. A mother brings her 5-year-old child to the hospital after the child collapses at home. The mother states the child has been having diarrhea for the last 3 days. She has tried to get him to drink fluids. Upon further questioning, the mother states the child has had 12 loose stools a day for the last 3 days. Examination reveals the child to be responsive, but lethargic and dehydrated. The child is admitted to the hospital and mom is very involved in the child's care. While mom is there, the child is improving slightly, but still having multiple loose stools. When the mother had to leave to go to work, the child responded well to treatment without any further episodes of diarrhea. What is the most likely diagnosis?

    (A) Munchausen syndrome
    (B) schizophrenia
    (C) malingering
    (D) Munchausen by proxy
    (E) factitious disorder

49. Which of the following criteria is considered to be a high risk factor for "successful" suicide?

    (A) people who live in climates with limited amount of sun
    (B) lower socioeconomic status
    (C) male
    (D) committed religious beliefs

50. QT interval delay may occur in which antipsychotic medication?

    (A) risperidone
    (B) olanzapine
    (C) ziprasidone
    (D) quetiapine
    (E) aripiprazole

51. A patient describes a desire for close relationships and to be more successful at work. However, she views herself as being undesirable and inferior. Because of these feelings she avoids social activities and extra occupational projects out of fear of criticism, rejection, and embarrassment. Which diagnosis would best fit this description?

    (A) avoidant personality disorder
    (B) borderline personality disorder
    (C) histrionic personality disorder
    (D) schizoid personality disorder

52. What type of schizophrenia is characterized by self-injury, harm to others, mutism, or rigidity?

    (A) paranoid
    (B) undifferentiated
    (C) disorganized
    (D) catatonic
    (E) schizophreniform

53. Which disorder is characterized by episodes of hypomania and depression for greater than 2 years?

    (A) dysthymia
    (B) major depressive disorder
    (C) cyclothymia
    (D) bipolar
    (E) mood disorder

54. Which laboratory test determines recent alcohol consumption in patients who have committed to abstinence?

    (A) carbohydrate-deficient transferring (CDT)
    (B) ethyl glucuronide testing (EtG)
    (C) aspartate aminotransferase (AST)
    (D) alanine aminotransferase (ALT)

55. A 32-year-old male presents to your office with the complaint of low back pain for 7 months. The patient states he was initially injured on the job while trying to lift a 50-pound barrel off a truck. He denies any paresthesias or bowel/bladder problems associated with the low back pain. The patient states that he had been given NSAIDs and a muscle relaxer, followed by physical therapy treatments. X-rays that were taken 5 months ago were reported as normal. He was placed on light duty at that time. The patient has seen many practitioners who have "not helped him." Another person who works with this patient was at the clinic and stated the patient has had problems with one of his other coworkers. You consider trying the patient on an antidepressant first and then possibly sending him to a pain clinic if there is no success. What is the most likely diagnosis?

    (A) somatoform disorder
    (B) hypochondriasis
    (C) drug addiction
    (D) somatoform pain disorder
    (E) schizophreniform

56. Which problem shows up as a medical complication of cocaine?

    (A) hypertension
    (B) mood disorder
    (C) cardiomyopathy
    (D) cardiac dysrhythmias
    (E) ischemic heart disease

57. What is a commonly shared feature of bipolar disorder and ADHD in pediatric patients?

    (A) disruptive
    (B) obsessed with ideas
    (C) behavior problems
    (D) impaired concentration
    (E) insomnia

58. A child who has oppositional defiant disorder is at high risk for developing which disorder?

    (A) mood disorder
    (B) personality disorder
    (C) conduct disorder
    (D) ADHD
    (E) developmental disorder

59. A 24-year-old woman comes to your office complaining of anxiety. The patient had witnessed a traumatic event 3 days earlier that made her feel fearful. She has not been able to tell her family about this experience. She now feels like she is numb and in a dazed, dreamlike state with poor concentration, and difficulty sleeping. She experienced a flashback of the event yesterday. What is the most likely diagnosis?

    (A) post-traumatic stress disorder
    (B) dissociative fugue
    (C) psychosis
    (D) acute stress disorder
    (E) depersonalization

60. Which symptom would be found in amphetamine withdrawal?

    (A) fatigue
    (B) arrhythmias
    (C) confusion
    (D) seizure
    (E) tension

61. Sleepwalking disorders occur during what part of the night?

    (A) first one-third
    (B) second half

    (C) second one-third
    (D) last third
    (E) first half

62. What laboratory test should be run to rule out other causes in children who have ADHD?

    (A) thyroid levels
    (B) LDH
    (C) ferritin
    (D) folic acid
    (E) CBC

63. What would be an adverse effect of amphetamine use?

    (A) headache
    (B) profuse sweating
    (C) cyanosis
    (D) stomach cramps

64. Which pharmacologic agent most frequently causes postural hypotension?

    (A) quetiapine
    (B) risperidone
    (C) olanzapine
    (D) ziprasidone

65. A 6-month-old is brought to your office by his mother due to failure to thrive. The child was eating fine until a month ago when he started regurgitating the food. What is the most likely diagnosis?

    (A) pica
    (B) rumination
    (C) oppositional defiant disorder
    (D) mental retardation

66. What sleep changes occur in patients older than 65 years?

    (A) redistribution of REM sleep
    (B) less REM episodes
    (C) longer REM episodes
    (D) more total REM sleep

67. Which SSRI has a less sedating effect and is most likely to cause insomnia in some patients?

    (A) fluoxetine
    (B) sertraline
    (C) paroxetine
    (D) fluvoxamine
    (E) citalopram

68. Which of the following do the majority of patients with dissociative identity disorder also meet diagnostic criteria for?

    (A) schizophrenia
    (B) post-traumatic stress disorder
    (C) bipolar II disorder
    (D) major depressive disorder

69. Which nonnicotine related agent has been approved by the FDA as a first-line medication in the treatment of smoking cessation?

    (A) nortriptyline
    (B) clonidine
    (C) bupropion
    (D) fluoxetine

70. When admitting a patient for anorexia nervosa, what laboratory finding would you expect to see?

    (A) metabolic acidosis
    (B) hyperkalemia
    (C) decreased serum bicarbonate level
    (D) leukopenia

Answers and Explanations

1. **(D)** A patient with ambivalence toward sexual relationships, no close contacts, and no desire for either, along with anhedonism and flat affect are typical for this disorder. The preference for solitary activities and use of fantasy furthers this picture. The lack of aggressiveness and risk-taking behavior lessons the antisocial diagnosis. The patient denied any precipitating event that would lend the problem to an adjustment disorder and the lack of variance, seasonal or otherwise, lessens the seasonal affective disorder diagnosis. *(Eisendrath and Lichtmacher, 2009, pp. 925-926; Sadock and Sadock, 2008, p. 378)*

2. **(E)** Osteoporosis is found in anorexia nervosa due to a lack of calcium intake, decreased estrogen, and increase in cortisol. Bulimia nervosa has multiple medical complications in the cardiovascular, dental, dermatologic, endocrine, gastrointestinal, and neurologic systems. There are also associated dehydration and electrolyte disorders. Salivary gland hypertrophy, reversible cerebral atrophy, petechial hemorrhages, and hypokalemia are all part of the complications. *(Gwirtsman et al., 2008, p. 465; Baron, 2010, p. 1139)*

3. **(E)** Dissociative identity disorder is also called multiple personality disorder. There are usually at least two personalities both distinct in their own rights. The dominant personality at the time determines the behavior and attitudes. *(Eisendrath and Lichtmacher, 2009, pp. 914-918; Sadock and Sadock, 2008, p. 299)*

4. **(A)** Diagnostic criteria for anorexia nervosa include a weight loss to 85% of the required body weight. Homosexual orientation in men, not women, is considered a predisposing factor.

Anorexia is associated with amenorrhea and decreased interest in sex. *(Baron, 2010, pp. 1138-1139; Sadock and Sadock, 2008, pp. 334-335)*

5. **(A)** The combination of taking a calcium channel inhibitor with lithium can potentially cause a fatal neurotoxicity. The potassium-sparing diuretics may increase serum lithium levels while loop diuretics do not affect the lithium levels. Patients taking ACE inhibitors require a 50% to 75% reduction in lithium to maintain therapeutic levels. *(Sadock and Sadock, 2008, p. 518)*

6. **(B)** It is estimated that as many as three-quarters of the prison population has antisocial personality disorder. It has been found to be more common in males especially those from large families in poor urban areas. Although they may appear charming, they are otherwise known for their failure to conform to social norms and having a lack of remorse for their actions. Substance abuse, theft, lying, and aggressiveness are all common features as well. *(Sadock and Sadock, 2008, p. 380)*

7. **(B)** A delusional disorder presents with non-bizarre delusions for at least a month. The disorder does not present with any other symptoms related to schizophrenia or a mood disorder. A brief psychotic disorder has symptoms that last for 1 day to 1 month. Schizophreniform has symptoms that last at least a month, but no longer than 6 months. In schizoaffective disorders, depression or mania develop along with schizophrenic symptoms. *(Sadock and Sadock, 2008, p. 171)*

8. **(A)** Tangentiality is a disturbance in thought causing the person to start a train of thought, but

never getting to the point. Circumstantiality is seen in someone who eventually gets to the point after a delay in the thought process. Word salad is a mixture of words and phrases that are incoherent. Looseness of association is when the ideas shift between subjects that are totally unrelated to each other. Neologisms are the creation of new words. *(Nurcombe and Ebert, 2008, p. 48)*

9. **(C)** Patients with this diagnosis will resort to any means to remain the center of attention. They are commonly seen as emotionally shallow and obsessed with their physical appearance. Impressionistic speech, tantrums, and accusations are commonly employed. They commonly believe relationships to be much deeper and more solid than they actually are even after limited contact and interaction. *(Eisendrath and Lichtmacher, 2009, p. 925-926; Sadock and Sadock, 2008, p. 383)*

10. **(B)** The scenario represents a typical "snapshot" of this diagnosis. These persons typically have fantasies of unlimited success and have a strong need for admiration from others. They can be jealous of others but commonly assume that others are extremely jealous of them. Treatment is made difficult as they do not accept criticism or any attack on their "narcissistic supply." *(Eisendrath and Lichtmacher, 2009, p. 925-926; Sadock and Sadock, 2008, p. 384)*

11. **(C)** Hypochondriacs feels there is something wrong with their body. Patients seek reassurance and make frequent visits for medical care. Hypochondriacs can mimic obsessive compulsive disorder obsessions. The difference between the two diagnoses is that hypochondriacs limit their obsessions to their body. *(Hewlett, 2008, p. 388)*

12. **(B)** Dissociative or psychogenic fugue is precipitated by a stressful event that causes the patient to develop amnesia, leave home, and assume another identity. *(Sadock and Sadock, 2008, p. 297; Eisendrath and Lichtmacher, 2009, p. 915)*

13. **(E)** A response to a stressor that disturbs the mood of the patient causes impairment in function. The symptoms occur within 3 months of the stressor and last no longer than 6 months. Anxiety, depression, or combination is associated with adjustment disorders. *(Eisendrath and Lichtmacher, 2009, p. 912; Sadock and Sadock, 2008, p. 371)*

14. **(D)** The *Diagnostic and Statistical Manual* (*DSM*) is a classification system developed by the American Psychiatric Association. Each axis provides different types of information in order to assist providers in improving their treatment of patients and for coding purposes. Axis IV lists the psychosocial and environmental stressors in a person's life. These stressors may be positive or negative related to occupation, housing, education, economic, or support problems. This axis also includes difficulty accessing health care services. *(Sadock and Sadock, 2008, p. 37)*

15. **(C)** It is sometimes difficult to tell if shaken baby syndrome has occurred or a child is having a viral illness unless identifiable signs of fractures, traumatic brain injury, optic nerve edema, retinal hemorrhages, or subdural hemorrhage can be found. The presentation can also include irritability, change in mental status, emesis, and cardiac arrest. *(Braverman, 2009, p. 404)*

16. **(D)** The diagnosis is indicated in this case due to the age of the patient, age of onset, and the deliberate and frequent attempts to counter well-known adult authority. It is differentiated from adjustment disorder because there is no reported precipitating change in his environment or life circumstances. Disruptive behavior disorder is made less likely in that his indifference is primarily applied to adults and that he is not violating the rights of others and not completely parting from age-appropriate societal norms. *(Sadock and Sadock, 2008, p. 623)*

17. **(A)** Patients who are malingerers do not want to improve until their goal is met. Goals may be financial, occupational, or legal. These patients will act differently when they think they are not being observed. They may fake their symptoms in order to be admitted to a hospital or to obtain drugs. These patients have an antisocial personality disorder. *(Ford, 2008, p. 417; Sadock and Sadock, 2008, pp. 421-422)*

18. **(A)** Echolalia and stereotyped words and phrases are commonly used by autistic children with little understanding of what is being vocalized. This is due to a decreased and/or delayed receptive language development. *(Sadock and Sadock, 2008, p. 607)*

19. **(B)** The lack of language and communication skill deficits is the main factor that differentiates these two, otherwise, very similar disorders. The remaining choices are shared diagnostic criteria for both of these disorders. *(Sadock and Sadock, 2008, p. 614; Volkmar, 2008, p. 568)*

20. **(C)** The mental status exam is able to evaluate appearance, affect, mood, speech, activity, and behavior, thought processes, cognition, fund of knowledge, judgment, content of thought, and insight. You can obtain a basic knowledge of the level of intelligence based on information provided by the patients and their behavior. Intelligence quotient is measured through IQ tests. *(Nurcombe and Ebert, 2008, p. 40; Sadock and Sadock, 2008, pp. 5–9)*

21. **(B)** Patients who have delusions of persecution often feel that people are taking pictures and tape recording them. Patients often believe that external agencies or relatives are attempting to harm them. *(Sadock and Sadock, 2008, p. 185; Shelton, 2008, p. 294)*

22. **(A)** The screening test of alcohol abuse is called CAGE. The four questions to ask for the screening test are: "Have you ever felt the need to cut down on drinking?" "Have you ever felt annoyed by criticism of your drinking?" "Have you ever felt guilty about your drinking?" and "Have you ever taken a morning eye opener?" If a patient responds yes to two of the questions, it is considered to be positive for abuse. *(Pignone and Salazar, 2009, p. 19)*

23. **(A)** Patients who have a phobia realize it is an irrational fear and try to avoid whatever they have the fear of. In attempts to avoid the "problem," patients can develop anxiety or panic attacks. *(Sadock and Sadock, 2008, p. 250; Shelton, 2008, p. 361)*

24. **(A)** The main historical component that points to this diagnosis is the long-term (equal to or greater than 2 years), unfluctuating symptoms without mention of manic or hypomanic symptoms that would be typical of cyclothymic disorders. No variances with menstrual cycles are mentioned. Major depressive disorder is generally associated with more intense symptoms, including suicidal ideation, and only requires a 2-week duration of symptoms to diagnose. *(Loosen and Shelton, 2008, p. 328; Sadock and Sadock, 2008, p. 226)*

25. **(A)** The two differentiating factors between mania and hypomania are the duration of symptoms (mania: at least a week or longer; hypomania: at least 4 days) and their severity. Manic episodes cause a marked disturbance in function, generally resulting in hospitalization, while hypomania results in noticeable but functional changes in behavior and lacks any psychotic attributes. *(Sadock and Sadock, 2008, p. 206)*

26. **(E)** The hallmark of mania is irritability. At times, the patient can have a euphoric mood, which can result in denial of their illness. *(Loosen and Shelton, 2008, p. 333; Sadock and Sadock, 2008, p. 215)*

27. **(A)** Orthostatic hypotension is the most frequent side effect with MAOIs. Weight gain, edema, insomnia, and sexual dysfunction can also occur. *(Sadock and Sadock, 2008, p. 522)*

28. **(C)** Fluvoxamine, paroxetine, and sertraline are all approved for the treatment of obsessive compulsive disorder. Use of an SSRI in combination with behavioral therapy is recommended. *(Hewlett, 2008, p. 391; Sadock and Sadock, 2008, p. 257)*

29. **(B)** Post-traumatic stress disorder is a type of anxiety disorder characterized by re-experiencing a traumatic event. Patients have difficulty concentrating, insomnia, illusions, nightmares about the event, and startle reactions. Treatment needs to begin as soon as possible, though sometimes the symptoms do not occur until quite a while after the initial

traumatic event. *(Johnson et al., 2008, p. 367; Sadock and Sadock, 2008, p. 258)*

30. **(C)** ECT is used for treating major depressive disorder. ECT can also be used in patients who do not respond to medication, have severe psychotic symptoms, or stupor, or are homicidal or suicidal. Severe bouts of depression with psychotic episodes do not respond as well to ECT. *(Sadock and Sadock, 2008, p. 562)*

31. **(D)** Patients intoxicated with cocaine present with mydriasis. In opioid intoxication, the pupils are constricted. PCP intoxication is associated with nystagmus. *(Eisendrath & Lichtmacher, 2010, p. 1398; Sadock and Sadock, 2008, p. 119, 143)*

32. **(E)** Fever, tremor, tachycardia, perceptual distortions, diaphoresis, perceptual distortions consisting of visual or tactile hallucinations, hypertension, as well as changes in the psychomotor activity levels are all symptoms of delirium tremens. *(Sadock and Sadock, 2008, p. 97)*

33. **(E)** The person denies reality from an external source so that it never existed or happened. Denial is a defense mechanism that can be benign or pathological. *(Sadock and Sadock, 2008, p. 24)*

34. **(B)** Vascular dementia is an abrupt onset in comparison to Alzheimer, which is slower in onset. Vascular dementia can be prevented by reduction of risk factors such as hypertension and diabetes. The disease typically occurs in males. Carotid bruits, cardiac chamber enlargement, and abnormalities on funduscopic exam may be found. *(Johnson and Yaffe, 2008, pp. 280-286)*

35. **(D)** The description is most befitting of obsessions. The sometimes-confused compulsions infer the repetitive behaviors performed to counter the obsessive thoughts. *(Eisendrath and Lichtmacher, 2009, p. 915; Sadock and Sadock, 2008, p. 29)*

36. **(C)** The recent combat exposure and implied loss of comrades qualifies as a significant traumatic event. Combat exposures are not the only such event, as rape, sexual abuse, and assault can also be precipitating events. Hyperarousal and avoidance are typical along with insomnia, anhedonia, poor concentration, and problem-solving skills. Feelings of isolation from even close friends and family is common as the patient feels they would not be able to understand or that they do not share a common ground. The lack of structure and the need to avoid aggressive responses can be difficult for service members to adjust to upon their return. Onset of symptoms may not develop for many months after the event or return to the civilian world. Whether an introverted or extroverted response occurs, family, relationship, occupational, and sometimes legal issues arise. *(Eisendrath and Lichtmacher, 2009, p. 913; Sadock and Sadock, 2008, p. 260)*

37. **(C)** Illusions are associated with external stimuli whereas hallucinations are not. Delusions are beliefs that are false based on wrong inference by the patient about what is happening in reality. *(Eisendrath and Lichtmacher, 2009, p. 928; Sadock and Sadock, 2008, p. 27)*

38. **(D)** A younger age of onset/diagnosis along with an insidious onset, social isolation, family history of schizophrenia, and negative symptoms (affective flattening, alogia, apathy, anhedonia) all portend a poor prognosis. To the contrary, acute onset, late diagnosis, positive symptoms (hallucinations, delusions, disordered thought processes, etc.), and a concomitant mood disorder actually lend to a better prognosis. *(Sadock and Sadock, 2008, p. 163)*

39. **(E)** Clanging is a disturbance in thought in which the person selects words that are similar by sound, but do not mean the same. Sometimes the person will rhyme the words. Flight of ideas is rapid transitioning between subjects, but tends to be connected. Looseness of association is when a person changes subjects, but there is no connection between the subjects. Circumstantiality is where the person has a point and eventually gets to that point, but with delay in the thought process. Word salad is a mixture of words that have no sense. *(Sadock and Sadock, 2008, pp. 23-32)*

40. (C) Fluoxetine has the longest half-life of 4 to 14 days. This pharmaceutical agent will not cause a discontinuation syndrome like the rest of the agents listed. *(Cole et al., 2008, p. 221)*

41. (D) Benzodiazepines are the first line of treatment for alcohol withdrawal. Dosage should start out high and titrate downward as the patient improves. Carbamazepine has also been found to be beneficial in the treatment of alcohol withdrawal in place of the benzodiazepines. *(Sadock and Sadock, 2008, p. 97)*

42. (C) Lithium impairs the ability to have an erection. Clomipramine may increase sex drive in some patients. Trazodone does not impair erection or ejaculation. Sympathomimetics increase libido. However, if on this type of agent for a prolonged period of time, men may have difficulty with erections and desire. Antianxiety agents diminish anxiety and thereby improve sexual function. *(Sadock and Sadock, 2008, p. 313)*

43. (B) Hypoactive sexual disorder can occur in both men and women and is a loss of desire for sexual activity. The clinician must take into consideration the patient's life stressors, medical condition, age, and desire for sexual activity prior to this event. *(Balon and Segraves, 2008, p. 430)*

44. (A) Circumstantiality is seen in someone who eventually gets to the point after a delay in the thought process. Tangentiality is a disturbance in thought causing the person to start a train of thought, but never getting to the point. Derailment is when a patient skips to another subject. This mainly occurs if a topic is brought up that the patient does not wish to discuss. *(Nurcombe and Ebert, 2008, p. 48)*

45. (E) Lithium affects the cutaneous, cardiac, endocrine, renal, neurological, and gastrointestinal systems. Symptoms can include decreased appetite, nausea, vomiting, diarrhea, polyuria, EKG changes, hyperthyroidism, hypothyroidism, tremor, cognitive changes, skin eruptions, and weight gain. *(Sadock and Sadock, 2008, pp. 516-517)*

46. (C) These patients are sensitive to any criticism and are constantly searching for any insult or mistreatments, no matter how small or unintentional they may be. Confrontation is to be avoided as it is only counterproductive and will reinforce their beliefs. This is commonly seen in paranoid personality disorders. *(Sadock and Sadock, 2008, p. 30)*

47. (D) Club drugs consist of MDMA, Rohypnol, GHB, and ketamine. MDMA is ecstasy and has both hallucinogenic and stimulant properties. People who ingest the drug while in areas that are confined can develop severe hyperthermia, dehydration, possible fibrillation, brain damage, and death. Rohypnol is considered to be a "date rape" drug. GHB has anabolic, euphoric, and sedative properties. This drug is called "liquid ecstasy." Ketamine has also been used as a date rape drug. It can be mixed into drinks, injected, or snorted. Another name for ketamine is special K. *(Ebert et al., 2008, p. 413; Eisendrath and Lichtmacher, 2009, p. 959; Sadock and Sadock, 2008, p. 109)*

48. (D) Munchausen by proxy is when a parent, usually the mother, exaggerates, induces, or creates an illness in their child. The parent remains very involved in the child's care. The problem seems to originate when the parent is around and disappears if the parent is away from the child for a period of time. *(Eisendrath and Lichtmacher, 2009, p. 919)*

49. (C) Risk factors for successful suicide include being male, prior suicide attempts, depression, unemployment, being single, divorced, or widowed; alcoholism, or older than 45 years old. *(Sadock and Sadock, 2008, pp. 428-430)*

50. (C) Ziprasidone has been found to induce a QT-interval delay in some patients. It is important to screen patients for cardiac risk factors. *(Eisendrath and Lichtmacher, 2009, p. 931)*

51. (A) An individual with avoidant personality disorder differs from schizoid in that they desire interaction and closeness but are unable to overcome their deep seated self-beliefs and fears. They tend to be less impulsive and more stable than borderline personality disorder patients and have less of a need to be the center of attention than those with histrionic personality disorders. *(Sadock and Sadock, 2008, p. 385)*

52. **(D)** Catatonic schizophrenia is characterized by self-injury or violence to others, mutism, posturing, and other motor symptoms such as rigidity. *(Sadock and Sadock, 2008, p. 164)*

53. **(C)** Cyclothymia is characterized by symptoms of depression and hypomania for at least 2 years. Symptoms are milder than a regular depressive or manic episode. Occasionally, patients will have regular depressive or manic symptoms at which time they need to be reclassified as bipolar. *(Loosen and Shelton, 2008, p. 326)*

54. **(B)** Ethyl glucuronide testing (EtG) will show recent use of alcohol, but not about the amount of consumption. GGT (γ-glutamyl transpeptidase) is the most sensitive laboratory test to determine the use of alcohol. The test will show heavy consumption of alcohol. Liver function tests can demonstrate the toxic effects from consuming alcohol. *(Martin, 2008, p. 248)*

55. **(D)** Somatoform pain disorder is a focus on pain for greater than 6 months. The subjective findings outweigh the objective findings. Pain in the neck, pelvic, or low back areas are frequent sites, as well as headaches. The disorder may be precipitated by an injury. The patient will have a history of seeing multiple providers and possibly many medical and surgical treatments. The patient is unresponsive to treatment. Stressors can aggravate or precipitate the pain. There may be an expectation of secondary gains. Age of onset is around 30s and 40s. Treatment consists of placing the patient on an antidepressant and sending the patient to a pain clinic. *(Ford, 2008, pp. 407-408; Sadock and Sadock, 2008, pp. 284-285)*

56. **(D)** Medical complications from cocaine include cardiac dysrhythmias, seizures, CVAs, headache, nasal septal perforations, chest pain, CHF, cardiovascular collapse, noncardiogenic pulmonary edema, and spontaneous pneumothorax. *(Olson, 2009, p. 1390)*

57. **(C)** Behavior problems are a commonly shared feature of pediatric ADHD and bipolar disease. Disruptive and impulsive behaviors are a shared feature of conduct disorder. Disruptive behavior and being annoying to others can be found with oppositional defiant disorder; impaired attention and concentration can be found in major depression. Bipolar patients are obsessed with ideas while ADHD and conduct disorder patients are not. *(Stafford et al., 2009, p. 183)*

58. **(C)** Oppositional defiant disorder is a less intense form of conduct disorder. Children who continue with the chronic behavior are at risk of developing conduct disorder. This disorder is most often seen in boys, with problems being worse at school. The behavior can occur at home and with peers. *(Sadock and Sadock, 2008, p. 622)*

59. **(D)** Acute stress disorder is characterized by experiencing or witnessing a traumatic event where the person felt threatened by death or injury or the people they witnessed. The person feels fearful and helpless. Symptoms usually occur within a month of the event, last 2 days, and resolve in a month. The person feels numb, has lack of awareness of surroundings, and sees everything in a dreamlike state. Sometimes they develop amnesia. Flashbacks or recurrent images can occur with acute stress disorder. Difficulty sleeping, poor concentration, anhedonia, irritability, and despair are associated with this disorder. If not treated at the early stages, the patient is at risk of developing PTSD. *(Johnson et al., 2008, pp. 377-378; Sadock and Sadock, 2008, p. 260)*

60. **(A)** Fatigue is found in amphetamine withdrawal. Arrhythmias, confusion, seizure, and tension are found in amphetamine intoxication. *(Sadock and Sadock, 2008, p. 107)*

61. **(E)** Sleepwalking disorders occur in the first half of the night. Nightmare disorders occur in the last third, sleep terrors in the first third, and REM sleep behavior disorders in the second half of the night. *(Eisendrath and Lichtmacher, 2009, p. 950)*

62. **(A)** Serum lead levels and thyroid function tests should be done to rule out other causes of the symptoms. *(Goldson and Reynolds, 2009, pp. 91-92)*

63. **(C)** Cyanosis is associated with adverse effects of amphetamine use. The rest of the symptoms listed are associated with amphetamine withdrawal. *(Sadock and Sadock, 2008, pp. 107-108)*

64. **(A)** Quetiapine is more frequently associated with postural hypotension as well as somnolence and dizziness. Ziprasidone has side effects that include nausea, lightheadedness, headache, dizziness, and somnolence. Weight gain is more prevalent in olanzapine. Risperidone is associated with anxiety, nausea, vomiting, erectile dysfunction, orgasmic dysfunction, increased pigmentation, and rhinitis. *(Sadock and Sadock, 2008, pp. 543-544)*

65. **(B)** Rumination is the rechewing or regurgitation of food by an infant or child. The child is usually seen due to failure to thrive. The condition usually starts after normal eating habits have been established which is approximately 3 months of age. The symptoms must be ongoing for at least a month. The problem can be attributed to medical conditions such as hiatal hernia or esophageal reflux. *(Sadock and Sadock, 2008, p. 630)*

66. **(A)** People older than the age of 65 have a redistribution of REM sleep. They also have more REM episodes, shorter REM episodes, and less total REM sleep. *(Sadock and Sadock, 2008, p. 696)*

67. **(A)** Fluoxetine has mild sedating properties, but has a high probability of insomnia. The rest of the SSRIs have a mild possibility of causing insomnia. *(Cole et al., 2008, p. 218)*

68. **(B)** Dissociative identity disorder (DID), formerly known as multiple personality disorder, is classified as a trauma spectrum disorder due to the strong link with early childhood trauma and/or maltreatment. As such, approximately 70% of DID patients also meet criteria for PTSD. *(Sadock and Sadock, 2008, pp. 299-300)*

69. **(C)** Bupropion SR has been approved by the U.S. Food and Drug Administration (FDA) for smoking cessation. The drug has been successful in doubling cessation rates. Side effects include dry mouth, agitation, insomnia, and headache. *(Rigotti, 2008, p. 166)*

70. **(D)** Leukopenia is seen in anorexia nervosa. Other laboratory values include an abnormal LH release, elevated liver function tests, serum bicarbonate, and cortisol. There is also hypercarotenemia, hypochloremia, hypokalemia, hypozincemia, and hypercholesterolemia along with low estrogen in females, low normal T_3, and low T_4. *(Gwirtsman et al., 2008, p. 458)*

REFERENCES

Balon R, Segraves RT. Sexual dysfunction and paraphilias. In: Ebert MH, Loosen PT, Nurcombe B, Leckman JF, eds. *Current Diagnosis and Treatment in Psychiatry.* New York: McGraw-Hill; 2008.

Baron RB. Nutritional disorders. In: McPhee SJ, Papdakis MA, eds. *Current Medical Diagnosis and Treatment,* 49th ed. New York: McGraw-Hill; 2010.

Braverman RS. Eye. In: Hay W, Levin M, Deterding R, Sondheimer J, eds. *Current Diagnosis and Treatment in Pediatrics.* New York: McGraw-Hill; 2009.

Cole SA, Christensen JF, Cole MR, et al. Depression. In: Feldman MD, Christensen JF, eds. *Behavioral Medicine in Primary Care: A Practical Guide,* 3rd ed. New York: McGraw-Hill; 2008.

Eisendrath SJ, Lichtmacher JE. Psychiatric disorders. In: McPhee SJ, Papdakis MA, eds. *Current Medical Diagnosis and Treatment,* 48th ed. New York: McGraw-Hill; 2009.

Ford, CV. Somatoform disorders. In: Ebert MH, Loosen PT, Nurcombe B, Leckman JF, eds. *Current Diagnosis and Treatment in Psychiatry.* New York: McGraw-Hill; 2008.

Goldson E, Reynolds A. Child development and behavior. In: Hay W, Levin M, Deterding R, Sondheimer J, eds. *Current Diagnosis and Treatment in Pediatrics.* New York: McGraw-Hill; 2009.

Gwirtsman HE, Mitchell JE, Ebert MH. Eating disorders. In: Ebert MH, Loosen PT, Nurcombe B, Leckman JF, eds. *Current Diagnosis and Treatment in Psychiatry.* New York: McGraw-Hill; 2008.

Hewlett WA. Obsessive-compulsive disorder. In: Ebert MH, Loosen PT, Nurcombe B, Leckman JF, eds. *Current Diagnosis and Treatment in Psychiatry.* New York: McGraw-Hill; 2008.

Johnson B, Yaffee K. Dementia & Delerium. In: Feldman MD, Christensen JF, eds. *Behavioral Medicine in Primary Care: A Practical Guide,* 3rd ed. New York: McGraw-Hill; 2008.

Johnson DC, Krystal JH, Southwick SM. Posttraumatic stress disorder and acute stress disorder. In: Ebert MH, Loosen PT, Nurcombe B, Leckman JF, eds *Current Diagnosis and Treatment in Psychiatry.* New York: McGraw-Hill; 2008.

Loosen PT, Shelton RC. Mood disorders. In: Ebert MH, Loosen PT, Nurcombe B, Leckman JF, eds. *Current Diagnosis and Treatment in Psychiatry.* New York: McGraw-Hill; 2008.

Martin PR. Substance-related disorders. In: Ebert MH, Loosen PT, Nurcombe B, Leckman JF, eds. *Current Diagnosis and Treatment in Psychiatry.* New York: McGraw-Hill; 2008.

Nurcombe B, Ebert MH. The psychiatric interview. In: Ebert MH, Loosen PT, Nurcombe B, Leckman JF, eds. *Current Diagnosis and Treatment in Psychiatry.* New York: McGraw-Hill; 2008.

Olson KR. Poisoning. In: McPhee SJ, Papdakis MA, eds. *Current Medical Diagnosis and Treatment,* 48th ed. New York: McGraw-Hill; 2009.

Pignone M, Salazar R. Disease prevention and health promotion. In: McPhee SJ, Papdakis MA, eds. *Current Medical Diagnosis and Treatment,* 48th ed. New York: McGraw-Hill; 2009.

Rigotti NA. Smoking. In: Feldman MD, Christensen JF, eds. *Behavioral Medicine in Primary Care: A Practical Guide,* 3rd ed. New York: McGraw-Hill; 2008.

Sadock BJ, Sadock VA. *Concise Textbook of Clinical Psychiatry,* 3rd ed. Philadelphia, PA: Lippincott, Williams & Wilkins; 2008.

Shelton RC. Other psychotic disorders. In: Ebert MH, Loosen PT, Nurcombe B, Leckman JF, eds. *Current Diagnosis and Treatment in Psychiatry.* New York: McGraw-Hill; 2008.

Stafford B, Hagman J, Dech B. Child and adolescent psychiatric disorders and psychosocial aspects of pediatrics. In: Hay W, Levin M, Deterding R, Sondheimer J, eds. *Current Diagnosis and Treatment in Pediatrics.* New York: McGraw-Hill; 2009.

Volkmar FR. Autism and the pervasive developmental disorders. In: Ebert MH, Loosen PT, Nurcombe B, Leckman JF, eds. *Current Diagnosis and Treatment in Psychiatry.* New York: McGraw-Hill; 2008.

SECTION VI
Surgery

CHAPTER 17

Emergency Medicine

Cynthia D. Ferguson, MHS, PA-C

DIRECTIONS: Each of the numbered items or incomplete statements in this section is followed by answers or by completion of the statement. Select the ONE lettered answer or completion that is BEST in each case.

1. Which of the following interventions is the most important factor in surviving an out-of-hospital cardiac arrest?

    (A) immediate airway control with intubation
    (B) early defibrillation
    (C) aggressive management of hypotension
    (D) epinephrine usage
    (E) rapid transport to appropriate facility

2. A 27-year-old Rh-negative 14-week gestation woman presents to the emergency department (ED) with vaginal bleeding and passage of "clots." The patient is suspected of undergoing a spontaneous abortion. Which of the following is the most appropriate dose of RhoGAM?

    (A) 50 μg
    (B) 75 μg
    (C) 100 μg
    (D) 300 μg
    (E) 600 μg

3. A 65-year-old ill-appearing woman presents to the ED with tachycardia, tachypnea, and an arterial pH of 7.10. What is the most *likely* cause of her high anion gap metabolic acidosis?

    (A) diabetic ketoacidosis (DKA)
    (B) lactic acidosis
    (C) alcoholic ketoacidosis
    (D) nonketotic hyperosmolar acidosis
    (E) aspirin poisoning

4. A 64-year-old woman presents to the ED with dyspnea and exertional fatigue. There is a high clinical suspicion for pulmonary embolism. The ventilation/perfusion ($\dot{V}/\dot{Q}$) lung scan was read as "low probability" for a pulmonary embolism. Of the following, which would be the most appropriate next step?

    (A) Obtain a pulmonary angiogram if the lower extremity ultrasound is negative for deep vein thrombosis (DVT).
    (B) Initiate intravenous (IV) heparin without further testing.
    (C) Send the patient home with instructions to follow up with her physician the next day for further outpatient work-up.
    (D) Obtain an echocardiogram to assess right atrial pressures.
    (E) Repeat the $\dot{V}/\dot{Q}$ lung scan.

5. The most reliable clinical assessment tool to confirm endotracheal intubation is which of the following?

(A) endotracheal tube condensation

(B) symmetrical chest expansion

(C) breath sounds auscultated equally over the chest

(D) no breath sounds auscultated over the stomach

(E) use of a carbon dioxide (CO_2) detection device

6. A 76-year-old woman (60 kg) with organic brain syndrome presents to the ED with a serum sodium level of 180 mg/dL. What is the approximate calculation of the water deficit in this hypernatremic patient?

(A) 4 L

(B) 6 L

(C) 8 L

(D) 11 L

(E) 14 L

7. A 65-year-old man with chronic obstructive pulmonary disease (COPD) taking chronic theophylline therapy presents to the ED with palpitations, chest pain, and the feeling that his heart is beating irregularly after starting erythromycin for bronchitis. What is the likely dysrhythmia?

(A) multifocal atrial tachycardia (MAT)

(B) atrial fibrillation (AF)

(C) atrial flutter

(D) sinus bradycardia

(E) Mobitz type II heart block

8. A 58-year-old man with multiple myeloma presents to the ED with altered mental status, hypertension, back pain, and constipation. These findings are suggestive of which of the following medical conditions?

(A) hyperkalemia

(B) hypercalcemia

(C) hypomagnesemia

(D) hypoglycemia

(E) hyponatremia

9. Which of the following diagnoses is associated with a non–anion gap acidosis?

(A) renal tubular acidosis

(B) methanol poisoning

(C) ketoacidosis

(D) uremia associated with renal failure

(E) ethylene glycol poisoning

10. A 16-year-old long-distance runner suffered an external rotation injury to the ankle. Which of the following ligaments is most likely injured?

(A) anterior talofibular

(B) posterior talofibular

(C) deltoid

(D) calcaneofibular

(E) tibiofibular

11. A 68-year-old man with a medical history of coronary artery disease presents to the ED with a 2-day history of intermittent chest tightness. The pain was not relieved with three nitroglycerin sublingual tablets. What would be the initial assessment if the electrocardiogram (ECG) demonstrated 2 mm ST-segment elevations in leads II, III, and aVF?

(A) acute anterior wall myocardial infarction

(B) acute lateral wall myocardial injury

(C) subendocardial inferior wall myocardial infarction

(D) subendocardial anterior wall myocardial ischemia

(E) acute inferior wall myocardial injury

12. A 64-year-old woman presents to the ED with complaints of left-sided headache, low-grade fever, malaise, pain with chewing, and decreased vision in her left eye. Which of the following would be the most appropriate measure in managing this patient?

(A) aspirin therapy

(B) lumbar puncture

(C) muscle relaxants

(D) intravenous steroids

(E) oxygen (O_2) therapy

13. A 28-year-old pregnant woman in her third trimester presents with a blood pressure (BP) of 164/98 mm Hg. Which of the following medications is the agent of choice in this scenario?

    (A) nitroglycerin
    (B) magnesium
    (C) hydralazine
    (D) captopril
    (E) hydrochlorothiazide

14. Cardiac enzymes in a patient with a 2-hour history of chest pain secondary to an acute myocardial infarction would commonly demonstrate which of the following findings?

    (A) normal creatine kinase (CK-MB) and troponin I levels
    (B) elevated troponin I and normal CK-MB levels
    (C) elevated CK-MB and normal troponin I levels
    (D) normal myoglobin with elevated CK-MB levels
    (E) elevated myoglobin, troponin I, and CK-MB levels

15. Which of the following is considered the most specific myocardial injury enzyme marker?

    (A) CK-MB
    (B) myoglobin
    (C) troponin I
    (D) troponin T
    (E) lactate dehydrogenase (LDH)

16. Which of the following is the most appropriate indication for IV thrombolytic therapy in a patient with acute coronary syndrome?

    (A) 0.5 mm ST-segment elevation in the inferior wall leads resolving with two sublingual nitroglycerins
    (B) posterior wall myocardial infarction duration of 12 to 14 hours
    (C) right bundle branch block
    (D) 2 mm of ST-segment elevation in the anterior/lateral wall
    (E) 3 mm of ST-segment depression

17. A 42-year-old woman was brought to the ED from a psychiatric facility for an evaluation following a brief "seizure." The psychiatric staff reports that she has been confused and complaining of thirst for the past 5 days. What is the most likely diagnosis?

    (A) idiopathic hypoglycemia
    (B) psychogenic polydipsia
    (C) brain tumor
    (D) new-onset epilepsy
    (E) psychogenic cerebritis

18. A 44-year-old AIDS patient being treated for *Pneumocystis jiroveci* pneumonia presents to the ED with an acute onset of confusion, pallor, diaphoresis, and tachycardia. What is the most likely cause of the patient's symptoms?

    (A) hypoglycemia
    (B) meningitis
    (C) subarachnoid hemorrhage (SAH)
    (D) hypoxemia
    (E) mucous plugging

19. Of the following ECG findings, which is most likely associated with hypokalemia?

    (A) shortened QT interval
    (B) ST-segment elevation
    (C) flattened T waves
    (D) prolonged PR interval
    (E) tall-peaked T waves

20. A 72-year-old woman is brought to the ED after being found on her kitchen floor comatose with a BP of 280/150 mm Hg and pinpoint reactive pupils. What is the most likely diagnosis?

    (A) thalamic hemorrhage
    (B) cerebellar hemorrhage
    (C) pontine hemorrhage
    (D) subarachnoid hemorrhage
    (E) intracerebral left occipital hemorrhage

21. A 68-year-old patient presents to the ED with palpitations and dizziness. The ECG demonstrates three or more differently shaped P waves; varying PP, PR, and RR intervals; and atrial rhythm usually between 100 and 180. What is the most likely dysrhythmia?

    (A) MAT
    (B) AF
    (C) ventricular tachycardia (VT)
    (D) sinus dysrhythmia
    (E) supraventricular tachycardia

22. A 58-year-old man presents to the ED with palpitations and chest pain. The ECG reveals a narrow complex tachycardia at 180 beats per minute (bpm). Which of the following medications is the most appropriate therapeutic agent for this scenario?

    (A) amiodarone
    (B) lidocaine
    (C) adenosine
    (D) alprazolam
    (E) bretylium

23. The most immediate management priority in a patient with septic shock is:

    (A) empiric antimicrobial therapy
    (B) inotropic support
    (C) oxygenation and ventilation
    (D) fluid therapy
    (E) acid–base status

24. Which of the following drugs represents the most appropriate antidotal agent for benzodiazepine overdose?

    (A) naloxone
    (B) activated charcoal
    (C) ketamine
    (D) flumazenil
    (E) flutamide

25. A 25-year-old patient presented to the ED with a 3 cm linear left palmar hand laceration from a broken glass bottle container. Which of the following would be the most appropriate initial management of the hand injury?

    (A) Allow the wound to close by secondary intention after irrigation.
    (B) Explore the wound and place the patient on prophylactic antibiotics.
    (C) Obtain a hand radiograph, explore wound, and suture the wound if no foreign body is observed.
    (D) Obtain a hand radiograph and consult a hand surgeon.
    (E) Suture the wound and place the patient on prophylactic antibiotics.

26. A 19-year-old woman presents to the ED with a 4-day history of a warm, swollen, erythematous hand following a cat bite. Which of the following is the most likely causative pathogen in this scenario?

    (A) *Staphylococcus intermedius*
    (B) *Haemophilus aphrophilus*
    (C) *Eikenella corrodens*
    (D) *Pasteurella multocida*
    (E) *S aureus*

27. A 59-year-old cancer patient presents to the ED with fever, pneumonia, hypotension, and tachycardia. Investigative studies include hyperkalemia, hyponatremia, and hypoglycemia. What is the most likely concomitant diagnosis in this scenario?

    (A) adrenal insufficiency
    (B) syndrome of inappropriate antidiuretic hormone (SIADH)
    (C) Cushing syndrome
    (D) hypothyroidism
    (E) hyperparathyroidism

28. Which of the following is the most common cause of nontraumatic cardiac tamponade?

    (A) metastatic malignancy
    (B) uremia
    (C) acute idiopathic pericarditis
    (D) hemorrhage (anticoagulant use)
    (E) bacterial or tubercular pericarditis

29. Which of the following best defines the peripheral wedge-shaped consolidation on the pleural surface observed in a patient with a pulmonary embolism?

    (A) Hampton hump
    (B) pleural effusion
    (C) atelectatic lesion
    (D) Westermark sign
    (E) reticular pattern

30. Which of the following is the most compelling indication for thrombolytic therapy in a patient with acute pulmonary embolism?

    (A) severe dyspnea
    (B) poor tissue perfusion
    (C) right ventricle dysfunction
    (D) circulatory collapse and refractory hypoxemia
    (E) severe right heart pressures

31. The drug of choice for treating hypertensive encephalopathy in the nonpregnant patient is

    (A) sodium nitroprusside
    (B) labetalol
    (C) esmolol
    (D) IV nitroglycerin
    (E) hydralazine

32. Which of the following signs and symptoms best describes the presentation of a dissecting thoracic aortic aneurysm?

    (A) syncope, abdominal pain, back pain, and shock
    (B) severe quadriplegia and coma
    (C) abrupt and severe pain in the chest or between the scapulae
    (D) lower back pain with radiation into the legs
    (E) headache, neck pain, and vomiting accompanied by an inability to walk or stand

33. A 46-year-old patient was diagnosed 8 days ago with a DVT of his right leg. He now presents with a white leg with absent dorsalis pedis and posterior tibial pulses. Which of the following is the most likely diagnosis?

    (A) phlegmasia alba dolens
    (B) phlebitis areta
    (C) phlegmasia cerulea dolens
    (D) phlebitis fulminans

34. An 89-year-old female patient from a nursing home presents to the ED with abdominal pain and distention. The abdominal radiograph demonstrates multiple air-fluid levels and dilated large bowel loops consistent with a large bowel obstruction (LBO). What is the most likely cause of the obstruction?

    (A) diverticulitis
    (B) abdominal wall hernias
    (C) carcinoma
    (D) sigmoid volvulus
    (E) adhesions

35. A 28-year-old man presents to the ED with a back injury following an all-terrain vehicle (ATV) crash. The examination reveals a sensory deficit at the nipples. The spinal cord injury level is most likely at which of the following levels?

    (A) T1
    (B) T2
    (C) T3
    (D) T4
    (E) T5

36. *Pseudomonas* pneumonia is most likely associated with which of the following patient populations, signs, symptoms, and diagnostic findings?

    (A) immunocompromised patients such as alcoholics with an acute onset of fevers, rigors, and chest pain

    (B) minimal cough, mild fever, and minimal radiographic chest radiographic findings

    (C) prevalence in patients with chronic lung disease, insidious onset with low-grade fevers, dyspnea, and sputum production

    (D) prevalence in very young and old, high fever, bloody sputum, and chest pain

    (E) severe cyanosis, confusion, signs of systemic illness, and chest radiographic findings of bilateral lower lobe infiltrates and occasional empyema

37. In community-acquired pneumonia, which of the following bacterial organisms is most likely to be implicated?

    (A) *Klebsiella pneumoniae*
    (B) *Mycoplasma pneumoniae*
    (C) *Neisseria meningitidis*
    (D) *Streptococcus pneumoniae*
    (E) *Pseudomonas aeruginosa*

38. Using a scoring system such as the Pneumonia (PORT) Severity Index to determine the risk of mortality, which of the following patients could be appropriately managed with outpatient treatment for community-acquired pneumonia?

    (A) 49-year-old male nursing home resident with congestive heart failure, a serum blood urea nitrogen (BUN) level of 35 mg/dL and bilateral pleural effusions

    (B) 51-year-old woman with breast cancer, a temperature of 41°C, and blood glucose level of 260 mg/dL

    (C) 75-year-old woman with liver disease and altered mental status

    (D) 86-year-old man with a respiratory rate of 32/min

    (E) 86-year-old woman with a respiratory rate of 28/min and a history or chronic renal insufficiency

39. Which of the following extrapulmonary findings is most likely to be associated with *M pneumoniae*?

    (A) bullous myringitis
    (B) conjunctivitis
    (C) lymphangitis
    (D) otitis externa
    (E) guttate psoriasis eruption

40. Which of the following signs and symptoms is most likely to be indicative of acute myocardial ischemia or infarction?

    (A) dyspnea
    (B) left arm numbness and tingling
    (C) referred back pain
    (D) retrosternal chest discomfort
    (E) sternal chest pain

41. A tall, thin, 26-year-old woman presents to the ED with an acute onset of right-sided pleuritic chest pain and dyspnea. What is the most likely diagnosis?

    (A) right tension pneumothorax
    (B) left pneumothorax
    (C) right pleural effusion
    (D) right spontaneous pneumothorax
    (E) left atelectasis

42. A patient presents with an acute asthmatic attack. Multiple doses of inhaled adrenergic agents are used but the patient continues to have bronchospasms. Which of the following medications is most paramount in the treatment of bronchospasms?

    (A) corticosteroids
    (B) anticholinergics
    (C) theophylline
    (D) magnesium
    (E) leukotriene modifiers

43. A 21-year-old woman presents to the ED with a several-hour history of abdominal pain that has localized to the right lower quadrant (RLQ), with associated nausea, vomiting, diarrhea, and anorexia. For suspected appendicitis,

which of the following would be the diagnostic study of choice?

(A) abdominal pelvic ultrasound

(B) plain abdominal radiograph

(C) abdominopelvic helical computed tomography (CT) unenhanced CT abdomen/pelvis

(D) magnetic resonance imaging (MRI)

(E) focused appendiceal helical CT with oral and colonic contrast CT abdomen/pelvis

44. Which of the following is the most common etiology of upper gastrointestinal (GI) bleeding?

(A) diverticulosis

(B) erosive gastritis

(C) Mallory–Weiss syndrome

(D) peptic ulcer disease

(E) inflammatory bowel disease

45. A 51-year-old man presents to the ED with complains of colicky right upper quadrant and epigastric pain radiating to his back about 3 hours after eating. Which of the following would be the diagnostic study of choice?

(A) helical CT with rectal contrast

(B) right upper quadrant ultrasound

(C) chest CT with IV contrast

(D) acute abdominal plain radiographs

(E) cardiac stress test with echocardiogram

46. Which of the following is the most likely underlying source of an adult food bolus impaction?

(A) angiodysplasia

(B) bezoars

(C) Boerhaave syndrome

(D) Mallory–Weiss syndrome

(E) Schatzki ring

47. Which of the following clinical conditions would the focused assessment sonography for trauma (FAST) be most useful in confirming the suspected diagnosis?

(A) suspected ectopic pregnancy

(B) right upper quadrant pain

(C) suspected retroperitoneal bleeding

(D) right calf swelling and pain

(E) blunt abdominal injury

48. Which of the following is the most common cause of erosive esophagitis?

(A) radiation therapy

(B) gastrointestinal reflux

(C) candida

(D) herpes simplex virus

(E) pills

49. A 2-year-old child was brought to the ED after swallowing a button battery from a watch. Which of the following statements is true regarding button battery ingestion?

(A) A button battery lodged in the esophagus is a true emergency because of the extremely rapid action of the alkaline substance on the mucosa.

(B) Button battery ingestion is essentially a benign ingestion because of the unlikelihood of the battery dissolving.

(C) Button battery ingestion is a minor emergency that can often be treated with a Foley balloon technique extraction.

(D) Most button batteries, even if symptomatic, can be left to pass through the GI tract naturally by peristalsis.

(E) Surgical removal of the button battery is always indicated, even if the patient is asymptomatic.

50. A 62-year-old patient presents to the ED with generalized abdominal pain, nausea, vomiting, and abdominal distention. The radiographs demonstrate multiple loops of dilated small bowel, air-fluid levels, and a string of pearls sign. What is the most likely cause of this clinical scenario?

(A) neoplasm

(B) incarceration of abdominal hernias

(C) gallstone ileus

(D) bezoars

(E) adhesions following abdominal surgery

51. A patient presents to the ED with frequent, mucoid, watery stools, nausea, and lower abdominal pain. The patient has been on a cephalosporin-type antibiotic for about 3 months. The most likely diagnosis would be

(A) diverticulitis
(B) anal fissures
(C) pseudomembranous enterocolitis
(D) anorectal tumor
(E) ulcerative colitis (UC)

52. A 48-year-old patient presents to the ED with tachycardia, palpitations, and restlessness. The diagnosis of thyroid storm is confirmed and general supportive care is provided. Which of the following is the correct sequence of medications to treat thyroid storm?

(A) propylthiouracil (PTU)—propranolol—iodide
(B) propranolol—PTU—iodide
(C) propranolol—iodide—PTU
(D) iodide—propranolol—PTU
(E) iodide—PTU—propranolol

53. A 6-year-old child (20 kg) presents to the ED after being struck by a car. The child suffered chest, head, and abdominal trauma. The vital signs demonstrate a blood pressure of 80/40 mm Hg, a pulse of 170/min, and a respiratory rate of 40/min. After the airway is managed, which is the most appropriate initial fluid therapy?

(A) dextrose 5% water at 100 mL/h
(B) normal saline 5 mL/kg bolus, then 100 mL/h
(C) lactated Ringer's 20 mL/kg bolus
(D) lactated Ringer's at 20 mL/h
(E) normal saline 200 mL bolus

54. A patient presents to the ED with a dislocated shoulder. Nitrous oxide is the drug selected for sedation and analgesia during reduction. Which of the following is true with regard to the administration of nitrous oxide for short-term painful procedures in the ED?

(A) A 50:50 concentration of nitrous and oxygen should be used.
(B) Never administer oxygen with nitrous oxide.
(C) Nitrous oxide concentrations should always be less than 30%.
(D) Higher altitudes require lower concentrations of nitrous oxide.
(E) Nitrous oxide is not approved for ED use.

55. A 1-month-old infant presents to the ED with lethargy, tachycardia, fever, rash, and leukocytosis. The diagnosis of bacterial meningitis is suspected and a lumbar puncture was performed. What organisms should the antibiotic cover in this case?

(A) *Listeria monocytogenes*, group B streptococcus, and *Escherichia coli*
(B) *E coli*, *Klebsiella*, and *Pseudomonas*
(C) group B streptococcus, enterococcus, and chlamydia
(D) *Listeria*, *Staphylococcus*, and *Campylobacter* species
(E) group A streptrococcus and *Salmonella* species

56. A pregnant woman, at 25 weeks' gestation, is involved in a motor vehicle accident. She suffers blunt abdominal trauma. The vital signs are a pulse of 100/min, a respiratory rate of 40/min, and a BP of 78/40. Which of the following is a true statement regarding the management of trauma in pregnancy?

(A) Intubation should be avoided in the mother because of barotrauma complications.
(B) The first resuscitative efforts should be directed toward the mother.
(C) The fetus is less susceptible to hypoxia because of uterine reserve.
(D) A stat C-section should be considered in every patient.
(E) Fetal distress is not easily recognized.

57. Which of the following disorders may present with a patient experiencing anxiety, tremors, palpitations, fatigue, and hemiplegia?

(A) hyperglycemia

(B) euglycemia

(C) ketoacidosis

(D) hyperglycemic hyperosmolar nonketotic coma

(E) hypoglycemia

58. A 45-year-old woman presents to the ED with acute painless loss of vision, photophobia associated with a smaller unilateral pupil on the involved side. Which of the following is the most likely diagnosis?

(A) central retinal artery occlusion

(B) central retinal vein occlusion (CRVO)

(C) iritis/uveitis

(D) retrobulbar hemorrhage or hematoma

(E) hyphema

59. Which of the following patient population is at the greatest risk for an epidural hematoma (EDH) following head trauma?

(A) infants

(B) young adults

(C) young children

(D) elderly patients

60. Subdural hematomas are most likely characterized by which of the following findings?

(A) may result from a skull fracture across the middle meningeal artery

(B) formed deep within the brain tissue and usually caused by shearing or tensile forces that mechanically stretch and tear deep small-caliber arterioles

(C) are associated with traumatic blood within the cerebrospinal fluid (CSF) and meningeal intima caused by small tears of subarachnoid vessels

(D) a collection of clear, xanthochromic blood-tinged fluid in the dural space

(E) a rupture of superficial bridging vessels with rapid movement of the head, as in acceleration–deceleration injuries

61. Which of the following therapeutic interventions is the most beneficial in lowering increased intracranial pressure (ICP) associated with a subarachnoid hemorrhage?

(A) nimodipine

(B) mannitol

(C) hyperventilation

(D) corticosteroids

(E) phenobarbital

62. Which of the following maneuvers would be the most helpful in diagnosing an Achilles tendon rupture?

(A) pivot shift

(B) Thompson–Doherty test

(C) Lachman test

(D) anterior drawer test

(E) posterior drawer test

63. Which of the following diagnostic studies is the most reliable marker of rhabdomyolysis?

(A) urine myoglobin

(B) creatinine kinase

(C) creatinine kinase-MB

(D) lactate dehydrogenase (LDH)

(E) aldolase

64. Le Fort I facial fracture is best described as

(A) a fracture involving the maxilla, the nasal bones, and the medial aspects of the orbits

(B) a fracture involving the maxilla at the level of the nasal fossa

(C) a fracture involving the maxilla, zygoma, nasal bones, ethmoids, vomer, and all lesser bones of the cranial base

(D) A fracture involving frontal bones and bones of the midface

65. Maxillofacial trauma in a 35-year-old woman is most likely associated with

(A) falls

(B) motor vehicle collision (MVC)

(C) work related

(D) sports related

(E) domestic violence

66. Which of the following conventional or plain radiographic views of the face is most beneficial for evaluating trauma of the midface?

    (A) panorex
    (B) submental-vertex
    (C) Towne view
    (D) Caldwell view
    (E) Waters view

67. A 42-year-old man presents to the ED with a right-sided facial injury after an assault with a wooden club. The patient complains of diplopia and pain to the right side of the face. The examination reveals enophthalmos, impaired ocular motility, and infraorbital hypoesthesias. What is the most likely diagnosis?

    (A) maxilla fracture involving the superior orbital ridge
    (B) orbital blowout fracture with herniation of contents into the frontal sinus
    (C) maxillary blowout fracture with herniation into the soft palate
    (D) orbital blowout fracture with herniation of contents into the maxillary sinus
    (E) orbital blowout fracture without herniation

68. A patient is involved in a motor vehicle accident and suffered a fractured neck. The fracture lines extend through the pedicles of C2. Which of the following describes this unstable hyperextension fracture to the cervical spine?

    (A) Jefferson fracture
    (B) extension teardrop fracture
    (C) clay-shoveler fracture
    (D) Johnson fracture
    (E) hangman fracture

69. A 68-year-old woman presents to the ED with an exacerbation of chronic low-back pain. Which of the following indicates the patient has developed cauda equina syndrome?

    (A) lower leg weakness, paresthesias to both legs, and incontinence
    (B) loss of deep tendon reflexes bilaterally and urinary retention

    (C) bilateral leg weakness, loss of peripheral pulses, and incontinence
    (D) bilateral leg pain, saddle anesthesia, urinary incontinence, and fecal incontinence
    (E) anesthesia to entire leg, bilateral leg weakness, and loss of deep tendon reflexes

70. A 64-year-old man presents to the ED with decreased visual acuity, red eye, and a "steamy" or hazy cornea. What is the most likely diagnosis?

    (A) acute narrow-angle glaucoma
    (B) iritis/uveitis
    (C) orbital cellulitis
    (D) allergic conjunctivitis
    (E) episcleritis

71. A 6-year-old boy presents to the ED with abdominal pain, blood in the stools, and arthritis. The examination reveals multiple dark erythematous lesions on his legs and buttocks. These findings are characteristic of which disease?

    (A) Kawasaki disease
    (B) meningococcemia
    (C) erythema nodosum
    (D) Henoch–Schonlein purpura
    (E) pneumococcal meningitis

72. A 71-year-old woman presents to the ED with malaise, acute headache, and a rapidly decreasing visual acuity. Which of the following best describes this condition?

    (A) glaucoma
    (B) multiple sclerosis
    (C) temporal arteritis
    (D) myasthenia gravis
    (E) viral encephalitis

73. A 40-year-old man presents to the ED with acute blunt chest and abdominal trauma following a motor vehicle crash. The patient presented with jugular venous distention,

decreased BP, and muffled heart tones. Which of the following is the most likely diagnosis?

(A) pericardial tamponade
(B) tension pneumothorax
(C) myocardial rupture
(D) aortic rupture
(E) myocardial contusion

74. Spontaneous esophageal rupture following forceful vomiting after overindulging in food and alcohol is known as:

(A) bezoar
(B) Boerhaave syndrome
(C) Burger sign
(D) Brudzinski sign

75. A patient presents to the ED after suffering a significant pelvic injury following a fall. The patient has a grade III pelvic fracture and blood at the tip of the urethral meatus. How should one proceed in evaluating urethra and/or bladder injuries?

(A) Gently pass a 14- or 16-Fr Foley catheter.
(B) Gently pass a 14- or 16-Fr Coudé catheter.
(C) Notify the urologist for immediate cystoscopy.
(D) Gently pass a 10- or 12-Fr (pediatric) Foley catheter.
(E) Perform a retrograde urethrogram.

76. A 34-year-old male patient presents to the ED following an episode of "rough" sex with his girlfriend. He complains of a painful swollen penis. Which of the following descriptions best defines a penile rupture?

(A) rupture of the corpus cavernosum when the tunica albuginea is torn
(B) rupture of the dorsal penile artery into the tunica albuginea
(C) rupture of the corpus spongiosum from a tear in the dorsal penile vein
(D) rupture of the tunica albuginea from a tear into the corpus cavernosum
(E) rupture of the corpus cavernosum when the corpus spongiosum is torn

77. A 41-year-old man injures his finger while playing basketball. He is unable to extend the distal interphalangeal (DIP) joint. The radiograph shows an avulsion fracture to the proximal dorsal region of the distal phalanx. What is the diagnosis?

(A) Bennett fracture
(B) Rolando fracture
(C) mallet finger fracture
(D) swan neck deformity

78. A child falls on an outstretched hand. She complains of pain and swelling to the wrist. The radiograph demonstrates a buckling of the cortex to the distal radius. What is your diagnosis?

(A) torus fracture
(B) greenstick fracture
(C) complete fracture
(D) plastic deformation

79. A 40-year-old man slips on the ice, injuring his left arm. He complains of pain and swelling to the midshaft humeral region. The physical examination reveals a wrist drop on the injured side. Which nerve is most likely injured?

(A) ulnar
(B) radial
(C) median
(D) axillary
(E) subclavian

80. After viewing the picture in Fig. 17-1, identify the proper nomenclature of this elbow injury.

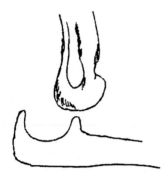

Figure 17-1. Elbow dislocation

(A) anterior elbow dislocation
(B) posterior elbow dislocation
(C) anterior humeral dislocation
(D) posterior humeral dislocation

81. A 7-year-old child presents to the ED with fever, neck pain, and a "duck-like" voice. Which of the following is the most likely diagnosis?

(A) peritonsillar abscess
(B) streptococcus pharyngitis
(C) epiglottitis
(D) Ludwig angina
(E) retropharyngeal abscess

82. What is the mechanism of injury for an anterior shoulder dislocation?

(A) shoulder internal rotation and adduction
(B) shoulder internal rotation with abduction
(C) shoulder external rotation with adduction
(D) shoulder external rotation with abduction
(E) fall on an outstretched hand

83. Which of the following medications is responsible for the most drug-related deaths?

(A) benzodiazepines
(B) tricyclic antidepressants (TCAs)

(C) stimulants
(D) monoamine oxidase inhibitors
(E) lithium

84. A 30-year-old male patient presents to the ED with an acute change in mental status. The examination reveals a patient who is sleepy but arousable to loud verbal stimuli. His airway is intact and the vital signs are stable. Investigative studies indicate an alcohol level of 150 mg/dL, an anion gap of 30 meq/L, a metabolic acidosis, an osmolar gap of 20, and calcium oxalate crystalluria. What is the most likely diagnosis?

(A) methanol poisoning
(B) ethanol poisoning
(C) ethylene glycol poisoning
(D) isopropanol poisoning
(E) buspirone poisoning

85. A 20-year-old man presents to the ED following a lethal overdose of acetaminophen. What is the antidote for acetaminophen toxicity?

(A) flumazenil
(B) narcan
(C) vitamin K
(D) *N*-acetylcysteine (NAC)
(E) ethanol

86. Which of the following clinical findings differentiates periorbital from orbital cellulitis?

(A) erythema
(B) fever
(C) lid edema
(D) worsening pain with eye movements
(E) development of a rash on the face

87. A 47-year-old man presents to the ED comatose after ingesting an unknown liquid substance. Investigative studies include the following: pH, 7.45; Na, 140; Cl, 110; HCO$_3$, 19; glucose, 180; BUN, 30; Cr, 1.5; ETOH, 0.0; high serum ketones; and a measured osmolality of 380. These findings are most consistent with which of the following toxin ingestions?

(A) methanol

(B) ethylene glycol

(C) diabetic ketoacidosis

(D) isopropanol

(E) alcoholic ketoacidosis

88. A 58-year-old man presents to the ED hypothermic after an environmental exposure to cold weather and snow. The patient's core temperature is 85.5°F. Which of the following is the most accurate statement regarding this scenario?

(A) Shivering is common.

(B) An Osborne (J) wave is pathognomic for hypothermia.

(C) Rough handling can produce serious dysrhythmias.

(D) A nasogastric tube should be inserted to protect the airway from regurgitation.

(E) The patient is in an excitation phase of hypothermia.

89. A patient presents to the ED after being bitten by an unknown "insect" while camping. The pain began as a pinprick sensation at the bite site and spread quickly to include the entire bitten extremity. The bite wound became erythematous 45 minutes after the bite. The bite evolved into a target lesion and the patient complains of muscle cramp-like spasms in the large muscle groups. Which of the following is the most likely cause?

(A) black widow spider

(B) hobo spider

(C) brown recluse spider

(D) tarantula

(E) scorpion

90. Which of the following is the most important treatment option in a patient with moderate acute mountain sickness (AMS)?

(A) oxygen therapy

(B) dexamethasone

(C) hyperbaric therapy

(D) acetazolamide

(E) immediate descent

91. A patient presents to the ED after being trapped in a house fire. The patient suffered partial thickness burns over the entire anterior chest and abdomen, entire right arm, and the entire right leg. Using the rule of nines, what is the estimated percentage of burn?

(A) 36%

(B) 45%

(C) 48%

(D) 54%

(E) 72%

92. Which of the following is the most common cause of death by hemorrhage in patients with hemophilia A?

(A) gastrointestinal hemorrhage

(B) retroperitoneal hemorrhage

(C) pulmonary hemorrhage

(D) renal hemorrhage

(E) intracranial hemorrhage

93. A 29-year-old logger was struck in the back with a load of logs. The evaluation reveals absence of patellar reflexes. This finding is consistent with an injury at which of the following dermatome levels?

(A) C7

(B) L1

(C) L4

(D) S1

(E) S4

94. A 79-year-old man presents to the ED with a heart rate of 50 bpm, second degree A–V block Mobitz at 50 bpm, BP of 90/60 mm Hg, potassium level of 5.8 mEq/L, and a digoxin level of 6.9 ng/mL. What is the treatment of choice in this scenario?

(A) calcium chloride

(B) potassium infusion

(C) atropine

(D) magnesium

(E) digoxin immune Fab fragments

95. A 39-year-old woman presents to the ED with agitation, tremors, visual hallucinations, fever, and tachycardia. The eye examination reveals nystagmus and a sixth cranial nerve palsy. Which of the following conditions best describes this clinical scenario?

(A) Korsakoff psychosis
(B) Wernicke encephalopathy
(C) acute dystonia
(D) acute cocaine toxicity
(E) trigeminal neuralgia

96. In addition to dental referral, which of the following represents the most appropriate standard therapy for a routine periodontal abscess in the ED setting?

(A) intravenous penicillin and topical analgesics
(B) intravenous penicillin and incision and drainage (I/D)
(C) oral penicillin and oral analgesics
(D) oral penicillin and saline rinses
(E) oral clindamycin and topical analgesics

97. Which of the following demographic groups below would be most likely to suffer from a primary tuberculosis (TB) infection presenting as extrapulmonary tuberculosis meningitis?

(A) elderly
(B) children younger than 2 years
(C) young adults
(D) alcoholics
(E) HIV patients with CD4 counts higher than $350/\mu L$

98. A patient is being evaluated for cough, fever, night sweats, and sputum production. On the basis of the history, the patient is suspected to have active tuberculosis. Which of the following is most significant in the ED setting for management of a patient with suspected active TB infection?

(A) hospital admission for multidrug resistant tuberculosis (MDRTB)
(B) respiratory isolation in negative pressure room

(C) health care providers should wear N-95 particulate respirators or mask
(D) reporting to local public health department
(E) all of the above

99. Air contrast enema is diagnostic in approximately what percentages of intussusception cases of less than 24 hours of duration?

(A) 1%
(B) 10%
(C) 30%
(D) 70%
(E) 95%

100. A 4-week-old infant presents with several hours of persistent crying. A markedly red and edematous left third toe is found upon examination. What anatomical location of the affected digit would be the most appropriate site to perform an emergent surgical release of the strangulation?

(A) anterior
(B) dorsal
(C) lateral
(D) proximal
(E) superficial

101. A 3-month-old infant presents with low-grade fevers, rhinorrhea, cough, wheezing, mild retractions, and no difficulty feeding for 3 days. The oxygen saturation was greater than 93%. The medical history is noted for 35 weeks' gestation at birth. Immunizations are up to date. Otherwise, the infant has been healthy. The infant was diagnosed with respiratory syncytial virus (RSV). Which of the following clinical rationales would most likely warrant hospital admission?

(A) evaluation for additional coexisting respiratory infections
(B) intravenous antimicrobial therapy
(C) intravenous steroid therapy
(D) monitoring for episodes of apnea or respiratory failure
(E) parent education

102. A 16-year-old man presents with fever, sore throat, malaise and fatigue, and cervical adenopathy for 5 days. His primary care physician (PCP) had placed him on an antimicrobial medication 2 days ago. The adolescent now presents to the ED with a diffuse widespread maculopapular rash and petechiae on the soft palate. Which of the following medications was likely prescribed by the PCP and caused the reaction?

    (A) acyclovir
    (B) azithromycin
    (C) amoxicillin
    (D) rifampin
    (E) tetracycline

103. A 19-year-old man presents with delirium, dilated pupils, tachycardia, urinary retention, and hyperthermia. Which of the following classes of drugs is suspected to be the offending agent the patient ingested?

    (A) anticholinergic
    (B) caffeine
    (C) heroin
    (D) salicylate
    (E) acetaminophen

104. A 32-year-old man presents in police custody for an evaluation of bizarre behavior. The patient is disheveled, paranoid, and agitated. After his initial medical screening examination and initial diagnostic screening, he becomes combative. His toxicology screen was negative. Which of the following is the most appropriate medication to administer in the ED setting?

    (A) haloperidol or ziprasidone HCl
    (B) risperidone
    (C) clomipramine
    (D) lithium
    (E) lorazepam

105. Which of the following complications has a high likelihood of developing in ED management of venomous snakebites to the extremities?

    (A) delayed serum sickness
    (B) dislodged teeth contaminating the wound
    (C) compartment syndrome
    (D) delayed absorption of antivenom
    (E) immediate death after venomous snakebite

Answers and Explanations

1. **(B)** Survival of prehospital cardiac arrest is most notably improved by defibrillation and good cardiopulmonary resuscitation (CPR). Emergent airway management, the use of epinephrine, prompt treatment of hypotension, and rapid transport to the most appropriate facility only moderately increase survival rates when compared with early defibrillation or CPR. *(Ornato, 2004, p. 65)*

2. **(D)** Rh-negative women who are exposed to Rh-positive blood through pregnancy, delivery, threatened or spontaneous hemorrhage, surgery for ectopic pregnancy, or amniocentesis may become sensitized and require anti-D immunoglobulin (RhoGAM). Patients who are Rh-negative should be administered RhoGAM in threatened or spontaneous abortions. Rh-negative women in the setting of ectopic pregnancies, threatened abortions, and/or complete abortions should be given 50 μg if they are at less than 12 weeks' gestation and 300 μg if they are at 12 or more weeks' gestation. *(Houry and Abbott, 2006, p. 2752)*

3. **(B)** Metabolic acidosis is characterized by increased production of acids, decreased excretion of acids, or loss of bicarbonate. The etiology of metabolic acidosis is divided into those with a normal anion gap and those associated with an increased anion gap. Metabolic acidosis with an increased anion gap includes lactic acidosis, ketoacidosis, and renal failure. Lactic acidosis, the most common cause of nonhospitalized, nondiabetic metabolic acidosis is due to decreased oxygen delivery to tissues and associated anaerobic metabolism, which results in an increased production of lactate. This lactate production accompanies severe metabolic acidosis. Low tissue perfusion, characteristic of lactic acidosis, may include shock and sepsis. Metabolic acidosis with a normal anion gap is known as hyperchloremic metabolic acidosis. The primary causes of normal anion gap acidosis include renal loss of bicarbonate through proximal tubular acidosis, distal tubular acidosis, hyperkalemic renal tubular acidosis, renal insufficiency, or carbonic anhydrase inhibition and gastrointestinal loss of alkali through diarrhea, pancreatic fistulas, or ureterosigmoidostomy. *(Collings, 2006, pp. 1922-1932)*

4. **(A)** Pulmonary thromboembolism (PTE) is primarily the result of clot migration from DVT. Even with current technology, the diagnosis of DVT and PTE is rather evasive and difficult. Ventilation/perfusion scanning ($\dot{V}/\dot{Q}$) is relatively nondiagnostic in most cases of PTE. Only 41% of patients with PTE confirmed through pulmonary angiography will have a high-probability lung scan. In general, a patient has a less than 5% chance of having a PTE if the scan is read as "normal." A "high-probability" scan has a more than 85% chance that a PTE is present. A scan interpreted as "low probability" or "nondiagnostic" will have a 15% to 85% chance of having a PTE. Therefore, a nondiagnostic or low-probability scan is useless in ruling in or ruling out a PTE. Computed tomography offers a relatively good way of diagnosing PTE; however, the sensitivity ranges from 40% to 65% and the negative predictive value is around 82% when compared with pulmonary angiography. The pulmonary angiogram is considered the last resort for diagnosing a PTE. A "positive" angiogram provides

essentially 100% certainty of the diagnosis of PTE. A "negative" angiogram provides more than 90% certainty that PTE is excluded. However, technical and patient factors such as dye concerns and movement can significantly alter the diagnostic ability of angiogram. *(Kline and Runyon, 2006, pp. 1371-1381)*

5. **(E)** Direct visualization of the endotracheal tube passing through the vocal cords is the most reliable indicator for endotracheal tube placement. The next most reliable is an end CO_2 device. Auscultation of the chest and epigastric areas may reveal transmitted sounds from the endotracheal tube in the stomach. Condensation in the tube can be an unreliable indicator of proper endotracheal tube placement. *(Danzl and Vissers, 2004, pp. 108-109)*

6. **(C)** The definition of hypernatremia is a serum sodium level more than 145 mEq/L. Hypernatremia is classified as isovolemic (diabetes insipidus, skin loss through hyperthermia, and iatrogenic), hypervolemic (administration of hypernatremic solutions, mineralocorticoid excess as in Conn or Cushing syndrome, and salt ingestion), and hypovolemic (renal losses through diuretics or glycosuria, GI, respiratory, or skin losses, and adrenal deficiencies). Water deficit in hypernatremic patients is calculated by the following formula:

In Women:

Water deficit (L) = [0.5 (body weight, kg)] × (measured serum sodium/normal serum sodium) − 1

Water deficit = 0.5 (60) = 30 [(180/140) − 1] = 30 (0.2857) = 8.6 L.

(Gibbs and Tavel, 2006, pp. 1935-1937)

7. **(A)** MAT is defined as a chaotic, irregular rhythm with atrial rates of 100 to 150 bpm. Typically, there are more than two foci of impulse formation with at least three distinctly different P waves with varying P″ R, RR, and P′ P′ intervals. MAT is commonly associated with COPD, theophylline toxicity, and β-adrenergic agonist therapy. AF is a totally chaotic atrial rhythm with multiple microreentry circuits of atrial rates from 300 to 600 impulses/min. The most common causes of AF include ischemic heart disease, valvular heart disease, pericarditis, and hyperthyroidism. Atrial flutter is characterized by regular atrial depolarization rates of 250 to 350 bpm, with varying degrees of atrioventricular block. Common causes of atrial flutter include atherosclerotic heart disease, myocardial infarction, thyrotoxicosis, pulmonary embolism, mitral valve disease, congestive heart failure, and metabolic derangements. Sinus bradycardia is a regular rhythm with atrial and ventricular rates of less than 60 bpm with normal P-wave morphology and PR duration. Sinus bradycardia can be found in healthy adults or it may be associated with pathologic conditions such as hypothermia, excessive parasympathetic tone, carotid sensitivity, or myocardial infarction. A type II second-degree AV block or Mobitz II block is characterized by a sudden interruption of AV conduction without prior prolongation of the PR interval. Mobitz II is often associated with a variety of acute and chronic diseases such as anterior wall ischemia. *(Yearly and Delbridge, 2006, pp. 1228-1229)*

8. **(B)** Hypercalcemia associated with malignancies is commonly due to increased bone resorption through osteoclastic factors, parathyroid hormone (PTH) factors, prostaglandins, peptides, steroids, and direct erosion by tumor cells. Common neoplasms include multiple myeloma, lymphosarcoma, adult T-cell lymphoma, and Burkitt lymphoma. Symptoms of hypercalcemia are variable depending on the degree elevation. Typical symptoms include constipation, anorexia, vomiting, confusion, obtundation, psychosis, nephrolithiasis, renal insufficiency, myopathy, back pain, weakness, and hypertension. Hyperkalemia may produce manifestations of weakness, irritability, paresthesias, paralysis, cardiac arrhythmia, and decreased deep tendon reflexes. Hypomagnesemia symptoms include weakness, fasciculations, tremors, convulsions, delirium, coma, hyperreflexia, and cardiac arrhythmias. Hypoglycemia commonly presents with varying degrees of diaphoresis, anxiety, tremors, tachycardia, palpitations, fatigue, syncope, headache, visual disturbances,

hemiplegia, and seizures. Hyponatremia may present as confusion, muscle cramps, anorexia, nausea, lethargy, seizures, and coma depending on the degree and rapidity of onset. *(Gibbs and Taval, 2006, pp. 1944-1947)*

9. **(A)** Renal tubular acidosis is an example of a normal anion gap acidosis in which there is an increase in chloride and a loss of bicarbonate. The other choices of diagnoses are associated with a high anion gap metabolic acidosis or a metabolic alkalosis. *(Morris, 2008, p. 831)*

10. **(C)** The medial ankle support comprises the deltoid ligaments, which include tibionavicular, anterior tibiotalar, tibiocalcaneal, and posterior tibiotalar parts. The most common mechanism of injury is an external rotational force. The lateral portion of the ankle is supported by the anterior talofibular, anterior inferior tibiofibular, interosseous, posterior tibiofibular, and the calcaneofibular ligaments. Approximately two-thirds of all ankle injuries are isolated anterior talofibular ligament injuries. About 20% involve both anterior talofibular and calcaneofibular ligament injuries. Less than 5% of the ankle injuries are isolated deltoid ligament sprains. *(Ho and Abu-Laban, 2006, pp. 808-820)*

11. **(E)** The ECG criterion used to define an acute myocardial injury pattern is ST-segment elevation of 1 mm or more above the baseline. This should be measured 0.04 seconds past the J point. ST-segment depression and T wave changes are indicative of myocardial ischemia. Abnormal Q waves are consistent with myocardial infarction. Q waves that are 2 mm wide or 25% of the height of the R wave in that lead are indicative of dead heart muscle. The following are the anatomical sites of coronary ischemia related to the ECG leads: anterior septal wall is leads V1 to V4; high lateral wall is leads V5, V6, plus I, and aVL; inferior wall are leads II, III, and aVF; posterior wall leads demonstrate marked depression in leads V1 to V4 (mirror image of anterior wall); and right ventricular infarction will demonstrate ST-segment changes in lead V4R. *(Cummins, 1999, pp. 9-30)*

12. **(D)** The patient in this scenario has clinical signs and symptoms associated with temporal arteritis or giant cell arteritis. The most appropriate course of action is to treat with intravenous steroids and obtain ophthalmology consultation when patient has visual loss. Lumbar puncture would be an appropriate intervention if meningitis was suspected. Oxygen therapy is a customary intervention for treating cluster headaches. Nonsteroidal anti-inflammatory drugs (NSAIDs) are indicated for tension headaches *(Tobleman and Stone, 2004, p. 288, 291-294)*

13. **(C)** Pregnancy-induced hypertension (PIH) is defined as a blood pressure (BP) reading of 140/90 mm Hg or higher. The subtypes of PIH include hypertension without proteinuria or edema, preeclampsia (hypertension with proteinuria or edema), and eclampsia (seizures in the pregnant patient with signs of preeclampsia). PIH occurs in about 5% of pregnancies and eclampsia occurs in less than 1 in 2,000 deliveries. Hydralazine is the most common antihypertensive used in PIH. The typical dose is 5 mg IV and repeated in a dose of 5 to 10 mg IV every 20 minutes as needed to keep the diastolic BP less than 110 mm Hg. Other agents used with some degree of success include nifedipine, nitroprusside, and labetalol. Magnesium sulfate is used primarily in pregnancy to terminate ongoing seizures and prevent further seizures. This is usually accomplished by keeping the serum magnesium levels at 4 to 7 mg/dL. In general, nitroglycerin and hydrochlorothiazide are not indicated in PIH. *(Newton and Calder, 2006, pp. 2762-2765)*

14. **(A)** Two hours after the onset of an acute myocardial infarction, the cardiac enzymes would most commonly demonstrate a normal troponin and CK-MB levels. Cardiac troponin I and CK-MB levels elevate in 3 to 12 hours after the onset of myocardial infarction. Serum myoglobin level elevates 1 to 4 hours after the onset of myocardial infarction. *(Hollander and Dierks, 2004, p. 361)*

15. **(C)** Myocardial necrosis can be identified with a great degree of specificity by troponin I,

particularly in settings of cocaine use, recent surgery, and chronic renal failure. Troponin T and serum myoglobin have a very high sensitivity, but the specificity is poor with regard to myocardial injury. *(Green and Hill, 2004, pp. 336-338)*

16. **(D)** Indications for IV thrombolytic therapy include acute myocardial infarction less than 6 to 12 hours old, new or presumed new left bundle branch block, and an ECG that has at least 1 mm of ST-segment elevation in two or more contiguous leads. Additional indications include chest pain and ST elevation unresolved with nitroglycerin. ST-segment depression is not an indication for thrombolytic therapy. Known absolute and relative contraindications to use of thrombolytics must always be taken in consideration. *(Hollander and Dierks, 2004, pp. 352-353; Humphries, 2008, pp. 561-562)*

17. **(B)** In this scenario, the patient's sodium level dropped severely and rapidly secondary to excessive water intake. In this setting, patients may present with confusion, muscle cramps, lethargy, anorexia, nausea, seizures, and coma. Other causes of euvolemic hyponatremia include syndrome of inappropriate secretion of antidiuretic hormone (SIADH), renal failure, glucocorticoid deficiency (hypopituitarism), hypothyroidism, and multiple medications such as thiazide diuretics. *(Gibbs and Taval, 2006, p. 1934)*

18. **(A)** The symptoms described are due to hypoglycemia caused by pentamidine isethionate. Pentamidine is a common treatment for pneumocystis in the AIDS patient. Pentamidine is an antiprotozoal agent that inhibits synthesis of DNA, RNA, phospholipids, and proteins. Common side effects include hypoglycemia, renal impairment, leukopenia, hepatotoxicity, nausea, anorexia, hypotension, fever, and rash. Monitor metabolic parameters such as BUN level, creatinine level, glucose level, CBC, platelet count, liver function tests, and calcium level regularly while on pentamidine therapy. *(Rothman et al., 2006, p. 2079)*

19. **(C)** Hypokalemia is associated with serum potassium levels of less than 3.5 mEq/L. The ECG findings of hypokalemia include the following: flattened T waves, U waves, and ST-segment depressions. Hyperkalemia relates to serum potassium levels of more than 5.5 mEq/L. Serum potassium levels in the 6.5 to 7.5 mEq/L typically result in tall peaked T waves and short QT interval. Prolonged PR interval is seen with 7.5 to 8.0 mEq/L serum potassium level. QRS widening, flattening of the P wave, is associated with serum potassium levels of 10 to 12 mEq/L—prolonged QT interval is also associated with hypocalcemia *(Londner et al., 2004, pp. 172-174)*

20. **(C)** The typical presentation of pontine hemorrhage is coma, pinpoint reactive pupils, impaired lateral ocular motility, and quadriplegia with decerebrate posturing. Thalamic hemorrhage characteristically leads to impaired consciousness, contralateral motor and sensory loss, and gaze preference to the side of the hemorrhage. Cerebellar hemorrhages typically present with impaired gait, vertigo, limb ataxia, impaired consciousness, and cranial nerve palsies. Subarachnoid hemorrhage presents as a severe acute onset of a headache with associated neurological deficits of varying degrees depending on the extent and location of the hemorrhage. Lobar hemorrhages may present with symptoms of headache, nausea, vomiting, change in mental status, visual disturbance, seizures, and coma, depending on the extent and location of the bleed. *(Zivin, 2007, pp. 2769-2775)*

21. **(A)** MAT is associated with the following ECG characteristics: (1) three or more differently shaped P waves; (2) varying PP, PR, and RR intervals; and (3) atrial rhythm usually between 100 and 180. AF is associated with the following ECG characteristics: (1) fibrillatory waves of atrial activity, best seen in leads V1, V2, V3, and aVF and (2) irregular ventricular response, usually around 170 to 180 in patients with a healthy AV node. Ventricular tachycardia is associated with the following ECG characteristics: (1) wide QRS complexes; (2) rate greater than 100; (3) usually regular rhythm; and (4) a constant QRS axis. A sinus dysrhythmia is associated with the following ECG characteristics: (1) normal sinus P waves and PR intervals, (2)

1:1 AV conduction, and (3) variation of at least 0.12 second between the shortest and longest PP interval. Supraventricular tachycardia usually occurs at a rate of 100 to 250 bpm with a regular rhythm. *(Bolton, 2004, pp. 181-191)*

22. **(C)** Adenosine 6 mg, rapid IV push over 1 to 3 seconds, is the first-line drug for paroxysmal supraventricular tachycardia. If conversion to NSR is unsuccessful after 1 to 2 minutes, an additional dose of adenosine 12 mg, rapid IV over 1 to 3 seconds, may be given. The first-line therapy for VT is lidocaine. If the patient is free of carotid bruits, vagal maneuvers such as carotid sinus massage may be tried. In patients with ischemic heart disease, ice water immersion could be detrimental and should be avoided. *(Cummins; AHA, 1-32-1-35)*

23. **(C)** The first priority in the management of septic shock is assessment of the airway, oxygenation, and ventilation. Oxygen should be administered at 100% via mask or endotracheal tube. Fluid resuscitation is the second priority in the patient with septic shock. Tissue and organ perfusion can be assessed by parameters such as the patient's mental status, blood pressure, respiratory rate, pulse rate, skin color and temperature, central venous pressure, and urine output more than 30 mL/h (1 mL/kg/h in pediatric patients). Other important areas of assessment and management include acid–base status and antimicrobial therapy. *(Jui, 2004, pp. 236-241)*

24. **(D)** Flumazenil competitively blocks the effects of benzodiazepines on GABAnergic pathway–mediated inhibitors in the central nervous system (CNS). Naloxone HCl (Narcan) is a narcotic antagonist. Ketamine is a rapid-acting general anesthetic. Flutamide is a nonsteroidal, antiandrogenic agent used for prostate carcinoma. *(Bosse, 2004, pp. 1055-1056)*

25. **(D)** Organic material is generally not visible on plain radiographs. Glass and metal that are a reasonable size of at least 2 mm should be visible on plain radiographs. After imaging and wound exploration, if no foreign body is located, it is highly unlikely to be present in the wound. If the wound was at high risk of infec-

tion, a delayed wound closure would be indicated. *(Hollander and Singer, 2004, p. 287-288)*

26. **(D)** The most common pathogen found in infected cat bite wounds is *P multocida*. Pathogens like *S intermedius*, *E corrodens*, and *S aureus* are commonly seen in infected dog bite wounds. Infection with *Capnocytophaga canimorsus* infection is a rare occurrence secondary to dog bites that can lead to a widespread virulent bacterial infection. *H aphrophilus* infection is more common after tongue piercings. *(Schwab and Powers, 2004, p. 327)*

27. **(A)** Primary adrenocortical insufficiency (Addison disease) is characterized by inadequate secretion of cortisol, aldosterone, or both most frequently resulting from autoimmune-induced destruction of the adrenal glands. Other causes of Addison disease include tuberculosis, viral infections, carcinomatous destruction of the adrenals, adrenal infarction from arteritis or thrombosis, and adrenal hemorrhage. Laboratory results characteristically include hyperkalemia, hyponatremia, hypochloremia, hypoglycemia, elevated BUN/creatinine ratio (prerenal azotemia), anemia, decreased 24-hour urinary cortisol, 17-hydroxycorticosteroid, and 17-ketosteroids and increased ACTH (adrenocorticotropic hormone; primary adrenocortical insufficiency). SIADH is a syndrome of antidiuretic hormone (ADH) excess, which causes water retention and sodium loss. Common causes of SIADH include malignant tumors, intracranial hemorrhage, hydrocephalus, meningitis, brain abscess, chlorpropamide, thiazide diuretics, desmopressin, and chemotherapeutic agents. Laboratory values of SIADH include hyponatremia, urinary osmolarity greater than serum osmolarity, and urinary sodium level usually higher than 30 mEq/L. Cushing syndrome is characterized by glucocorticoid excess secondary to exaggerated adrenal cortisol production or chronic glucocorticoid therapy. Causes of primary glucocorticoid excess include idiopathic, tuberculosis, fungal infections, adrenal hemorrhage, congenital adrenal hyperplasia, sarcoidosis, amyloidosis, HIV/AIDS, and metastatic diseases. Common laboratory results include hypokalemia, hypochloremia, metabolic

alkalosis, hyperglycemia, and hypercholesterolemia. Primary hypothyroidism (ie, thyroid gland dysfunction) causes most cases of hypothyroidism. Secondary hypothyroidism includes pituitary dysfunction, postpartum necrosis, neoplasm, and infiltrative diseases causing a deficiency of thyroid-stimulating hormone (TSH or **thyrotropin**). Tertiary causes of hypothyroidism include hypothalamic diseases such as granuloma, neoplasm, or irradiation causing deficiency of thyroid releasing hormone. Common laboratory results of hypothyroidism are increased TSH, hyponatremia, increased cholesterol triglycerides, and liver function tests. Primary hyperparathyroidism is the result of oversecretion of PTH, which in turn causes hypercalcemia. A parathyroid adenoma is the primary etiology of hyperparathyroidism. Laboratory findings include hypercalcemia, hypophosphatemia, hyperchloremia, elevated serum alkaline phosphatase level, and hypercalcuria *(Ausiello et al., 2004, pp. 1900-1902; Gibbs and Taval, 2006, p. 1934; Ladenson and Kim, 2004, pp. 1700-1703; Niemann, 2004, pp. 1713-1720; Skorecki and Ausiello, 2004, pp. 831-834)*

28. **(A)** The most common cause of nontraumatic cardiac tamponade is metastatic malignancy. Common symptoms include dyspnea and profound exercise intolerance. Physical examination findings include tachycardia, low systolic arterial BP with a narrow pulse pressure, and pulsus paradoxus. Less common causes of nontraumatic tamponade include acute or chronic idiopathic pericarditis, uremia, bacterial or tubercular pericarditis, hemorrhage (from anticoagulant use), systemic lupus erythematosus, radiation treatments, and myxedema. *(Niemann, 2004, pp. 383-386)*

29. **(A)** A Hampton hump generally represents a focal area of hemorrhage within the lung or an actual pulmonary infarction. It is a wedge-shaped, dense, consolidated area on the pleural surface of the chest wall. A Westermark sign is a regional area of decreased pulmonary vascularity. Other more common findings of pulmonary embolism on a chest radiograph include atelectasis, elevated hemidiaphragm, patchy consolidation, and pleural effusions. *(Kline and Runyon, 2006, pp. 1371-1373)*

30. **(D)** Use of thrombolytic agents in the clinical setting of pulmonary embolism is steep in controversy. In evaluation of the benefits to risk ratio, the situation of a massive pulmonary embolism associated with sustained severe hypotension characterized as a systolic pressure of less than 80 mm Hg, refractory hypoxemia, and circulatory collapse should receive a thrombolytic agent such as alteplase. Thrombolytics have proven to be effective in normalizing pulmonary artery pressures, improving right ventricular dysfunction, stabilizing hemodynamics, and correcting hypoxia. The use of fibrinolytic agents such as urokinase and streptokinase and alteplase have been proven to be effective and are approved by the U.S. Food and Drug Administration. *(Kline and Runyon, 2006, pp. 1371-81)*

31. **(A)** Most of the medications listed are a good option for hypertensive emergencies. Sodium nitroprusside is the most widely used/available, is a rapidly acting arterial and venous dilator, and is the drug of choice for most hypertensive emergences unless there is severe kidney disease. Labetalol is an excellent drug for hypertensive emergencies. It is a competitive, selective alpha - 1-blocker and a competitive, nonselective β-blocker, with the β-blocking action four to eight times that of alpha blocking. Esmolol is an ultrashort-acting $β_1$ selective adrenergic blocker with rapid distribution and elimination. Nitroglycerin causes both arterial and venous dilation, with a greater effect on the venous system. The onset of action with nitroglycerin is almost immediate when given IV, and the half-life is 4 minutes. Hydralazine is a direct arterial dilator, with the onset of action within 10 minutes when given IV and duration of action 4 to 6 hours. *(Wu and Chanmugam, 2004, pp. 399-402)*

32. **(C)** Severe, abrupt chest pain that also may be located between the scapulas is common in aortic dissection. Pain in the anterior chest or back may represent involvement of the ascending or descending aorta. In the setting of symptoms of

severe back or abdominal pain accompanied by shock, a dissecting abdominal aneurysm is strongly likely. Rapid onset of stroke, inability to move muscles (except the lateral gaze), and quadriplegia are indicative of basilar artery occlusion. Headache, neck pain, and vomiting accompanied by the sudden onset of an inability to walk or stand are associated with cerebellar infarction. *(Prince and Johnson, 2004, pp. 1384-1385)*

33. **(C)** Phlegmasia alba dolens, "milk leg," is an uncommon presentation of DVT in which there is massive iliofemoral thrombosis. The leg is usually white or pale secondary to associated arterial spasm. When the dorsalis pedis and posterior pulses are diminished or absent, a false diagnosis of arterial occlusion may be made. A patient with phlegmasia cerulea dolens presents with an extensively swollen, cyanotic leg from venous engorgement due to massive iliofemoral thrombosis. This high-grade obstruction can compromise perfusion to the foot from high compartment pressures and lead to venous gangrene. *(Chopra, 2004, pp. 411-414)*

34. **(C)** Carcinoma of the colon is the most common cause of LBOs in adults. Diverticulitis can also cause LBOs, and patients often give a history of intermittent left lower quadrant pain. Sigmoid volvulus is a less common cause of LBO. It is seen most often in the elderly with poor bowel habits and chronic constipation. *(Chang et al., 2008, pp. 693-696)*

35. **(D)** The thoracic T4 dermatome runs across the nipple line. T2 dermatome involves the upper medial bicep region. T3 runs just above the nipple line, and T5 runs just below the nipple line. *(Ferri, 2005, pp. 5-6)*

36. **(E)** *Pseudomonas* pneumonia is commonly associated with hypoxia, confusion, fever, sepsis, and signs of systemic illness and lower lobe infiltrate on chest radiograph. *(Moffa and Emerman, 2004, p. 447)*

37. **(D)** Pneumococcus is the most commonly implicated bacteria in community-acquired pneumonia, except for *Mycoplasma* pneumonia, which is classified as an atypical pneumo-

nia. The other organisms are not frequently classified as community acquired. *(Moffa and Emerman, 2004, pp. 445-447)*

38. **(D)** Using the Pneumonia PORT, severity criteria points are assigned by gender, age, nursing home resident, underlying disease, and alterations of hemodynamic and abnormal diagnostic findings. Scores greater than 91 tend to have higher risk of mortality with recommendations to hospitalize *(Jaffe and Morris, 2004, pp. 763-766)*

39. **(A)** *Mycoplasma* pneumonia is most prevalent in older children, young adults, and the elderly. Bullous myringitis, rash (erythema multiforme), neurologic symptoms, arthritis, and arthralgia are common extrapulmonary symptoms found in patients with *Mycoplasma* pneumonia. *(Moffa and Emerman, 2004, pp. 448-449)*

40. **(D)** Retrosternal chest discomfort that is best described as pressure or squeezing as opposed to a pain is most likely to indicate myocardial ischemia or infarction. *(Field, 2006, p. 69)*

41. **(D)** Spontaneous pneumothorax most commonly affects tall, thin men, between the ages of 20 and 40 years, who are heavy cigarette smokers. The pain is usually pleuritic and localizes to the affected side. Most patients have decreased breath sounds on the affected side, but few have a significant tachypnea or tachycardia. *(Young and Humphries, 2004, pp. 462-464)*

42. **(A)** Corticosteroids remain one of the keystones of treatment for asthma. Steroids are thought to decrease airway inflammation and restore β-adrenergic responsiveness. The peak onset of inflammatory effects is delayed at least 4 to 8 hours following oral or intravenous administration. Theophylline is no longer considered a first-line therapy for acute asthma because of its high risk for toxicity, especially when combined with β-adrenergic drugs. Magnesium does have some bronchodilating effects and can be used in the management of acute asthma. Magnesium should be used only after standard therapy has been unsuccessful. Leukotriene modifiers decrease inflammation,

edema, mucous secretion, and bronchoconstriction, thereby diminishing the need for short-acting β_2 agonists; however, their role in the ED setting has not proven to be of significant benefit in the setting of acute bronchospasms. *(Cydulka, 2004, pp. 469-473)*

43. **(E)** In evaluation of suspected appendicitis a focused appendiceal helical CT with oral and colonic contrast has a sensitivity and specificity of 100% and 95%, respectively. Abdominal pelvic ultrasound has a sensitivity and specificity of 84% and 96%, respectively. Plain films have a sensitivity and specificity of 48% and 58%, respectively. An unenhanced abdominopelvic helical CT has slightly decreased sensitivity of 91% and specificity of 95%. MRI yields sensitivity of 97% and 92% specificity but is not frequently utilized for such evaluation. *(Gallagher, 2004, p. 491-492)*

44. **(D)** The most common etiology of upper GI bleeding (60%) is peptic ulcer disease. This includes gastric, duodenal, and stomal ulcers. Diverticular bleeding usually results from erosion into a penetrating artery of the diverticulum. The GI bleeding associated with diverticular bleeding is usually painless and profuse. Recurrent episodes of retching can cause longitudinal tears in the cardioesophageal portion of the stomach. GI bleeding associated with this tear is known as Mallory–Weiss syndrome. *(Overton, 2004, p. 505)*

45. **(B)** Ultrasound has been established as the most appropriate initial diagnostic imaging study in the ED for suspected biliary tract disease. Imaging studies for evaluation of biliary tract disease have parameters of the following specificity and sensitivity (cholethiasis): abdominal CT has a sensitivity of 91% and specificity of 97%; sensitivity and specificity ultrasound have been established at 91% and 97%, respectively; plain films are noted to have a sensitivity of 64% and specificity of 68%. *(Gallagher, 2004, pp. 491-492)*

46. **(E)** Partially chewed meat and esophageal abnormalities such as strictures, esophageal spasms, and Schatzki rings are commonly implicated in adult food bolus impactions. *(Humphries, 2008, p. 624)*

47. **(E)** The focused abdominal sonography for trauma (FAST) has most notably been useful in evaluation of trauma patients utilizing the noninvasive diagnostic modality of ultrasonography. The FAST examination consists of four standard views. It is helpful in identifying those patients in need of emergent laparotomy as it is able to detect blood in the peritoneal cavity. Retroperitoneal bleeding may not be visualized with FAST evaluation. Ultrasonography is useful in evaluating patients in the first trimester of pregnancy; however, the FAST examination approach is not typically applied when assessing pathology of the extremity venous system and the right upper quadrant of the abdomen. *(Melanson and Heller, 2004, pp. 1874-1876)*

48. **(B)** Gastroesophageal reflux disease (GERD) has been established as the most widespread etiology of inflammation of the esophagus, also known as esophagitis. Additional commonly occurring sources of esophagitis comprise pill esophagitis, esophageal damage and inflammation associated with the effects of alkaline or acidic ingestions, radiation, and infectious agents. It is suspected that the true incidence of pill esophagitis is underreported. Candida is one of the primary infectious pathogens for the infection of the esophagus. As more individuals in immunocompromised immune states receive preventative therapy for opportunistic fungal infections, viral esophagitis has increased in prevalence. Herpes simplex I (HSV) and cytomegalovirus (CMV) have been established as the most common viral agents. *(Lowell, 2006, pp. 1386-1388)*

49. **(A)** Button battery ingestion may cause significant complications in as little as 4 to 6 hours due to the rapid action of alkaline in the battery. Severe burns of the esophagus or perforation may occur. A plain radiograph of the abdomen should be obtained first to localize the battery. A battery lodged in the esophagus should be removed emergently with endoscopy. A surgical consult may be indicated for symptomatic

ingestions past the esophagus. *(Gaasch and Barish, 2006, pp. 515-516)*

50. **(E)** Small bowel obstruction (SBO) is most often due to adhesions following surgery. Incarcerated groin hernias are the second most common cause of SBOs. Other hernias that are responsible for SBOs are umbilical, femoral, and obturator foramen. Less common causes of SBOs are polyps, lymphoma, and adenocarcinoma. Bezoars (undigested vegetable matter) represent an intraluminal obstruction in those having undergone prior surgeries such as pyloric resection. Gallstone ileus is an unusual cause of intraluminal SBO. The most common cause of LBO is neoplasm. *(Vicario and Price, 2004, pp. 524-526)*

51. **(C)** Pseudomembranous enterocolitis is an inflammatory bowel disorder caused by *Clostridium difficile*. The disorder is associated with antibiotic use and is marked by membrane-like plaques of exudates that overlie and replace necrotic intestinal mucosa. The use of broad-spectrum antibiotics, notably clindamycin, cephalosporins, and ampicillin/amoxicillin, is a common cause of *C difficile* colonization. The treatments of choice include supportive measures and antibiotics such as metronidazole and vancomycin. Inflammation of the diverticulum, or diverticulitis, a common disorder of industrialized nations most commonly presents as pain and may be associated with changes in bowel habits. Crohn disease usually presents with abdominal pain, decrease in appetite, fever, and diarrhea; the ileum is the most commonly affected region of the bowel. Ulcerative colitis (UC) is a progressive chronic inflammatory bowel condition that usually affects the colon. UC has a variable presentation and is frequently associated with rectal bleeding. With the exception of pseudomembranous enterocolitis, none of the preceding diseases are precipitated by the use of antimicrobial agents. *(Werman et al., 2004, pp. 530-537)*

52. **(B)** Thyroid storm is characterized by an abrupt, severe, exacerbation of hyperthyroidism. Hyperthyroidism (ie, thyrotoxicosis, thyrotoxic crisis, and thyroid storm) refers to varying degrees of thyroid hyperfunction.

Common causes of thyroid storm include major stress (eg, infection, surgery, DKA, myocardial infarction) in a patient with undiagnosed hyperthyroidism and inadequate therapy in a hyperthyroid patient. Patients typically present with fever, anxiety, agitation, psychosis, hyperhidrosis, heat intolerance, weakness, muscle wasting, palpitations, diarrhea, and vomiting. Laboratory findings show an increased free T4 level and/or a decreased TSH level. Initial therapy is aimed at reducing the peripheral effects of thyroid hormone with β-blockers such as propranolol 80 to 120 mg po every 4 to 6 hours. The next objective in thyroid storm is to inhibit hormonal synthesis of thyroid by administering propylthiouracil (PTU) 400 to 600 mg initially, then 400 to 600 mg po every 8 hours. Last, iodide is given to inhibit the release of stored thyroid hormone. Iodide is typically given as sodium iodide 250 mg IV every 6 hours or as potassium iodide (SSKI), 5 gtt po every 8 hours. Always administer PTU 1 hour before the iodide to prevent the oxidation of iodide and its incorporation in the synthesis of additional thyroid hormone. *(Sternlicht and Wogan, 2006, pp. 1985-1989)*

53. **(C)** A crystalloid fluid bolus of 20 mg/kg is recommended for initial resuscitation in hypovolemic pediatric trauma patients. If 40 mg/kg of crystalloid fluids does not lead to improvement of the hypovolemic state, administration of packed red blood cells should be initiated. *(Cantor, 2006, p. 331)*

54. **(A)** Nitrous oxide may be used for both sedation and analgesia in the emergency department, as long as it is mixed with at least 30% oxygen to prevent hypoxia. Therapeutic concentrations of nitrous oxide include those in the 30% to 50% range (maximum 70%). Concentrations lower than 30% may not be effective in this setting. Higher concentrations of nitrous oxide are required at higher altitudes. Younger children (younger than 8 years) may not gain a therapeutic effect from nitrous oxide. *(Chudnofsky and Lozon, 2006, pp. 2940-2941)*

55. **(A)** The most common causes of bacterial meningitis in the infants aged 0 to 4 weeks

include group B streptococci, *E coli*, and *L monocytogenes*. Pathogens commonly infecting infants 4 to 12 weeks include group B streptococci, *E coli*, *L monocytogenes*, *H influenzae*, and *S pneumoniae*. Pathogens infecting children and young adults 3 months through 17 years include *S pneumoniae* and *N meningitidis*. With the introduction of the conjugate vaccine for *H influenzae*, dramatic reductions in incidences of *H influenzae* meningitis has been seen. Finally, likely pathogens in adults 18 years and older include *S pneumoniae* and *N meningitides* and less frequently *L monocytogenes*. (*Rubin, 2006, p. 2657*)

56. **(B)** The first priority is resuscitation of the mother. A secure airway is very important because aspiration is common. Oxygen therapy is critical because of the reduced oxygen reserve and increased oxygen consumption in the mother. A trauma patient can quickly become hypoxic, making the fetus very vulnerable to any reduction in oxygen delivery. (*Neufield, 2006, pp. 321-323*)

57. **(E)** Hypoglycemia is defined as a plasma glucose level less than 50 mg/dL; however, the criteria for the diagnosis should include the presence of symptoms, low plasma glucose level in a symptomatic patient, and relief of symptoms after ingestion of carbohydrates. Contributing factors to symptoms of hypoglycemia include the rate at which the glucose decreases patient's overall size, underlying health conditions, and previous hypoglycemic reactions. Common symptoms include anxiety, diaphoresis, tremors, tachycardia, palpitations, fatigue, syncope, headache, mental status changes, visual disturbances, and hemiplegia. Patients with ketoacidosis are noted to frequently have Kussmaul respirations, changes in BP, and increased respirations and heart rate. These patients may also have ketone or acetone breath odor. Patients with new-onset hyperglycemia may present with increased thirst, increased urination, and increased appetite. Euglycemia refers to normal blood glucose levels; subsequently, patient should be asymptomatic. Hyperglycemic hyperosmolar nonketotic coma (HHNC) relates to a disorder that affects elderly diabetic patients with findings of

increased osmolarity, blood glucose level, and dehydration. These patients have a spectrum of changes in mentation from confusion to frank coma. (*Cydulka and Pennington, 2006, pp. 1960-1973*)

58. **(A)** Central retinal artery occlusion is characterized by acute visual loss usually attributed to ischemic or thrombus to the major retinal arterial blood supply. Typically, the patient presents with sudden, painless onset of markedly decreased unilateral loss of vision. Physical examination findings include significant decrease in visual acuity, relative afferent pupillary defect (ie, Marcus Gunn pupil), and a pale retina with a red spot that is visible on funduscopic examination. Central retinal vein occlusion (CRVO) is characterized by painless, unilateral vision loss of varying severity, slower onset of decreased vision than with arterial occlusion, retinal hemorrhages, cotton wool spots, and macular edema. Physical examination findings include ciliary flush (ie, circumcorneal perilimbal injection of the episcleritis and scleral vessels) conjunctival injection and cells may be present in the anterior chamber. The pupil on the affected side is often small and irregular. Direct and consensual light reflex will cause pain on the affected side to increase. Retrobulbar hemorrhage is associated with decreased ocular range of motion, decreased vision, ptosis of the lid, and increased pressure in the globe raising intraocular pressure. The high pressure decreases retinal artery perfusion, which results in retinal ischemia. The patient presents with decreased visual acuity, proptosis, and a dilated nonreactive pupil. A hyphema is caused by bleeding from the vasculature of the iris usually precipitated by trauma. Blood is often visualized in the anterior chamber and can be seen via slit lamp evaluation. Symptoms usually consist of pain, photophobia, and decreased vision. Intraocular pressures may increase as well. The major clinical consideration is the potential of reoccurring bleeding. (*Brunette, 2006, pp. 1046-1060*)

59. **(B)** Young adults are the population at the greatest risk for epidural hematomas (EDHs) following head trauma. Direct force on the skull's temporal and parietal bones fracture

can lead to lacerations of the middle meningeal artery or the dural sinus. These specific vessel lacerations account for 80% of the incidence of EDH. Subsequently, arterial hemorrhage occurs, leading to blood clotting in the space between the skull's inner table and the dura. This specific type of head injury rarely occurs in the elderly population because of the anatomical close attachment of the dura to periosteum of the inner skull's table. The dura is also closely adhered in the pediatric skull with infrequent occurrences of EDH seen in children younger than 2 years. *(Heegaard and Biros, 2006, pp. 374-375)*

60. **(E)** Subdural hematomas are usually the result of venous bleeding, causing blood clots to form between the dura and the brain. The most common mechanisms are acceleration–deceleration injuries, which usually cause the superficial bridging vessels to rupture. Subarachnoid hemorrhage caused by trauma is secondary to small tears of the subarachnoid vessels. Blood will collect within the CSF and meningeal intima. A subdural hygroma is formed by clear xanthochromic dural space fluid. Although the pathogenesis is unknown, it is thought to be from a tear in the arachnoid space that permits CSF to escape into the dural space. Intracerebral hematomas are the result of mechanical stretching and tearing of deep small-caliber arterioles of the brain. These mechanical forces usually are the result of the brain being propelled against irregular surfaces in the cranial vault. Most of the intracerebral hematomas are in the frontal and temporal lobes. *(Heegaard and Biros, 2006, pp. 375-377; Kothari, 2006, pp. 1610-1611; Kwiatkowski and Alagappan, 2006, pp. 1635-1637)*

61. **(A)** In treating subarachnoid hemorrhage (SAH), the use of nimodipine has established parameters of reducing disability and death by 55% as compared with the placebo. Mannitol is a good therapeutic agent for reducing ICP, however, not specific to SAH. Although hyperventilation is noted to reduce ICP, it is no longer recommended as a preventative measure in the initial period after a traumatic brain injury (TBI). Steroids have no clinical indications in the treatment of TBI or increased ICP. Use of a

barbiturate coma is not indicated in the ED setting, although there is evidence of its benefit in stable patients who have failed to respond to other ICP-lowering treatment modalities. *(Kirsch and Lipinski, 2004, p. 1565)*

62. **(B)** The most beneficial maneuver in evaluating a patient with an Achilles tendon injury is the Thompson–Doherty test or the Thompson test. This maneuver is performed by squeezing the patient's calf of the affected lower extremity while the patient is lying in a prone position. An intact Achilles is noted by visualizing plantar flexion of the foot while applying the preceding described maneuver. The Lachman test is the more sensitive and specific for establishing anterior cruciate ligament (ACL) injuries. Anterior drawer test and the pivot shift test are also used to evaluate ACL injuries. The posterior drawer test is used to evaluate injuries to the posterior cruciate ligament. *(Haller, 2004, 1735-1737; Steele and Glaspy, 2004, pp. 1729-1730)*

63. **(B)** Measuring serum levels of the enzyme creatine phosphokinase (CK or CPK) is the most sensitive marker for evaluating muscle damage as associated with rhabdomyolysis. In rhabdomyolysis, the isoenzyme CK-MB would not be more than 5% of the total CK or CPK. Myoglobin is also associated with muscle injury; however, it is a less sensitive marker than CPK. LDH and aldolase are additional laboratory tests that can be used in evaluating rhabdomyolysis. However, both are less specific than CPK. *(Counselman, 2004, pp. 1749-1750)*

64. **(B)** Le Fort I fractures involve the maxilla at the level of the nasal bones. A Le Fort II fracture involves several facial bones, including the maxilla, the nasal bones, and the medial aspects of the orbits. A Le Fort III fracture includes aspects of the maxilla, zygoma, nasal bones, ethmoids, vomer, and lesser bones of the cranial base. It can also be described as a craniofacial dysfunction. *(McKay, 2006, pp. 393-394)*

65. **(E)** The source of facial injuries varies by city or rural settings. There is a high incidence of domestic violence associated with a female patient presenting with an orbital fracture.

Statistics reports that about 25% of facial injuries seen in the ED are associated with domestic violence. Facial injuries associated with falls are seen more frequently with the elderly and pediatric populations. Rural hospitals see higher rates of facial trauma associated with MVC and sports-related injuries. *(Hasan and Colucciello, 2004, p. 1583)*

66. **(E)** In evaluating facial trauma of the midface region, the Waters view has been established as the most sensitive of plain radiographs. The Waters view is useful in evaluation of the presence of orbital rim fractures and air-fluid levels in the maxillary sinuses. The most appropriate plain radiograph to evaluate the upper face is the Caldwell or posteroanterior view. To evaluate the base of the skull and zygoma, the submental view is the most appropriate plain radiograph. Although not available at all institutions, when available, the Panorex is the best imaging study for evaluation for suspected fracture of the mandible fractures. To evaluate the mandible ramus and condyles, the Towne view is the best imaging view. *(Hasan and Colucciello, 2004, p. 1586)*

67. **(D)** Direct and compressive forces to the eye may cause a blowout fracture to the orbital floor with herniation of the contents into the maxillary sinus. Blowout fractures may produce enophthalmos, diplopia, impaired ocular motility, and infraorbital hypoesthesias. Many orbital floor fractures resolve spontaneously and require only close follow-up with consultants. A decision to operate may be delayed 10 to 14 days, depending on persistent diplopia or enophthalmos. *(McKay, 2006, p. 393)*

68. **(E)** An unstable, hyperextension fracture through the pedicles of C2 is known as a hangman fracture. Fortunately, cord damage is usually minimal because the anteroposterior diameter of the neural canal is greatest at the C2 level. Furthermore, less neurological damage occurs because bilateral pedicle fractures tend to decompress themselves, allowing more space for the spinal cord. A Jefferson fracture of C1 is produced by an axial loading injury to the cervical spine, transmitting a force through the

occipital condyles to the superior articular surfaces of the lateral masses of the atlas. A clay-shoveler fracture is an avulsion fracture of the spinous process of the lower cervical vertebrae. This oblique fracture of the base of the spinous process, classically C7, derived its name in the 1930s when Australian miners lifted a heavy shovelful of clay causing an abrupt flexion of the head, in opposition to the stabilizing force of the strong supraspinous muscle, resulting in an avulsion fracture of the spinous process. An extension teardrop fracture involves a hyperextension injury in which the anterior longitudinal ligament avulses the inferior portion of the anterior vertebral body at its insertion. The second cervical vertebra is the most common location for an extension teardrop fracture. *(Hockberger et al., 2006, pp. 401-413)*

69. **(D)** The most severe neurological dysfunction, as a result of inadequate or delayed treatment of disk herniation, is cauda equina syndrome. The most common presenting symptoms are saddle anesthesia, bilateral leg pain, urinary incontinence or retention, and fecal incontinence or retention. Most cases of cauda equina syndrome and cord compression develop over a matter of hours. If the symptoms are delayed, these patients are at high risk for chronic neurological deficits. *(Stettler and Pancioli, 2006, pp. 1678-1679)*

70. **(A)** Acute narrow-sangle glaucoma should be recognized as an ophthalmic emergency. It is characterized by a sudden onset of severe pain localized to the affected eye. Common associated visual symptoms include halos around lights, blurriness, and scotomas. Other associated symptoms include nausea and vomiting. The typical physical examination findings reveal a red eye with fixed, mid-dilated pupil, corneal clouding, and a shallow anterior chamber. Anterior uveitis is inflammation of the anterior segment of the eye. Anterior uveitis includes iritis (inflammation that involves only the iris) and iridocyclitis (inflammation of both the iris and ciliary body). Physical examination findings include ciliary flush (ie, circumcorneal perilimbal injection of the episcleritis and scleral vessels) conjunctival injection, and cells may

be present in the anterior chamber. The pupil on the affected side is often small and irregular. Direct and consensual light reflex will cause pain on the affected side to increase. Orbital cellulitis is recognized as a soft tissue infection that extends deep into the fascia and eye orbit. Clinical findings include ocular pain, limitation of eye movement, lid edema, and proptosis, tenderness of the globe, decreased visual acuity, increased ocular pressure, and pupillary paralysis. Allergic conjunctivitis is most common signs and symptoms include red or injected conjunctiva, chemosis, eye drainage, and pruritus. It is mediated by a hypersensitivity exposure. Episcleritis is the inflammation of the connective tissue between the sclera and the conjunctiva. Episcleritis is commonly described as an irritation rather than a true pain. In addition, the orbital vessels blanch with topical neosynephrine. *(Dutton, 2008, pp. 1460-1461; Forster, 2008 pp. 783-788; Goldstein and Tessla, 2008, p. 255; Rubenstein and Virasch, 2008, pp. 237-240; See and Chew, 2008, pp. 1164-1167)*

71. **(D)** Henoch–Schonlein purpura is characterized by the triad of abdominal pain, arthritis, and nonthrombocytopenic purpura. This condition is typically immunologically mediated vasculitis by a stimulus that often cannot be identified. However, at least half of the affected patients had an upper respiratory tract infection. Occasionally, a drug or bacterial agent can be identified as the source. Patients characteristically develop a slightly raised symmetrical petechial rash, which is most prominent on the lower extremities. In addition, patients develop colicky abdominal pain, bloody diarrhea, intussusception, and migratory large joint arthritis. Renal manifestations may present in the form of hematuria, proteinuria, and nephrosis. Therapy is directed at identifying and treating the underlying problem. Kawasaki disease is an inflammatory vasculitis characterized by fever for 5 days and four out of five of the following criteria: conjunctival injection (bilateral), strawberry tongue and mouth fissures, desquamation and swelling of the fingers and toes, erythematous rash starting on the palms and soles, and enlarged lymph nodes. Erythema nodosum is an inflammatory disease of the skin and sub-

cutaneous tissue characterized by tender red nodules. Etiologies include bacterial infections (deep fungal infections, e.g., histoplasmosis, coccidioidomycosis), viral upper respiratory tract infection drugs, and idiopathy. The rash is described as multiple raised, warm, tender nodules with bluish discoloration that most commonly involve the pretibial region; however, the forearms or thighs may be involved as well. Pneumococcal meningitis does not typically present with a petechial rash or purpura. Meningococcemia is caused by encapsulated gram-negative diplococci that present with 1 to 2 mm petechiae to full-blown ecchymoses. *(Backin and Zukin, 2006, pp. 2509-2512; McCollough and Sharieff, 2006, pp. 1816-1817)*

72. **(C)** Temporal arteritis is a vasculitis usually occurring in the elderly involving the temporal and external carotid artery. Left untreated, temporal arteritis may result in bilateral blindness. Patients typically present with unilateral, excruciating, burning pain over the affected artery. The disease is often associated with polymyalgia rheumatica and may present with systemic involvement including fever, polymyalgia, malaise, weight loss, and anorexia. Patients complain of decreased visual acuity, and the examination reveals a tender, inflamed temporal artery. Acute narrow angle glaucoma is characterized by a sudden onset of severe pain localized to the affected eye with halos around lights, blurriness, scotomas, and sometimes nausea and vomiting. Typical physical examination findings reveal a red eye with fixed, mid-dilated pupil, corneal clouding, and a shallow anterior chamber. Multiple sclerosis is a demyelinating disease that affects the CNS and is characterized by recurrent attacks of focal and multifocal neurologic deficits. Multiple sclerosis may manifest as an optic neuritis, which is an inflammatory condition of the optic nerve. Optic neuritis typically manifests as eye pain and visual impairment. Myasthenia gravis is characterized by episodic muscle weakness caused by loss or dysfunction of acetylcholine receptors. Common symptoms related to ocular muscle involvement include ptosis, diplopia, and muscle fatigability after exercise. Viral encephalitis is an acute inflammatory disease of the brain caused by

direct viral invasion (eg, arbovirus, poliovirus, echovirus, and coxsackie virus). Common symptoms include fever, malaise, headache, vomiting, stiff neck, seizures, and cranial nerve abnormalities. *(Sercombe, 2006, pp. 1813-1814)*

73. **(A)** Any patient who has sustained a penetrating wound or blunt trauma to the thorax or upper abdomen should be suspected of having a diagnosis of pericardial tamponade. The most common signs of pericardial tamponade are hypotension and tachycardia-associated elevation in central venous pressure. Beck triad of pericardial tamponade consists of hypotension, distended neck veins, and distant heart sounds. A tension pneumothorax is an accumulation of air under pressure within the pleural cavity. The air under pressure shifts the mediastinum to the opposite hemithorax and compresses the contralateral lung and great vessels. A myocardial rupture refers to an acute traumatic perforation of the ventricles and atria. Acute myocardial rupture also includes rupture of the interventricular septum, pericardium, chordae, interatrial septum, and papillary muscles and valves. The most common vessel injured in an acute blunt trauma is the thoracic aorta. Deceleration injuries most commonly injure the thoracic aorta because the descending aorta is relatively fixed by the attachments of the intercostal arteries and ligamentous arteriosum. Myocardial contusion will usually demonstrate direct areas of hemorrhage in the anterior wall of the right ventricle and atria. *(Eckstein, 2006, pp. 461-478)*

74. **(B)** Boerhaave syndrome, postemetic rupture, and spontaneous esophageal rupture are synonymous terms. The most common site of injury is the distal esophagus, which demonstrates a longitudinal tear occurring in the left posterolateral aspect. Most cases occur in middle-aged men after they have overindulged in food and alcohol. Burger sign is defined as a physical examination finding of advanced peripheral vascular disease. Brudzinksi sign is a physical examination diagnostic maneuver in which hip flexion occurs with passive flexion of the neck and is interpreted as a positive meningeal sign. Bezoars (undigested vegetable matter) represent an intraluminal obstruction

in those having undergone prior surgeries such as pyloric resection. *(Aufderheide, 2006, pp. 1346, 1714; Vicario and Price, 2004, pp. 524-526; Zun and Singh, 2006, pp. 201-202)*

75. **(E)** A retrograde urethrogram should be performed prior to invasive interventions such as urethral catheterization if there is any possibility of urethral disruption. Signs of urethral disruption include a high riding prostate and the presence of blood at the tip of the meatus. Sixty milliliters (or 0.6 mL/kg) of full-strength or half-strength iothalmate meglumine (Conray II) is injected over 30 to 60 seconds. A radiograph is taken during the last 10 mL of contrast material. Retrograde flow through the urethra and into the bladder without extravasation ensures continuity of the urethra and absence of urethral injury. *(Schneider, 2006, pp. 517-520)*

76. **(A)** A penile rupture is a traumatic rupture of the corpus cavernosum when the tunica albuginea is torn. During vigorous sexual intercourse, a patient commonly will hear a snapping sound followed by localized pain, detumescence, and slowly progressive penile hematoma. *(Schneider, 2004, pp. 615-616)*

77. **(C)** Mallet finger is a disruption of the distal tendon, resulting in a flexion deformity at the **Distal interphalangeal joint (DIP)**. It is the most common zone I injury. Bennett fracture is a combination of a dislocated carpometacarpal joint and the thumb's **metacarpophalangeal joint** (MCP) that is fractured intra-articularly. Rolando fracture is defined as a comminuted fracture involving the base of the thumb's MCP. A Boutonniere deformity involves deformity of the index finger. The swan neck deformity does not represent an acute finding but rather is associated with an untreated mallet finger. *(Lyn and Antosia, 2006, pp. 599-607)*

78. **(A)** The developing bones of the child are more pliable and flexible than an adult mature bone. In a torus fracture, there is a buckling of the cortex of the bone without complete disruption of the cortical segment. Multiple radiographic views may be necessary to make the

diagnosis in small, nondisplaced fractures. *(Woolfrey and Eisenhaver, 2006, pp. 644-645)*

79. **(B)** The most common nerve injured with a humeral shaft fracture is the radial nerve. The radial nerve runs in close proximity to the posterior midhumeral shaft. A radial nerve injury is evident by a wrist drop. *(Geiderman, 2006a, p. 655)*

80. **(B)** A dislocation is described by comparing the most distal portion of the joint dislocated to the most proximal. The mechanism for a posterior elbow dislocation is a fall on an outstretched hand or wrist, the elbow being either extended or hyperextended at the time of impact. These patients hold the elbow in flexion at approximately 45° and have marked prominence of the olecranon. *(Geiderman, 2006b, pp. 664-666)*

81. **(E)** Retropharyngeal abscess is an infected fluid collection in the fascial plane between the posterior pharyngeal muscles and the paraspinous muscles. Primarily, retropharyngeal abscess is a pediatric problem because there are lymph nodes in the retropharyngeal space that can become suppurative. Clinical manifestations include an ill-appearing child with fever, sore throat, neck pain, and voice changes (ie, "duck-like voice"). A CT scan with IV contrast of the soft tissues of the neck and upper chest is the best diagnostic test. Peritonsillar abscess is an infected fluid collection in the pharyngeal pillar. The most common etiology is β-hemolytic streptococcus. Symptoms include fever, sore throat (unilateral), and odynophagia. In addition, the patient drools and finds it hard to handle his/her own secretions. Streptococcal pharyngitis is an infection of the pharynx and tonsils due to group A β-hemolytic streptococci. Clinical features include sudden onset of fever and sore throat with enlargement of the cervical lymph nodes. Headache, vomiting, abdominal pain, meningismus, and torticollis can occur as well. Epiglottitis is an inflammatory disorder of the supraglottic laryngeal region. Etiologies of epiglottitis include bacterias, viruses, chemical damage (eg, aspiration of fuel), and mechanical damage (eg, trauma, burns). Symptoms include sore throat, fever, a muffled voice, dysphagia, and respiratory distress. Clinical features include drooling, dyspnea, tachypnea, inspiratory stridor, tripod position (ie, patient leans forward, supporting himself/herself with both hands), and toxic appearance. Ludwig angina is an abscess formation of the submaxillary, sublingual, and submental spaces accompanied by elevation of the tongue. The cause is due to an infection of the lower second and third molars usually due to β-hemolytic streptococcus, staphylococcus, and mixed anaerobic and aerobic infections. Patients commonly present with swelling beneath the chin. The tongue is displaced up and posteriorly. Trismus often makes opening the mouth for examination difficult. *(Manno, 2006, pp. 2522-2523, 2530; Melio, 2006, pp. 1109-1110)*

82. **(D)** The most common mechanism of injury for an anterior shoulder dislocation is abduction, extension, and external rotation. The lateral edge of the acromion process is prominent and the arm is held in slight abduction and external rotation by the opposite extremity. Anterior shoulder dislocations account for 95% to 97% of all glenohumeral dislocations. Falls onto an outstretched hand as mechanism of injury is more common in older patient population. *(Daya, 2006, pp. 687-693)*

83. **(B)** The class of prescription medications responsible for the most drug-related deaths is TCAs. The clinical toxicity is due to the complex pharmacologic activity, low therapeutic index, and general availability. The clinical toxicity is quite variable, ranging from mild antimuscarinic activity to severe cardiotoxicity. Benzodiazepine related overdoses account for few deaths; however, in combination with other agents, they account for significant deaths and disability due to additive effects. Although not reflected in death rates, monoamine oxidase inhibitors have greater toxicity than the newer antidepressants. The toxic effects of lithium are frequently related to drug interactions. Stimulants are associated with significant side effects. *(Mills, 2004, pp. 1025-1066; Perrone and Hoffman, 2004, p.1075; Schneider and Cobaugh, 2004, pp. 1048-1049, 1055)*

84. **(C)** Patients with ethylene glycol ingestion usually present with an acute change in mental

status, high anion gap metabolic acidosis, osmolar gap, and calcium oxalate crystals in the urine. Ethylene glycol is commercially available as preservatives, glycerine substitutes, and antifreeze. Ethylene glycol may be ingested in suicide attempts, accidentally by children, and by alcoholics as an alcohol substitute. The toxic metabolites formed by ethylene glycol metabolism are primarily formaldehyde, formic acid, and oxalic acid. When noteworthy acidosis is present, ethanol is most likely not the underlying source of intoxication. Isopropyl alcohol ingestion usually has abnormal anion gap. Methanol is noted to have a delay in presentation of toxic-related symptoms. *(Berk and Herndersh, 2004, pp. 1065-1070)*

85. **(D)** Treatment priorities of acetaminophen toxicity consist of supportive care, gastrointestinal decontamination, and the use of the antidote *N*-acetylcysteine (NAC). No additional therapies are recognized for intervention in acetaminophen overdoses. If given early (less than 8 hours after ingestion), NAC can prevent toxicity by inhibiting the binding of the toxic metabolite *N*-acetyl-*p*-benzoquinoneimine to hepatic proteins. In acetaminophen toxicity, more than 24 hours after ingestion, NAC diminishes hepatic necrosis by nonspecific mechanisms. The standard 72-hour oral NAC regimen used in the United States is a loading dose of 140 mg/kg followed by maintenance doses of 70 mg/kg every 4 hours for 17 doses. *(Hung and Nelson, 2004, pp. 1091-1093)*

86. **(D)** Periorbital cellulits is characterized by warmth, redness, swelling, and tenderness over the affected eye, along with conjunctival injection, eyelid swelling, chemosis, and fever. Orbital cellulitis includes all the symptoms of periorbital (preseptal) cellulitis with the addition of ocular pain and limitation of eye movement. Other physical examination findings may include lid edema, proptosis, marked tenderness to the globe, decreased visual acuity, and pupillary paralysis. *(Meislin and Guisto, 2006, pp. 2197-2198)*

87. **(D)** Isopropyl alcohol (isopropanol), commonly referred to as rubbing alcohol, is a solvent and disinfectant used in many household items such as hair and skin products, antifreeze, and window cleaning solutions. The toxic dose is 1 mL/kg of a 70% solution. Isopropanol is metabolized to acetone. Mild acidosis may occur because of the formation of acetate and formate. This toxicity is associated with high serum and urine ketone levels. However, a distinguishing factor is that there is no increase in the osmolal gap or anion gap acidosis. Methanol, also referred to as wood alcohol, is commonly used in products such as solvents, antifreeze, windshield washer fluid, and varnishes. The lethal ingested dose is approximately 15 to 30 mL in adults. Methanol is oxidized in the liver to formaldehyde and formate, subsequently a severe lactic acidosis develops. These metabolites concentrate in the vitreous humor and optic nerve, causing ocular toxicity and blindness. This toxicity is associated with an osmolal gap and an anion gap acidosis but no ketosis. Ethylene glycol is frequently implicated in overdoses of antifreeze. Clinical findings include increase in serum potassium level and the presence of a wide anion gap metabolic acidosis. Diabetic Ketoacidosis (DKA) is a disorder found in insulin-dependent diabetes patients that is characterized by hyperglycemia, ketonemia, and acidosis. Serum glucose levels are typically higher than 300 mg/dL. Metabolic acidosis is demonstrated by a serum bicarbonate concentration of less than 15 mEq/L and a pH of less than 7.2. Ketonemia results from β-hydroxybutyrate and acetoacetate. This toxicity results in an anion gap acidosis, a ketotic state, but no osmolal gap. Alcoholic ketoacidosis is typically seen in alcoholic patients who are forced to stop drinking shortly after a drinking binge. β-Hydroxybutyric acid is the predominant ketone formed in alcoholic ketoacidosis. A metabolic acidosis may occur from vomiting, dehydration, and respiratory alkalosis. Therefore, this toxicity is characterized by an anion gap acidosis and a high ketone level but an osmolal gap is not found. *(Cydulka, 2006, pp. 1962-1965; McMicken and Finell, 2006, pp. 2872-2873; White and Kosnick, 2006, pp. 2395-2396)*

88. **(C)** Mild hypothermia is defined as a temperature from 32°C to 35°C (89.6°F–95°F). In mild hypothermia, the body responds by increasing

metabolic activity to produce heat. This is known as the excitation or the responsive phase. When the temperature drops to less than 32°C (89.6°F), bodily functions slow down, giving way to the adynamic phase. As metabolism slows, there is a decrease in both oxygen utilization and carbon dioxide production. As the body temperature falls to less than 30°C to 32°C (86°F–89.6°F), shivering will cease. Hypothermia may induce life-threatening dysrhythmias and ECG changes. A characteristic, but not pathognomonic, ECG finding in hypothermia is the Osborne (J) wave. This abnormal wave is a slow, positive deflection at the end of the QRS complex. (*Bessen, 2004, pp. 1179-1180*)

89.   **(A)** The black widow spider (*Latrodectus*) is found in many areas of the United States. Its bite produces immediate pain and pinprick sensations that soon encompass the entire extremity. Erythema of the bitten area develops usually within 1 hour and in about half of the cases quickly evolves into a target pattern. Patients frequently complain of cramp-like spasms in the large muscle groups. The physical examination rarely exhibits muscle rigidity, and serum creatine kinase concentrations usually are not elevated significantly. The brown recluse (*Loxosceles*) spider bites are difficult to identify. The bite lesion is usually mildly erythematous and may become firm and heal with little scarring over several days to weeks. Occasionally, the lesion may become necrotic over 3 to 4 days with subsequent eschar formation. The hobo spider (*Tegenaria*) usually causes a painless local reaction similar to that of the brown recluse spider. Blisters eventually develop that rupture, leaving an encrusted cratered wound. A tarantula bite typically causes pain and local swelling at the site. Treatment consists of local wound care. Scorpions (Scorpionida) present with a multitude of local and systemic manifestations. Some of these manifestations include pain, paresthesia, cranial nerve and somatic motor dysfunction, uncontrolled jerking, restlessness, pharyngeal incoordination, and respiratory compromise. (*Clark and Scheir, 2004, pp. 1193-1197*)

90.   **(E)** The three principles of treatment regarding acute mountain sickness (AMS) are (1) to stop the ascent, (2) to descend to lower altitude, and (3) to treat immediately in the presence of change in normal mental status, ataxia, or pulmonary edema. Emergent treatments include oxygen, acetazolamide, nifedipine, dexamethasone, hyperbaric therapy, and continuous positive airway pressure. (*Hackett, 2004, pp. 1265-1267*)

91.   **(B)** The answer is 44% burn. The rule of nines to estimate percentage of burns is as follows: head 9%, anterior trunk 18%, posterior trunk 18%, each leg 18%, each arm 9%, and perineum 1%. (*Schwartz and Balakrishnam, 2004, pp. 1221-1222*)

92.   **(E)** Hemophilias A and B are X-linked recessive disorders that are deficiencies in factor VIII and factor IX, respectively. Approximately 85% of patients with hemophilia have hemophilia A. Severity of the disorder depends on the level of factor deficiency. Common clinical findings include hemarthroses, soft tissue bleeding, muscular hematomas, and intracranial bleeding. Intracranial bleeding is the leading cause of death in people with hemophilia. Gastrointestinal bleeding is rare. (*Janz and Hamilton, 2006, pp. 1900-1902*)

93.   **(D)** An L4 injury may present as weakness or paralysis to the quadriceps and thigh adductor muscles, sensory loss to the medial leg, and loss of the patellar reflexes. An injury to C7 may manifest as decreased sensation in the middle finger and the loss of the triceps reflexes and thumb extension. An injury to L1 would involve loss of the cremasteric reflex, decreased sensation in groin area, and loss of hip flexion. An injury to S1 would more likely be indicated by loss of sensation of the lateral dorsal and plantar aspect of the foot, loss of Achilles reflex, and loss plantar flexion. S4 deficits may present with a loss of the anal reflex (wink), loss of perineal area sensation, and loss of voluntary control of the pelvic floor. (*Cleveland and Rock, 2008, pp. 391-398*)

94.   **(E)** Digoxin toxicity results in enhanced excitability and contractility in myocardial muscle and decreased conduction velocity in conduction tissue. Therapy is directed at airway management, cardiovascular resuscita-

tion, and continuous cardiac monitoring. Ventricular ectopy is treated with lidocaine or phenytoin, and symptomatic bradycardia is treated with atropine. Antidote treatment is with digoxin-specific antibodies, which consist of Fab fragments that bind digoxin, removing it from cardiac receptors and reversing toxicity. Indications include life-threatening dysrhythmias, a serum potassium level higher than 5.0 mEq/L, a serum digoxin level higher than 10 to 15 ng/mL, and advanced age. Potassium replacement would be contraindicated in acute toxicity with elevation of the serum potassium level; calcium chloride may worsen the arrhythmia. Variable results such as bradycardia and heart block are noted with the use of atropine. Magnesium is best indicated for tachyarrhythmias associated with digoxin toxicity. *(Roberts, 2006, pp. 2368-2373)*

95. **(B)** Wernicke encephalopathy is a potentially fatal neurologic disorder found in alcoholics with poor nutritional status that is caused by chronic vitamin B_6 deficiency. Alcoholism interferes with gastrointestinal absorption of vitamin B_6 and impairs conversion of vitamin B_6 to its active metabolite. In many patients, concomitant liver disease impairs storage of vitamin B_6. The administration of glucose to an alcoholic patient with an inadequate supply of thiamine may precipitate this disorder. Clinical features include the triad of abnormal mental status, ophthalmoplegia, and gait ataxia. Patients are often disoriented, forgetful, and unable to recognize familiar objects. With prompt therapy, the ophthalmoplegia usually resolves within hours and the coma resolves in hours to days, but the memory deficit may never resolve. Thiamine 100 mg administered intravenously is the treatment of choice. Thiamine 100 mg intravenous administration is continued daily until the patient has achieved proper oral nutritional status. It is essential that thiamine be given prior to the administration of glucose. *(McMicken and Finell, 2004, p. 2869)*

96. **(C)** In the emergency medicine setting, treatment of small dental abscess or periapical abscess with oral antibiotics is warranted. The most appropriate antimicrobial agents include Penicillin VK 500 mg PO QID, clindamycin 300 mg PO QID, or erythromycin 500 mg QID. Small periodontal abscess may respond to antibiotic therapy as described earlier along with the application of warm saline rinses. Larger abscesses warrant incision and drainage. It is crucial to provide sufficient analgesic therapy for dental abscesses. Analgesic therapy may include NSAIDs and/or short courses of opioid medications. Definitive therapy for dental abscesses is provided by a dentist. *(Beaudreau, 2004, pp. 1484-1485)*

97. **(B)** Six percent of the cases of extrapulmonary TB affect the CNS. The peak incidence of extrapulmonary CNS TB are seen in the pediatric age range of birth to 4 years. Among children younger than 4 years, about 25% will develop extrapulmonary TB manifestations. In recent years, military TB (acute disseminated TB) has become more common in the elderly and those with HIV infections; previously this form of TB was more common in children. The multisystem or miliary form of TB is also seen in chronic alcoholics and those with cirrhotic liver disease. *(Sokolove and Chan, 2006, pp. 2145-2171)*

98. **(E)** Active multidrug resistant TB (MDRTB) warrants hospital admission. Limiting exposure to these patients, who are likely infectious, is best accomplished by early identification and placement in a negative airflow room (respiratory isolation). Staff working in the ED should be accustomed to using respiratory protective equipment, specifically protective masks, with the more advanced staff using the N-95 particulate respirators. *(Sokolove and Chan, 2006, pp. 2146-2171)*

99. **(D)** In evaluating a pediatric patient for suspected intussusception, air contrast enema has proven to be diagnostic and therapeutic in approximately 60% to 80% of cases. Contrast enema utilizing air is preferred to barium because of greater management of colonic pressures when performing the reduction when compared with the barium technique. An additional benefit in the case of bowel perforation is that there is no risk of spillage of barium contrast into the peritoneum. The patient should

be stable and well resuscitated before undergoing the contrast enema procedure. *(Albanese and Sylvester, 2008, pp. 1301-1302)*

100. **(B)** An infrequent injury of the digits seen in infancy is known as the hair tourniquets syndrome, in which a strand of hair inadvertently gets wrapped around a digit (usually toes). Local tissues of the affected digit become strangulated and ischemia subsequently develops. To resolve vascular compromise, the hair must be completely excised to restore perfusion to the affected digit. A midline longitudinal incision on the extensor surface (dorsal) of the digit deep enough to cut the extensor ligament is considered to customary approach to accomplish reperfusion. Complete removal of any remaining hair strands should be attempted with the use of forceps without teeth. *(Reisdorff, 2006, pp. 316-317)*

101. **(D)** RSV pulmonary infections in young infants can be accompanied by apneic episodes as well as chlamydia and pertussis infections. Mucous plugging results from necrosis of the respiratory epithelium and destruction of ciliated epithelial cells. This and submucosal edema lead to peripheral airway narrowing and variable obstruction mechanism inducing RSV-related apnea in young infants is not completely understood but may be related to hypoxemia and upper airway obstruction. Infants at the highest risk are those younger than 6 weeks and those who have a history of prematurity, apnea of prematurity, and low O_2 saturation on admission. It is difficult to predict apneic events. Steroids are not recommended as studies have failed to prove benefit unless underlying asthma; in addition, they can be administered in the oral formulation. Hospital admission is recommended for children with clinically defined hypoxia and RSV diagnosis; the frequently chosen parameter is pulse oximetry of less than 90% to 93%. Ribavirin (antiviral) is clinically indicated for RSV infections in high-risk patients and comes in oral and aerosol formulations. Educating the parents on the clinical course of RSV infection and signs and symptoms or respiratory distress is critical in disposition of pediatric patients.

Children with mild symptoms who are tolerating fluids can be released in the care of capable caregivers with good follow-up. Additional home care options can include home health nursing visits and discharging the patient with nebulizer machines if medically necessary. *(Kou and Mayer, 2004, pp. 795-797)*

102. **(C)** In acute mononucleosis infection, there is a 5% incidence of an associated generalized erythematous maculopapular rash. In addition, there may be petechiae on the soft palate. When patients are treated with ampicillin or an ampicillin-based antibiotic, the incidence of the rash reaches almost 100%. As the underlying etiology of mononucleosis is the Epstein–Barr virus, the treatment should be mainly supportive. *(Weinstock and Rosenau, 2004, p. 873)*

103. **(A)** Anticholinergic overdose is often characterized by the following: "blind as a bat, hot as Hades, red as a beet, dry as a bone, mad as a hatter." Other frequently encountered clinical findings include tachycardia, gastrointestinal ileus, urinary retention, seizures, delirium, and hallucinations. Caffeine at higher doses (1 g) is noted to have symptoms of gastrointestinal disturbance, similar to theophylline toxicity. Additional findings associated with very high levels of caffeine are tachycardia, agitation, tachypnea, and electrolyte disturbances. Heroin overdose is accompanied by findings of respiratory depression, changes in mental status, hypotension, somnolence, nausea and emesis, urinary retention, and histamine release–related complaints. Salicylate overdose is associated with nausea and vomiting and multiple acid–base disturbances. Acetaminophen overdose initially is associated with minimal clinical signs and symptoms. Later in the course of the drug's effects of toxicity, hepatic failure, coagulation disturbance, metabolic acidosis, renal failure and GI symptoms will develop. *(Dovon, 2004, p. 1090; Perrone and Hoffman, 2004, p. 1078; Wax, 2004, p. 1145; Yip, 2004, p. 1085)*

104. **(A)** Haloperidol is the most appropriate pharmaceutical agent to choose in the ED setting to manage agitated or psychotic behavior in patients. The antipsychotic medications are

useful in managing psychotic symptoms whether the result of a psychiatric disorder, the manifestation of a medical disorder, or due to an ingestion of a psychotic symptoms–inducing substance. Benzodiazepines are frequently selected to treat agitation associated with alcohol withdrawal and cocaine abuse. The antihistamine agent diphenhydramine has a side effect of sedation, which is utilized therapeutically. Other properties of diphenhydramine include anticholinergic, antitussive, antiemetic, and local anesthetic properties. There are rare indications for prescribing antidepressants and lithium by emergency medicine prescribers. Both of these psychiatric therapeutics have long delays in onset of action, have multiple side effects, and require ongoing continuous monitoring. *(Nockowitz and Rund, 2004, pp. 1812, 1819, 1820-1822)*

105. **(C)** Crotaline or pit viper venomous poisoning is noted by the following clinical findings: localized pain, the spreading of edema in the affected area, and the presence of at least one fang mark. The development of compartment syndrome of a snake-bitten extremity is a noted complication. The clinical symptoms of the compartment syndrome are noted by severe localized pain that is unrelieved with narcotic medications. Delayed serum sickness after Fab AV antivenom treatment occurs only in 5% of patients and is treated with oral steroids. Dislodged teeth contaminating a wound are often associated with bites from the midwestern Gila monsters. Delayed absorption of the antivenom is not an expected complication as intramuscular injection in not recommended in lieu of venom-induced hypovolemia in the snake-bitten patient. Intravenous infusion of the Fab AV antivenom is the recommended method of therapy. Rapid collapse and death are associated with the bite of the Australian brown snake (elapids) as its venom causes severe cardiovascular depression. *(Dart and Daly, 2004, pp. 1200-1205)*

REFERENCES

Albanese CT, Sylvester KG. Pediatric surgery. In: Doherty GM, Way LW, eds. *Current: Surgical Diagnosis and Treatment.* 12th ed. Maidenhead, United Kingdom: McGraw-Hill; 2006.

Ausiello D, Wysolmerski JJ, Insogna KL. The parathyroid glands, hypothalamus, and hypocalcemia. In: Goldman L, Ausiello D, eds. *Cecil Textbook of Medicine.* 22nd ed. Philadelphia, PA: Saunders; 2004.

Aufderheide T. Peripheral arteriovascular disease. In: Marx JA, Hockberger RS, Walls RM, et al., eds. *Rosen's Emergency Medicine: Concepts and Clinical Practice.* 6th ed. Philadelphia, PA: Mosby; 2006.

Backin RM, Zukin PP. Fever. In: Marx JA, Hockberger RS, Walls RM, et al., eds. *Rosen's Emergency Medicine: Concepts and Clinical Practice.* 6th ed. Philadelphia, PA: Mosby; 2006.

Brunette DD. Ophthalmology. In: Marx JA, Hockberger RS, Walls RM, et al., eds. *Rosen's Emergency Medicine: Concepts and Clinical Practice.* 6th ed. Philadelphia, PA: Mosby; 2006.

Beaudreau RW. Oral and dental emergencies. In: Tintinalli JE, Kelen GD, Stapczynski JS, et al., eds. *Emergency Medicine: A Comprehensive Study Guide.* 6th ed. New York, NY: McGraw-Hill; 2004.

Berk WA, Herdersch WV. Alcohols. In: Tintinalli JE, Kelen GD, Stapczynski JS, et al., eds. *Emergency Medicine: A Comprehensive Study Guide.* 6th ed. New York, NY: McGraw-Hill; 2004.

Bessen H. Hypothermia. In: Tintinalli JE, Kelen GD, Stapczynski JS, et al., eds. *Emergency Medicine: A Comprehensive Study Guide.* 6th ed. New York, NY: McGraw-Hill; 2004.

Bolton E. Disturbances of cardiac rhythm and conduction. In: Tintinalli JE, Kelen GD, Stapczynski JS, et al., eds. *Emergency Medicine: A Comprehensive Study Guide.* 6th ed. New York, NY: McGraw-Hill; 2004.

Bosse GM. Benzodiazepines. In: Tintinalli JE, Kelen GD, Stapczynski JS, et al., eds. *Emergency Medicine: A Comprehensive Study Guide.* 6th ed. New York, NY: McGraw-Hill; 2004.

Cantor RM. Pediatric trauma. In: Marx JA, Hockberger RS, Walls RM, et al., eds. *Rosen's Emergency Medicine: Concepts and Clinical Practice.* 6th ed. Philadelphia, PA: Mosby; 2006.

Chang GJ, Shelton AA, Welton ML. Large Intestine" (Chapter). In: Doherty GM, ed. *Current Diagnosis & Treatment: Emergency Medicine.* 6th ed. New York, NY: McGraw-Hill; 2008.

Chang GJ, Shelton AA, Welton ML. "Chapter 30. Large Intestine" (Chapter). In: Doherty GM, ed. *Current Diagnosis & Treatment: Surgery.* 13th ed. http://www.accessmedicine.com/content.aspx?aID=5309393.

Chopra A. Thrombophlebitis and occlusive arterial disease. In: Tintinalli JE, Kelen GD, Stapczynski JS, et al., eds. *Emergency Medicine: A Comprehensive Study Guide.* 6th ed. New York, NY: McGraw-Hill; 2004.

Chudnofsky CR, Lozon MM. Procedural sedation and analgesia. In: Marx JA, Hockberger RS, Walls RM, et al., eds. *Rosen's Emergency Medicine: Concepts and Clinical Practice.* 6th ed. Philadelphia, PA: Mosby; 2006.

Cleveland JE, Rock TC. Vertebral column & spinal cord trauma. In: Stone CK, Humphries RL, eds. *Current Diagnosis & Treatment: Emergency Medicine.* 6th ed. New York, NY: McGraw-Hill; 2008.

Collings JL. Acid-base disorders. In: Marx JA, Hockberger RS, Walls RM, et al., eds. *Rosen's Emergency Medicine: Concepts and Clinical Practice.* 6th ed. Philadelphia, PA: Mosby; 2006.

Counselman FL. Rhabdomyolysis. In: Tintinalli JE, Kelen GD, Stapczynski JS, et al., eds. *Emergency Medicine: A Comprehensive Study Guide.* 6th ed. New York, NY: McGraw-Hill; 2004.

Clark RF, Scheir AB. Arthopods bites and stings. In: Tintinalli JE, Kelen GD, Stapczynski JS et al., eds. *Emergency Medicine: A Comprehensive Study Guide.* 6th ed. New York, NY: McGraw-Hill; 2004.

Cummins R. *Textbook of Advanced Cardiac Life Support— Emergency Cardiovascular Care Programs.* Dallas, TX: American Heart Association; 1999.

Cydulka RK. Acute asthma in adults. In: Tintinalli JE, Kelen GD, Stapczynski JS, et al., eds. *Emergency Medicine: A Comprehensive Study Guide.* 6th ed. New York, NY: McGraw-Hill; 2004.

Cydulka RK, Pennington J. Diabetes mellitus and disorders of glucose homeostasis. In: Marx JA, Hockberger RS, Walls RM, et al., eds. *Rosen's Emergency Medicine: Concepts and Clinical Practice.* 6th ed. Philadelphia, PA: Mosby; 2006.

Danzl DF, Vissers RJ. Tracheal intubation and mechanical ventilation. In: Tintinalli JE, Kelen GD, Stapczynski JS, et al., eds. *Emergency Medicine: A Comprehensive Study Guide.* 6th ed. New York, NY: McGraw-Hill; 2004.

Dart RC, Daly FFS. Reptile bites. In: Tintinalli JE, Kelen GD, Stapczynski JS, et al., eds. *Emergency Medicine: A Comprehensive Study Guide.* 6th ed. New York, NY: McGraw-Hill; 2004.

Daya M. Shoulder. In: Marx JA, Hockberger RS, Walls RM, et al., eds. *Rosen's Emergency Medicine: Concepts and Clinical Practice.* 6th ed. Philadelphia, PA: Mosby; 2006.

Dovon S. Opioids. In: Tintinalli JE, Kelen GD, Stapczynski JS, et al., eds. *Emergency Medicine: A Comprehensive Study Guide.* 6th ed. New York, NY: McGraw-Hill; 2004.

Dutton JJ. Orbital diseases. In: Yanoff M, Duker JS, eds. *Ophthalmology.* 3rd ed. Baltimore, MD: Mosby; 2008.

Eckstein ME. Thoracic trauma. In: Marx JA, Hockberger RS, Walls RM, et al., eds. *Rosen's Emergency Medicine: Concepts and Clinical Practice.* 6th ed. Philadelphia, PA: Mosby; 2006.

Ferri F, eds. *Ferri's Clinical Advisor: Instant Diagnosis and Treatment.* St Louis, MO: Mosby; 2005.

Field JM. *Advanced Cardiac Life Support: Provider Manual.* Dallas, TX: American Heart Association; 2006.

Forster DJ. General approach to the uveitis patient and treatment strategies. In: Yanoff M, Duker JS, eds. *Ophthalmology.* 3rd ed. Baltimore, MD: Mosby; 2008.

Gaasch WR, Barish RA. Swallowed foreign bodies. In: Marx JA, Hockberger RS, Walls RM, et al., eds. *Rosen's Emergency Medicine: Concepts and Clinical Practice.* 6th ed. Philadelphia, PA: Mosby; 2006.

Gallagher EJ. Gastrointestinal emergencies. In: Tintinalli JE, Kelen GD, Stapczynski JS, et al., eds. *Emergency Medicine: A Comprehensive Study Guide.* 6th ed. New York, NY: McGraw-Hill; 2004.

Geiderman JM. General principles of orthopedic injuries. In: Marx JA, Hockberger RS, Walls RM, et al., eds. *Rosen's Emergency Medicine: Concepts and Clinical Practice.* 6th ed. Philadelphia, PA: Mosby; 2006a.

Geiderman JM. Humerus and elbow. In: Marx JA, Hockberger RS, Walls RM, et al., eds. *Rosen's Emergency Medicine: Concepts and Clinical Practice.* 6th ed. Philadelphia, PA: Mosby; 2006b.

Gibbs MA, Tavel VS. Electrolyte disturbances. In: Marx JA, Hockberger RS, Walls RM, et al., eds. *Rosen's Emergency Medicine: Concepts and Clinical Practice.* 6th ed. Philadelphia, PA: Mosby; 2006.

Goldstein DE, Tessler, HH. Episcleritis and scleritis. In: Yanoff M, Duker JS, eds. *Opthalmology.* 3rd ed. Baltimore, MD: Mosby; 2008.

Green GB, Hill PM. Approach to chest pain. In: Tintinalli JE, Kelen GD, Stapczynski JS, et al., eds. *Emergency Medicine: A Comprehensive Study Guide.* 6th ed. New York, NY: McGraw-Hill; 2004.

Hackett PH. High altitude medical problems. In: Tintinalli JE, Kelen GD, Stapczynski JS, et al., eds. *Emergency Medicine: A Comprehensive Study Guide.* 6th ed. New York, NY: McGraw-Hill; 2004.

Haller PR. Leg injuries. In: Tintinalli JE, Kelen GD, Stapczynski JS, et al., eds. *Emergency Medicine: A Comprehensive Study Guide.* 6th ed. New York, NY: McGraw-Hill; 2004.

Hasan N, Colucciello SA. Maxillofacial trauma. In: Tintinalli JE, Kelen GD, Stapczynski JS, et al., eds. *Emergency Medicine: A Comprehensive Study Guide.* 6th ed. New York, NY: McGraw-Hill; 2004.

Heegaard WG, Biros MH. Head. In: Marx JA, Hockberger RS, Walls RM, et al., eds. *Rosen's Emergency Medicine: Concepts and Clinical Practice.* 6th ed. Philadelphia, PA: Mosby; 2006.

Ho K, Abu-Laban RB. Ankle and foot. In: Marx JA, Hockberger RS, Walls RM, et al., eds. *Rosen's Emergency Medicine: Concepts and Clinical Practice.* 6th ed. Philadelphia, PA: Mosby; 2006.

Hollander JE, Singer AJ. Emergency wound management. In: Tintinalli JE, Kelen GD, Stapczynski JS, et al., eds. *Emergency Medicine: A Comprehensive Study Guide.* 6th ed. New York, NY: McGraw-Hill; 2004.

Hockberger RS, Kaji AH, Newton EJ. Spinal injuries. In: Marx JA, Hockberger RS, Walls RM, et al., eds. *Rosen's Emergency Medicine: Concepts and Clinical Practice.* 6th ed. Philadelphia, PA: Mosby; 2006.

Hollander JE. Acute coronary syndromes: acute myocardial infarction and unstable angina. In: Tintinalli JE, Kelen GD, Stapczynski JS, et al., eds. *Emergency Medicine: A Comprehensive Study Guide.* 6th ed. New York, NY: McGraw-Hill; 2004.

Hollander JE, Dierks DB. Intervention strategies for acute coronary syndromes. In: Tintinalli JE, Kelen GD, Stapczynski JS, et al., eds. *Emergency Medicine: A Comprehensive Study Guide.* 6th ed. New York, NY: McGraw-Hill; 2004.

Houry DE, Abbott JT. Acute complications of pregnancy. In: Marx JA, Hockberger RS, Walls RM, et al., eds. *Rosen's Emergency Medicine: Concepts and Clinical Practice.* 6th ed. Philadelphia, PA: Mosby; 2006.

Humphries RL. Cardiac emergencies. In: Stone KE, Humphries RL, eds. *Current Medical Diagnosis and Treatment.* 6th ed. New York, NY: McGraw-Hill; 2008.

Hung OL, Nelson LS. Acetaminophen. In: Tintinalli JE, Kelen GD, Stapczynski JS, et al., eds. *Emergency Medicine: A Comprehensive Study Guide.* 6th ed. New York, NY: McGraw-Hill; 2004.

Jaffe J, Morris JE. Infectious disease emergencies. In: Tintinalli JE, Kelen GD, Stapczynski JS, et al., eds. *Emergency Medicine: A Comprehensive Study Guide.* 6th ed. New York, NY: McGraw-Hill; 2004.

Janz TG, Hamilton GC. Disorders of hemostasis. In: Marx JA, Hockberger RS, Walls RM, et al., eds. *Rosen's Emergency Medicine: Concepts and Clinical Practice.* 6th ed. Philadelphia, PA: Mosby; 2006.

Jui J. Septic shock. In: Tintinalli JE, Kelen GD, Stapczynski JS, et al., eds. *Emergency Medicine: A Comprehensive Study Guide.* 6th ed. New York, NY: McGraw-Hill; 2004.

Kirsch TD, Lipinski CA. Head injury. In: Tintinalli JE, Kelen GD, Stapczynski JS, et al., eds. *Emergency Medicine: A Comprehensive Study Guide.* 6th ed. New York, NY: McGraw-Hill; 2004.

Kline JA, Runyon MS. Pulmonary embolism and deep venous thrombosis. In: Marx JA, Hockberger RS, Walls RM, et al., eds. *Rosen's Emergency Medicine: Concepts and Clinical Practice.* 6th ed. Philadelphia, PA: Mosby; 2006.

Kothari RU, Todd J, Crocco TJ, Barsan WG. Stroke. In: Marx JA, Hockberger RS, Walls RM, et al., eds. *Rosen's Emergency Medicine: Concepts and Clinical Practice.* 6th ed. Philadelphia, PA: Mosby; 2006.

Kou M, Mayer T. Pediatric asthma and bronchiolitis. In: Tintinalli JE, Kelen GD, Stapczynski JS, et al., eds. *Emergency Medicine: A Comprehensive Study Guide.* 6th ed. New York, NY: McGraw-Hill; 2004.

Kwiatkowski TE, Alagappan K. Headache. In: Marx JA, Hockberger RS, Walls RM, et al., eds. *Rosen's Emergency Medicine: Concepts and Clinical Practice.* 6th ed. Philadelphia, PA: Mosby; 2006.

Ladenson P, Kim D. Thyroid. In: Goldman L, Ausiello D, eds. *Cecil Textbook of Medicine.* 22nd ed. Philadelphia, PA: Saunders; 2004.

Londner M, Hammer D, Kelen GD. Fluid and electrolyte problems. In: Tintinalli JE, Kelen GD, Stapczynski JS, et al., eds. *Emergency Medicine: A Comprehensive Study Guide.* 6th ed. New York, NY: McGraw-Hill; 2004.

Lowell MJ. Esophagus, stomach and duodenum. In: Marx JA, Hockberger RS, Walls RM, et al., eds. *Rosen's Emergency Medicine: Concepts and Clinical Practice.* 6th ed. Philadelphia, PA: Mosby; 2006.

Lyn E, Antosia RE. Hand. In: Marx JA, Hockberger RS, Walls RM, et al., eds. *Rosen's Emergency Medicine: Concepts and Clinical Practice.* 6th ed. Philadelphia, PA: Mosby; 2006.

Manno M. Pediatric respiratory emergencies: upper airway obstruction and infection. In: Marx JA, Hockberger RS, Walls RM, et al., eds. *Rosen's Emergency Medicine: Concepts and Clinical Practice.* 6th ed. Philadelphia, PA: Mosby; 2006.

McCollough ME, Sharieff G. Renal and GU tract disorders. In: Marx JA, Hockberger RS, Walls RM, et al., eds. *Rosen's Emergency Medicine: Concepts and Clinical Practice.* 6th ed. Philadelphia, PA: Mosby; 2006.

McKay MP. Facial trauma. In: Marx JA, Hockberger RS, Walls RM, et al., eds. *Rosen's Emergency Medicine: Concepts and Clinical Practice.* 6th ed. Philadelphia, PA: Mosby; 2006.

McMicken DB, Finell JT. Alcohol-related disease. In: Marx JA, Hockberger RS, Walls RM, et al., eds. *Rosen's Emergency Medicine: Concepts and Clinical Practice.* 6th ed. Philadelphia, PA: Mosby; 2006.

Melanson SW, Heller MB. Principles of emergency department sonography. In: Tintinalli JE, Kelen GD, Stapczynski JS, et al., eds. *Emergency Medicine: A Comprehensive Study Guide.* 6th ed. New York, NY: McGraw-Hill; 2004.

Melio FR. Upper respiratory tract infection. In: Marx JA, Hockberger RS, Walls RM, et al., eds. *Rosen's Emergency Medicine: Concepts and Clinical Practice.* 6th ed. Philadelphia, PA: Mosby; 2006.

Meislin HW, Guisto JA. Soft tissue infections. In: Marx JA, Hockberger RS, Walls RM, et al., eds. *Rosen's Emergency Medicine: Concepts and Clinical Practice.* 6th ed. Philadelphia, PA: Mosby; 2006.

Mills KC. Monoamine oxidase inhibitors. In: Tintinalli JE, Kelen GD, Stapczynski JS, et al., eds. *Emergency Medicine: A Comprehensive Study Guide.* 6th ed. New York, NY: McGraw-Hill; 2004.

Mills KC. New antidepressant and serotonin syndrome. In: Tintinalli JE, Kelen GD, Stapczynski JS, et al., eds. *Emergency Medicine: A Comprehensive Study Guide.* 6th ed. New York, NY: McGraw-Hill; 2004.

Mills KC. Tricyclic antidepressants. In: Tintinalli JE, Kelen GD, Stapczynski JS, et al., eds. *Emergency Medicine: A Comprehensive Study Guide.* 6th ed. New York, NY: McGraw-Hill; 2004.

Moffa DA Jr, Emerman CL. Bronchitis, pneumonia, and pleural empyema. In: Tintinalli JE, Kelen GD, Stapczynski JS, et al., eds. *Emergency Medicine: A Comprehensive Study Guide.* 6th ed. New York, NY: McGraw-Hill; 2004.

Morris JE. Fluid: electrolyte and acid-base emergencies. In: Stone KE, Humphries RL, eds. *Current Medical Diagnosis and Treatment.* 6th ed. New York, NY: McGraw-Hill: 2008.

Nockowitz RA, Rund DA. Psychotropic medications. In: Tintinalli JE, Kelen GD, Stapczynski JS, et al., eds. *Emergency Medicine: A Comprehensive Study Guide.* 6th ed. New York, NY: McGraw-Hill; 2004.

Neufield JDG. Trauma in pregnancy. In: Marx JA, Hockberger RS, Walls RM, et al., eds. *Rosen's Emergency Medicine: Concepts and Clinical Practice.* 6th ed. Philadelphia, PA: Mosby; 2006.

Newton EJ, Calder KK. Chronic medical illness during pregnancy. In: Marx JA, Hockberger RS, Walls RM, et al., eds. *Rosen's Emergency Medicine: Concepts and Clinical Practice.* 6th ed. Philadelphia, PA: Mosby; 2006.

Niemann JT. The Cardiomyopathies, myocarditis, and pericardial disease. In: Tintinalli JE, Kelen GD, Stapczynski JS, et al., eds. *Emergency Medicine: A Comprehensive Study Guide.* 6th ed. New York, NY: McGraw-Hill; 2004.

Ornato P. Sudden cardiac deaths. In: Tintinalli JE, Kelen GD, Stapczynski JS, et al., eds. *Emergency Medicine: A Comprehensive Study Guide.* 6th ed. New York, NY: McGraw-Hill; 2004.

Overton DT. Gastrointestinal bleeding. In: Tintinalli JE, Kelen GD, Stapczynski JS, et al., eds. *Emergency Medicine: A Comprehensive Study Guide.* 6th ed. New York, NY: McGraw-Hill; 2004.

Perrone J, Hoffman RS. Cocaine amphetamines, caffeine and nicotine. In: Tintinalli JE, Kelen GD, Stapczynski JS, et al., eds. *Emergency Medicine: A Comprehensive Study Guide.* 6th ed. New York, NY: McGraw-Hill; 2004.

Prince LA, Johnson GA. Aortic dissection and aneurysms. In: Tintinalli JE, Kelen GD, Stapczynski JS, et al., eds. *Emergency Medicine: A Comprehensive Study Guide.* 6th ed. New York, NY: McGraw-Hill; 2004.

Reisdorff EJ. Lacerations of the leg and foot. In: Tintinalli JE, Kelen GD, Stapczynski JS, et al., eds. *Emergency Medicine: A Comprehensive Study Guide.* 6th ed. New York, NY: McGraw-Hill; 2004.

Roberts DJ. Cardiovascular drugs. In: Marx JA, Hockberger RS, Walls RM, et al., eds. *Rosen's Emergency Medicine: Concepts and Clinical Practice.* 6th ed. Philadelphia, PA: Mosby; 2006.

Rothman R, Marco CA, Yang S, et al,. AIDS and HIV. In: Marx JA, Hockberger RS, Walls RM, et al., eds. *Rosen's Emergency Medicine: Concepts and Clinical Practice.* 6th ed. Philadelphia, PA: Mosby; 2006.

Rubenstein JB, Virasch V. Allergic conjunctivitis. In: Yanoff M, Duker JS, eds. *Opthalmology.* 3rd ed. Baltimore, MD: Mosby; 2008.

Rubin D. Bacterial meningitis. In: Marx JA, Hockberger RS, Walls RM, et al., eds. *Rosen's Emergency Medicine: Concepts and Clinical Practice.* 6th ed. Philadelphia, PA: Mosby; 2006.

Schneider SM, Cobaugh DJ. Lithium. In: Tintinalli JE, Kelen GD, Stapczynski JS, et al., eds. *Emergency Medicine: A Comprehensive Study Guide.* 6th ed. New York, NY: McGraw-Hill; 2004.

Schneider RE. Genitourinary system. In: Marx JA, Hockberger RS, Walls RM, et al., eds. *Rosen's Emergency Medicine: Concepts and Clinical Practice.* 6th ed. Philadelphia, PA: Mosby; 2006.

Schneider RE. Male genital problems. In: Tintinalli JE, Kelen GD, Stapczynski JS, et al., eds. *Emergency Medicine: A Comprehensive Study Guide.* 6th ed. New York, NY: McGraw-Hill; 2004.

Schwab RA, Powers RD. Puncture wounds and mammalian bites. In: Tintinalli JE, Kelen GD, Stapczynski JS, et al., eds. *Emergency Medicine: A Comprehensive Study Guide.* 6th ed. New York, NY: McGraw-Hill; 2004.

Schwartz LR, Balakrishnam C. Thermal burns. In: Tintinalli JE, Kelen GD, Stapczynski JS, et al., eds. *Emergency Medicine: A Comprehensive Study Guide.* 6th ed. New York, NY: McGraw-Hill; 2004.

See J, Chew P. Angle-closure glaucoma In: Yanoff M, Duker JS, eds. *Ophthalmology.* 3rd ed. Baltimore, MD: Mosby; 2008.

Sercombe CT. Systemic lupus erythematosus and vasculitides. In: Marx JA, Hockberger RS, Walls RM, et al., eds. *Rosen's Emergency Medicine: Concepts and Clinical Practice.* 6th ed. Philadelphia, PA: Mosby; 2006.

Skorecki K, Ausiello D. Disorders of sodium or water homeostasis. In: Goldman L, Ausiello D, eds. *Cecil Textbook of Medicine*. 22nd ed. Philadelphia, PA: Saunders; 2004.

Steele MT, Glaspy JN. Knee injuries. In: Tintinalli JE, Kelen GD, Stapczynski JS, et al., eds. *Emergency Medicine: A Comprehensive Study Guide*. 6th ed. New York, NY: McGraw-Hill; 2004.

Sternlicht JE, Wogan JM. Thyroid and adrenal disorders. In: Marx JA, Hockberger RS, Walls RM, et al., eds. *Rosen's Emergency Medicine: Concepts and Clinical Practice*. 6th ed. Philadelphia, PA: Mosby; 2006.

Stettler BE, Pancioli AM. Spinal cord disorders. In: Marx JA, Hockberger RS, Walls RM, et al., eds. *Rosen's Emergency Medicine: Concepts and Clinical Practice*. 6th ed. Philadelphia, PA: Mosby; 2006.

Sokolove PE, Chan D. Tuberculosis. In: Marx JA, Hockberger RS, Walls RM, et al., eds. *Rosen's Emergency Medicine: Concepts and Clinical Practice*. 6th ed. Philadelphia, PA: Mosby; 2006.

Tobleman R, Stone K. Headache. In: Stone KE, Humphries RL, eds. *Current Medical Diagnosis and Treatment*. 6th ed. New York, NY: McGraw-Hill: 2008.

Vicario SJ, Price TG. Intestinal obstruction. In: Tintinalli JE, Kelen GD, Stapczynski JS, et al., eds. *Emergency Medicine: A Comprehensive Study Guide*. 6th ed. New York, NY: McGraw-Hill; 2004.

Wax PM. Anticholinergic toxicity. In: Tintinalli JE, Kelen GD, Stapczynski JS, et al., eds. *Emergency Medicine: A Comprehensive Study Guide*. 6th ed. New York, NY: McGraw-Hill; 2004.

Weinstock MS, Rosenau AM. Pediatric exanthems. In: Tintinalli JE, Kelen GD, Stapczynski JS, et al., eds. *Emergency Medicine: A Comprehensive Study Guide*. 6th ed. New York, NY: McGraw-Hill; 2004.

Werman HA, Mekhjian HS, Rund DA. Ileitis, colitis, and diverticulitis. In: Tintinalli JE, Kelen GD, Stapczynski JS, et al., eds. *Emergency Medicine: A Comprehensive Study Guide*. 6th ed. New York, NY: McGraw-Hill; 2004.

White SR, Kosnick J. Toxic alcohols. In: Marx JA, Hockberger RS, Walls RM, et al., eds. *Rosen's Emergency Medicine: Concepts and Clinical Practice*. 6th ed. Philadelphia, PA: Mosby; 2006.

Woolfrey KG, Eisenhaver MA. Wrist & forearm. In: Marx JA, Hockberger RS, Walls RM, et al., eds. *Rosen's Emergency Medicine: Concepts and Clinical Practice*. 6th ed. Philadelphia, PA: Mosby; 2006.

Wu MM, Chanmugam A. Hypertension. In: Tintinalli JE, Kelen GD, Stapczynski JS, et al., eds. *Emergency Medicine: A Comprehensive Study Guide*. 6th ed. New York, NY: McGraw-Hill; 2004.

Yearly DM, Delbridge TR. Dysrhythmias. In: Marx JA, Hockberger RS, Walls RM, et al., eds. *Rosen's Emergency Medicine: Concepts and Clinical Practice*. 6th ed. Philadelphia, PA: Mosby; 2006.

Yip L. Salicylates. In: Tintinalli JE, Kelen GD, Stapczynski JS, et al., eds. *Emergency Medicine: A Comprehensive Study Guide*. 6th ed. New York, NY: McGraw-Hill; 2004.

Young WF Jr, Humphries RL. Spontaneous and iatrogenic pneumothorax. In: Tintinalli JE, Kelen GD, Stapczynski JS et al., eds. *Emergency Medicine: A Comprehensive Study Guide*. 6th ed. New York, NY: McGraw-Hill; 2004.

Zivin JA. Hemorrhagic cerebrovascular disease. In: Goldman L, Ausiello DA, et al., eds. *Goldman: Cecil Medicine*. 23rd ed. Philadelphia, PA: Saunders; 2008.

Zun LS, Singh A. Nausea and vomiting. In: Marx JA, Hockberger RS, Walls RM, et al., eds. *Rosen's Emergency Medicine: Concepts and Clinical Practice*. 6th ed. Philadelphia, PA: Mosby; 2006.

CHAPTER 18

General and Vascular Surgery

Michel Statler, MLA, PA-C

Frank A. Acevedo, MS, PA-C, DFAAPA

Jennie Hocking, MPAS, PA-C

DIRECTIONS: Each of the numbered items or incomplete statements is followed by answers of completion of the statement. Select the ONE-lettered answer or completion that is BEST in each case.

1. Which of the following physiologic responses characterizes the proliferative phase of wound healing?

    (A) Migration of neutrophils to the wound
    (B) Platelet activation
    (C) Production of collagen
    (D) Neovascularization

2. A patient who has been on chronic prednisone for rheumatoid arthritis is scheduled for a total knee replacement. Which of the following interventions is recommended to promote wound healing for this patient?

    (A) Vitamin A
    (B) Vitamin C
    (C) Zinc replacement
    (D) Hyperbaric oxygen

3. A paraplegic patient developed a sacral decubitus ulcer secondary to sitting in wheelchair for prolonged periods of time. Initial treatment included debridement and saline dressing changes. There is no evidence of infection or necrotic tissue in the wound. Which of the following interventions would be recommended to promote rapid closure of the wound?

    (A) Occlusive dressings
    (B) Topical 1% silver nitrate
    (C) Application of platelet-derived growth factor
    (D) Negative pressure wound vacuum device

4. Which of the following surgical procedures would be classified as a clean-contaminated case?

    (A) Inguinal herniorrhaphy
    (B) Repair of a perforated gastric ulcer
    (C) Open cholecystectomy with common bile duct exploration
    (D) Resection of necrotic bowel

5. A patient is scheduled for a mitral valve replacement. Which of the following pharmacologic agents would be recommended for surgical prophylaxis? There are no known drug allergies.

    (A) Cefazolin
    (B) Vancomycin
    (C) Ciprofloxacin
    (D) Nafcillin

6. Which pulmonary function parameter is the most helpful in predicting potential postoperative complications, including the inability to wean from ventilatory support?

(A) Tidal volume
(B) Functional residual capacity
(C) Expiratory reserve volume
(D) Forced expiration volume in 1 second

7. A 35-year-old man is postoperative day 4–status post exploratory laparotomy for a gunshot wound to the abdomen. At the time of exploration, a perforation to the left colon was found and he underwent repair with proximal colostomy. He now is confused, agitated, and has developed oliguria over the past 8 hours. His vital signs are temperature 104°F, respiratory rate 24/min, heart rate 134/min, blood pressure 85/60 mm Hg. Which of the following types of shock is most likely in this situation?

(A) Hypovolemic
(B) Cardiogenic
(C) Septic
(D) Neurogenic

8. A 22-year-old man is brought to the emergency department by paramedics after having sustained a single stab wound along the left sternal border at the fourth intercostal space. Upon arrival to the emergency department, he was hypotensive and tachycardic. The neck veins were distended and heart sounds were muffled. Which of the following interventions is the most appropriate first-line management of this patient?

(A) Left tube thoracostomy
(B) Pericardiocentesis
(C) Fluid resuscitation
(D) Immediate intubation

9. A 32-year-old lactating female presents to the surgical clinic with a fluctuant mass of her left breast. The area directly above the lesion is erythematous and tender to touch. You make the diagnosis of localized breast abscess. Which of the following pathogens is the most likely cause of the patient's symptoms?

(A) *Staphylococcus aureus*
(B) Viridens *streptococcus*
(C) *Pseudomonas aeruginosa*
(D) *Escherichia coli*

10. Which of the following type of gallstones is the most common in the United States?

(A) Mixed
(B) Calcium
(C) Brown pigmented
(D) Black pigmented

11. Which population has the highest incidence of gallstones in the United States?

(A) Caucasian women older than 50 years
(B) Hispanic men older than 50 years
(C) African American men younger than 50 years
(D) Native American women before the age of 60 years

12. A 52-year-old woman presents with the acute onset of right upper quadrant pain that is associated with fever, nausea, and vomiting. Which of the following best describes the underlying pathology associated with her diagnosis?

(A) Intermittent obstruction of the cystic duct without inflammation
(B) Sustained obstruction of the cystic duct with inflammation
(C) Obstruction of the common bile duct without inflammation
(D) Obstruction of the common bile duct with inflammation

13. A 63-year-old white male is seen in the ambulatory outpatient clinic with complaints of midepigastric pain, weight loss, and jaundice. On examination, he is jaundiced and his sclerae are icteric. On palpation of the abdomen, you find a distended nontender gallbladder. Which of the following is the most likely diagnosis?

(A) Gastric carcinoma

(B) Chronic pancreatitis

(C) Pancreatic carcinoma

(D) Choledocholithiasis

14. A 48-year-old woman presented with the new onset of jaundice and right upper quadrant abdominal pain. Which of the following findings on abdominal ultrasound would be consistent with choledocholithiasis?

(A) Pericholecystic fluid

(B) Thickened gallbladder wall

(C) Dilated hepatic ducts

(D) Air in the lumen of the gallbladder

15. A 46-year-old African American male is seen in the emergency department with upper right quadrant pain that radiates to the right infrascapular area. The pain is colicky and was precipitated by a meal of fried fish and French fries. Which of the following diagnostic studies is the initial study of choice for this patient?

(A) Plain abdominal x-ray

(B) Ultrasonography

(C) Radionuclide scan (HIDA scan)

(D) Computed tomography (CT)

16. A 73-year-old jaundiced female is noted to have a posthepatic obstruction on ultrasound. Which of the following tests will best determine the level of obstruction and type of pathology present?

(A) Plain abdominal x-ray

(B) Radionuclide scan (HIDA scan)

(C) Computed tomography

(D) Intravenous cholangiography

17. A 58-year-old man presents with the acute onset of abdominal pain associated with fever and shaking chills. The patient is hypotensive and febrile with a temperature of 102.2°F. Although he is confused and disoriented, he complains of right upper quadrant pain during palpation of the abdomen. His sclerae are icteric and the skin is jaundiced. Which of the following is the most likely diagnosis?

(A) Acute cholecystitis

(B) Choledocholithiasis

(C) Acute pancreatitis

(D) Ascending cholangitis

18. A 43-year-old Native Indian female presents with a 3-month history of recurrent episodes of right upper quadrant pain that occur a few hours after eating. The episodes are associated with dyspepsia but no fever or chills. Ultrasound is consistent with cholelithiasis. Which of the following interventions is the treatment of choice for this patient?

(A) Follow-up ultrasound in 6 months

(B) ERCP with sphincterotomy

(C) Laparoscopic cholecystectomy

(D) Extracorporeal shock wave lithotripsy

19. A 54-year-old man with a history of chronic alcohol abuse presents to the emergency department with complaints of a subjective fever and severe epigastric pain radiating to the back. The pain has been present for the past 8 hours and is associated with nausea and vomiting, which has not relieved the pain. Laboratory data reveal a WBC of 14,000/mm^3 and a serum amylase of 500 U/L (reference range 0–286 U/L). Plain films of the abdomen were unremarkable. Which of the following is the most likely diagnosis?

(A) Perforated duodenal ulcer

(B) Acute cholecystitis

(C) Acute pancreatitis

(D) Mesenteric ischemia

(E) Choledocholithiasis

20. Patients with acute pancreatitis may present with varying degrees of severity. In order to triage patients appropriately, what is the most commonly used scale of prognostic indicators?

(A) Charcot's triad

(B) Ranson's criteria

(C) Glasgow scale

(D) Child–Turcotte–Pugh score

21. A 54-year-old man complains of persistent midepigastric abdominal pain 2 weeks following the diagnosis of acute pancreatitis. The patient also complains of anorexia but no fever or chills. There is a palpable mass in the midepigastrium; bowel sounds are normal in all four quadrants. Which of the following is most likely diagnosis?

    (A) Adynamic ileus
    (B) Pancreatic carcinoma
    (C) Infected pancreatic necrosis
    (D) Pancreatic pseudocyst

22. Which of the following physical examination findings is associated with Courvoisier's sign?

    (A) Periumbilical ecchymosis
    (B) Palpable, nontender gallbladder
    (C) Flank ecchymosis
    (D) Inspiratory arrest on palpation of the abdomen

23. What is the most important factor in determining overall survival rates for patients with breast cancer?

    (A) Tumor size
    (B) Estrogen receptor status
    (C) Tumor histology
    (D) Axillary lymph node status

24. Which of the following signs and symptoms is associated with the abdominal pain secondary to chronic intestinal ischemia?

    (A) Guarding and rigidity
    (B) Fear of eating
    (C) Nausea and vomiting
    (D) Bloody diarrhea
    (E) Positive obturator and psoas signs

25. What features are commonly associated with lower extremity ulcers that are due to chronic arterial insufficiency?

    (A) Ulcers are associated with hyperpigmentation changes in the skin
    (B) Ulcers are most commonly seen around the medial and lateral malleoli

    (C) Ulcers have a "punched out" appearance with a pale or necrotic base
    (D) Ulcers are associated with painless lower extremity edema

26. A 22-year-old obese white female is seen with a complaint of a mass in the upper outer quadrant of the left breast. The lesion is smooth, firm, and freely movable, approximately 3 cm in size. Which of the following is the most likely diagnosis?

    (A) Breast cyst
    (B) Lipoma of the breast
    (C) Fibroadenoma
    (D) Fibrocystic changes

27. A 63-year-old woman presented with a painless left breast mass. The mass was approximately 3 cm in size and there were two palpable nodes in the left axilla. CT scans of the chest and abdomen were negative for metastatic disease. What would be the TNM (tumor, node, metastasis) staging for this patient?

    (A) T1N0M0
    (B) T2N0M0
    (C) T2N1M0
    (D) T3N1M0

28. Which symptom associated with an acute arterial occlusion to the lower extremities is most associated with the time of occlusion?

    (A) Pain
    (B) Pallor
    (C) Paresthesias
    (D) Paralysis

29. A 62-year-old man presents to the office concerned about an abdominal aortic aneurysm (AAA). He has had no symptoms but states that his father died from an aortic dissection at the age of 50 and his brother was diagnosed last week with an AAA. What is the most appropriate screening tool in this situation?

    (A) Abdominal radiograph
    (B) Computed tomographic angiography (CTA)

(C) Palpation

(D) Ultrasound

(E) Aortography

30. A 56-year-old woman presents to the office with complaint of left lower extremity pain, particularly in the evening. She states that she can walk six to eight blocks without difficulty. Examination reveals a 3 × 4 cm ulceration on the medial aspect of her left lower leg, proximal to the medial malleolus. The ulcer base is erythematous with good granulation tissue, and it is surrounded by a border of induration. Varicosities are identified along the distribution of the greater saphenous vein. What is the most likely diagnosis?

(A) Arteriosclerosis

(B) Diabetes mellitus

(C) Scleroderma

(D) Venous stasis

(E) Deep venous thrombosis

31. A 66-year-old man, with a 20-year history of hypertension and 80 pack-year smoking history, presents with progressive claudication affecting both lower extremities. Recently, he has begun to waken at night with leg pain. What would be the expected ankle/brachial index for this patient?

(A) Greater than 1.0

(B) 0.8 to 1.0

(C) 0.6 to 0.8

(D) 0.4 to 0.6

(E) less than 0.4

32. What is the most common embolic source of acute arterial occlusion in the lower extremities?

(A) Atrial fibrillation

(B) Aortic aneurysm

(C) Myocardial infarction

(D) Prosthetic cardiac valve

(E) Iliac artery thrombus

33. A 50-year-old man presents with persistent hypertension that has been difficult to control with medications. On examination, there is evi-dence of hypertensive retinopathy on fundoscopic examination and bilateral flank bruits. What is the most common likely of his renovascular hypertension?

(A) Atherosclerosis

(B) Fibromuscular dysplasia

(C) Renal artery dissection

(D) Cardiac emboli

34. A 6-year-old girl presents to the emergency department with abdominal distension of 1-day duration. She has not had a bowel movement or passed flatus in 72 hours. Examination reveals markedly diminished bowel sounds with tympany to percussion. She has also passed bloody mucus from her rectum. There is no evidence of hernia, and surgical history is negative. Which of the following is the most likely diagnosis?

(A) Regional enteritis

(B) Pyloric stenosis

(C) Meckel diverticulum

(D) Acute appendicitis

35. Which are the most common symptoms of Crohn disease?

(A) Abdominal pain, diarrhea, and weight loss

(B) Bloody diarrhea, anal fistulas, and fever

(C) Weight loss, fever, and melena

(D) Abdominal pain, rectal bleeding, and fever

36. A 58-year-old man with a 20-year history of gastroesophageal reflux disease (GERD) presents with progressive dysphagia for 5 months associated with a 20-lb weight loss. Results from a barium swallow are pictured below (Figure 18.1). Which of the following is the most likely diagnosis?

(A) Achalasia

(B) Esophageal leiomyoma

(C) Uncomplicated reflux esophagitis

(D) Esophageal carcinoma

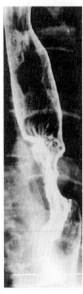

Figure 18-1
(Reproduced, with permission, from Fauci AS, Braunwald E, Kasper DL, et al. Harrison's Principles of Internal Medicine, 17th ed. New York: McGraw-Hill, 2008:1849.)

37. A patient presents with abdominal distension associated with nausea and vomiting. Which of the following findings is consistent with a paralytic ileus?

(A) Crampy abdominal pain
(B) Hyperactive bowel sounds
(C) Obstipation and failure to pass flatus
(D) Gas in small intestine only on KUB (kidney, ureter, bladder)

38. A 56-year-old man presents with abdominal distension associated with nausea and vomiting. On examination, the abdomen is distended with tympany on percussion. Bowel sounds are hyperactive. Past medical history (PMH) reveals an exploratory laparotomy for a ruptured appendix 20 years ago. Which of the following interventions is the most appropriate first-line management of this patient?

(A) Correction of fluid and electrolyte abnormalities
(B) Emergency surgery
(C) Obtaining barium radiograph studies
(D) Scheduling a sigmoidoscopy

39. A 64-year-old man has been experiencing intermittent left lower abdominal pain associated with alternating diarrhea and constipation. The pain has been increasing over the past 24 hours and is now associated with a fever. The abdomen is tender with evidence of peritoneal signs. Which of the following diagnostic studies is most appropriate to evaluate this patient?

(A) Barium enema
(B) Computed tomography (CT)
(C) Sigmoidoscopy
(D) Colonoscopy

40. Which of the following conditions is the most common cause of massive lower gastrointestinal bleeding?

(A) Hemorrhoids
(B) Colon cancer
(C) Diverticular disease
(D) Upper gastrointestinal hemorrhage
(E) Meckel diverticulum

41. Which of the following patients would be recommended for an elective surgical repair for treatment of symptoms due to diverticular disease?

(A) Patient with an initial presentation of left lower quadrant pain
(B) Patient who is refractory to medical management of their symptoms
(C) Patient with fever and a left lower quadrant abscess
(D) Patient with a rigid abdomen and free air on a KUB

42. Which of the following types of colon polyps should be treated by surgical excision because of a high risk of malignant degeneration?

(A) Hamartoma
(B) Inflammatory
(C) Hyperplastic
(D) Villous

43. Which of the following guidelines for screening colonoscopy would be recommended for a 40-year-old woman whose father was diagnosed with colon cancer at the age 58?

   (A) She should undergo an air contrast barium enema at 50 years of age and repeat every 10 years.

   (B) She should have a flexible sigmoidoscopy every 1 to 2 years starting at age 30.

   (C) She should undergo a screening colonoscopy every 5 years starting at age 48.

   (D) She should have a flexible sigmoidoscopy and air contrast barium enema every 10 years starting at age 50.

44. An 82-year-old woman presents to the office with a complaint of right lower quadrant pain, a 15-lb weight loss over the past month, and fatigue. Examination reveals conjunctival pallor, and a palpable mass in the right lower quadrant. Which of the following is the most likely diagnosis?

   (A) Sigmoid volvulus
   (B) Cecal carcinoma
   (C) Acute appendicitis
   (D) Incarcerated hernia
   (E) Pancreatic carcinoma

45. A 57-year-old woman underwent a hemicolectomy for adenocarcinoma of the colon. Which of the following recommendations is part of postoperative monitoring for a potential recurrence?

   (A) Annual fecal occult blood testing
   (B) Annual chest radiograph
   (C) Annual CA 19-9 testing
   (D) Annual flexible sigmoidoscopy
   (E) Annual colonoscopy

46. A patient presented with intermittent rectal bleeding associated with decreased caliber in the size of his stool. On examination, there were no palpable abdominal masses, but the fecal occult testing was positive. A barium enema was obtained with the results pictured below. What is the most likely diagnosis for this patient?

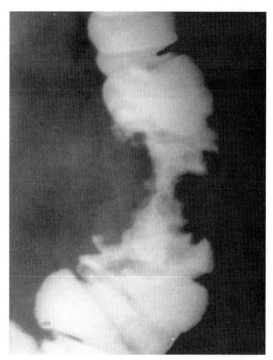

Figure 18-2
(Reproduced, with permission, from Fauci AS, Braunwald E, Kasper DL, et al. Harrison's Principles of Internal Medicine, 17th ed. New York: McGraw-Hill, 2008:577.)

   (A) Diverticular disease
   (B) Crohn disease
   (C) Colorectal carcinoma
   (D) Intussusception

47. A 56-year-old woman has had a left hemicolectomy for resection of an adenocarcinoma of the colon. Pathology reveals that the lesion has penetrated into but not through the muscularis propia of the bowel wall. Positive lymph nodes are also identified. According to the Dukes–Astler–Coller system what is the stage for this lesion?

   (A) Stage A
   (B) Stage B1
   (C) Stage B2
   (D) Stage C1
   (E) Stage C2

48. Which of the following pathologic findings is associated with ulcerative colitis?

(A) Transmural inflammation

(B) Rectal involvement

(C) Perianal fistulas

(D) Presence of skip lesions

49. A 32-year-old woman with a history of Crohn's disease presents with an acute flare-up of worsening abdominal pain associated with diarrhea. Which of the following pharmacologic agents is indicated for this patient?

(A) Prednisone

(B) Azathioprine

(C) Metronidazole

(D) Sulfasalazine

50. A 55-year-old man has a history of ulcerative colitis for the past 22 years, and colonoscopy has now revealed a low-grade dysplasia in the left colon. Which of the following surgical procedures would be recommended for this patient?

(A) Subtotal colectomy with ileoproctostomy

(B) Proctocolectomy with ileoanal pull-through

(C) Local resection of the lesion with 2 cm margins

(D) Total proctocolectomy with a permanent ileostomy

51. A 66-year-old woman presents to the emergency department with a complaint of abdominal pain and distension for the past 3 days. Examination reveals a protuberant abdomen with diminished bowel sounds and tympany to percussion. Flat and upright abdominal radiographs reveal distended loops of bowel with prominent haustral markings. Which of the following etiologies is the most likely cause of the patient's condition?

(A) Volvulus

(B) Adenocarcinoma

(C) Diverticular disease

(D) Strangulated hernia

(E) Adhesions

52. Which of the following radiographic findings is consistent with a large bowel obstruction?

(A) Distended proximal colon with air-fluid levels

(B) Free air under the diaphragm

(C) Large volume of rectal air

(D) Loss of haustral markings

53. A 54-year-old man presents to the emergency department with crampy abdominal pain, nausea, and vomiting. The patient has not passed gas or had a bowel movement for at least 10 hours. On examination, the abdomen is distended and there are high-pitched bowel sounds with rushes. A plain radiograph of the abdomen reveals cecal distension to 12 cm. What is the most appropriate definitive management for this patient?

(A) Intravenous fluids

(B) Nasogastric suction

(C) Observation

(D) Surgical exploration

54. An 80-year-old male nursing home patient is brought to the emergency department with abdominal distension. A plain film of the abdomen is pictured below. Which of the following is the most likely diagnosis?

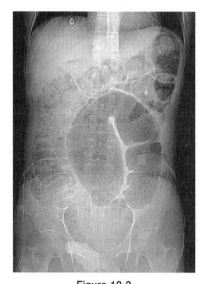

Figure 18-3
(Reproduced, with permission, from Fauci AS, Braunwald E, Kasper DL, et al. Harrison's Principles of Internal Medicine, 17th ed. New York: McGraw-Hill, 2008:1842.)

(A) Small bowel obstruction

(B) Cecal volvulus

(C) Sigmoid volvulus

(D) Toxic megacolon

55. A 34-year-old woman presents to the office complaining of bleeding per rectum in association with defecation. Examination reveals a large internal hemorrhoid that required manual manipulation for reduction. Which of the following classifications best describes this type of hemorrhoid?

(A) First degree

(B) Second degree

(C) Third degree

(D) Fourth degree

56. A 10-year-old boy with rectal pain is brought by his mother into the office. The boy says that pain is worse when he has a bowel movement. He has noticed bright red blood on the toilet paper after wiping himself. Which of the following is the most likely diagnosis?

(A) Perianal abscess

(B) Pilonidal cyst

(C) Fistula in ano

(D) Anal fissure

57. Which of the following is an absolute contraindication to surgical resection of lung cancer?

(A) $FEV_1 < 1L$ (<80% of predicted)

(B) Solitary brain metastasis

(C) Myocardial infarction in last 6 months

(D) Malignant pleural effusion

58. A 45-year-old nonsmoking female is found to have a 2-cm mass in the periphery of the left lung on a routine chest radiograph. She has no significant medical history, known exposures, or contributory family history. A subsequent biopsy confirms malignancy. Which of the following is the most likely underlying cell type?

(A) Squamous cell

(B) Large cell

(C) Adenocarcinoma

(D) Small cell

59. What is the treatment of choice for an otherwise healthy (low surgical risk) patient with stage IA nonsmall cell lung cancer?

(A) Lobectomy

(B) Pneumonectomy

(C) Wedge resection and chemotherapy

(D) Radiation

(E) Radiofrequency ablation

60. Which of the following is considered first-line surgical treatment for achalasia?

(A) Nissen fundoplication

(B) Esophagectomy

(C) Myotomy

(D) Vagotomy with pyloroplasty

61. A 19-year-old basic training cadet presents with 3 days of pain in his right hand and forearm after having an IV placed for hydration following an intense training exercise. Examination is significant for a warm, palpable cord originating on the dorsum of the right hand; there is no associated cellulitis or purulence. A Doppler examination reveals thrombosis of the cephalic vein without extension into the deep veins. Which of the following is the most appropriate next step in management?

(A) Heparin

(B) Warfarin

(C) Nonsteroidal anti-inflammatory drugs

(D) Antibiotics

62. Which of the following etiologies is the most common cause of nontraumatic subarachnoid hemorrhage (SAH)?

(A) Cerebral aneurysm

(B) Poorly controlled hypertension

(C) Anticoagulant use

(D) Arteriovenous malformation

63. A 58-year-old man presents with to the emergency department with the acute onset of the "worst headache of his life," which was associated with a brief loss of consciousness. The patient is complaining of increased pain with movement of his neck as well as photophobia. What is the recommended first-line study to evaluate this patient?

(A) Lumbar puncture
(B) Noncontrast CT scan of the head
(C) Magnetic resonance imaging (MRI) of the brain
(D) Four-vessel angiogram

64. A 74-year-old woman presented with the new onset of seizures. An MRI with gadolinium showed a parasagittal mass with homogenous enhancement and a "dural tail." What is the appropriate management of this patient?

(A) Radiation therapy
(B) Chemotherapy
(C) Surgical resection
(D) Surgical resection with chemotherapy

65. A 65-year-old man presented with the acute onset of a severe headache. The patient has nuchal rigidity on examination but no focal neurologic deficits. Noncontrast CT scan of the head showed blood in the lateral and interhemispheric fissures. Subsequent four-vessel angiogram showed the presence of an anterior communicating artery aneurysm. What is the recommended management of this patient?

(A) Observation for rebleeding
(B) Endovascular embolization
(C) Craniotomy with clipping of the aneurysm
(D) Coiling of the aneurysm via interventional radiology

66. A 58-year-old woman presented with signs and symptoms consistent with nephrolithiasis. During workup for the underlying etiology, the patient was found to have a serum calcium of 13.2 mg/dL (reference range 8.5–11.0 mg/dL) and an elevated PTH. Which of the following interventions is recommended for this patient?

(A) alendronate (Fosamax)
(B) raloxifene (Evista)
(C) Parathyroidectomy
(D) Cervical thymectomy

67. Which of the following is the most common serious complication following a parathyroidectomy?

(A) Persistent hypercalcemia
(B) Hypophosphatemia
(C) Hypoparathyroidism
(D) Bilateral recurrent laryngeal nerve injury

68. A 28-year-old woman presents with nervousness and palpitations associated with heat intolerance. On examination, there is no evidence of thyromegaly, but there is a palpable nodule that is "hot" on a thyroid scan. The TSH was low and T3 and T4 were both elevated. Which of the following is the recommended treatment for this patient?

(A) Propylthiouracil (PTU)
(B) Thyroid lobectomy
(C) Total thyroidectomy
(D) Radioiodine ablation

69. A 60-year-old man presented with a mass in the left lobe of the thyroid. Fine needle aspiration was consistent with papillary carcinoma. There was no evidence of locally invasive or metastatic disease. Which of the following treatments is recommended for this patient?

(A) Chemotherapy
(B) External beam radiation
(C) Preoperative radioiodine ablation
(D) Total thyroidectomy

70. A 58-year-old man presented with a history of episodic fluctuations in his blood pressure associated with anxiety, palpitations, and flushing. Urinary tests were positive for elevated metanephrine levels. Which of the following interventions is the first step in preparing the patient for surgical resection?

(A) β-Blockers to control the heart rate

(B) α-Blockers to control the blood pressure

(C) Nitrates for vasodilation

(D) Cortisol replacement for adrenal insufficiency

71. A patient who is 6 days status post a left inguinal herniorrhaphy develops redness and pain at the operative site. His vital signs are stable, but he does have a temperature of 99.7°F. There is erythema and induration around the skin edges with purulent discharge from the wound. What is the most important step in the management of this patient?

(A) Warm compresses to the operative site

(B) Bedrest with elevation of the left leg

(C) A 10-day course of intravenous antibiotics

(D) Reopening the wound with evacuation of purulent material

72. A 58-year-old man is in the hospital postoperative day 3 after a laparoscopic right colon resection. Your morning labs reveal a serum potassium level of 2.9 mEq/L (normal 3.5–5.0 mEq/L) despite aggressive potassium replacement during the previous shift. At this time you should check which of the following laboratory values?

(A) Magnesium

(B) Calcium

(C) Phosphorous

(D) Sodium

(E) Albumin

73. A patient with peritonitis secondary to a ruptured appendix was admitted to the intensive care unit with hypotension and tachycardia. Which of the following crystalloid solutions would be recommended for the fluid resuscitation of this patient?

(A) 5% Dextrose water

(B) 5% Dextrose water with 0.45% sodium chloride

(C) 0.9% Sodium chloride

(D) Lactated Ringer's solution

74. A patient is admitted to the intensive care unit in hypovolemic shock secondary to a splenic injury sustained in a motor vehicle collision. What is the most objective means of assessing that the intravascular volume is being adequately replaced during fluid resuscitation?

(A) Measurement of patient weight

(B) Maintenance of urinary output

(C) Resolution of orthostatic changes

(D) Normalization of peripheral perfusion

75. What is the most appropriate step following the placement of a nasoenteric feeding tube?

(A) Obtain a radiograph

(B) Check position of the tube by instillation of air

(C) Instill sterile saline prior to tube feedings

(D) Check gastric residuals

76. A 23-year-old man, unrestrained driver, is brought to the emergency department by ambulance after having been involved in an automobile accident. His vitals are BP: 99/54 mm Hg, P: 112/min, R: 18/min, oxygen saturation: 99%, T: 99.8°F. Examination reveals mild abdominal tenderness with pain radiating to the right shoulder. What is the most appropriate diagnostic test to order initially?

(A) Computed tomography of the abdomen and pelvis

(B) Diagnostic peritoneal lavage

(C) Flat and upright abdominal radiographs

(D) Diagnostic ultrasound

77. Which of the following treatment options is recommended for a patient with a grade I splenic laceration on CT scan who is otherwise hemodynamically stable?

(A) Exploratory laparotomy and splenectomy

(B) Exploratory laparotomy and splenorrhaphy

(C) Exploratory laparotomy and partial splenectomy

(D) Nonoperative management with splenic preservation

(E) Splenic autotransplantation into the omentum

78. A 39-year-old man presents to the emergency department with massive hematemesis. His physical examination reveals slight jaundice, palmar erythema, spider angiomas, and marked ascites. Vitals at the time of presentation are as follows: BP: 85/44 mm Hg, P: 122/min, R: 16/min, oxygen saturation: 96%, and T: 99.8°F. Which of the following is the most likely cause of the massive hematemesis?

(A) Peptic ulcer disease
(B) Mallory–Weiss tear
(C) Gastric carcinoma
(D) Arteriovenous malformation
(E) Esophageal varices

79. Which of the following procedures is the most effective treatment for a patient with complete intrahepatic portal vein thrombosis?

(A) End-to-side portocaval shunt
(B) Side-to-side portocaval shunt
(C) Distal splenorenal shunt
(D) Transjugular intrahepatic portosystemic shunt
(E) Esophagogastric devascularization

80. Which of the following is the most common indication for a splenectomy?

(A) Sickle cell disease
(B) Hereditary spherocytosis
(C) Traumatic injury
(D) Myeloproliferative disorders
(E) Thalassemia

81. What is the most common site of an acute arterial occlusion due to embolic disease?

(A) Iliac artery
(B) Aortic bifurcation
(C) Mesenteric arteries
(D) Femoral artery
(E) Popliteal artery

82. A 59-year-old woman presents to the emergency department with an acute upper gastrointestinal hemorrhage. Her medical history is pertinent for peptic ulcer disease for the past 5 years and hypertension. A nasogastric tube is inserted and bright red blood is seen. Her vital signs are BP: 110/70 mm Hg, P: 94/min, R: 14/min, oxygen saturation: 97%, T: 99°F. Which of the following diagnostic studies would be the most appropriate next step to determine the site of bleeding?

(A) Abdominal and pelvic computed tomography
(B) Abdominal ultrasound
(C) Upper gastrointestinal series with barium
(D) Bleeding scan
(E) Upper endoscopy

83. A 21-year-old man presents to the emergency department with a low-grade fever, anorexia, and right lower abdominal pain that began approximately 24 hours ago. Which of the following etiologies is the most common cause of the patient's symptoms?

(A) Fecalith
(B) Intussusception
(C) Lymphoid hyperplasia
(D) Cecal volvulus

84. Which of the following is the appropriate age for closing an asymptomatic umbilical hernia in a child?

(A) 12 months
(B) 2 years
(C) 5 years
(D) 7 years
(E) There is no indication for repair in this case

85. A 45-year-old man presents with progressive painless dysphagia and regurgitation of undigested food. The patient has tried drinking large amounts of fluids with meals in an attempt to wash down his food. What is the most likely diagnosis?

(A) Achalasia

(B) Esophageal leiomyoma

(C) Reflux esophagitis

(D) Esophageal carcinoma

86. What is the characteristic finding seen on a contrast study of the esophagus for a patient diagnosed with achalasia?

(A) String sign

(B) Apple core lesion

(C) Bird beak deformity

(D) Lead pipe deformity

87. A 64-year-old man has been experiencing signs and symptoms compatible with diverticular disease for the past 3 weeks. He now presents to the emergency department malnourished with severe left-sided lower abdominal pain. After appropriate workup and hydration, he is taken to the operating room where a perforated sigmoid colon is discovered with gross contamination. What is the most appropriate surgical intervention at this time?

(A) Left colectomy with primary anastomosis

(B) Hartmann procedure

(C) Proctocolectomy

(D) Abdominoperineal resection

(E) Low anterior resection

88. Which of the following patient education recommendations is most likely to decrease the incidence of diverticular disease?

(A) Weight loss

(B) Annual colonoscopy

(C) Annual fecal occult blood testing

(D) High fiber diet

(E) Use of stool softeners on a regular basis

89. What is the most important risk factor for the development of colon cancer?

(A) Dietary content

(B) Ulcerative colitis

(C) Age

(D) Cigarette smoking

(E) Positive family history

90. A 56-year-old man is diagnosed with a carcinoma of the sigmoid colon by colonoscopy. Which of the following tests should be performed as part of the preoperative evaluation for distant metastasis?

(A) Carcinoembryonic antigen level

(B) CT of the chest

(C) Endorectal ultrasound

(D) CT scan of the abdomen

(E) Bone scan

91. A 45-year-old man presents to the office with the complaint of perianal pain and bleeding. Examination reveals an anal/perianal mass complex. Biopsy is taken and the results are positive for epidermoid carcinoma of the anus. Which of the following treatment options would be the most appropriate therapy for this patient?

(A) Local resection, chemotherapy, and external beam radiation

(B) Abdominoperineal resection

(C) Chemotherapy only

(D) Local resection only

(E) Radiation only

92. Which of the following etiologies is the most common cause of an incisional hernia?

(A) Obesity

(B) Prior surgery

(C) Deep wound infections

(D) Chronic steroid use

93. A 53-year-old woman presents to the emergency department with acute abdominal pain of 2 hours duration. She has a medical history of peptic ulcer disease and gout. During intake history you find out that she had been experiencing some epigastric discomfort that awakened her from sleep over the past couple of days. This morning the pain all of a sudden worsened and was felt "all over her abdomen." Pain is described as "excruciating" and is associated with rebound tenderness. Which of the following is the most likely diagnosis?

(A) Dumping syndrome

(B) Upper gastrointestinal bleeding

(C) Intractable pain

(D) Perforated ulcer with peritonitis

(E) Gastric outlet obstruction

94. Which of the physical examination findings is pathognomonic of advanced gastric carcinoma?

(A) Palpable umbilical nodule

(B) Palpable Virchow node

(C) Weight loss

(D) Acanthosis nigricans

(E) Blumer shelf palpable on rectal examination

95. Which of the following diagnostic tests is the imaging study of choice in patients suspected of having Zollinger–Ellison syndrome?

(A) Transabdominal ultrasound

(B) Computed tomography of the abdomen

(C) Magnetic resonance imaging

(D) Somatostatin receptor scintography

(E) Endoscopic ultrasonography

Answers and Explanations

1. **(C)** The initial phase of wound healing is characterized by coagulation and inflammation, which are associated with platelet activation and migration of white blood cells to the wound. Neovascularization also begins with the inflammatory phase. The proliferative phase of wound healing is characterized by the production of collagen. The inflammatory phase typically lasts the first 4 days following a traumatic injury or surgical wound; the proliferative phase typically begins by day 4 and continues for approximately 3 weeks; the final phase of wound healing, or the remodeling phase, continues for several months. Wounds have typically achieved approximately 50% of their tensile strength at 6 weeks following the injury. *(Bauer, 2006, pp. 102-107)*

2. **(A)** Vitamin A in doses of 25,000 IU orally is helpful for patients who have thin, fragile skin secondary to chronic steroid therapy. Vitamin C and zinc are helpful for patients with poor nutrition; hyperbaric oxygen may be helpful for chronic wounds. *(Bauer, 2006, p. 109)*

3. **(D)** A negative pressure wound vacuum device or Wound VAC (vacuum-assisted closure system, Kinetic Concepts, Inc., San Antonio, TX) is a porous sponge that is packed into the wound cavity and then connected to negative pressure. The negative pressure stimulates rapid wound healing by removing edematous fluid and promoting new tissue growth with contraction of the wound. Use of a Wound VAC is contraindicated in any wounds with an active infection or because of the presence of necrotic or devitalized tissue. While occlusive dressings can be helpful, there is a risk of bacterial overgrowth. Topical growth factors and silver nitrate are beneficial for chronic wound care, but the Wound VACs provide more rapid wound healing. *(Talboy, 2006, pp. 158-160)*

4. **(C)** A clean-contaminated case involves an operative procedure of the respiratory, gastrointestinal (GI), or genitourinary (GU) tracts where those areas are entered in a controlled fashion and there is no intraoperative contamination. An inguinal herniorrhaphy is a clean case since there is no entry into the respiratory, GI, or GU tracts. Wounds with gross spillage from the GI tract, that is, a perforated ulcer, would be considered a contaminated wound; resection of necrotic bowel would be considered a dirty case. *(Leshnower, 2006, p. 57)*

5. **(A)** Cefazolin is used as prophylaxis for the majority of clean surgical procedures. For cases in which there is an increased likelihood of encountering gram-negative organisms or anaerobic bacteria, a second-generation cephalosporin is recommended to provide broader coverage. Vancomycin is an alternative if the patient has an allergy to cephalosporin antibiotics. *(Leshnower, 2006, p. 57)*

6. **(D)** Forced expiration volume in 1 second (FEV_1) is the amount of air exhaled in 1 second during a forced expiration. It is a parameter used to evaluate for problems with ventilation and intrinsic lung disease. FEV_1 values less than 1 are indicative of an increased risk of postoperative pulmonary complications and ventilator dependence. *(Eddy, 2006, p. 26)*

7. **(C)** The clinical scenario reveals contamination of the abdomen at the time of injury with a potential source of gram-negative bacteria. Causes of septic shock may include traumatic injuries, infections, and systemic inflammatory response syndrome. Vasoactive mediators that are released cause a decrease in vascular tone, which leads to a relative hypovolemia resulting in hypotension and decreased cardiac output. Therapy will require empiric antibiotic use guided by knowledge of the source of infection and most likely pathogens. Although hypovolemic or hemorrhagic shock is the most commonly encountered clinical cause of shock in the surgical/trauma patient, the timelines and clinical presentation rule it out. Cardiogenic shock represents pump failure and is inconsistent with the clinical presentation. Neurogenic shock is usually found in association with spinal cord injuries at the cervical or high thoracic region. *(Jackson, 2006, p. 266)*

8. **(B)** Cardiac tamponade is classically described by the triad of jugular venous distension (JVD), arterial hypotension, and muffled heart sounds. In the emergency department, suspicion of this clinically entity is usually confirmed by ultrasonography and is acutely treated by pericardiocentesis, which will be diagnostic, therapeutic, and buy time until a definitive procedure can be done. A left tube thoracostomy may be indicated in this patient but would not relieve symptoms. Fluid resuscitation though applied to all trauma patients would help stabilize the patient until more therapeutic interventions could be completed. Immediate intubation, even if indicated, would require a prophylactic tube thoracostomy to prevent the development of tension pneumothorax in the event of an unrecognized lung injury. Emergency thoracotomy will relieve the signs and symptoms associated with cardiac tamponade and allow for repair of any underlying cardiac injuries. *(Dolich, 2006, p. 191)*

9. **(A)** A breast abscess is commonly seen in conjunction with lactation. The most common bacterial pathogen is *Staphylococcus aureus*. While antibiotics are the treatment of choice, the patient should be instructed to continue breast feeding in order to promote drainage of the breast. If the abscess does not respond to antibiotics, then an aspiration should be considered. *(Morrow, 2006, p. 1266)*

10. **(A)** Approximately 75% of the gallstones found in Western civilization are of the mixed variety. The mixed variety contains cholesterol and calcium. Most of the mixed stones do not contain enough calcium to be appreciated on plain films. Black-pigmented stones account for 20% of the stones and are often associated with hemolysis and cirrhosis. Brown-pigmented stones are most commonly associated with infected bile. *(Danzinger, 2006, pp. 337-338)*

11. **(D)** Native Americans have the highest incidence of gallstones. By the age of 60 years, the Native American male runs a rate of 50%, whereas the female of the same age and population will develop gallstones 80% of the time. The prevalence rate in white females younger than 50 years is 5% to 15%, and for those older than 50 years, the prevalence rate is 25%. For white males younger than 50 years, the prevalence rate is 4% to 10%, and for those older than 50 years, it is 10% to 15%. *(Danziger, 2006, p. 338)*

12. **(B)** The case described is consistent with acute cholecystitis that results from sustained obstruction of the cystic duct from cholelithiasis resulting in right upper quadrant (RUQ) pain, fever, and leukocytosis. Biliary colic is characterized by intermittent obstruction without inflammation resulting in intermittent episodes of RUQ pain without fever or elevation in the white blood cell count. Choledocholithiasis is characterized by jaundice secondary to obstruction of the common bile duct; in ascending cholangitis, the common bile duct obstruction is complicated by infection resulting in RUQ pain, jaundice, fever, and leukocytosis. *(Danziger, 2006, pp. 343-345)*

13. **(C)** Pancreatic carcinoma presents with weight loss, jaundice, and midepigastric pain. A palpable, nontender gallbladder (Courvoisier sign) is more often associated with a pancreatic malignancy than cholelithiasis, especially if the tumor is in the head of the pancreas. In acute

cholecystitis, the obstruction in the cystic duct is associated with inflammation, resulting in a tender gallbladder on palpation of the right upper quadrant (Murphy sign); obstruction of the common bile duct in choledocholithiasis will result in jaundice but not weight loss. Gastric carcinoma will present with midepigastric pain and weight loss but not jaundice or a palpable gallbladder. Midepigastric pain is the most common symptom seen in chronic pancreatitis, and weight loss may be seen in association with malabsorption secondary to exocrine insufficiency. *(Danziger, 2006, pp. 343-345; Paige, 2006, p. 264; Sharp, 2006, pp. 361-362)*

14. **(C)** The abdominal ultrasound will show dilated intrahepatic and extrahepatic ducts secondary to obstruction of the common bile duct in choledocholithiasis. Ultrasound findings of a thickened gallbladder wall and pericholecystic fluid are seen with acute cholecystitis. Air in the lumen of the gallbladder is seen in acute emphysematous cholecystitis. *(Danziger, 2006, pp. 343, 345)*

15. **(B)** Ultrasonography is the first-line study in the evaluation of patients presenting with signs and symptoms of biliary disease. The sensitivity and specificity is 95%. It can detect stones, dilation of biliary ducts, thickening of the gallbladder, and pericolic collections of fluid and can also provide information pertaining to associated liver or pancreatic pathology. *(Danziger, 2006, p. 339)*

16. **(C)** Computed tomography is an excellent noninvasive procedure to determine not only the level of obstruction but also the pathologic process. In the event a carcinomatous condition is identified, this procedure will also aid in the staging of the disease as well as guide the surgeon in evaluating the resectability of the condition. *(Danziger, 2006, pp. 341-342)*

17. **(D)** The presenting symptoms associated with ascending cholangitis include fever, chills, right upper quadrant pain, and jaundice (Charcot's triad); the symptoms are secondary to an infected obstruction of the common bile duct. With spread of the infection, the patient may also develop hypotension and mental status changes; these additional symptoms in conjunction with Charcot's triad are known as Reynolds' pentad. Additional symptoms of common bile duct obstruction include light-colored stools and dark, tea-colored urine. *(Danziger, 2006, pp. 344-345)*

18. **(C)** Once cholelithiasis is confirmed in patients with biliary colic, the treatment of choice is an elective cholecystectomy, which is performed laparoscopically in most cases. *(Danziger, 2006, p. 343)*

19. **(C)** Acute pancreatitis typically presents with severe, steady midepigastric abdominal pain that radiates through to the back; pain is associated with fever, nausea, and vomiting. The most common causes of acute pancreatitis are gallstones and alcohol. Laboratory studies will show elevated WBC and serum amylase levels. Amylase elevations are nonspecific and can be elevated with perforated ulcers and mesenteric ischemia. A perforated ulcer will show evidence of free air on plain film; mesenteric ischemia will not present with fever or an elevated WBC unless there is the presence of infarcted bowel at which point the patient would appear septic. Acute cholecystitis may be associated with elevations in amylase but they are typically only a modest increase. *(Sharp, 2006, pp. 355-357)*

20. **(B)** Ranson's criteria were developed to grade the severity of pancreatitis by utilizing laboratory and clinical findings. These are measured when the patient is admitted. Within the next 48 hours, in addition to the original five criteria, an additional six variables are employed. Upon admission, the patient's age, WBC, glucose, LDH, and aspartate aminotransferase (AST) are evaluated. Within the next 48 hours, the HCT, BUN, calcium, P_{O_2} on room air, base deficit, and estimated fluid sequestration are measured. When less than two Ranson's signs are present, mortality is virtually zero; however, it increases to more than 50% when seven or more are present. While Ranson's criteria are the most commonly used predictive criteria for the severity of acute pancreatitis, final

predictions cannot be assessed until 48 hours following admission. The Acute Physiology and Chronic Health Evaluation II (APACHE II) is another classification of severity of disease, which can be assessed at any time. This system evaluates variables in temperature, mean arterial pressure, heart rate, respiratory rate, oxygenation, arterial pH, serum sodium, serum potassium, serum creatinine, hematocrit, WBC, and Glasgow Coma Scale (neurologic evaluation). Charcot's triad is the classic presentation of ascending cholangitis (fever, RUQ pain, and jaundice); Child–Turcotte-Pugh classification is used to assess liver failure. *(Dumon, 2006, p. 488)*

21. **(D)** Pancreatic pseudocysts are the most common complication associated with acute pancreatitis. A pseudocyst should be suspected for a patient who has continued abdominal pain, the development of an abdominal mass, and continued elevations of amylase or lipase levels following an episode of acute pancreatitis. An adynamic ileus would be associated with abdominal distension and changes in bowel sounds; an infected area of necrosis within the pancreatic gland would be associated with fever. Pancreatic cancer may be seen in conjunction with chronic pancreatitis. *(Sharp, 2006, p. 359)*

22. **(B)** A palpable, nontender gallbladder in a patient with jaundice is known as Courvoisier's sign. This finding is seen in patients with pancreatic carcinoma, especially with lesions involving the head of the pancreas. Flank ecchymosis (Grey Turner sign) and periumbilical ecchymosis (Cullen's sign) are seen in association with acute hemorrhagic pancreatitis. Pain in the RUQ associated with inspiratory arrest is known as Murphy's sign. *(Sharp, 2006, pp. 356, 362)*

23. **(D)** Axillary lymph node status is the most important prognostic factor in breast cancer. Patients with evidence of spread of disease have a significant decrease in 5-year survival; patients with stage I disease have a 96% five-year survival rate compared with patients with stage III disease and evidence of lymph node involvement who have a 53% five-year survival rate. The next most important factors are estrogen receptor status and tumor size. *(Dunnington, 2006, p. 397)*

24. **(B)** The clinical symptoms associated with chronic intestinal ischemia include severe epigastric pain following meals, which results in weight loss and fear of eating. Nausea, bloody diarrhea, and vomiting as well as guarding and rigidity are consistent with acute intestinal ischemia. Obturator and psoas signs are indicative of acute appendicitis. *(McKinsey, 2006, p. 457; Shelton, 2006, p. 678)*

25. **(C)** Ulcers secondary to chronic arterial insufficiency are painful and have a punched-out appearance with a pale or necrotic base. Arterial ulcerations may occur on the toes, heel, or dorsum of the foot as the result of minor trauma. By contrast, venous ulcers that occur at the level of the malleoli are associated with significant lower extremity edema and pigmentation changes due to chronic venous insufficiency (CVI). In addition, venous ulcerations have granulation tissue at the base. Diabetic ulcerations are painless, secondary to diabetic neuropathy. *(McKinsey, 2006, p. 451)*

26. **(C)** Fibroadenomas are among the most common benign lesions found in young female patients. They occur usually from the late teens into the early 30s, although they have been found to a lesser degree in all age groups. This lesion is firm, ovoid, freely movable, and usually 1 to 3 cm in size. In most instances when the lesion is greater than 3 cm, observation is recommended since in the younger patient many of these lesions will have spontaneous resolution. Surgery is recommended, after fine-needle aspiration, on those lesions that increase in size on observation. Fibrocystic disease usually occurs between the ages of 30 and 50 years. Breast cysts and lipomas are soft. *(Dunnington, 2006, p. 392)*

27. **(C)** The American Joint Committee on Cancer established the TNM system for the clinical staging of cancer. Utilizing this system, T relates to tumor size, N to nodal involvement,

and M for the presence of distant metastasis. A tumor that is greater than 2 cm but less than 5 cm in size would be a T2 tumor; evidence of 1–3 suspicious lymph nodes would be N1; MO would indicate no evidence of distant metastasis. Treatment is designed according to the staging of a lesion along with its cell type. *(Dunnington, 2006, p. 395)*

28. **(A)** The acute onset of pain seen with ischemia in an acute arterial occlusion is associated with the time of occlusion in 80% patients. Pain is often followed by paresthesias, pallor, and paralysis. *(Rapp, 2006, p. 806)*

29. **(D)** Ultrasonography is cost-effective and is the most commonly utilized screening modality for AAAs. It can be utilized for initial detection of a nonruptured AAA and for monitoring of progression. Anteroposterior and lateral abdominal radiographs may reveal calcification of an AAA as an incidental finding but are nonsensitive/nonspecific. CTA scans are used in monitoring for progression of AAA size and preoperatively to assess aortic anatomy. Abdominal palpation on physical examination may be reliable in thin patients but cannot accurately provide information about the presence or absence of aneurysms in all patients. Aortography is an expensive and invasive procedure traditionally used in preoperatively planning of AAA repair; however, it has largely been supplanted by multiplanar CTA scans. *(Rapp, 2006, pp. 810-811)*

30. **(D)** Chronic venous insufficiency (CVI) can result in many characteristic skin changes to the affected limb. Typically, patients will develop edema, induration, pigmentation, and ulceration. Although arterial disease typically results in ulcerations located on the distal toes or lateral aspect of the affected extremity, CVI will most commonly produce ulcers proximal to the medial malleolus. *(Wakefield, 2006, p. 859)*

31. **(E)** An ankle/brachial index of 1.0 is considered to be normal; values less than 1.0 are consistent with chronic occlusive disease. Values less than 0.7 are consistent with claudication. Rest pain is associated with values less than 0.3. Rest pain is an indicator of advanced arterial insufficiency and may also be associated with tissue necrosis. *(Rapp, 2006, p. 799)*

32. **(A)** The heart accounts for 80% of all emboli, with atrial fibrillation making up 70% of that. Aortic aneurysms are frequently lined with thrombus but infrequently embolize; aneurysmal disease only accounts for 6% of all acute arterial occlusion. Acute myocardial infarction (especially those associated with left ventricular thrombus) accounts for 25% of cardioembolism, with peripheral embolization often the first sign of a previously "silent" MI. Prosthetic cardiac valves make up a still small but increasingly prevalent source of emboli. Peripheral arterial thrombi account for only 3% of acute occlusion. *(Belkin, 2007, p. 1955-1956)*

33. **(A)** Atherosclerosis accounts for 67% of the cases of renovascular hypertension, which is seen more commonly in males older than 45 years; it can be bilateral in 95% of cases. Fibromuscular dysplasia accounts for 33% of cases and can also be bilateral (50%); however, it is seen predominately in women and the hypertension develops before the age of 45. Rare causes of renovascular hypertension include renal artery aneurysms, dissections, emboli, and hypoplastic renal arteries. *(Rapp, 2006, p. 829)*

34. **(C)** Meckel diverticulum is prevalent in 2% of the population, has a 2:1 male:female predominance, and is usually located 2 ft from the ileocecal valve. The most common clinical presentations are bleeding, intestinal obstruction, and inflammation. Bright red or maroon bleeding is the most frequent complication in children younger than 2 years of age. Obstruction may develop secondary to a volvulus that occurs at the site of the diverticulum or from an intussusception with the diverticulum acting as the lead point. An air contrast barium enema may be able to reduce intussusceptions in children. *(Mellinger, 2006, p. 287)*

35. **(A)** Although certain clinical features are more commonly associated with specific locations of the disease along the gastrointestinal tract,

most Crohn disease patients have the triad of abdominal pain, diarrhea, and weight loss. Abdominal pain is the most common presenting symptom. It may be intermittent or constant. Perianal involvement with fistulas is common with Crohn disease, but bleeding is uncommon. Bloody diarrhea is more commonly associated with ulcerative colitis. Rectal bleeding is commonly associated with colorectal carcinoma and hemorrhoidal disease. *(Mellinger, p. 2006, 291; Dayton, 2006, pp. 317, 323, 328)*

36. **(D)** Dysphagia on a background of GERD is an alarm signal for cancer, since GERD is related to increased risk for esophageal adenocarcinoma. Esophageal cancer is associated with a progressive course of dysphagia, first to bulky foods, then softer foods, and then liquids as the tumor invades the esophagus; significant weight loss is almost universal at the time of presentation. Barium swallow demonstrates narrowing at the tumor site with normal appearance of the remainder of the esophagus. Achalasia is a motor disorder characterized by dysphagia to both liquids and solids as well as regurgitation of food. Patients with achalasia typically drink large amounts of liquids to force their food down and have problems with aspiration pneumonia. Barium swallow in achalasia typically shows a dilated esophagus with a narrowing at the lower esophageal sphincter (bird's beak). Leiomyomas are generally asymptomatic. Patients with reflux esophagitis will complain of epigastric or substernal pain that is worse when supine or leaning forward. *(Patti, 2006, pp. 469-471; Goyal, 2008, pp. 1848-1850)*

37. **(C)** Obstipation and failure to pass flatus are actually symptoms of both paralytic ileus and a small bowel obstruction (SBO). However, patients with a paralytic ileus usually have minimal abdominal pain and hypoactive or absent bowel sounds due to hypomotility. Patients with an SBO will have crampy abdominal pain and increased bowel sounds with high-pitched sounds and rushes due to increased peristalsis. Plain films in paralytic ileus will show gas throughout the small and the large bowel on plain films as opposed to air

confined to the small intestine only in SBO. *(Mellinger, 2006, pp. 297-299)*

38. **(A)** The first priority in proven or suspected small bowel obstruction is the correction of fluid and electrolyte abnormalities. Often, large volumes of fluid must be infused. The patient must be given sufficient fluid not only for maintenance requirements but also to correct losses from vomiting and nasogastric output and third-space loss. Urine output should be closely monitored for the adequacy of hydration. If the patient has a partial small bowel obstruction, no detectable hernia on examination, and a history of operation, resolution may occur with fluid replacement and nasogastric tube placement, making an operation unnecessary. If the patient has no apparent etiology for obstruction, a cause should be determined by upper gastrointestinal and small bowel radiograph series. Laboratory data cannot confirm the diagnosis of bowel obstruction but are useful to rule out other diagnoses. A patient with a complete small bowel obstruction should undergo operation at the earliest opportunity, once the fluid and electrolyte repair is sufficient to establish adequate urine output. *(Mellinger, 2006, pp. 299-300)*

39. **(B)** For a patient with diverticular disease, the preferred study to evaluate complications, such as a perforation or abscesses, is a CT scan. A barium enema or endoscopic procedure is contraindicated due to increased risk of perforation during an acute exacerbation. *(Su, 2006, p. 208; Otterson, 2006, p. 1133)*

40. **(C)** Although hemorrhoids are a common cause of lower gastrointestinal hemorrhage, they do not cause massive hemorrhage. Massive lower gastrointestinal hemorrhage is most commonly due to diverticular disease. Upper gastrointestinal hemorrhage may present as massive lower hemorrhage due to the cathartic effect of blood. Colon cancer usually presents with occult bleeding. Meckel diverticulum may also present significant lower gastrointestinal hemorrhage, but it affects only approximately 2% of the population and is therefore not as common. *(Mellinger, 2006, p. 286; Dayton, 2006, p. 314)*

41. **(B)** Most patients with diverticular disease respond to medical therapy with antibiotics. Patients who have required admission for two episodes of diverticulitis are recommended to undergo elective surgical resection to avoid complications. Patients with complications such as obstruction, perforation, or abscess require emergent surgery. Patients with bleeding require surgical intervention only if bleeding does not stop spontaneously or with medical interventions. *(Dayton, 2006, pp. 313-314)*

42. **(D)** Villous adenomas may contain cancer in 33% of cases, and when greater than 2 cm in size, this risk goes up to 50%. Hamartomas, or juvenile polyps, lack malignant potential, but they can serve as a lead point for an intussusceptions so they can be removed electively. Hyperplastic polyps are not associated with malignant potential; however, they are hard to distinguish from adenomas and should be biopsied. Inflammatory polyps can be seen with inflammatory bowel disease, but they are not associated with a risk for malignancy. *(Dayton, 2006, pp. 314-315; Su, 2006, p. 212)*

43. **(C)** A patient with a first-degree relative who is diagnosed with colorectal cancer before the age of 60 years puts the patient in the moderate risk category. Accordingly, she should undergo a screening colonoscopy at age 40 or 10 years younger than the age her family member was first diagnosed with colorectal cancer. Colonoscopy should be repeated every 5 years for patients in the moderate risk category. *(Chang, 2006, pp. 1114-1115)*

44. **(B)** Right-sided colon lesions can grow to large sizes due to the liquid characteristic of stool in this region. Large exophytic lesions can result in occult blood loss with the subsequent development of iron deficiency anemia. The triad of weight loss, anemia, and a palpable mass in the right lower quadrant should raise suspicion for right colon carcinoma. *(Dayton, 2006, p. 317)*

45. **(E)** Routine follow-up after surgical resection of a colon cancer includes annual colonoscopy not sigmoidoscopy, which only assesses the distal colon. The tumor marker for colon cancer is carcinoembryonic antigen (CEA) not carbohydrate antigen 19-9 (CA 19-9), which is used for pancreatic cancer. There is no role for annual chest films or fecal occult blood testing to monitor for a recurrence. *(Chang, 2006, p. 1126)*

46. **(C)** Barium enema finding of carcinoma of the sigmoid colon causing high-grade obstruction shows the classic "apple core" lesion. Crohn's disease is typically associated with the string sign, which is an area of stricture or stenosis that shows up as a narrow line of contrast, giving the appearance of a string associated with the stricture. Diverticular disease is associated with outpouchings from the colon that will be filled with barium. *(Chang, 2006, p. 1111; Mellinger, 2006, p. 291; Dayton, 2006, p. 313)*

47. **(D)** The Dukes–Astler–Coller system of staging colon cancer uses the depth of tumor penetration and lymph node involvement as predictors of 5-year survival rates. Stage A tumors are confined to mucosal penetration, and both stages B1 and B2 have negative lymph nodes, with B1 tumors penetrate into but not through the muscularis propia, whereas B2 tumors penetrate through the muscularis propia. Both stages C1 and C2 have positive lymph nodes; C1 tumors penetrate into but not through the muscularis propia and C2 tumors penetrate through the muscularis propia. Stage D denotes distant metastasis. Five-year survival rate for stage A is 85% to 90%; for stage B1, survival rate is 70% to 75%; for stage B2, survival rate is 60% to 65%; for stage C1, survival rate drops to 30% to 35%, with the presence of positive lymph nodes; for stage C2, survival rate is 25%; for stage D tumors with evidence of distant metastasis, the five-year survival is less than 5%. *(Dayton, 2006, p. 321)*

48. **(B)** Ulcerative colitis is characterized by inflammation that is confined to the mucosal and submucosal layers of the colon. The rectum is involved in at least 90% of patients with continuous distribution. Crohn's disease is characterized by transmural inflammation that can involve any part of the gastrointestinal tract. Crohn's disease is associated with segmental involvement with skip lesions. Strictures and

perianal fistulas are also commonly seen with Crohn's disease and rare in ulcerative colitis. Both diseases are characterized by exacerbations and remissions. *(Dayton, 2006, pp. 323-324)*

49. **(A)** Acute exacerbations of Crohn's disease are best treated with systemic corticosteroids. Prednisone is used for patients who can take oral medications; for patients who cannot tolerate oral medications, intravenous methylprednisolone is given. Patients should be tapered from steroids to avoid long-term complications. For patients who cannot be removed from steroid therapy, sulfasalazine is considered a first-line agent for treating mild-to-moderate inflammatory bowel disease. While some evidence exists to support the use of antibiotics like metronidazole for the purpose of decreasing intraluminal bacteria, metronidazole is not effective with active disease. Immunosuppressive agents, such as azathioprine, are used for patients who have failed salicylate therapy and/or are refractory or dependent on corticosteroids. *(Michelassi, 2006, pp. 793-795)*

50. **(B)** Total proctocolectomy with a permanent ileostomy was previously the standard management of low-grade dysplasia in patients with ulcerative colitis. The current procedure of choice is a proctocolectomy with ileo-anal pull through which will preserve anal sphincter function and avoid a permanent ileostomy. A subtotal colectomy with ileoproctostomy can be utilized if the patient has minimal rectal disease, but it does not cure the disease, so the patient is at risk for recurrent symptoms or developing a malignant lesion in the remaining portion of the colon. A local resection is inadequate due to continuous involvement of the colon. *(Dayton, 2006, p. 324)*

51. **(B)** Large bowel obstructions are most commonly caused by an adenocarcinoma (65%). This is followed in decreasing incidence by diverticular scarring and volvulus. Adhesions are the most common cause of small-bowel obstruction but are rare as a cause of large bowel obstruction. The presence of haustral markings on radiographic evaluation helps differentiate between small and large bowel involvement. *(Dayton, 2006, pp. 325-326)*

52. **(A)** Large bowel obstruction appears radiographically as proximal colonic distention with air–fluid levels and absence of air seen in the distal rectum. With distension of the colon, haustral markings become more prominent; loss of haustral markings or a "lead pipe" appearance is seen with ulcerative colitis. Free air under the diaphragm may be seen with any perforation of a hollow viscus. *(Dayton, 2006, pp. 323, 325)*

53. **(D)** Massive distention of the cecum, as detected on plain radiograph, is typically seen in "closed loop" obstructions where the ileocecal valve is competent. When distention approaches 12 cm, there is an increased risk of perforation and/or gangrene. Expedient surgical intervention is indicated. Although observation with intravenous fluids and nasogastric decompression are important adjuncts to management, surgical exploration is the only way to rapidly address this emergent situation. *(Dayton, 2006, pp. 325-326)*

54. **(C)** A volvulus is an obstruction of the colon due to a loop of bowel that has rotated more than 180 degrees on its axis with the mesentery. The most common site for a volvulus is the sigmoid colon (65%). A sigmoid volvulus is associated with abdominal pain and distension. Plain films of the abdomen would show a characteristic "bent inner tube" appearance. Sigmoidoscopy can be used to decompress the bowel by gently releasing the area of obstruction. Following decompression, a rectal tube is inserted to act as a stent to prevent the bowel from twisting upon itself again. *(Saund, 2006, p. 781)*

55. **(C)** Hemorrhoids are classified as external (distal to the dentate line and covered with anoderm) and internal (proximal to the dentate line and covered with insensate anorectal mucosa). Internal hemorrhoids are further classified on the basis of their extent of prolapse. First-degree hemorrhoids bulge into the anal canal and may prolapse in association with straining. Second-degree hemorrhoids prolapse

through the anus but reduce spontaneously. Third-degree hemorrhoids prolapse through the anal canal and require manual manipulation for reduction. Fourth-degree hemorrhoids prolapse and cannot be reduced, as such they are at increased risk for strangulation. *(Dayton, 2006, p. 329)*

56. **(D)** Anal fissures are linear tears in the lining of the anal canal. They are painful due to their location below the dentate line. Pain is worse with defection and associated with steaks of bright red blood on the stool or on the paper with wiping. Examination of the area is often difficult because of increased pain and sphincter spasm. Anal fissures are treated conservatively with mild analgesic medications, laxatives or stool softeners, and Sitz baths. For patients with refractory symptoms, a lateral internal sphincterotomy will release the sphincter spasm and allow the fissure to heal. There is a small risk of fecal incontinence following a sphincterotomy. A perianal abscess will present with localized swelling associated with pain, redness, and fever. Fistula-in-ano will present with chronic drainage. *(Dayton, 2006, pp. 330-331)*

57. **(D)** Malignant pleural effusion is classified as surgically unresectable disease. Impaired pulmonary function conveys a high morbidity rate that constitutes a relative (not absolute) contraindication to surgical resection. Patients with solitary brain or adrenal metastasis are surgical candidates as studies have shown prolonged survival. Myocardial infarction in last 3 months is absolute contraindication, given less than 20% risk of peri- or postoperative reinfarction, but at 6 months surgery may be considered. *(Minna, 2008, p. 557)*

58. **(C)** While adenocarcinoma, like other lung cancer types, is more likely to appear in smokers; it is the most common lung cancer seen in nonsmokers, particularly women and younger patients. It generally originates in the periphery of the lung. All other answers are associated with significant smoking history and, with the exception of large cell carcinoma, originate centrally. *(Minna, 2008, p. 552)*

59. **(A)** Lobectomy with sampling of contiguous hilar nodes is the standard of care for early stage lung cancer. Pneumonectomy is reserved for cancer that involves the bronchus or crosses a major fissure because of its effect on total lung function. Wedge (segmental) resections are associated with increased local recurrence and are reserved for patients who would not tolerate lobectomy or for later stage disease combined with adjuvant chemotherapy. Radiofrequency ablation is a good option with the patient is at high risk for a surgical intervention. Combination chemotherapy and radiation without surgical intervention is reserved for later stage disease. *(Theodore, 2006, pp. 382-385)*

60. **(C)** Myotomy or pneumatic dilatations are treatments of choice in otherwise healthy individuals with achalasia. Nissen fundoplication is used for gastroesophageal reflux and is relatively contraindicated in achalasia. Esophagectomy is reserved for treatment of refractory or endstage achalasia. Medical treatment, consisting of calcium channel blockers and botulinum injections can also be used but has not been found to provide the long-term relief of symptoms achieved with myotomy. Vagotomy with pyloroplasty has been used historically for peptic ulcer disease; its use has now been largely replaced by proton pump inhibitors. *(Patti, 2006, p. 457)*

61. **(C)** Superficial thrombophlebitis is not uncommon following needle or IV infiltration. Appropriate initial management includes warm compresses/compression sleeves or hose and anti-inflammatory medications. Anticoagulation is not indicated because there is no evidence of deep vein thrombosis. Antibiotics are not indicated because there is no evidence of infection. *(Freischlag, 2008, p. 2017)*

62. **(A)** Congenital cerebral aneurysms or Berry aneurysms account for 75% to 80% of nontraumatic subarachnoid hemorrhages (SAHs). Poorly controlled hypertension and anticoagulant use are more commonly associated with intracerebral hemorrhages (ICH). AVMs can cause either SAH or ICH. *(Heuer, 2006, p. 21)*

63. (B) The initial study to diagnose a subarachnoid hemorrhage is a noncontrast CT scan of the head. If the CT scan is nondiagnostic for a SAH and the clinical suspicion is high, then proceed with a lumbar puncture for the presence of red blood cells in the cerebrospinal fluid; xanthochromia can be seen with an old SAH. *(Heuer, 2006, p. 21)*

64. (C) The clinical presentation is consistent with a meningioma. Meningiomas are commonly located in the parasagittal region, the convexity of the brain, sphenoid ridge, or posterior fossa. Radiographic features on MRI include homogenous enhancement and evidence of a "dural tail" indicating the origin of the tumor. Since meningiomas are a benign tumor, the primary treatment is surgical removal. In the event of a subtotal resection or if the meningioma is found to be malignant, surgical resection is followed by radiation therapy. *(Leveque, 2006, pp. 2049-2051)*

65. (C) A patient with a moderate-severe headache and nuchal rigidity but no focal neurologic deficits is considered to have a Hunt and Hess Grade II subarachnoid hemorrhage which is treated surgically within 72 hours of the bleed. Surgical treatment includes a craniotomy with clipping of the neck of the aneurysm. For higher grade bleeds, the patient is treated medically until stabilized and safe to treat surgically. Coiling of aneurysms is done by interventional radiology for high grade bleeds (Grades III and IV) or for aneurysms that are surgically inaccessible. Endovascular embolization is done prior to surgical resection of an arteriovenous malformation. *(Leveque, 2006, pp. 2056-2057)*

66. (C) A parathyroidectomy is indicated for treatment of a patient with symptoms of primary hyperparathyroidism. Surgical options include a minimally-invasive radioguided resection using either radioactivity to identify abnormal tissue or monitoring intraoperative PTH levels to insure adequate resection. Bisphosphonates and selective estrogen receptor modulators are ineffective in primary hyperparathyroidism. Cervical thymectomy is indicated for secondary hyperparathyroidism. *(Borman, 2006, pp. 411-412)*

67. (D) A unilateral recurrent laryngeal nerve injury will result in paralysis of the vocal cord on that side causing hoarseness and difficulty with phonation. Bilateral recurrent laryngeal nerve injuries can result in abduction of both vocal cords, which can cause complete obstruction of the airway requiring an emergent intubation or tracheostomy. *(Borman, 2006, p. 412; Karakousis, 2006, p. 460)*

68. (B) In Graves' disease, the thyroid is diffusely enlarged in contrast to a toxic adenoma in which the thyroid is normal sized but with a palpable nodule. Surgery is the treatment of choice for a toxic adenoma. Surgical treatment of a toxic adenoma is a thyroid lobectomy and isthmusectomy. A subtotal or total thyroidectomy is indicated for toxic multinodular goiters or Plummer disease. Thionamides and radioiodine ablation are not effective therapies for toxic adenomas. *(Coe, 2006, pp. 404-406)*

69. (D) Papillary carcinoma is the most common type of thyroid malignancy. Treatment includes a thyroid lobectomy and isthmusectomy or total thyroidectomy. The decision regarding the extent of the surgery is based on the extent of the disease, the tumor size, and histologic grade. A poor prognosis is seen in males, patients older than 50 years of age, primary tumors greater than 4 cm in size, tumors that are less well differentiated, or evidence of locally invasive or metastatic disease. Accordingly, the recommended treatment for this patient is a total thyroidectomy. Radioiodine ablation is recommended postoperatively. *(Coe, 2006, pp. 407-408)*

70. (B) α-Blockade is the first step in preparing a patient for resection of a pheochromocytoma. While β-blockers are also indicated to control the heart rate, they should only be started once the α-blockers have been initiated. Secondary to the effects of the pheochromocytoma, patients are severely vasoconstricted with an increased systemic vascular resistance (SVR). The heart rate and stroke volume are increased in order to compensate for the increased SVR. If β-blockers are initiated first, then cardiovascular collapse may occur because of the loss of the compensatory mechanisms. Cortisol is not indicated for a unilateral pheochromocytoma unless the patient was already taking steroids preoperatively. *(Rao, 2006, pp. 419-420)*

71. **(D)** The most important step in the management of a postoperative wound infection is reopening the incision and evacuating any purulent discharge. Antibiotics are indicated only if there are systemic signs of sepsis, such as temperature >38°C, tachycardia, a WBC >12,000/mm^3, or evidence of invasion into the subcutaneous or fascial tissue. *(Dellinger, 2006, pp. 169-170)*

72. **(A)** Hypokalemia is a common electrolyte disturbance in surgical patients. It can be caused by enhanced losses, hyperaldosteronism, inappropriate replacement, and intracellular shifts caused by alkalosis. Symptoms of hypokalemia may include constipation, neuromuscular weakness, diminished tendon reflexes, paralysis, and distinctive electrocardiographic changes. Concomitant deficiencies in magnesium can contribute significantly to the development of hypokalemia as well as hypocalcemia. In the surgical patient with persistent hypokalemia refractory to potassium administration, one should check magnesium levels and correct as appropriate. *(Shires, 2010, p. 62)*

73. **(D)** Third-space fluid losses that occur with inflammatory conditions such as peritonitis result in an isotonic volume depletion; the recommended intravenous fluid used to replace those losses is lactated Ringer's solution, which is a balanced salt solution that contains 130 mEq/L of sodium, 109 mEq/L of chloride, 4.0 mEq/L of potassium, 3.0 mEq/L of calcium, and 28 mEq/L of lactate. *(Kaiser, 2006, p. 48)*

74. **(B)** The most objective means of assessing the adequacy of volume replacement for fluid losses is by following the urinary output, which should be at a minimum of 0.5 mL/kg/h. Other objective measures include normalization of hemoglobin and hematocrit values as well as BUN and creatinine levels. Following the patient weight as well as intake and output can provide valuable information about the patient's volume status over time. *(Kaiser, 2006, p.51)*

75. **(A)** The use of nasoenteric feeding is usually reserved for patients who have an intact mental status examination and have intact protective aspiration reflexes. All tubes that are placed for feeding must be verified by a radiograph. The instillation of air is inaccurate to document position of nasoenteric feeding tubes. After a radiograph is obtained, the results should be documented in the chart prior to the start of tube feedings. *(Jan, 2010, p. 43)*

76. **(D)** The initial evaluation of blunt abdominal trauma is by the performance of a FAST (focused assessment with sonography for trauma) ultrasound, which is performed by an emergency department physician or surgeon. CT scan remains an adjunct test in hemodynamically stable patients or in patients in whom further assessment of solid intra-abdominal organs is required. *(Cothren, 2010, p. 155)*

77. **(D)** Nonoperative management in hemodynamically stable patients with splenic injuries is preferred. This modality of therapy avoids a laparotomy and its associated complications and preserves splenic function. Although infections postsplenectomy with encapsulated bacteria are more common in the pediatric age group, in immunocompromised adults, they are nevertheless a concern. *(Cothren, 2010, p. 177)*

78. **(E)** The most common cause of massive upper gastrointestinal bleeding in patients with cirrhosis is esophageal varices. Although 20% of patients with portal hypertension will have bleeding from other causes (peptic ulcer disease, Mallory–Weiss tears, or gastritis), endoscopic evaluation in patients with portal hypertension is necessary for diagnosis and initial therapy. *(Geller, 2010, p. 1113)*

79. **(A)** Patients with complete intrahepatic portal vein thrombosis are best managed with the end-to-side portocaval shunt because of its easier technical considerations and better decompression of the portal system. Selective shunts such as the distal splenorenal shunt are more appropriate in nonalcoholic patients in whom liver function is preserved. *(Geller, 2010, p. 1115)*

80. **(C)** Although all of the conditions listed involve the spleen, by far the most common cause of surgical splenectomy is trauma. Traumatic injury to the spleen resulting in splenectomy is a common surgical condition, as the spleen is the most commonly injured solid intra-abdominal organ. *(Park, 2010, p. 1249)*

81. **(D)** The most common site for an acute embolic occlusion is the femoral artery. Other common sites include the axillary, popliteal, and iliac arteries as well as the aortic bifurcation and mesenteric vessels. The majority (80%) of arterial embolic originate in the heart in patients with atrial fibrillation or from mural thrombi in the left ventricle from an akinetic or dyskinetic portion of the myocardium following a myocardial infarction. *(Lin, 2010, p. 752)*

82. **(E)** Patients who present with hematemesis and shock requiring multiple transfusions in 24 hours are at high risk for mortality from gastrointestinal bleeding. The hematemesis in this patient warrants further investigation with upper gastrointestinal endoscopy to both determine the site of bleeding and provide potential therapy by endoscopic electrocautery or injection. *(Dempsey, 2010, p. 916)*

83. **(C)** Obstruction of the lumen of the appendix is the underlying pathophysiology for the development of acute appendicitis; the most common cause of the luminal obstruction is lymphoid hyperplasia, which occurs in 60% of patients; the second most common cause is a fecalith. *(Mellinger, 2006, p. 296, 301, 327)*

84. **(C)** Umbilical hernias are typically asymptomatic and prompt attention when the family is concerned about cosmetic appearance, symptoms develop, or the rare event of incarceration. Asymptomatic umbilical hernias can be observed until the age of 4 or 5 years, and if they have not spontaneously closed, then surgical intervention is indicated. *(Seymour, 2010, p. 1273)*

85. **(A)** Achalasia is characterized by progressive dysphagia, which is painless in contrast to esophageal cancer, which is characterized by odynophagia. While patients with achalasia have regurgitation of food, there is minimal loss of weight. Esophageal cancer is associated with anorexia and weight loss. Patients with achalasia typically drink large amounts of liquids to force their food down and have problems with aspiration pneumonia. Patients with reflux esophagitis will complain of epigastric or substernal pain that is worse when supine or leaning forward. Leiomyomas are generally asymptomatic. *(Jobe, 2010, pp. 850-851)*

86. **(C)** Patients with achalasia have constriction at the level of the distal esophagus, leading to progressive dilation of the proximal esophagus. On contrast study, this has a bird's beak appearance. The bird's beak appearance can also be seen in patients with a sigmoid volvulus. Apple core lesions are commonly seen with colorectal carcinoma; and lead pipe deformity is seen with loss of normal haustral marking in ulcerative colitis. String sign is seen in association with small bowel obstruction in Crohn disease. *(Jobe, 2010, p. 852)*

87. **(B)** This vignette is consistent with an emergent resection in an unprepared patient. The most appropriate therapy for an acute perforation is a Hartmann procedure, which includes resection of the affected portion of the bowel, a temporary diverting colostomy, and oversewing of the distal rectal stump; the second stage of the procedure will involve taking down the colostomy with anastomosis to the rectal stump. A colectomy with a primary anastomosis should not be done when the bowel is unprepared due to the significant risk of infection and leakage of the bowel at the site of the anastomosis. Abdominoperineal resection is used in the treatment of malignant disease of the lower rectum. In this procedure, a permanent colostomy is created and the entire rectum, anal canal, and anus are removed. In the management of benign disease of the lower rectum, a proctocolectomy is appropriate to preserve anal function. *(Bullard, 2010, pp. 1024-1028; Dayton, 2006, p. 314)*

88. **(D)** The only factor that appears to decrease the incidence of diverticular disease is the

eating of a diet high in fiber. A commonly accepted theory in the formation of diverticula is that high intraluminal pressure causes herniation of the mucosa and muscularis mucosa at the point where vessels penetrate the colon. Lack of dietary fiber results in diminished stool volume, which in turn requires higher intraluminal pressures and wall tension for distal propulsion. Fecal occult blood testing and colonoscopy have been shown to accurately screen and detect for colon cancer. *(Bullard, 2010, pp. 1044-1046)*

89. **(C)** Colon cancer is the most common malignancy of the gastrointestinal tract. Although individuals of any age can develop colon cancer, increasing age is the most dominant risk factor associated with its development. Only 20% of colon cancers are found in patients with a known family history of colorectal carcinoma. Ulcerative colitis is associated with an increased risk of 1% to 2% per year after having the disease for 10 years. Cigarette smoking has been identified as conveying an increased risk for the development of colonic adenomas as do diets high in animal fat and low in fiber. *(Bullard, 2010, pp. 1041-1044; Dayton, 2006, p. 324)*

90. **(D)** Abdominal/pelvic CT scans and chest radiographs should be obtained as part of the preoperative staging of colon carcinoma for the evaluation of distant metastasis. CT scan of the chest is indicated only if the chest radiograph is abnormal. Endorectal ultrasound is useful in further staging rectal carcinoma. Bone scan is not indicated as a routine diagnostic study in the preoperative staging of colon cancer. Although carcinoembryonic antigen levels are performed preoperatively, they are not helpful in staging and are useful only in the postoperative follow-up of patients to monitor for a recurrence. *(Bullard, 2010, pp. 1047-1048)*

91. **(A)** Epidermoid carcinoma of the anal canal is a slow-growing tumor that often presents as an anal or perianal mass. Wide excision, followed by 5-fluorouracil, mitomycin, and external beam radiation (Nigro Protocol), typically results in a greater than 80% cure rate. The presence of inguinal lymph node metastasis is a poor prognostic indicator. Management of recurrences is typically achieved by performing an abdominoperineal resection. *(Bullard, 2010, p. 1053)*

92. **(C)** Incisional or ventral hernias can occur at any surgical site where there has been an incision extending into the fascial layer; incisional hernias are most commonly associated with a deep wound infection. Other causes can include obesity and the history of chronic steroid use or previous surgical procedures. *(Neumayer 2006, p. 236)*

93. **(D)** Patients with perforated peptic ulcer disease present with acute abdominal pain and an examination that usually is indicative of diffuse peritonitis. The initial pain is usually due to a chemical irritation of the peritoneum by gastric and/or duodenal contents. As the disease progresses or as there is a delay in presentation, a bacterial peritonitis may develop. *(Dempsey, 2010, p. 921)*

94. **(A)** A physical examination that detects a palpable umbilical nodule (Sister Joseph node) is pathognomonic for gastric carcinoma. Other findings may be suggestive for carcinoma but are nonspecific. *(Dempsey, 2010, p. 932)*

95. **(D)** Although imaging tests such as CT scan, MRI, transabdominal ultrasound, and endoscopic ultrasound can be utilized with varying frequencies of sensitivity and specificity, the test of choice is the somatostatin receptor scintigraphy. This test has close to a 100% sensitivity and specificity. *(Fisher, 2010, p. 1218)*

REFERENCES

Bauer SM, Velazquez OC. Wound healing. In: Alturi P, Karakousis GC, Porrett PM, Kaiser LR, eds. *The Surgical Review: An Integrated Basic and Clinical Science Study Guide*. 2nd ed. Philadelphia, PA: Lippincott Williams & Wilkins; 2006.

Belkin M, Owens CD, Whittemore AD, et al. Peripheral arterial occlusive disease. In: Townsend CM, Beauchamp RD, Evers BM, Mattox K, eds. *Sabiston Textbook of Surgery: The Biological Basis of Modern Surgical Practice*. 18th ed. Philadelphia, PA: Elsevier Saunders; 2007:1941-1977.

Borman KR, Coe NPW. Surgical endocrinology: parathyroid glands. In: Lawrence PF, ed. *Essentials of General Surgery*. 4th ed. Philadelphia, PA: Lippincott Williams & Wilkins; 2006.

Bullard Dunn KM, Rothenberger DA. Colon, rectum and anus. In: Brunicardi FC, et al., eds. *Schwartz's Principles of Surgery*. 9th ed. New York, NY: McGraw-Hill; 2010.

Chang AE, Morris AM. Colorectal cancer. In: Mulholland MW, Lillemoe KD, Doherty GM, Maier RV, Upchurch GR, eds. *Greenfield's Surgery: Scientific Principles and Practice*. 4th ed. Philadelphia, PA: Lippincott Williams & Wilkins; 2006.

Coe NPW. Surgical endocrinology: thyroid gland. In: Lawrence PF, ed. *Essentials of General Surgery*. 4th ed. Philadelphia, PA: Lippincott Williams & Wilkins; 2006.

Cothren CC, Biffl WL, Moore EE. Trauma. In: Brunicardi FC, et al. eds. *Schwartz's Principles of Surgery*. 9th ed. New York, NY: McGraw-Hill; 2010.

Danzinger RG, Nauta R, Park J. Biliary tract. In: Lawrence PF, ed. *Essentials of General Surgery*. 4th ed. Philadelphia, PA: Lippincott Williams & Wilkins; 2006.

Dayton MT, Tradel JL. Colon, rectum, and anus. In: Lawrence PF, ed. *Essentials of General Surgery*. 4th ed. Philadelphia, PA: Lippincott Williams & Wilkins; 2006.

Dellinger EP. Surgical infections. In: Mulholland MW, Lillemoe KD, Doherty GM, Maier RV, Upchurch GR, eds. *Greenfield's Surgery: Scientific Principles and Practice*. 4th ed. Philadelphia, PA: Lippincott Williams & Wilkins; 2006.

Dempsey DT. Stomach. In: Brunicardi FC, et al., eds. *Schwartz's Principles of Surgery*. 9th ed. New York, NY: McGraw-Hill; 2010.

Dolich MO, Chipman JG. Trauma. In: Lawrence PF, ed. *Essentials of General Surgery*. 4th ed. Philadelphia, PA: Lippincott Williams & Wilkins; 2006.

Dumon K, Rosato E. The pancreas. In: Alturi P, Karakousis GC, Porrett PM, Kaiser LR, eds. *The Surgical Review: An Integrated Basic and Clinical Science Study Guide*. 2nd ed. Philadelphia, PA: Lippincott Williams & Wilkins; 2006.

Dunnington GL, Kaiser S, Peralta E, et al. Breast. In: Lawrence PF, ed. *Essentials of General Surgery*. 4th ed. Philadelphia, PA: Lippincott Williams & Wilkins; 2006.

Eddy VA, Bell RM. Perioperative management of surgical patients. In: Lawrence PF, ed. *Essentials of General Surgery*. 4th ed. Philadelphia, PA: Lippincott Williams & Wilkins; 2006.

Fisher WE, Anderson DK, Bell RH, et al. Pancreas. In: Brunicardi FC, et al., eds. *Schwartz's Principles of Surgery*. 9th ed. New York, NY: McGraw-Hill; 2010.

Freischlag JA, Heller JA. Venous disease. In: Townsend CM, Beauchamp RD, Evers BM, Mattox K, eds. *Sabiston Textbook of Surgery: The Biological Basis of Modern Surgical Practice*. 18th ed. Philadelphia. Elsevier Saunders; 2008.

Geller DA, Goss JA, Tsung A. Liver. In: Brunicardi FC, et al., eds. *Schwartz's Principles of Surgery*. 9th ed. New York, NY: McGraw-Hill; 2010.

Goyal RK. Diseases of the esophagus. In: Fauci AS, Kasper DL, Longo DL, Braunwald E, Hauser SL, Jameson JL, Loscalzo J, eds. *Harrison's Principles of Internal Medicine*. 17th ed. New York, NY: McGraw-Hill; 2008.

Heuer G, Reiter GT, Stiefel MF, et al. Neurosurgery. In: Alturi P, Karakousis GC, Porrett PM, Kaiser LR, eds. *The Surgical Review: An Integrated Basic and Clinical Science Study Guide*. 2nd ed. Philadelphia, PA: Lippincott Williams & Wilkins; 2006:1-31.

Jackson BM, Gale SC, Schwab CW. Trauma evaluation and resuscitation, shock, and acid-base disturbances. In: Alturi P, Karakousis GC, Porrett PM, Kaiser LR, eds. *The Surgical Review: An Integrated Basic and Clinical Science Study Guide*. 2nd ed. Philadelphia, PA: Lippincott Williams & Wilkins; 2006.

Jan BV, Lowry SF. Systematic response to injury and metabolic support. In: Brunicardi FC, et al., eds. *Schwartz's Principles of Surgery*. 9th ed. New York, NY: McGraw-Hill; 2010.

Jobe BA, Hunter JG, Peters JH. Esophagus and diaphragmatic hernia. In: Brunicardi FC, et al., eds. *Schwartz's Principles of Surgery*. 9th ed. New York, NY: McGraw-Hill; 2010.

Kaiser S, Corwin C, Sanfey H, et al. Fluids, electrolytes, and acid-base balance. In: Lawrence PF, ed. *Essentials of General Surgery*. 4th ed. Philadelphia, PA: Lippincott Williams & Wilkins; 2006.

Karakousis GC, Kelz, RR, Fraker DL. Thyroid, parathyroid, and adrenal glands. In: Alturi P, Karakousis GC, Porrett PM, Kaiser LR, eds. *The Surgical Review: An Integrated Basic and Clinical Science Study Guide*. 2nd ed. Philadelphia, PA: Lippincott Williams & Wilkins; 2006.

Leshnower BG, Gleason TG. Surgical infectious diseases. In: Alturi P, Karakousis GC, Porrett PM, Kaiser LR, eds. *The Surgical Review: An Integrated Basic and Clinical Science Study Guide.* 2nd ed. Philadelphia, PA: Lippincott Williams & Wilkins; 2006.

Leveque J, Hoff JT. Neurosurgery. In: Mulholland MW, Lillemoe KD, Doherty GM, Maier RV, Upchurch GR, eds. *Greenfield's Surgery: Scientific Principles and Practice.* 4th ed. Philadelphia, PA: Lippincott Williams & Wilkins; 2006.

Lin PH, Kouglas P, Bechara C, et al. Arterial disease. In: Brunicardi FC, et al., eds. *Schwartz's Principles of Surgery.* 9th ed. New York, NY: McGraw-Hill; 2010.

Mayer RJ. Gastrointestinal tract cancer. In: Fauci AS, Braunwald E, Kasper SL, Longo DL, Jameson JL, Loscalso J, eds. *Harrison's Principles of Internal Medicine,* 17th ed. New York: McGraw-Hill; 2008.

McKinsey JF, Lawrence PF, Gewertz BL. Diseases of the vascular system. In: Lawrence PF, Bell RM, Dayton MT, Ahmed MI, eds. *Essentials of General Surgery.* 4th ed. Philadelphia, PA: Lippincott Williams & Wilkins; 2006.

Mellinger JD, Macfadyen BV, Mercer DW, et al. Small intestine and appendix. In: Lawrence PF, ed. *Essentials of General Surgery.* 4th ed. Philadelphia, PA: Lippincott Williams & Wilkins; 2006.

Michelassi F, Hurst RD, Fichera A. Crohn disease. In: Mulholland MW, Lillemoe KD, Doherty GM, Maier RV, Upchurch GR, eds. *Greenfield's Surgery: Scientific Principles and Practice.* 4th ed. Philadelphia, PA: Lippincott Williams & Wilkins; 2006.

Minna JD, Schiller JH. Neoplasms of the lung. In: Fauci AS, Kasper DL, Longo DL, Braunwald E, Hauser SL, Jameson JL, Loscalzo J, eds. *Harrison's Principles of Internal Medicine.* 17th ed. New York, NY: McGraw-Hill; 2008.

Morrow M, Khan S. Breast disease. In: Mulholland MW, Lillemoe KD, Doherty GM, Maier RV, Upchurch GR, eds. *Greenfield's Surgery: Scientific Principles and Practice.* 4th ed. Philadelphia, PA: Lippincott Williams & Wilkins; 2006.

Neumayer L, McGregor DB, Mann B. Abdominal wall, including hernia. In: Lawrence PF, ed. *Essentials of General Surgery.* 4th ed. Philadelphia, PA: Lippincott Williams & Wilkins; 2006.

Otterson MF, Korus GB. Diverticular disease. In: Mulholland MW, Lillemoe KD, Doherty GM, Maier RV, Upchurch GR, eds. *Greenfield's Surgery: Scientific Principles and Practice.* 4th ed. Philadelphia, PA: Lippincott Williams & Wilkins; 2006.

Paige J, O'Leary JP. Stomach and duodenum. In: Lawrence PF, ed. *Essentials of General Surgery.* 4th ed. Philadelphia, PA: Lippincott Williams & Wilkins; 2006.

Park AE, Godinez CD Jr. Spleen. In: Brunicardi FC, et al., eds. *Schwartz's Principles of Surgery.* 9th ed. New York, NY: McGraw-Hill; 2010.

Patti MG, Pietro T, Way LW. Esophagus and diaphragm. In: Doherty GM, Way LM, eds. *Current Surgical Diagnosis & Treatment.* 12th ed. New York, NY: Lange Medical Books/McGraw-Hill; 2006.

Rao R, Wait RB. Surgical endocrinology: adrenal glands. In: Lawrence PF, ed. *Essentials of General Surgery.* 4th ed. Philadelphia, PA: Lippincott Williams & Wilkins; 2006.

Rapp JH, MacTaggart J. Arteries. In: Doherty GM, Way LM, eds. *Current Surgical Diagnosis & Treatment.* 12th ed. New York, NY: Lange Medical Books/McGraw-Hill; 2006.

Saund M, Soybel DI. Ileus and bowel obstruction. In: Mulholland MW, Lillemoe KD, Doherty GM, Maier RV, Upchurch GR, eds. *Greenfield's Surgery: Scientific Principles and Practice.* 4th ed. Philadelphia, PA: Lippincott Williams & Wilkins; 2006.

Seymour NE, Bell RL. Abdominal wall, omentum, mesentery, retroperitoneum. In: Brunicardi FC, et al., eds. *Schwartz's Principles of Surgery.* 9th ed. New York, NY: McGraw-Hill; 2010.

Sharp KW, Goldin SB, Lomis KD. Pancreas. In: Lawrence PF, ed. *Essentials of General Surgery.* 4th ed. Philadelphia, PA: Lippincott Williams & Wilkins; 2006.

Shelton AA, Chang G, Welton ML. Small intestine. In: Doherty GM, Way LM, eds. *Current Surgical Diagnosis & Treatment.* 12th ed. New York, NY: Lange Medical Books/McGraw-Hill; 2006.

Shires GT III. Fluid and electrolyte management of the surgical patient. In: Brunicardi FC, et al., eds. *Schwartz's Principles of Surgery.* 9th ed. New York, NY: McGraw-Hill; 2010.

Su LT, Fry R. The colon, rectum and anus. In: Alturi P, Karakousis GC, Porrett PM, Kaiser LR, eds. *The Surgical Review: An Integrated Basic and Clinical Science Study Guide.* 2nd ed. Philadelphia, PA: Lippincott Williams & Wilkins; 2006.

Talboy GE, Gordon I. Wounds and wound healing. In: Lawrence PF, ed. *Essentials of General Surgery.* 4th ed. Philadelphia, PA: Lippincott Williams & Wilkins; 2006.

Theodore PR, Jablons D. Thoracic wall, pleura, mediastinum and lung. In: Doherty GM, Way LM, eds. *Current Surgical Diagnosis & Treatment.* 12th ed. New York, NY: Lange Medical Books/McGraw-Hill; 2006.

Wakefield TW, Rectenwald JR, Messina LM. Veins and lymphatics. In: Doherty GM, Way LM, eds. *Current Surgical Diagnosis & Treatment.* 12th ed. New York, NY: Lange Medical Books/McGraw Hill; 2006.

Wong-Kee-Song LM, Topazian M. Gastrointestinal endoscopy. In: Fauci AS, Braunwald E, Kasper SL, Longo DL, Jameson JL, Loscalzo J, eds. *Harrison's Principles of Internal Medicine,* 17th ed. New York: McGraw-Hill; 2008.

CHAPTER 19

Orthopedics

Thomas A. Woods, DHSc, PA-C

DIRECTIONS: Each of the numbered items or incomplete statements in this section is followed by answers or completion of the statement. Select the ONE lettered answer or completion that is BEST in each case.

1. Approximately 90% of ankle injuries result from which mechanism of injury?

   (A) eversion
   (B) inversion
   (C) plantar flexion
   (D) eversion and plantar flexion
   (E) inversion and plantar flexion

2. A 33-year-old man complains of left anterior shoulder pain for 4 weeks. The pain is made worse with overhead activities. On examination, you note maximal pain in the shoulder with palpation between the greater and lesser tubercle. Pain in the shoulder is exacerbated when the arm is held at the side, elbow flexed to 90° and the patient is asked to supinate and flex the forearm against your resistance. On the basis of this presentation, what is the most likely diagnosis?

   (A) rotator cuff tendonitis
   (B) myocardial infarction
   (C) anterior shoulder dislocation
   (D) rotator cuff tear
   (E) bicipital tendonitis

3. A 62-year-old man presents complaining of progressively worse right shoulder pain for 5 weeks. The pain is located anterolaterally and is aggravated by overhead activities. The patient notes significant pain when trying to sleep with his arm in a forward-flexed position and his hand behind his head. The patient notes weakness of the right arm and states that he has noticed that he uses the arm less because of the pain. On physical examination, you elevate the patient's arms to 90°, abduct to 30°, and internally rotate the arms with the thumbs pointing downward. You note weakness and drooping of the right arm with this maneuver that is exacerbated when you apply downward pressure to the right arm. On the basis of this presentation, what is the most likely injured structure?

   (A) infraspinatus tendon
   (B) supraspinatus tendon
   (C) teres minor tendon
   (D) subscapularis tendon
   (E) bicipital tendon

4. A 73-year-old woman presents to the emergency department following a fall in her home. She tripped over a throw rug, fell forward, and landed with her arms extended and hands outstretched. She presents complaining of left wrist pain. Radiographs reveal a dorsally angulated and displaced distal radius metaphyseal fracture. What is the most likely diagnosis?

(A) Barton fracture
(B) Colles fracture
(C) Smith fracture
(D) boxer fracture

5. Idiopathic osteonecrosis of the femoral head is the most likely diagnosis in which of the following patients?

(A) Five-year-old boy who complains of significant hip and knee pain
(B) Six-year-old boy who reports a limp and aching in the groin and proximal thigh
(C) Seven-year-old obese girl who manifests a painless limp
(D) Twelve-year-old girl who complains of progressively worsening hip pain, fever, and chills
(E) Eighteen-year-old boy who complains of bilateral hip pain that is worse in the morning and is relieved with activity

6. A 22-year-old female person was playing basketball when she tripped and landed on the pavement with her hands outstretched. She presents complaining of abrasions on the right thenar eminence and "wrist pain." Physical examination reveals tenderness to palpation between the extensor pollicis longus and the extensor pollicis brevis. Assessment of the median, ulnar, and radial nerves reveals no sensor or motor changes when compared with the left hand. Radial and ulnar pulses are 2+ bilaterally with capillary refill less than 2 seconds on all five fingers of the right hand. Posterior–anterior view radiographs of the wrist and posterior–anterior wrist radiographs with the wrist in ulnar deviation reveal no fractures or dislocations. What is the appropriate management for this patient at this time?

(A) immediate orthopedic referral
(B) cock-up splint until symptoms resolve
(C) physical therapy referral for assessment and treatment
(D) thumb spica splint and repeat radiographs in 3 weeks
(E) No further treatment is necessary because the radiographs were negative and no vascular or neurological abnormalities were noted on examination.

7. A 53-year-old patient of Scandinavian descent presents with pain in the ring finger of the right hand. The patient states that he/she has pain when he/she extends his/her finger after making a fist. The finger will not extend on its own, requiring the patient to manually extend the finger, a maneuver that produces both an audible snap and considerable pain. What is the most likely diagnosis?

(A) jersey finger
(B) trigger finger
(C) Dupuytren contracture
(D) gamekeeper finger
(E) ganglion cyst

8. A 37-year-old flight attendant presents complaining of worsening foot pain for 3 weeks. The pain is located on the plantar surface of her forefoot and is described as severe, "burning" pain. The pain also radiates into her third and fourth toes. The patient states that, at first, she thought she had a pebble in her shoe, but when she removed her shoe, she could not find any obvious offending agent in her shoe. On physical examination, you are able to reproduce the pain by grasping the medial and lateral aspect of the foot in your hand and squeezing the metatarsal heads together. What is the appropriate treatment strategy for this patient?

(A) No intervention is necessary for this patient because it is a self-limited condition.
(B) Lifestyle modifications including shoe choice is the appropriate first step.

(C) A series of lidocaine and corticosteroid injections should be initiated.

(D) Referral for surgical intervention is necessary at this time.

(E) Magnetic resonance imaging (MRI) of the foot should be ordered before any interventions are employed.

9. A 27-year-old woman with no significant medical history presents complaining of left elbow pain for 3 days. The patient states that over the last 3 days, her left elbow has become increasingly red, swollen, and painful. The patient is left-hand-dominant. The patient is employed as a chiropractor, she is sexually active but denies a history of sexually transmitted infections. The patient is currently having her menses, denies any recent foreign travel, and acknowledges that while she regularly plays tennis, she does not recall any history of elbow trauma. On physical examination, you discover an elbow joint that is markedly erythematous, warm to touch, and tender to palpation. Range of motion is decreased secondary to edema and pain. Radiograph of the elbow reveals only soft tissue swelling but no fracture or dislocation. Joint aspiration is performed and a gram-negative diplococcus is identified on cytological examination. What is the most likely cause of this patient's septic arthritis?

(A) *Staphylococcus aureus*

(B) *Escherichia coli*

(C) *Neisseria gonorrhoeae*

(D) *Pseudomonas aeruginosa*

(E) Methicillin-resistant *Staphylococcus aureus*

10. A 53-year-old woman presents with pain in her right wrist. The pain is aggravated by movement of the thumb and when she makes a fist. She also notes that when she moves her thumb, there is an occasional locking sensation in the radial aspect of her wrist. Physical examination of the wrist reveals swelling and tenderness over the distal radius, and full flexion of the thumb into the palm, with ulnar deviation of the wrist, produces pain. Radiographic evaluation of the wrist shows no bone abnormalities.

Which of the following would be the treatment of choice in this patient presentation?

(A) immobilization of the wrist with a thumb spica splint

(B) tendon sheath corticosteroid injection

(C) operative treatment to restore functionality

(D) prompt neurological evaluation

(E) proceed to bone scan to evaluate the area of pain

11. Which of the following most accurately describes the physical examination findings suggestive of a boutonniere deformity?

(A) hyperextension of the proximal interphalangeal joint with fixed flexion of the distal interphalangeal joint

(B) persistent extension of the proximal interphalangeal joint with hyperflexion of the distal interphalangeal joint

(C) hyperextension of the distal interphalangeal joint with flexion of the proximal interphalangeal joint

(D) persistent flexion of the proximal interphalangeal joint with hyperextension of the distal interphalangeal joint

(E) hyperextension of the distal interphalangeal joint with extension of the proximal interphalangeal joint

12. A 62-year-old man complains of low back pain that radiates from his back down into his buttock and into his right leg. On physical examination, you note sensory loss on the lateral aspect of the right foot, decreased ability to perform a toe walk on the right side and a decreased Achilles reflex. The straight leg raise test elicits pain at 45° of elevation. On the basis of the information contained in this scenario, between which pairing of vertebrae is the disc herniation most likely to have occurred?

(A) L2–L3

(B) L3–L4

(C) L4–L5

(D) L5–S1

(E) S1–S2

13. You have been following a 52-year-old man with a complaint of back pain over the past 7 weeks. During the first 5 weeks of his condition, Abraham's back pain was steadily declining and his neurological findings on physical examination were decreasing. Over the past 2 weeks, Abraham has complained of worsening pain that is currently unrelenting, especially at night. On physical examination, Abraham demonstrates findings on both the straight leg raise and crossed straight leg raise tests. His muscle weakness has likewise accelerated over the past 2 weeks, and he is no longer able to heel walk using his left ankle. What is the most appropriate management strategy at this time?

(A) conservative therapy including application of ice and physical therapy referral for muscle stretching and strengthening
(B) plain radiographs of the spine
(C) computed tomography (CT) of the spine
(D) MRI of the spine

14. A 62-year-old man is postop day 2 from a right total hip replacement. He has been ambulating with physical therapy, and his diet has been advanced to full without any restrictions. On morning rounds, the patient admits to an acute onset of pain in his left first metatarsophalangeal joint. The joint is erythematous to inspection. Pain is elicited with range of motion, and the patient is unable to bear weight on his foot secondary to the pain. Aspiration of the joint reveals calcium pyrophosphate crystals. What is the most likely diagnosis?

(A) gout
(B) pseudogout
(C) septic joint
(D) bunion

15. A 27-year-old man with a history of intermittent gout, mild obesity, and alcohol dependency complains of lumbar back pain for 2 days. The patient is employed by a moving company. He admits that he does not enjoy all of the physical labor associated with loading and unloading trucks and hopes he is able to get a better job in the near future. On physical exam-

ination, you note a man who is in moderate distress. He is sitting still on the examination table. Vital signs reveal a temperature of 101.5°F orally, pulse of 88/min regular, respirations of 20/min unlabored, pulse oximetry of 99% on room air, body mass index (BMI) of 28.5. Lungs are clear to auscultation; heart demonstrates a regular rate and rhythm without murmurs. Abdominal examination reveals normoactive bowel sounds and no rigidity or guarding. There are areas of erythema and ecchymosis in the antecubital crease on his right arm with red streaking extending proximally from the antecubital crease. Examination of the back reveals no erythema or muscle spasm. You elicit pinpoint tenderness over the fourth lumbar vertebra to palpation. There is only mild discomfort to palpation in the paraspinous muscles in the lumbar region. The patient has full range of motion to flexion and extension at the waist. Straight leg raise test elicits pain in the hamstring region at 80° on the right leg but the cross straight leg raise test is negative. There are no sensory changes noted in the lower extremities bilaterally and the deep tendon reflexes (DTRs) are 2+ in the patellar and Achilles bilaterally. Anal sphincter tone is within normal limits. What is the best treatment choice for this patient at this time?

(A) conservative management, including nonsteroidal anti-inflammatory drugs (NSAIDs) and a work excuse for 3 days
(B) narcotic pain medication plus physical therapy referral
(C) ciprofloxacin 750 mg once a day for 14 days
(D) parenteral antibiotics for 4 to 6 weeks
(E) parenteral antibiotics weekly for 6 months

16. A 10-year-old boy is brought to the emergency department after falling during the recess at school. The patient states that he was running with a football when two of his classmates tackled him. He complains of pain in his right wrist. Radiographs reveal a fracture to the right radius. The fracture line runs diagonally from the epiphysis through the metaphyseal bone.

By definition, how would you classify this patient's fracture?

(A) Salter–Harris type I
(B) Salter–Harris type II
(C) Salter–Harris type III
(D) Salter–Harris type IV
(E) Salter–Harris type V

17. A 25-year-old man was involved in a motor vehicle accident (MVA) and complains of right leg pain. The car was traveling approximately 50 miles per hour when the driver lost control of the vehicle, causing it to leave the road and run head-on into a tree. At the time of the accident, he was sitting in the passenger side of the front seat. The force of the collision caused the dashboard to be driven violently back against the patient's knees. On the basis of this mechanism of injury, what would you expect to find when you inspect the right leg?

(A) flexed, abducted, and externally rotated
(B) shortened, abducted, and externally rotated
(C) shortened, abducted, and internally rotated
(D) shortened and externally rotated
(E) shortened, adducted, and internally rotated

18. A 42-year-old automobile mechanic presents complaining of neck pain that radiates down the lateral aspect of his arm and into his left hand. The patient states that the pain has become progressively more constant over the past 3 weeks. He feels that he is "loosing strength" in his left hand and that parts of his left hand are feeling numb. He states that his symptoms seem to lessen when he places his hand on top of his head. Physical examination reveals vital signs that are within normal limits; no muscle atrophy or spasm are noted in the neck or upper extremities bilaterally. Sensory ability is diminished in the long finger on the left hand. Triceps muscle strength is 5/5 on the right and 4/5 on the left. Bicep strength is 5/5 bilaterally. Biceps and brachioradialis reflexes are +2 bilaterally, right-sided triceps reflex is 2+, and left-sided triceps reflex is 1+. On the basis of this presentation, what spinal root is most likely involved?

(A) C5
(B) C6
(C) C7
(D) C8
(E) T1

19. Nonsteroidal anti-inflammatory agents are frequently utilized in treating the patient with osteoarthritis. In addition to the potential for bleeding and gastrointestinal effects, the primary concern, especially in the elderly patient, is irreversible damage to which of the following?

(A) eyes
(B) heart
(C) kidneys
(D) peripheral vascular system
(E) central nervous system

20. A 7-year-old boy is brought to the emergency department after sustaining a fall onto his outstretched hand. He complains of pain involving the entire arm and refuses to move his arm, which is held in anatomical position with the elbow flexed at 90°. On physical examination, there is notable tenderness over the elbow with associated swelling and pain on attempted rotation. There is no apparent tenderness to palpation involving the wrist or shoulder. The child refuses to participate with range of motion evaluation. Radiographic evaluation of the elbow shows the presence of a positive posterior fat pad sign. What is the most likely diagnosis with this patient's presentation?

(A) nursemaid elbow
(B) lateral epicondylitis
(C) medial epicondylitis
(D) radial head dislocation
(E) occult fracture of the radial head

21. A 35-year-old man presents with complaints of swelling and pain in left knee. The patient states that he sustained a twisting injury in a basketball game 3 days ago. The injury did not take him out of the game; he was able to participate with minimal difficulty. Over the last 2 days, the pain has progressed. He notes a catching sensation and pain that is more medially located. On physical examination, the patient is found to have tenderness over the medial joint line and limited range of motion. Forced flexion and circumduction of the joint causes a painful click. What is the most likely diagnosis in this patient presentation?

    (A) anterior cruciate ligament tear
    (B) medial meniscus tear
    (C) pes anserine bursitis
    (D) tibial plateau fracture
    (E) medial collateral ligament tear

22. Which of the following motor, sensory, and reflex finding are most likely to be found in a patient with lumbar radiculopathy of the L4–L5 disc?

    (A) weakness of the anterior tibialis, numbness of the shin, and an asymmetric knee reflex
    (B) weakness of the great toe flexor and gastrocsoleus, inability to sustain tiptoe walking, and an asymmetrical ankle reflex
    (C) weakness of the great toe extensor, numbness on the top of the foot and first web space, no reflex findings
    (D) perianal numbness, urinary and bowel incontinence
    (E) ankle clonus

23. Which of the following characteristics help to distinguish the "pseudoclaudication" of a patient with spinal stenosis from true claudication?

    (A) insidious onset of symptoms
    (B) worsening of pain by lumbar flexion
    (C) radiation of pain to the upper back
    (D) preservation of pedal pulses

    (E) localizing maximum area of discomfort to the lower back

24. A 15-year-old boy was playing football and was hit during a play, causing an abduction injury of his left lower leg. He locates the pain along the medial aspect of the knee, and there is a minimal level of joint effusion. Which of the following tests would assess for stability of the medial collateral ligament?

    (A) valgus stress test
    (B) varus stress test
    (C) apprehension sign
    (D) Lachman test
    (E) anterior drawer sign

25. A 12-year-old obese boy presents with pain in the right thigh and medial knee. The pain has been over a 6-week period. The pain is described as aching in nature. Over the last month, the patient has had a limp present. On physical examination, the right knee is found to be unremarkable, but there is a slight limp noted with gait. Radiographs of the right knee are normal. Which of the following is the most appropriate step in the evaluation of this patient?

    (A) examine and x-ray the right hip
    (B) x-ray the left knee for comparison
    (C) obtain a CT scan of the right knee
    (D) obtain a magnetic resonance image of the right knee
    (E) reassure the parents and observe the patient for progression

26. Treatment of scoliosis is usually employed for patients with curvature beyond which of the following curve magnitudes:

    (A) 20°
    (B) 30°
    (C) 40°
    (D) 50°
    (E) 60°

27. A 24-year-old man presents with low back pain of 2 days' duration. The patient is a manual

laborer and reports lifting a heavy box while at work the previous day. Initially, the patient had no complaints, but the following day, stiffness and pain began. The patient denies radiation of the pain, numbness, or difficulty with urination. He denies previous complaints of back pain or injury. On physical examination, there is noted paravertebral muscle spasm and slight decrease in range of motion of the spine. Deep tendon reflexes are equal bilaterally, and no sensory deficits are noted. Which of the following is the most appropriate intervention?

(A) MRI of the lumbar spine

(B) plain radiographs of the lumbar spine

(C) return the patient to work with no limitations

(D) refer the patient for trigger point injections

(E) initiate a short period of rest, analgesia, and progressive functional program

28. Which of the following is most diagnostic of a septic joint?

(A) synovial fluid analysis

(B) plain radiograph

(C) ultrasound of the joint

(D) CT scan of the joint

(E) MRI of the joint

29. An 8-year-old boy presents with complaint of a painful right wrist of 2 days' duration. The mother of the child reports that the child jumped off of a swing landing on his outstretched arms. He immediately complained of pain in the right wrist and now has some mild swelling on the radial aspect of the wrist. Radiographic evaluation of the wrist presents an area of impaction on the distal radius, with a slight bend in the opposing cortex. Which of the following best describes this type of pediatric fracture?

(A) greenstick fracture

(B) torus fracture

(C) plastic deformation

(D) radial neck fracture

(E) Monteggia fracture

30. A 39-year-old woman presents with complaints of pain in her left foot of 4 weeks' duration. The patient works as a cashier in a department store, which requires her to be on her feet for long periods. She notes that the pain is most severe on the bottom of her foot and is worse upon arising in the morning and then it subsides with ambulation. The patient has a benign medical history and no other complaints. Which of the following is the most likely diagnosis of this patient?

(A) heel spur

(B) Achilles tendonitis

(C) tarsal tunnel syndrome

(D) plantar fascitis

(E) posterior tibial nerve entrapment

31. A 17-year-old boy presents with complaints of pain located in his fifth digit. He was involved in an altercation and states that his hand was injured from punching someone. On physical examination of the patient's hand, there is tenderness, swelling, and pain with extension. The patient is diagnosed with a "boxer fracture." What radiographic finding would be present to diagnose this patient?

(A) spiral fracture of the third metacarpal

(B) fracture of the fourth metacarpal

(C) fracture of the fifth metacarpal

(D) comminuted fracture of the distal phalanx of the fifth digit

(E) comminuted fracture of the distal phalanx of the fourth digit

32. Which of the following best defines the deformity that causes a "mallet finger"?

(A) rupture or avulsion of the insertion of the extensor tendon at the base of the distal phalanx

(B) rupture or avulsion of the insertion of the flexor tendon at the base of the distal phalanx

(C) fracture of the distal phalanx

(D) dislocation of the distal interphalangeal joint

(E) fracture of the proximal phalanx

33. A 10-year-old boy presents to the emergency department status post a fall from his bicycle. The patient complains of pain located in his right knee with an associated 2 cm × 2 cm abrasion just inferior to the patella. There is no swelling noted of the knee. The child is not cooperative with examination of the extremity. Radiographs are taken of the right knee, and there is no finding of fracture or joint changes. Incidentally, a lesion is noted at the distal femur, described as a pedunculated bone mass capped in cartilage. With this finding, what is the most likely diagnosis?

(A) osteoid osteoma
(B) chondroblastoma
(C) osteosarcoma
(D) osteochondroma
(E) Ewing sarcoma

34. A 39-year-old woman presents with complaints of left anterior knee pain of 4 weeks' duration. She has noted difficulty with going up and down the staircase. The patient also notes increased pain in the knee upon arising after being seated for a period. The pain may then improve with walking. The patient denies joint crepitus or locking sensation. On physical examination, there is no swelling or obvious joint distortion. The pain is reproduced with placing the knee in slight flexion and gentle pressure placed on the patella as the patient contracts the quadriceps. The knee appears stable, with no signs of crepitus, joint laxity, or internal derangement. Radiographs of the left knee are essentially benign. What course of treatment is best for this patient?

(A) crutches for 6 weeks, keeping the joint nonweight bearing
(B) cortisone injection
(C) physical therapy to strengthen the quadriceps
(D) physical therapy to strengthen the lower back
(E) progress to orthopedic evaluation for consideration of internal derangement of the knee

35. A 17-year-old basketball player complains of acute onset of right ankle pain. During a game, she jumped up for a rebound and when she landed, her foot came down on the foot of another player causing her ankle to invert. The patient heard a "pop" at the time of the injury and immediately experienced pain and edema on the lateral aspect of the ankle. What structure is most likely to have been compromised?

(A) deltoid ligament
(B) calcaneofibular ligament
(C) anterior talofibular ligament
(D) posterior talofibular ligament
(E) syndesmosis ligament

Answers and Explanations

1. **(E)** Approximately 90% of ankle injures result from forced inversion with the ankle in plantar flexion. The anterior talofibular ligament is the most commonly injured ligament. *(Van-Huysen et al., 2008, pp. 543-544)*

2. **(E)** Bicipital tendonitis is an inflammation of the long head of the biceps tendon and the tendon sheath causes anterior shoulder pain that resembles and often accompanies coexisting rotator cuff tendonitis. Tenderness with bicipital tendonitis is reproduced with Yergason test. During Yergason test, the shoulder pain is exacerbated when the arm is held at the side, elbow flexed to 90°, and the patient asked to supinate and flex the forearm against your resistance. Rotator cuff injuries often accompany bicipital tendonitis, and bicipital tendonitis can occur secondary to compensation for rotator cuff disorders or labral tears. In this case, the pain is clearly reproduced in a pattern suggestive of bicipital tendonitis. Myocardial infarction can present as shoulder pain and should always be considered in patients, especially those with known cardiac risk factors. *(Bickley and Szilagyi, 2009, p. 647)*

3. **(B)** The maneuver described is commonly referred to as the supraspinatus strength test or the "empty the can" test. Weakness in this maneuver is suggestive of injury to supraspinatus tendon. The teres minor and infraspinatus tendons are external rotators and are often tested with the arm at 90° of elbow flexion with the patient attempting to externally rotate against resistance. The subscapularis is also tested at 90° of elbow flexion with resistance applied as the patient attempts to internally rotate against resistance. *(Bickley and Szilagyi, 2009, p. 598)*

4. **(B)** Distal radius fractures are commonly associated with falls, especially falls on an outstretched hand. Middle-aged and elderly patients, especially those with osteoporosis, are susceptible to these injuries. A Colles fracture is classically described as dorsally angulated and displaced distal radius metaphysical fracture. A Smith fracture, sometimes referred to as a reverse Colles fracture, is an extra-articular metaphysical fracture of the radius with volar angulation and displacement. Barton fracture is a displaced unstable articular fracture-subluxation of the distal radius with volar displacement. A boxer fracture classically involves the fifth metacarpal bone and is associated with a closed hand trauma. *(Tay et al., 2006, p. 1124)*

5. **(B)** Legg–Calve–Perthes disease is idiopathic osteonecrosis of the femoral head in children. The condition typically affects children between the ages of 4 and 8 years, but the range of onset is 2 to 12 years of age. It is unilateral in 90% of patients and four times more common in male population. Typically, the patient presents with a limp that worsens with activity and is thus more noticeable at the end of the day. If the child reports pain, it is typically an aching in the groin or proximal thigh. *(Griffin, 2005, pp. 900-902)*

6. **(D)** The scaphoid bone is based in the proximal row of carpal bones but extends into the distal row, making it more vulnerable to injury when a patient falls on an outstretched hand. The scaphoid bone is the most frequently injured carpal bone, accounting for 60% to 70% of all

carpal fractures. At the time of initial injury, 10% to 15% of scaphoid fractures may not be visible on plain radiographs. Patients with pain in the anatomical snuffbox to palpation or axial loading, even with normal radiographs, should be treated as though they have a scaphoid fracture and placed in a thumb spica splint. Repeat radiographs should be taken after 2 to 3 weeks. If radiographs are still normal but tenderness over the scaphoid bone persists, a bone CT scan or MRI can be ordered. Fractures of the scaphoid have a high incidence of nonunion and osteonecrosis because the major blood supply enters in the distal segment of the bone and can be disrupted with injury/fracture and thus conservative management is warranted. *(Griffin, 2005, pp. 358-361)*

7. **(B)** Trigger finger is a painless nodule in the flexor tendon in the palm near the metacarpal head. The nodule is too large to easily enter the tendon sheath during extension of the finger. When the finger is extended, an audible snap can be palpated or heard as the nodule enters the tendon sheath. *(Bickley and Szilagyi, 2009, p. 650)*

8. **(B)** The symptom profile points toward a diagnosis of Morton neuroma. Morton neuroma is a perineural fibrosis of the common digital nerve as it passes between the metatarsal heads. It commonly occurs between the third and fourth toes and is associated with dysesthesias into the affected toes. Many patients state that they feel as though they are "walking on a marble" or that they feel as if they have a pebble in their shoe. Symptoms are made worse by wearing high-heeled or tight, restrictive shoes. Treatment should initially be conservative, including advising the patient to wear low-heeled, well-cushioned shoes with a wide toe box. Metatarsal pads to spread the metatarsal heads can also take pressure off of the nerve. Lidocaine and corticosteroid injection just proximal to the metatarsal heads can be diagnostic and therapeutic but multiple injections should be avoided. Surgical excision of the neuroma is warranted if symptoms persist or recur. *(Bickley and Szilagyi, 2009, p. 652; Griffin, 2005, pp. 655-657)*

9. **(C)** Gonococcal arthritis usually occurs in otherwise healthy individuals, is two to three times more common in women than in men, is especially common during menses and pregnancy, and is rare after age 40. There are two forms of gonococcal arthritis. Septic arthritis, the purulent monarthritis form, occurs approximately 40% of the time; and the bacteremic form, characterized by a triad of migratory polyarthritis, tenosynovitis, and dermatitis, occurs approximately 60% of the time. Septic monarthritis most frequently involves the knee, elbow, wrist, or ankle. Less than one-fourth of patients have any genitourinary symptoms. Patients with septic arthritis complain of pain, swelling, and redness beginning days to weeks after gonococcal infection. Staphylococcus aureus is a gram-positive organism that is the most common cause of nongonococcal septic arthritis. *Escherichia coli* and *Pseudomonas aeruginosa* are the most common nongonococcal gram-negative isolates in adults. Gram-negative septic arthritis occurs with more frequency in injection drug users and immunocompromised patients. *(Hellmann and Imboden, 2008, pp. 750-752)*

10. **(A)** This patient presentation is most consistent with De Quervain tendonitis, inflammation or tenosynovitis of the abductor pollicis longus and extensor pollicis brevis, which results from thickening of the tendon sheath results in pain, swelling, and a triggering phenomenon of locking or sticking. This disorder is more common in middle-aged women and in repetitive motion injuries. On physical examination, the finding of a positive Finkelstein test, which is pain with full flexion of the thumb into the palm, with ulnar deviation of the wrist, is diagnostic of De Quervain tendonitis. Initial treatment is aimed at immobilization of the wrist to allow for pain and inflammatory relief. A course of nonsteroidal anti-inflammatory drugs (NSAIDs) is helpful for pain relief as well. Corticosteroid injection is reserved for patients who fail with immobilization and NSAID use. Operative treatment should be considered only if injections are not helpful. Radiographic evaluation is not helpful in the evaluation or treatment of this condition. *(Griffin, 2005, pp. 328-329)*

11. **(D)** A Boutonniere deformity classically presents as persistent flexion of the proximal interphalangeal joint with hyperextension of the distal interphalangeal joint. A swan neck deformity is also commonly found with patients who have rheumatoid arthritis. A swan neck deformity classically manifests as hyperextension of the proximal interphalangeal joint with fixed flexion of the distal interphalangeal joint. *(Bickley and Szilagyi, 2009, p. 649)*

12. **(D)** Disc herniation at the L5–S1 level will affect the S1 nerve root. S1 nerve root irritation causes sensory changes in the lateral aspect of the foot, motor weakness with plantar flexion, and a change in the Achilles reflex. Disc herniation at the L4–L5 level affects the L5 nerve, which causes sensory changes on the dorsal aspect of the foot, motor weakness with dorsiflexion of the ankle and great toe, but no deep tendon reflex changes. Disc herniation at the L3–L4 level affects the L4 nerve root, causing sensory changes over the medial aspect of the foot and motor weakness with knee extension. *(Kinkade, 2008, p. 583)*

13. **(D)** The patient's symptoms and signs have progressed over the past 2 weeks. In particular, he has experienced the following "red flags": failure to improve after 4 to 6 weeks of conservative therapy, unrelenting night pain, and progressive motor or sensory deficit. Conservative therapy is not warranted in the face of these red flags. Plain radiographs are not highly sensitive or specific. They are reasonably useful to identify compression fractures and degenerative changes in the spine. CT is relatively good for revealing most bony spinal pathology. MRI provides the most detailed images of the soft tissues of the disc and nerve roots. Since the symptom profile points toward a nerve root irritation more than a boney abnormality, MRI would be the appropriate choice at this time. *(Kinkade, 2008, pp. 582-583)*

14. **(B)** Pseudogout, like gout, frequently develops 24 to 48 hours after major surgery. Pseudogout involves the knee most frequently but can affect the ankle, wrist, and metatarsophalangeal joints. Identification of calcium pyrophosphate crystals in the joint aspirates is diagnostic of pseudogout. In patients with gout, serum uric acid level is elevated in 95% of patients and identification of sodium urate crystals in joint fluid aspiration is diagnostic. *(Hellmann and Imboden, 2008, p. 707)*

15. **(D)** The patient demonstrates an elevated temperature with evidence of infection and proximal lymphagnitis from wounds in the antecubital crease. Intravenous drug use should be suspected with this presentation. Osteomyelitis is a serious infection of the bone. Osteomyelitis resulting from bacteremia is a disease associated with injection drug users that commonly develops in the spine. Patients with osteomyelitis often present with sudden onset of fever, chills, and pain and tenderness over the involved bone. Traditionally, antibiotics have been administered parenterally for at least 4 to 6 weeks. The straight leg raise test is positive if pain in the sciatic distribution is reproduced between 30° and 70° passive flexion of the straight leg. *(Hellmann and Imboden, 2008, p. 753)*

16. **(B)** A Salter–Harris type II fracture runs from the epiphysis through the metaphysis. *(Tay et al., 2006, p. 1158)*

17. **(E)** The mechanism of injury suggests a posterior hip dislocation. In a posterior hip dislocation, the femur is dislocated posterior to the acetabulum when the thigh is flexed, as may occur in a head-on MVA when the patient's knee is violently impacted by the dashboard. The significant clinical findings of a posterior hip dislocation are an extremity that is shortened, adducted, and internally rotated. An anterior hip dislocation classically presents as a flexed, abducted, and externally rotated leg. A fractured femoral neck is classically externally rotated and shortened. *(Tay et al., 2006, pp. 1131-1135)*

18. **(C)** Cervical radiculopathy is referred neurogenic pain in the distribution of a cervical nerve root with or without associated numbness, weakness, or loss of reflexes. The usual cause in young adults is herniation of a cervical disk

that entraps the root as it enters the foramen. C7 nerve root irritation often presents with pain in the neck, shoulder, medial boarder of the scapula, lateral aspect of the arm, and dorsum of the hand. Sensory changes are in the longer finger and dorsum of the hand. Muscle weakness is noted with triceps and finger extensors, and DTR changes are noted in the triceps. C5 radiculopathy presents with pain the neck, shoulder, and anterolateral aspect of the arm. Sensory changes are seen in the deltoid region; muscle atrophy is seen in the deltoid and biceps. DTR changes with a C5 root irritation are manifested in the biceps reflex. C6 root irritation manifests pain in the neck, shoulder, lateral aspect of the arm, and radial aspect of the forearm. Sensory changes are seen in the dorsolateral aspect of the thumb and index finger. Biceps and wrist extensors/pollicus longus are noted to have muscle weakness or atrophy. Biceps and brachioradialis DTRs manifest changes with C6 root irritation. *(Griffin, 2005, pp. 739-741)*

19. **(C)** Nonsteroidal anti-inflammatory drugs (NSAIDS) are metabolized in the liver and excreted via the kidneys. Elderly patients are more at risk of developing irreversible damage to the renal system. Renal function physiologically decreases with the advancing age. With decreased clearance of the medication, renal damage ensues and leads to accumulation of the drug and further renal damage. Renal function should be monitored in the elderly patient receiving high doses of any NSAIDS. Hepatic failure is also a concern with the use of NSAID, especially where there is potential for overdose. There is no documented evidence of damage to the eyes, heart, peripheral vascular system, or central nervous system. *(Hellmann and Imboden, 2008, p. 723)*

20. **(E)** The most likely diagnosis in this patient presentation is an occult fracture of the radial head. This is supported by the mechanism of injury, physical examination, and radiographic findings. On physical examination, tenderness over the radial head with local swelling and pain with rotation and flexion of the forearm is usually present. Fractures of the radial head

may be subtle on initial radiographs. The finding of an anterior fat pad may be a normal finding, but the finding of a posterior fat is pathological and usually indicates an occult fracture of the radial head. Nursemaid elbow is more commonly seen in children 1 to 3 years of age and is associated with injury that is pulling in nature on the hand with the elbow in full extension. Lateral and medial epicondylitis are typically overuse injuries that occur in patients 35 to 50 years of age. Radial head dislocation may be associated with fracture of the radial head; the supporting evidence in this case does not support dislocation. Radial head dislocation is typically posteriorly and evident on radiographs. *(Griffin, 2005, pp. 807-808; Polousky and Eilbert, 2009, p. 758)*

21. **(B)** This patient presentation is most consistent with a medial meniscus tear. Medial meniscus tears are more likely to present with a twisting injury of the knee. Patients usually are ambulatory after the injury, with pain and swelling progressing 2 to 3 days after the injury. The pain is usually located in the medial or lateral side of the knee and is associated with a catching or locking sensation caused by swelling or mechanical blockage from torn meniscus. On physical examination, there is tenderness over the medial or lateral joint line. The McMurray test is positive when forced flexion and circumduction of the joint causes a painful click. Anterior cruciate ligament can result from a twisting injury as well but would be more likely associated with hemarthrosis and a positive Lachman test or anterior drawer sign. Pes anserine bursitis more commonly presents with tenderness distal to the medial joint line and is more likely associated with overuse. Tibial plateau fracture would present with bony tenderness and a result of high-energy fracture. Medial collateral ligament tear would present with pain and instability with valgus stress on the joint. *(Griffin, 2005, pp. 523-526)*

22. **(C)** The radiculopathy found with L4–L5 disc herniation presents with weakness of the great toe extensor, numbness on the top of the foot and first web space, and no reflex findings. Radiculopathy of the L3–L4 disc presents with

weakness of the anterior tibialis, numbness of the shin, and an asymmetric knee reflex. Radiculopathy of the L5–S1 disc presents with weakness of the great toe flexor and gastrocsoleus, inability to sustain tiptoe walking, and an asymmetrical ankle reflex. Cauda equina syndrome is associated with perianal numbness and urinary and bowel incontinence. Ankle clonus is more likely to be associated with demyelinating conditions. *(Griffin, 2005, pp. 719)*

23. **(D)** The pain of spinal stenosis presents in the lower back, radiating to the buttocks and thighs, and is aggravated with walking and alleviated with rest or lumbar flexion. Distinguishing "pseudoclaudication" of a patient with spinal stenosis from true vascular insufficiency is best supported by the preservation of pedal pulses and the location of pain in the thighs. *(Griffin, 2005, pp. 774-776)*

24. **(A)** Evaluating the medial collateral ligament is best completed by applying valgus stress to the knee extended and then flexed at 25° and then evaluating the stability. If the knee shows exaggerated laxity, there is more likelihood that the medial collateral ligament is torn. Varus stress evaluates the integrity of the lateral collateral ligament. The apprehension sign evaluates for patellar instability. The Lachman test and anterior drawer sign are to evaluate for anterior cruciate ligament tears. *(Wilson and Penget, 2009, p. 785)*

25. **(A)** This patient presentation is most suggestive of slipped capital femoral epiphysis of the right hip. This condition is commonly seen during adolescence (11 to 13 years), and obesity is also a contributing factor. The patient more commonly presents with referred pain to the medial knee and thigh with an associated limp. The combination of a thickened growth plate from the influence of growth hormone causing a weaker bone, lack of sexual maturity to stabilize the physis, obesity adding mechanical stress, and the mechanics of the joint adds to the increased likelihood of slippage of the epiphysis. Examination of the hip along with radiographic studies is imperative to further

evaluate this patient. Hip examination would reveal loss of abduction and internal rotation of the hip. Radiographically, a frog-legged lateral view is best for detecting slippage. Establishing the degree of slippage is imperative to determining the treatment. In this patient presentation, a radiograph of the left knee is not necessary. Further radiographic evaluation of the knee with CT scan or MRI is not necessary. Reassuring the parents and observing this patient is not advisable, as prompt evaluation and treatment is imperative due to the progressiveness of this disease. *(Griffin, 2005, pp. 941-943; Wilson and Penget, 2009, p. 782)*

26. **(A)** The treatment of scoliosis depends on the magnitude of the curvature of the spine and the risk of progression. Curvatures less than 20° usually do not require intervention. Curvature at 20° to 40° in a skeletally immature patient may respond to bracing. Curvatures greater than 60° may require surgical intervention. *(Polousky and Eilbert, 2009, p. 754)*

27. **(E)** The initial treatment of a patient with low back pain without neurological deficit consists of conservative management despite the causation. Muscle strain, ligament sprain, or early disc disease are all treated with rest, analgesia, and progressive functional activities. Diagnostic evaluation to include radiographs, and MRI of the lumbar spine is reserved for the patient who does not respond to conservative management. Returning the patient to work, especially manual labor, would be counterproductive for the pain. Trigger point injections are not proven to show benefit in the treatment of acute low back pain. *(Griffin, 2005, pp. 757-759)*

28. **(A)** The evaluation of septic arthritis is best accomplished with synovial fluid analysis and culture. Radiological imaging can be normal. Ultrasound evaluation can demonstrate fluid in the joint but is not specific to the diagnosis. CT scan and MRI of the joint are not specific to the diagnosis. *(Tay et al., 2006, p. 1199)*

29. **(B)** This patient's scenario is consistent with a torus fracture of the radius. Torus fractures

commonly present as a "buckle" of the cortex and are due to force or compression of the bone. This type of fracture is more common to occur in a pediatric patient because of the "softer" nature of the bone. Torus fractures usually do not create alignment issues and heal within 3 weeks with simple immobilization. A greenstick fracture involves disruption of one side of the cortex with angulation of the bone; this type of fracture does not separate the ends of the bone. Plastic deformation is the change in the natural shape of the bone with a detectable suture line; there is no "buckle" with this type of fracture. Radial neck fracture would present with angulation of the radial head and is proximally located. Monteggia fracture refers to an ulnar fracture with associated radial head dislocation from the capitulum. *(Polousky and Eilert, 2009, p. 759)*

30. **(D)** This patient presentation is typical of the pain associated with plantar fascitis, where the pain is located on the bottom of the foot and more commonly is severe on initially getting up in the morning and lessens with ambulation. In most cases of plantar fascitis, there is maximal pain along the plantar medial aspect of the heel, corresponding to the origin of the plantar fascia at the medial calcaneal tuberosity. Heel spurs are more likely to be associated with continued pain. Achilles tendonitis is more likely to occur over the bony prominence of the calcaneus. Tarsal tunnel syndrome is associated with compression of the posterior tibial nerve and with diffuse pain, paresthesias, and burning of the medial ankle and is worse after walking and occurs at night. *(Griffin, 2005, pp. 667-669)*

31. **(C)** Boxer fracture refers to a fracture of the fifth metacarpal. This is the most common fracture of the hand and is seen with injuries associated with a closed fist striking an object. With all of the potential fractures, the patient will typically have a history of trauma, local tenderness, swelling, deformity, and/or decreased range of motion. *(Tay et al., 2006, p. 1129)*

32. **(A)** Mallet finger is caused by rupture or avulsion of the insertion of the extensor tendon. It is also known as baseball finger due to the cause of injury commonly associated with a ball striking the finger, causing sudden passive flexion of the actively extended distal interphalangeal joint. The presentation is a DIP joint that is unable to extend at the joint. Treatment of this extensor tendon injury is best accomplished with continuous splinting of the DIP joint in extension for 6 to 8 weeks. *(Griffin, 2005, p. 374)*

33. **(D)** This patient presentation is more consistent with osteochondroma, which is the most common bone tumor in children and is typically associated with a pain-free mass. The tumor appears as a pedunculated or sessile lesion that resembles a cartilaginous cap on a boney stalk. This tumor has a very rare malignant tendency and is excised only if it interferes with function. *(Polousky and Eilert, 2009, p. 765)*

34. **(C)** This patient presentation is most likely patellofemoral syndrome. The typical presentation includes anterior knee pain of vague location; the pain is increased by flexion load such as stair climbing and the patient has a positive "theater sign." Theater sign consist of pain after being seated for prolonged period. Treatment of patellofemoral syndrome is initially conservative and aimed at strengthening the quadriceps. Referral to physical therapy is helpful with regaining strength and implementing therapeutics. Injection of the joint with corticosteroid would be less likely associated with the initial approach and weight-bearing exercises should be avoided in the acute phase. Immobilizing the joint is counterproductive. *(Griffin, 2005, pp. 541-544)*

35. **(C)** An inversion injury to the ankle causes disruption of the lateral ligament complex that consists of the anterior talofibular ligament, calcaneofibular ligament, and the posterior talofibular ligament. The majority of inversion or varus ankle sprains first involve the anterior talofibular ligament. The calcaneofibular ligament is involved only in more serious injuries, and the posterior talofibular ligament is rarely injured. The deltoid ligament

is more likely to be injured with an eversion and rotational injury of the medial ankle. The syndesmosis ligament joins the tibia and fibula together and is more likely injured by an external rotational force to the foot, what commonly is known as a "high sprain." (*Hellmann and Imboden, 2008, p. 720; van-Huysen et al., 2008, pp. 543-545*)

REFERENCES

Bickley LS, Szilagyi, PG. *Bates' Guide to Physical Examination and History Taking*. 10th ed. Philadelphia, PA: Lippincott Williams & Wilkins; 2009.

Griffin LY. *Essentials of Musculoskeletal Care*. 3rd ed. Rosemont, IL: American Academy of Orthopaedic Surgeons; 2005.

Hellmann DB, Imboden JB. Arthritis & musculoskeletal disorders. In: Tierney LM, McPhee SJ, Papadakis MA, eds. *2008 Current Medical Diagnosis & Treatment*. 47th ed. New York, NY: McGraw-Hill; 2008.

Kinkade S. Low back pain. In: Sloane PD, Slatt LM, Ebell MH, Jacques LB, Smith MA, eds. 429*Essentials of Family Medicine*. 5th ed. Philadelphia, PA: Lippincott Williams & Wilkins; 2008.

Polousky JD, Eilert RE. Orthopedics. In: Hay WW, Levin MJ, Sondheimer JM, Deterding RR, eds. *Current Pediatric Diagnosis & Treatment*. 19th ed. New York: McGraw-Hill; 2009.

Tay KB, Colman WW, Berven S et al. Orthopedics. In: Doherty GM, Way WW, eds. *Current Surgical Diagnosis & Treatment*. 12th ed. New York, NY: Lange Medical Books; 2006.

Van-Huysen J, Blackwell D, Barry HC. Ankle and knee pain. In: Sloane PD, Slatt LM, Ebell MH, Jacques LB, Smith MA, eds. *Essentials of Family Medicine*. 5th ed. Philadelphia, PA: Lippincott Williams & Wilkins; 2008

Wilson PE, Penget KB. Sports medicine. In: Hay WW, Levin MJ, Sondheimer JM, Deterding RR, eds. *Current Pediatric Diagnosis & Treatment*. 19th ed. New York, NY: McGraw-Hill; 2009.

CHAPTER 20

Otolaryngology and Eye

Gary R. Uremovich, DMin, MPAS, PA-C, DFAAPA

DIRECTIONS: Each of the numbered items or incomplete statements in this section is followed by answers or completion of the statement. Select the ONE lettered answer or completion that is BEST in each case.

1. Melissa is a 7-year-old girl who is brought to her pediatrician by her mother for evaluation of a 2-day history of fever (temperature, 101°F), sore throat, and redness and tearing in both eyes. She denies any cough, nasal congestion, or any pain or photophobia in her eyes. Melissa has been taking swimming lessons 2 days a week for the past month. Findings on physical examination include copious watery discharge and scanty exudate in both eyes, prominent follicles present on both her conjunctiva and pharyngeal mucosa, and nontender preauricular lymphadenopathy. The most appropriate treatment for Melissa at this time is which of the following?

   (A) penicillin to be taken four times a day by mouth
   (B) topical or systemic antiviral such as acyclovir
   (C) only symptomatic treatment required
   (D) instillation of a mast cell stabilizer to each eye
   (E) culture of ocular exudate

2. A 35-year-old man presents to your office complaining of a painless, localized swelling of his left lower eyelid that has developed over a period of weeks. He comes in today because it is now producing a foreign body sensation in his left eye. On physical examination, his visual acuity is normal and there is no evidence of injection or discharge. There is a nontender, localized nodule on the lower eyelid. What is the likely diagnosis?

   (A) hordeolum
   (B) chalazion
   (C) pterygium
   (D) dacryocystitis
   (E) blepharitis

3. A 50-year-old man presents with an acute and painless onset of a bright red blood patch along the lateral part of his sclera. His visual acuity is normal and blood pressure is within normal limits. He has had a cough, which is getting better. What is the most appropriate treatment?

   (A) no treatment is needed
   (B) computed tomography (CT) scan to rule out intracranial hemorrhage
   (C) complete blood cell count and bleeding studies
   (D) emergent consultation with an ophthalmologist
   (E) a complete intraocular examination with dilation

4. A 43-year-old man presents with complaint of a 3-day history of localized pain, redness, and swelling of his upper eyelid. He denies fever, visual changes, or photophobia. On physical examination, the patient's eyelid is diffusely red, with a tender, localized area of swelling, which points outward. He appears to have an infection of the glands of the upper eyelid. The most common pathogen associated with this infection is which of the following?

    (A) *Staphylococcus aureus*
    (B) *Streptococcus pneumoniae*
    (C) *Haemophilus influenzae*
    (D) *Candida albicans*
    (E) *Aspergillus* species

5. A 38-year-old man presents to the emergency department complaining of persistent double vision after being hit in the left eye during a fistfight the night before. On physical examination, his left periorbital area is markedly edematous and ecchymotic. On the basis of his history, what other abnormal finding might you expect to find as you complete your ophthalmic examination, and what diagnostic study would you order to best confirm your diagnosis?

    (A) hyphema; Schiotz tonometer
    (B) hyphema; plain radiograph
    (C) restricted ocular movement; CT scan
    (D) restricted ocular movement; plain radiograph
    (E) ruptured globe; retinal angiography

6. A 45-year-old woman presents with sudden onset of excruciating pain in the right eye, blurred vision, nausea, and vomiting. Physical examination reveals decreased visual acuity, intraocular pressure of 70 mm Hg, shallow anterior chamber, steamy cornea, and a moderately dilated right pupil. Which of the following is the most likely diagnosis?

    (A) retinal detachment
    (B) retinal artery occlusion
    (C) uveitis
    (D) primary open angle glaucoma
    (E) primary acute angle closure glaucoma

7. What is the leading cause of permanent vision loss in people older than 65 years in the United States?

    (A) diabetic retinopathy
    (B) glaucoma
    (C) hypertensive retinopathy
    (D) cataracts
    (E) age-related macular degeneration (ARMD)

8. A 75-year-old man presents with painless, sudden loss of vision in one eye. A careful history reveals previous episodes of vision loss that resolved spontaneously. A workup for these previous episodes included a carotid ultrasound, which confirmed a diagnosis of bilateral carotid stenosis. Given this patient's current symptoms and medical history, which of the following findings would be expected on funduscopic examination?

    (A) retinal lines that have the appearance of a "ripple on a pond" or a "billowing sail"
    (B) a pale or milky retina with a cherry-red fovea
    (C) enlarged physiologic cup, occupying more than half of the disc's diameter
    (D) swollen disc with blurred margins; physiologic cup is not visible
    (E) yellowish-orange to creamy-pink disc with sharp margins and a centrally located physiologic cup

9. A 35-year-old woman presents with a history of a self-limited upper respiratory illness 3 weeks prior to this clinic visit. She now complains of persistent weakness and malaise, which worsens near the end of the day. She complains that she has a difficult time keeping her right eye open during the later part of the day. Taking a nap often helps. You notice that her right eyelid covers the top portion of her pupil. Pupillary reactions are normal. A complete neurological evaluation is otherwise negative. Which evaluation is most likely to confirm your preliminary diagnosis?

    (A) CT scan of the brain
    (B) lumbar puncture

(C) funduscopic examination

(D) Tensilon test

(E) psychiatric evaluation

10. A 26-year-old man presents with bilateral conjunctivitis, dysuria, and pain in his lower back and right Achilles tendonitis. What is the probable diagnosis?

   (A) ankylosing spondylitis

   (B) Reiter syndrome

   (C) Behçet disease

   (D) polyarteritis nodosa

   (E) gonococcal disease

11. A 2-year-old child presents with mild but obvious crossed-eyes since birth. Unless this is treated by an ophthalmologist, what is the likely outcome?

   (A) amblyopia

   (B) esotropia

   (C) exotropia

   (D) hypophoria

   (E) strabismus

12. A 40-year-old man presents with a history of having a fleck of metal getting into the eye while the patient was pounding on a piece of metal scrap. There is a significant subconjunctival hemorrhage with a central abrasion on the sclera. How can you rule out a perforation of the globe?

   (A) Apply gentle pressure to the globe to see if there is extrusion.

   (B) Perform a magnetic resonance imaging test.

   (C) Perform a Schiotz tonometry test.

   (D) Perform a test using fluorescein dye.

   (E) Do nothing until cleared by an ophthalmologist.

13. A 65-year-old woman fell down and bumped her head earlier in the evening. She now presents with a sensation of flashing lights and floaters in her right eye. She has a history of diabetic retinopathy. She now has decreased visual acuity and feels that there is a curtain over her visual field. Funduscopic examination is difficult and, therefore, nondiagnostic since the patient is on eye drops for glaucoma. What is the most appropriate disposition for this patient?

   (A) emergency referral to an ophthalmologist

   (B) fasting blood glucose level

   (C) CT scan of the head

   (D) neurologic evaluation

   (E) admission to the hospital for head injury observation

14. A 24-year-old man is working in a factory and felt a speck of material get into his eye, which was quite painful. He flushed out his eye at work but still complains of pain. He states that blinking makes the pain worse. The eye is very red. What is your next step?

   (A) patch the eye and refer to the ophthalmologist

   (B) flourescein staining

   (C) cycloplegics to reduce the patient's pain

   (D) slit-lamp examination

   (E) evert the upper eyelid

15. A 10-year-old boy presents with a fibrous nodule under his upper eyelid. It has been present for a couple of months. There is no drainage or pain. What is the most likely diagnosis?

   (A) chalazion

   (B) stye

   (C) chronic dacryocystitis

   (D) dacryocystocele

   (E) foreign body reaction

16. A 60-year-old man presents with long-standing poorly controlled hypertension. Which of the following is/are generally *not* associated with hypertensive retinopathy?

   (A) AV nicking with focal arteriolar damage

   (B) copper wire arterioles

   (C) decreased AV ratio

   (D) papilledema

   (E) microaneurysms and hard exudates

17. A 62-year-old woman presents with a 3-week history of progressively more painful and worsening external otitis. She is a type 2 diabetic patient and has been poorly controlled on oral hypoglycemics. Examination demonstrates a foul-smelling purulent drainage and the presence of granulation tissue within the auditory canal. The tympanic membrane (TM) appears to be normal and mobile to pneumatic testing. What is the most appropriate management decision at this time?

(A) Debride the canal and start on oral antipseudomonal antibiotics (eg, ofloxacin).

(B) Perform a Gram stain and culture of the discharge.

(C) Request an emergent CT of the head.

(D) Prescribe oral antibiotics, topical otic antibacterial drops, and effective pain management.

(E) Improve management of the diabetes to improve efficacy of conservative therapy.

18. A 16-year-old boy presents with a history of injury to his left pinna while competing at a wrestling match. The superior outer portion of the pinna is edematous and fluctuant to palpation (Figure 20-1). There is minimal

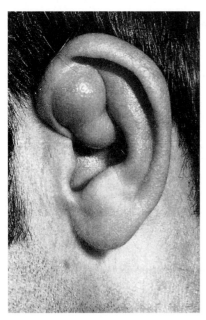

Figure 20-1
(*From Becker W, Naumann HH, Pfaltz CR, Buckingham RA, eds. Atlas of Ear, Nose and Throat Diseases. 2nd ed. New York, NY: Thieme; 1994, with permission.*)

tenderness to palpation. Which of the following management decisions is most appropriate?

(A) Refer the patient for incision and drainage (I&D) and pressure dressing.

(B) Have the patient return only if he develops a fever (temperature, 101°F).

(C) Apply a soft, bulky, and loose-fitting dressing to protect the pinna.

(D) Prescribe a 10-day course of amoxicillin and schedule for a clinic follow-up.

(E) Perform an I&D only if the pinna becomes red and tender.

19. A 65-year-old man with a history of diabetes mellitus presents with an acute episode of left facial paralysis. He is still able to wrinkle and elevate both sides of his forehead. He denies recent viral illness or ear pain. His diabetes has been well controlled. Examination of the tympanic membranes and the external pinnae are normal. The Weber and Rinné tuning fork assessments are normal. Visual acuity, extraocular movement, and pupillary responses are all normal and equal bilaterally. Which of the following is the most likely diagnosis?

(A) Bell palsy

(B) Ramsay–Hunt syndrome

(C) cerebrovascular accident

(D) peripheral facial nerve palsy

(E) diabetic neuropathy

20. A patient presents with a 3-day history of vertigo associated with turning over in bed, which lasts for several minutes. There are no other symptoms of the ear. Dix–Hallpike testing shows rotary nystagmus, which diminishes with repeated testing. Which of the following is the most likely diagnosis?

(A) central nervous system (CNS) lesion

(B) positional vertigo

(C) labyrinthitis

(D) Meniere disease

(E) vestibular neuronitis

21. A 33-year-old woman presents with episodes of vertigo lasting about 20 minutes and associated with fluctuating hearing loss and a low-frequency nonpulsatile tinnitus in the affected ear. After these episodes of vertigo, the patient states that her hearing improves and the tinnitus resolves. Which of the following illnesses is suggested by these symptoms?

    (A) Meniere disease
    (B) eustachian tube dysfunction
    (C) vestibular neuronitis
    (D) paroxysmal positional vertigo
    (E) none of the above

22. A 55-year-old woman patient presents with a lengthy history of chronic ear infections and episodic purulent drainage from the right ear canal. The patient is without symptoms at this time. Examination of the tympanic membrane shows it to be retracted with a pocket of white material within the pars flaccida (Figure 20-2). What is this finding called?

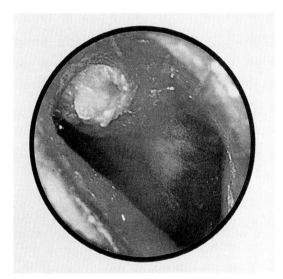

Figure 20-2
(*From Becker W, Naumann HH, Pfaltz CR, Buckingham RA, eds. Atlas of Ear, Nose and Throat Diseases. 2nd ed, New York, NY: Thieme; 1994, with permission.*)

    (A) tympanosclerosis
    (B) otosclerosis
    (C) cholesteatoma
    (D) keratosis obliterans
    (E) chronic otitis media

23. A 35-year-old man presents with a 1-week history of a marked decrease of hearing in his right ear. He denies trauma, otorrhea, or vertigo. The physical examination appears to be normal except for his tuning fork tests. The Weber test lateralizes to the better ear and the Rinné test shows air conduction to be better than bone conduction in both ears. After confirmation of your findings with an audiometric evaluation, what would be the most appropriate treatment?

    (A) broad-spectrum antibiotic
    (B) nasal steroids
    (C) decongestant
    (D) oral steroids
    (E) Antihistamines

24. A 60-year-old woman presents with an acute onset of left facial nerve paralysis. She has severe pain. You notice that she has vesicles on the pinna. What is the name of this syndrome?

    (A) Bell palsy
    (B) Ramsay–Hunt
    (C) Möbius
    (D) Millard–Gubler
    (E) Melkersson–Rosenthal

25. A 50-year-old woman presents with a progressive sense of decreased hearing in her right ear over several years. Her father had hearing problems at a young age but never was evaluated. She denies trauma, noise exposure, or ear disease as a child. Your examination demonstrates a completely normal-appearing tympanic membrane, which is mobile to pneumatic testing. Tuning fork tests show a Weber test that lateralizes to the affected (right) ear. Air conduction is greater than bone conduction of the left; on the right bone conduction is greater than air conduction. What is your diagnosis?

    (A) serous otitis media
    (B) otosclerosis
    (C) presbycusis
    (D) tympanosclerosis
    (E) idiopathic hearing loss

26. A 14-year-old boy presents with a history of "swimmer's ear," which was treated with Cortisporin Otic suspension 3 days prior. He now presents with increased erythema and crusting around the outer ear canal and a weeping somewhat vesicular area that extends below the tragus. His pain has increased. What is the likely diagnosis?

(A) *Pseudomonas* otitis externa
(B) mastoiditis
(C) Ramsay–Hunt syndrome
(D) neomycin allergy
(E) necrotizing otitis externa

27. A 59-year-old woman presents with severe right ear pain for the last week. She also complains that the ear hurts most when chewing. Her hearing has not been affected. Examination shows tenderness to palpation of the external canal meatus anteriorly. The tympanic membrane is clear. What is the most likely diagnosis?

(A) otitis externa
(B) otitis media
(C) temporomandibular joint dysfunction
(D) furuncle of the canal
(E) chondritis

28. Which of the following conditions is the most common for predisposing someone to developing acute sinusitis?

(A) viral infection of the upper respiratory tract
(B) dental infections
(C) intranasal foreign body
(D) barotrauma from deep-sea diving or airplane travel
(E) nasal steroid use

29. A 45-year-old man presents with decreased nasal flow from either nostril. He first noticed this when smoking and saw a decrease in the volume of air coming from one nostril and then reversing. Otherwise, he does not feel as if he is having problems breathing. He denies purulent drainage or facial pain. What treatment is most appropriate?

(A) nasal steroid sprays
(B) topical nasal decongestants
(C) oral decongestant
(D) saline irrigation
(E) no treatment necessary

30. A 3-year-old boy presents with a 2-week history of purulent rhinorrhea from his right nostril. Mother complains that the child's nose has a bad odor. What is the most likely diagnosis?

(A) maxillary sinusitis
(B) ethmoid sinusitis
(C) foreign body
(D) nasal polyp
(E) acute viral rhinitis

31. A young woman in her second trimester of pregnancy complains of chronic nasal congestion. She denies rhinorrhea, facial pain, or fever. She has not had previous problems with nasal symptoms until the last several weeks. It seems to be getting worse. Your examination of the nose and throat is normal. What is your diagnosis?

(A) allergic rhinitis
(B) perennial rhinitis
(C) vasomotor rhinitis
(D) rhinitis of pregnancy
(E) chronic rhinitis

32. Which nasal condition, if found in young children, is suggestive of cystic fibrosis?

(A) chronic rhinorrhea
(B) nasal polyps
(C) choanal atresia
(D) perennial allergic rhinitis
(E) acute sinusitis

33. Parents bring their 14-year-old son in for several severe nosebleeds from his left nostril over the past 2 weeks. There is a large reddish-brown mass within the left posterior nasal cavity. What is this mass?

(A) blood clot
(B) inverting papilloma
(C) hemorrhagic polyp

(D) septal hematoma

(E) juvenile angiofibroma

34. Which is the most common site of epistaxis in adults?

    (A) anterior septum

    (B) posterior septum

    (C) inferior turbinate

    (D) superior nasal vault

    (E) floor of nose

35. An elderly patient with a history of hypertension, diabetes mellitus, and supraventricular tachycardia presents with a brisk episode of epistaxis from the left nostril and a mild amount of bleeding from the right nostril. The bleeding first occurred last night and lasted for about 10 minutes and then stopped. It has now been continuously bleeding for about 20 minutes. You are in the emergency department and are unable to visualize the bleeding site because of the extent of bleeding from the left nostril. What is the most appropriate next step in your evaluation?

    (A) Get a detailed history of medications, prior surgery, prior episodes of epistaxis, and possible nasal disease. Review prior medical records if available.

    (B) Perform diagnostic laboratory work including complete blood cell counts and hemoglobin, hematocrit, and clotting factor levels. Prepare the patient for vitamin K administration.

    (C) Assess the hemodynamic state of the individual by obtaining blood pressures including a "tilt" test to rule out hypovolemia, pulse, and electrocardiogram and cardiac monitoring.

    (D) Start a large bore intravenous (IV) line and provide at least 1 L of lactated Ringer's solution. Start oxygen by mask with a flow of at least 2 L/min.

    (E) Focus your attention on the bleeding. Carefully insert a cotton pledget soaked in a topical vasoconstricter (eg, oxymetazoline) and pinching the nose. If this fails to slow down the bleeding, insert a nasal tampon or one of the many commercially prepared emergency nasal packs.

36. A 26-year-old healthy-appearing man presents with rhinorrhea since having a nondisplaced nasal fracture 3 weeks prior. According to the patient, his nose has completely healed and feels fine now. He complains of a short gushes of a clear salty tasting liquid out his right nostril several times a day. He states that he can sometimes precipitate the drainage by leaning his head forward. Which test should you run on this liquid?

    (A) "bull's-eye" test

    (B) specific gravity

    (C) Gram stain

    (D) culture and sensitivity

    (E) glucose dipstick

37. A 20-year-old male patient sustains a blow to his nose during a disagreement with some friends 5 or 6 days prior to his visit today. He complains that his breathing progressively worsened despite a decrease in external nasal swelling. Your examination shows soft fluctuant swelling of the septum bilaterally. This area is not tender to palpation. What is your treatment plan?

    (A) nasal steroids for a couple of weeks to reduce intranasal swelling

    (B) broad-spectrum antibiotic to prevent abscess formation

    (C) emergent referral to an ear, nose, and throat (ENT) provider

    (D) CT scan to rule out a complex nasal fracture

    (E) needle aspiration of the fluctuant area with cultures

38. The most common cause of chronic cough in adults is which of the following?

    (A) common cold

    (B) sinusitis

    (C) asthma

    (D) postnasal drip syndrome

    (E) gastroesophageal reflux disease

39. An elderly patient presents with slurred speech. You have her protrude her tongue and it deviates to the right. Which cranial nerve (CN) is involved?

    (A) left CN XII
    (B) right CN XII
    (C) left CN X
    (D) right CN X
    (E) left CN IX

40. A 45-year-old white man presents with a history of persistent fatigue throughout the day despite a full night of sleep. He complains of a sore throat and headache each morning. He has used short-acting sleeping pills, which only seem to worsen his symptoms. He is being treated for poorly controlled hypertension. The patient is morbidly obese. Which of the following conditions is most likely for this patient?

    (A) endogenous depression
    (B) diabetes mellitus
    (C) hypothyroidism
    (D) obstructive sleep apnea (OSA)
    (E) Cushing syndrome

41. A 14-year-old boy presents with a history of unilateral tonsillitis from a previous visit. His mother has noticed that his right tonsil has continued to rapidly enlarge over a period of 6 weeks despite a 10-day course of treatment with amoxicillin. The pharynx is normal except for a unilaterally enlarged tonsil on the right. There is no exudate or inflammation noted. Careful oral palpation and comparison of the tonsils demonstrates a firm nontender right tonsil that is 50% larger than the tonsil on the left. He has nontender right anterior cervical adenopathy. A complete blood cell count and differential is within normal limits. Which of the following is most appropriate in managing this patient?

    (A) Obtain an urgent surgical consult for tonsillectomy.
    (B) Prescribe an alternative antibiotic and schedule for routine follow-up.

    (C) Perform a monospot test.
    (D) Reassure the patient and his mother that this is normal after tonsillitis and that the tonsil will eventually decrease in size as the patient ages.
    (E) Request a soft tissue lateral radiograph to rule out a retropharyngeal abscess.

42. A patient presents with swelling and mild edema of the right ear canal after swimming. What is the most appropriate initial treatment?

    (A) oral antibiotics to prevent further swelling
    (B) insert an otowick into the canal to prevent the canal from closing
    (C) antibacterial ear drops
    (D) vigorous irrigation with saline to clean the ear
    (E) self-limited disorder requiring no treatment

43. A child with a history of a recent episode of acute otitis media presents with a painful swelling of the area behind the right ear. There is protrusion of the ear. The child is febrile and looks very ill. You notice that he has a right facial paresis. Your examination shows a hyperemic and bulging right tympanic membrane (TM) with a purulent effusion. The TM is immobile to pneumatic testing. What is your next step?

    (A) Insert an otowick and start the child on antibiotic otic drops to prevent further extension of the infection.
    (B) Admit the child to a pediatric service to watch and wait for additional CNS extension.
    (C) Consult ENT immediately for an emergent consult.
    (D) Prescribe high-dose amoxicillin (80 mg/kg/day in divided doses for 10 days).
    (E) Perform close outpatient follow-up the following day after prescribing oral antibiotics.

44. A 24-year-old woman patient presents with an acute onset of right facial paralysis. She woke with some discomfort behind the right ear and noted weakness of the face. She complains of a bitter taste in her mouth. Examination of the ear and face is completely normal. She has no history of rash, tick bites, or diabetes. What is the most appropriate treatment of this condition?

    (A) IV steroids
    (B) oral antibiotics alone
    (C) antiviral and antibiotic medications
    (D) eye precautions and saline eye drops
    (E) oral steroids and antiviral medications

45. A 60-year-old man presents with a 2-week history of sensation of spinning when turning over in bed at night. He occasionally has a spinning sensation when turning his head to the right. He denies tinnitus or decrease in his hearing. He also complains about ringing in his ear and notes that his wife complains about his inability to hear. He hears a pulsating sound in his right ear, which is worse at night. What is your diagnosis?

    (A) central vertigo
    (B) benign paroxysmal positional vertigo
    (C) labyrinthine neuronitis
    (D) viral labyrinthitis
    (E) basilar migraine

46. A febrile, 18-year-old boy presents with a 4-day history of sore throat that has suddenly become much worse. He complains of pain when attempting to eat or drink and has difficulty opening his mouth. He has a "hot potato" voice. On the basis of this clinical presentation, what is your diagnosis?

    (A) epiglottis
    (B) retropharyngeal abscess
    (C) croup
    (D) tonsillitis
    (E) peritonsillar abscess

47. A 70-year-old man presents to the emergency department with a 3-hour history of severe epistaxis from the right nostril. A bleeding site cannot be visualized. It is not controlled with a nasal decongestant, firm digital pressure of the nares, or anterior packing. Persistent bleeding is noted in the pharynx despite these measures. The patient is currently on a prophylactic antiplatelet medication. What is the most appropriate assessment or treatment while awaiting an ENT consultation?

    (A) CT scan of the sinuses
    (B) Foley catheter and anterior pack to stop a posterior bleed
    (C) sedation
    (D) transfusion
    (E) replace the anterior packing

48. A 45-year-old man presents with chronic nasal congestion. He has been using a topical 12-hour-duration nasal decongestant for the last several weeks, which has, up until recently, been very effective. Initially, he used it only a couple of times per day. Now, he states that he has to use it every 2 to 3 hours. If he does not use the nasal spray, he feels very congested and cannot breathe. He denies purulent drainage or epistaxis. What is your diagnosis?

    (A) deviated septum
    (B) allergic rhinitis
    (C) nasal polyps
    (D) rhinitis medicamentosa
    (E) chronic sinusitis

49. A patient presents with a history of a cold for the last 10 days or so. Initially, she thought she was getting better. However, during the last couple of days, she has had a fever, increasing right maxillary facial pain, and copious purulent drainage from the right nostril. What is the most appropriate next step?

   (A) Treat as an acute episode of sinusitis.
   (B) Order a CT scan to confirm a bacterial infection.
   (C) Treat symptomatically with decongestants and Tylenol.
   (D) Perform a culture on the drainage and await the results before treating.
   (E) Refer to an otolaryngologist.

50. A 15-year-old boy presents with an exudative tonsillitis. Anterior and posterior cervical lymph nodes are enlarged and tender. The rapid antigen test for strep is negative for group A β-hemolytic streptococcus. What is the most appropriate step in treating this disease?

   (A) Treat presumptively with penicillin.
   (B) Check for a history of recurrent tonsillitis.
   (C) Wait for confirmation of the disease with a formal culture.
   (D) Assume it is viral and, therefore, self-limited.
   (E) Perform a serum assay for mononucleosis.

Answers and Explanations

1. **(C)** Melissa's symptoms (fever, pharyngitis, and conjunctivitis) and findings on examination, particularly nontender preauricular lymphadenopathy, are characteristic of a viral conjunctivitis. This condition is found more commonly in children, and contaminated swimming pools are sometimes the source of infection. There is no specific treatment, but the conjunctivitis is self-limited, usually lasting about 10 days. Symptomatic treatment would include antipyretics such as acetaminophen. Application of topical antibiotics is occasionally recommended to prevent secondary infection. Penicillin, indicated for streptococcal pharyngitis, would not be appropriate because there are no physical examination findings such as pharyngeal erythema, tonsillar exudate, or tender cervical adenopathy to support the diagnosis. Acyclovir may be helpful in the treatment of herpes simplex virus conjunctivitis, which is a disease characterized by unilateral injection, irritation, mucoid discharge, pain, and mild photophobia. A mast cell stabilizer would be helpful in allergic conjunctivitis to alleviate symptoms of itching, a symptom that Melissa did not complain of. *(Ehlers et al., 2008, pp. 102-104)*

2. **(B)** A chalazion is a sterile granulomatous inflammation of a meibomian gland usually characterized by a hard, painless, localized swelling on the upper or lower eyelid that develops over weeks. It can be differentiated from hordeolum (stye) by the absence of acute, inflammatory signs. Most chalazia point toward the conjunctival surface and if large enough can produce a foreign body sensation and/or distort vision. A pterygium is a disorder of the conjunctiva, not the eyelid itself. Dacryocystitis also involves inflammation and is characterized as a warm, tender, localized infection of the lacrimal sac. Blepharitis is usually bilateral and involves inflammation of the entire lid margins. *(Ehlers et al., 2008, pp. 130-131, 137-138)*

3. **(A)** No treatment is needed for a subconjunctival hemorrhage. The sudden onset and bright red appearance can be quite alarming for the patient. The hemorrhage is caused by rupture of a small conjunctival vessel and may be associated with sneezing or coughing. The best treatment is reassurance. The blood is reabsorbed within 2 weeks. *(Ehlers et al., 2008, pp. 112-113)*

4. **(A)** The symptoms and findings described are associated with a hordeolum, which is most often caused by a staphylococcal infection, usually *S aureus*. *(Ehlers et al., 2008, pp. 130-131)*

5. **(C)** A history of facial/orbital trauma that results in diplopia is suggestive of an orbital blowout fracture causing entrapment. As a result, one would expect to find restriction of extraocular movements. Although plain radiographs may be helpful in the initial identification of bony injury, CT scanning with axial and coronal views provides the best assessment of orbital trauma. A hyphema is a possible abnormal finding in this patient as well but would not require radiographs or tonometry. *(Ehlers et al., 2008, pp. 28-30)*

6. **(E)** The patient's symptoms, abnormal findings noted on the eye examination, and her significantly elevated intraocular pressure of 70 mm Hg (normal range of intraocular pressure is

10–24 mm Hg) are all consistent with a diagnosis of acute angle closure glaucoma. This type of glaucoma is an ophthalmic emergency requiring immediate reduction in the intraocular pressure. Primary open angle glaucoma is the most common form of glaucoma; it is a chronic condition that is often asymptomatic until the disease is far advanced. Both retinal detachment and retinal artery occlusion are painless disorders with abnormal findings on examination that are different than those stated. (*Ehlers et al., 2008, pp. 198-202*)

7. **(E)** Age-related macular degeneration (ARMD) was formerly known as *macular degeneration*. It leads to loss of fine or central vision with sparing of lateral or peripheral vision. There is no cure for ARMD but occasional laser surgery can be helpful. Multivitamins with β-carotene and vitamin E have been shown to delay progression in some patients. (*Riordan-Eva, 2010, pp. 162-163*)

8. **(B)** A central retinal artery occlusion occurs as a result of a small emboli breaking loose from sclerotic plaque and lodging in retinal arterioles. The patient has a history of transient visual loss (amaurosis fugax), which often occurs with small recurrent emboli. Ophthalmoscopy reveals a pale retina with a cherry-red spot at the fovea. The funduscopic examination findings described in answer (A) are consistent with retinal detachment; in answer (C), the findings are consistent with glaucoma; in answer (D), the findings are consistent with papilledema; and in answer (E), the findings are normal. (*Ehlers et al., 2008, pp. 282-284*)

9. **(D)** Tensilon (edrophonium) testing will confirm that this patient has a classic presentation of myasthenia gravis. The usual adult test dose of 0.2 cm^3 edrophonium chloride is given intravenously. The eyelids are assessed for improvement in function. Additional dosing is provided in 0.2 cm^3 increments to total of 1.0 cm^3. Unilateral ptosis is often a presenting sign and worsens with fatigue and can improve with a nap. Often, the ptosis will become bilateral. The weakness increases and often shows diurnal variation. This disease most often affects young adults aged 20 to 40 years and

often occurs after an illness, stress, injury, or pregnancy. It involves cholinesterase destroying acetylcholine at the myoneural junction. It may be an autoimmune disease with the production of antiacetylcholine antibodies causing reduction in the replacement of acetylcholine. Cholinesterase-inhibiting drugs can reverse the ptosis and fatigue associated with myasthenia gravis. The differential diagnosis in this case could include multiple sclerosis and brain stem lesions. Respectively, absence of sensory deficits or pupil abnormalities rule against these. It is unlikely that a psychiatric etiology would result in unilateral ptosis and there are no signs suggesting infection of the spinal fluid. (*Ehlers et al., 2008, pp. 284-287*)

10. **(B)** Reiter syndrome is a disorder that consists of the triad of arthritis, conjunctivitis, and urinary tract symptoms. Reiter syndrome is sometimes referred to as a *reactive arthritis*, which is responding to an infection elsewhere in the body. Reiter syndrome develops in 1% to 3% of men after a nonspecific urethritis, up to 4% of persons after enteric infections caused by *Shigella, Salmonella,* and *Campylobacter;* and in a higher proportion of patients with *Yersinia* enteric infections. The major criteria include polyarthritis, conjunctivitis or anterior uveitis, urethritis or cervicitis, and balanitis circinata or keratoderma blennorrhagicum. The minor criteria include plantar fasciitis, Achilles tendonitis, lower back pain, sacroiliitis, and spondylitis; keratitis; cystitis and prostatitis; psoriasiform eruptions, oral ulcers, and nail changes; and diarrhea, leukocytosis, increased serum globulins, and evidence of inflammation in the synovial fluid. The diagnosis of Reiter syndrome is based on history and medical examination. (*Hellman and Imboden, 2010, p. 776*)

11. **(A)** Amblyopia is the permanent loss of visual acuity in a child from abnormal visual experience during the maturation phase of sight development. During this maturation phase, it is critical for the retina and central nervous system to become integrated. Strabismus ("crossed-eyes") or any disorder that causes a blurred retinal image in one or both eyes can lead to this permanent visual disorder. The eye

causing the blurred image is ignored by the central nervous system, thereby preventing neurological integration of that eye. Treatments center on forcing the ignored eye to be actively involved in perception. Interventions range from patching the good eye to force use of the amblyopic eye, use of special glasses, or surgical correction of the ocular muscles. The other answers are descriptions of muscles weakness. *(Ehlers et al., 2008, pp. 277-278)*

12. **(D)** Perform a special fluorescein dye examination of the eye. Since there is a possibility of globe penetration, the Seidel test should be performed. A moistened fluorescein dye strip is gently applied directly to the site of the injury. Slit-lamp examination is performed with cobalt blue light. If a perforation or leak is present, the fluorescein dye will be diluted by aqueous fluid from the injured site. It will appear as a dark (ie, diluted) stream within a pool of bright green (ie, concentrated) dye. This is known as the *Seidel sign* or a *positive Seidel test*. If globe rupture is suspected or confirmed, an eye shield should be immediately placed over the affected eye and further direct examination should be deferred to avoid putting pressure on the eye. Computed tomography of the head and orbits (coronal and axial views) is recommended. *(Pokhrel and Loftus, 2007, pp. 829-836)*

13. **(A)** Emergency referral to an ophthalmologist is the most appropriate disposition for this patient. Patients with retinal detachment often complain of unilateral photopsia (ie, sensation of flashing light), an increasing number of floaters in the affected eye signifying posterior vitreous detachment, decreased visual acuity, and metamorphopsia (ie, wavy distortion of an object). Floaters may move in and out of central vision. Vision loss may be curtain-like, filmy, or cloudy. If the macula or the central vision is involved, the patient may lose the ability to read, have loss of light perception, or may not be able to see a hand waved in front of his or her face. If retinal detachment is suspected from patient history alone, immediate referral to an ophthalmologist is warranted, especially for persons with known risk factors. *(Pokhrel and Loftus, 2007, pp. 829-836)*

14. **(E)** Everting the upper eyelid will help discover a foreign body. Conjunctival foreign bodies are very painful. Irrigation is important to remove debris from the eye. However, sometimes a speck of material can become lodged under the upper eyelid. The persistent presence of the foreign body continues to damage the cornea each time the patient blinks. The eyelid should be everted by using a cotton-tipped applicator. Carefully examine the area under the upper eyelid. Foreign bodies are usually 2 to 3 mm from the lid margin and are easily removed with a moistened cotton-tipped applicator. This should be done before applying analgesic drops or even staining the eye. *(Sullivan, 2008, p. 341)*

15. **(A)** A chalazion is a chronic inflammatory lesion of the eyelid not associated with conjunctivitis. It is a granulomatous reactionary lesion that may persist for weeks or even months. These lesions are usually rubbery and are nontender to palpation. Styes are often along the rim of the lid and cause discomfort. Lesions of the lacrimal system are medial to the lids and are fluctuant. Often, chalazia resolve without treatment. However, if they persist for more than 6 weeks, they probably should be removed to rule out an underlying sebaceous carcinoma. *(Horton, 2008, p. 184)*

16. **(E)** Microanyeursms and hard exudates are associated with diabetic retinopathy. There are two classification systems for hypertensive retinopathy. The Keith–Wagner–Barker Classification system considers vascular, retinal and disc changes rated I to IV. Groups I to III include the clinical findings of vascular changes (decreased caliber of arterioles, crossing changes), cotton-wool spots, and hemorrhages. Group 4 includes papilledema. *(Seidel et al., 2006, pp. 297-300)*

17. **(C)** The most pressing need at this time is to confirm the diagnosis of malignant external otitis (osteomyelitis of the skull base) by documenting osseous erosion with a CT scan. Persistent external otitis in a diabetic or any immunocompromised patient can evolve into osteomyelitis and extend into the skull base. Patients complain of a deep excruciating pain and foul drainage. Finding granulation tissue

within the ear canal and the presence of cranial nerve palsies are suggestive of this condition. Occasionally, surgical debridement of infected bone is needed if aggressive medical treatment does not control the infection. *(Grunstein et al., 2008, pp. 630-632)*

18. **(A)** The skin of the pinna is tightly bound to the perichondrium of the cartilage. The cartilage depends on the perichondrium for vascular nourishment. Blunt trauma to the pinna can result in a hematoma or seroma and can cause the perichondrium to become detached from the cartilage. The devascularized cartilage dies and can eventually cause a permanent "cauliflower" deformity of the pinna. Strict aseptic technique during the I&D and a tightly formed compressive dressing is necessary to allow effective blood supply to the cartilage of the pinna without the advent of a postoperative infection. Antibiotics are often prescribed after the procedure to prevent an infection since perichondritis worsens the cosmetic damage. *(Grunstein et al., 2008, pp. 628-629)*

19. **(C)** This patient has a central lesion causing facial paralysis instead of the typical peripheral lesion seen in Bell palsy. Sparing of forehead movement in patients with facial paralysis is evidence of a lesion superior to the nucleus of the VII cranial nerve (eg, a brain tumor or stroke). A central lesion causes paralysis of the lower face on the contralateral side with sparing of the forehead since ipsilateral fibers provide innervation of the forehead. When the facial paralysis is caused by a peripheral lesion (eg, middle ear infection), there is ipsilateral paralysis involving all subsections of the VII cranial nerve including the forehead. *(Beal and Hauser, 2008, pp. 2584-2585)*

20. **(B)** This patient has positional vertigo, which is assumed to be caused by movement of a small canalith within the inner ear. This is a benign process that is often self-limited. The Dix–Hallpike is positional testing that confirms this type of vertigo. Central lesions often have dissociation of the vertigo and nystagmus. The nystagmus in this condition is often vertical and without fatigability with repeated testing.

The other three options will all have vertigo that is not altered by position and have additional ear symptoms such as tinnitus or hearing loss. In benign paroxysmal positional vertigo, positional exercises are helpful in quickening its resolution. Canalith repositioning procedures are effective at resolving the vertigo in about 80% of cases with just one outpatient treatment. *(Johnson and Lalwani, 2008, pp. 713-716)*

21. **(A)** These symptoms are classically associated with Meniere disease (endolymphatic hydrops). Therefore, any patient presenting with episodic vertigo, tinnitus, and fluctuating hearing loss should have a complete otoneurologic evaluation. In vestibular neuronitis and paroxysmal positional vertigo, the patient will have normal hearing and does not complain of tinnitus. Eustachian tube dysfunction can cause a blocked sensation in the affected ear. Usually, there is no vertigo associated with this condition. Symptoms are resolved with valsalva as the pressure is equalized in the middle ear. The physical examination and laboratory tests are usually normal in Meniere disease except for vestibular and auditory tests. Treatment initially is dietary with a low-sodium diet and occasionally diuretics. *(Johnson and Lalwani, 2008, pp. 716-720)*

22. **(C)** A cholesteatoma is a squamous epithelium–lined sac that gradually increases in size and by pressure necrosis can eventually erode through bone (ie, ossicular chain) or nerves (ie, facial nerve). It often becomes infected and causes an intermittently draining ear. Eustachian tube dysfunction causes the tympanic membrane to become retracted and invaginate upon itself within the pars flaccida. Squamous epithelium becomes entrapped and gradually leads to the formation of a cholesteatoma. Cholesteatomas can also result from perforation of the tympanic membranes involving the margin or pars flaccida. Treatment includes marsupialization of the cyst and reconstructive surgery. *(Chang, 2008, pp. 666-672)*

23. **(D)** This patient has sudden neurosensory hearing loss. The neurosensory nature of this disorder is suggested by the tuning fork tests.

Weber testing lateralizing to the affected ear would be suggestive of a conductive hearing loss (otitis media or canal obstructed with cerumen). The etiology of sudden neurosensory hearing loss is unknown but may be viral or vascular. The only treatment that has shown effectiveness is the use of corticosteroids and antiviral medications as soon as possible after the onset of symptoms. Providing therapeutic doses of prednisone within 2 weeks of the hearing loss is important. *(Bhattacharya, 2009, p. 1379)*

24. **(B)** Ramsay–Hunt syndrome (herpes zoster oticus) is a syndrome of acute peripheral facial palsy associated with otalgia and varicella-like cutaneous lesions. It is defined by intense ear pain, pathognomonic vesicles on the pinna, and facial paralysis. It is caused by the herpes varicella virus producing a shingles type of cutaneous lesion. Treatment includes steroids, antiviral medications, and pain medication. *(Lustig and Niparko, 2008, pp. 847-861)*

25. **(B)** Otosclerosis is a genetic condition in which the bones of the inner ear soften and then harden. This causes the three bones of hearing to harden at the joints, preventing them from conducting vibrations into the cochlea. The diagnosis is made by observing a completely normal appearing tympanic membrane with conductive hearing loss as noted by tuning forks. Treatment is dependent on the amount of conductive loss and can be managed with hearing aids or by a surgical procedure called a stapedectomy. A middle ear effusion (serous otitis) would be apparent with pneumatic testing. Presbycusis is ruled out since the tuning fork testing indicates a conductive deficit. Tympanosclerosis is calcium defects in the tympanic membrane that rarely cause hearing loss. The last choice, idiopathic hearing loss, is another name for sudden neurosensory hearing loss that does not fit the tuning fork tests showing conductive hearing loss. *(Boahene and Driscoll, 2008, pp. 673-682)*

26. **(D)** Cortisporin contains neomycin for which 10% to 15% of the population have a topical sensitivity. The patient should have his ear drops changed to non–neomycin-containing drops,

such as Floxin or Ciprofloxacin. If the canal is too edematous for drops to enter, an otowick may need to be inserted. Occasionally, oral steroids are needed if the swelling and allergic reactions are severe. *(Bhattacharya, 2009, p. 1401)*

27. **(C)** Temporomandibular joint dysfunction (TMJ) is a common cause of referred ear pain. The cause may be inflammation induced by a recent dental procedure or grinding teeth at bedtime (bruxism). The diagnostic clues are that the patient has pain that is worsened with chewing and she has tenderness over the TMJ within the ear canal with an otherwise normal ear examination. Treatment involves a soft diet, warm compresses, and nonsteroidal anti-inflammatory medication. Dental evaluation is often needed in patients with chronic TMJ disorders. *(Goddard, 2008, pp. 389-392)*

28. **(A)** Upper respiratory infections are the most common disorder leading to acute sinusitis. The infection develops primarily because of ostial obstruction from mucosal edema. Initially, the patients feel as if they are getting over their viral infection when they then develop a worsening of their symptoms with an increase in purulent drainage, facial pain, and fever. *(Rubin et al., 2008, pp. 205-206; Shah et al., 2008, pp. 274-275)*

29. **(E)** No treatment is necessary. This is a normal physiological process called *nasal cycle*. Many people become aware of this cycle when sleeping. It allows the nasal mucosa to more effectively produce mucous that can trap particles. *(Wilson, 2004, p. 117)*

30. **(C)** Foreign bodies within the nose quickly create an unusually foul-smelling unilateral purulent drainage. The nose should be carefully decongested and anesthetized with topical solution. Care should be taken not to push the foreign body into the nasopharynx, where it can be aspirated. It is unusual to have unilateral sinusitis (such as from the maxillary or ethmoid sinuses) with purulent drainage just from one side. Acute viral rhinitis is typically thin serous drainage. Nasal polyps can create sinusitis. However, the main problem would be nasal congestion instead of purulent drainage. *(Wilson, 2004, p. 130)*

31. (D) Rhinitis of pregnancy is fairly common. Nasal congestion can peak in the third trimester. The rise in estrogen leads to a rise in hyaluronic acid in the nasal tissue, which can result in increasing nasal edema and congestion. Treatment can be recommended by the obstetrician depending on severity of symptoms and may include decongestants and nasal steroids. However, no treatment is usually required since this disorder resolves after delivery. *(Shah and Emanuel, 2008, p. 265)*

32. (B) Nasal polyps in a child should make the clinician suspicious for possible cystic fibrosis. Usually, this illness manifests itself in early childhood with predominantly lung involvement. Recurrent sinusitis and otitis media are also frequently seen. The onset of nasal polyps in these patients typically appears between the ages of 5 and 14 years. Diagnosis of cystic fibrosis is made by a sweat chloride test. *(Shah et al., 2008, pp. 262-263).*

33. (E) Juvenile angiofibromas are benign vascular tumors that tend to occur in postpubescent adolescent male persons (13–21 years of age). Typically, the patient presents with very brisk unilateral epistaxis. Biopsies are not performed in the outpatient clinic setting because of the risk of hemorrhage. *(Mandpe, 2008, pp. 289-290)*

34. (A) Anterior septal bleeding from Kiesselbach plexus is by far the most common site of epistaxis in children and adults. Often, there is a history of trauma (picking the nose) or hay fever. In adults, it is important to rule out clotting disorders, aspirin use, and a family history of epistaxis. Pinching the nose firmly, sitting upright, and leaning slightly forward is often helpful in stopping epistaxis. The site of bleeding should then be sought with a nasal speculum, topical nasal decongestant, and effective light source. Once the bleeding site is located, it could be cauterized with a silver nitrate stick. *(Wilson, 2004, pp. 146-147)*

35. (E) Stop the bleeding! Epistaxis can be life-threatening. Fortunately, most nosebleeds are mild and simple to treat; however, patients can still die from a severe nosebleed. While all of the other answers can be appropriate in the right setting, it is critical to stop a vigorous nasal bleed as soon as possible. This patient is at risk of a posterior arterial bleed because of being elderly, being a hypertensive, and taking blood thinners. If a nasal tampon or nasal packing is used, it should stay in place (as long as the bleeding is controlled) for at least 3 days. It should be removed by an ENT specialist in case bleeding recurs. Be sure to place the patient on a broad-spectrum antibiotic to prevent sinusitis (because of the blocked sinus ostia) or toxic shock syndrome from *S aureus*. *(Bhattacharya, 2009, pp. 1383-1386)*

36. (E) Glucose is present in cerebrospinal fluid (CSF) and can be detected with a urine glucose dipstick (50 to 80 mg/dL). Injuries in the region of the nasal bones and nasal process of the frontal bone may lead to a fracture through the cribiform or ethmoid bones. CSF drainage is most commonly unilateral and may be intermittent, coming in short, rapid gushes, or may present as a steady flow. A clue to a CSF leak can be gained from the characteristic "bull's-eye" test when the fluid is mixed with blood and allowed to dry on a white sheet. This is not helpful after the bleeding has stopped. Often, these leaks can seal off spontaneously by having the patient on bed rest, with the head elevated. Leaks that do not stop require more elaborate evaluation and surgical intervention. *(Wilson, 2004, pp. 155-156)*

37. (C) Emergency referral for definitive treatment of this septal hematoma is critical. The hematoma requires surgical drainage, evaluation of the septal cartilage, and use of a drain to prevent reaccumulation of the hematoma. Failure to treat a septal hematoma may lead to a septal abscess and a saddle deformity by destruction of the septal cartilage. *(Wilson, 2004, pp. 157-158)*

38. (D) Postnasal drip syndrome (PNDS) is the most common cause of a chronic cough in adults. In 30% to 60% of patients, sinusitis is postinfectious cause of the PNDS; another major cause is rhinitis of any etiology. Asthma is the second most common cause of chronic cough in adults, while gastroesophageal reflux disease is the third most common. *(Oliver, 2009, pp. 351-353)*

39. **(B)** The hypoglossal nerve (CN XII) controls movement of the tongue. A defect in this nerve will cause the tongue to deviate toward the side of the lesion. The increase in muscle tone of the innervated portion of tongue pushes it toward the weaker (contralateral) side. Further evidence of hypoglossal nerve damage can be documented by noting fasciculations and atrophy of the denervated portion of the tongue. Subtle defects can be detected by having the patient push his or her tongue against the inside of the cheek while the examiner feels the pressure exerted by the tongue against the outer cheek. The tongue muscles of the unaffected side will push more firmly against the contralateral cheek. *(Oghalai, 2008, p. 801)*

40. **(D)** Obstructive sleep apnea (OSA) syndrome is often the result of a structurally small upper airway combined with a loss of muscle tone, allowing the pharynx to collapse during inspiration. Most patients with OSA are obese, middle-aged men. Often, they have poorly controlled systemic hypertension. They frequently complain of daytime drowsiness, persistent fatigue, recent weight gain, and cognitive impairment. Use of alcohol or sedatives can worsen symptoms as seen in this patient. *(Oliver, 2009, pp. 372-376)*

41. **(A)** Unilateral tonsillar enlargement can be the presentation of lymphoma. Occasionally, one tonsil may appear larger than the other because one is more deeply placed within the tonsillar fossa. However, careful clinical examination and palpation can usually differentiate this from a truly enlarged tonsil. A malignant process is suggested by rapid growth and ipsilateral cervical adenopathy. A tonsillectomy should be performed to provide a biopsy of tissue for evaluation. Lymphoma and squamous cell carcinoma are the most common primary tonsillar neoplasms. A peritonsillar abscess is ruled out by the absence of trismus, peritonsilar swelling, and tenderness to palpation. *(Shnayder et al., 2008, pp. 343-346)*

42. **(C)** Antibacterial ear drops is the most appropriate initial treatment. The most common cause of pain in the external ear is acute otitis externa. Infections can be caused by bacteria or fungi. Water can macerate the skin of the auditory canal and raise the pH allowing for bacterial or fungal overgrowth. When a bacterial organism is suspected, treatment should include debridement of the canal and use of an antibacterial ear drop with or without steroids. The most common bacteria would be *Pseudomonas aeruginosa*, which is responsive to neomycin sulfate or fluoroquinolone drops. Neomycin preparations should not be used if there is a chance of a perforated tympanic membrane since it can be neuro-ototoxic. *(Lustig and Schindler, 2010, pp. 181-182)*

43. **(C)** An immediate emergency referral to an ENT surgeon is essential. Extension of the infection from the middle ear space into the mastoid air cells can lead to acute mastoiditis. The facial nerve courses through the middle ear and can become inflamed, leading to neuropraxia and facial paresis. An emergent ENT consult is essential for the treatment of this child. Besides requiring high-dose intravenous antibiotics, the child will probably require the insertion of a tympanostomy tube for drainage and perhaps an emergent mastoidectomy. *(Kelly et al., 2008, pp. 447-448)*

44. **(E)** Oral steroids and antiviral medications are indicated in the treatment of this patient. The patient has the typical symptoms of Bell palsy. This is an idiopathic inflammation of the VII cranial nerve (facial nerve). It is thought that it is most likely caused by a virus. The treatment for this condition is an antiviral medication and a 10-day course of a tapered-dose of steroids. *(Tiemstra and Khatkhate, 2007, pp. 1002-1004)*

45. **(B)** This patient has benign paroxysmal positional vertigo. It is stimulated by movement of the head. In the clinic, the clinician can perform a Dix–Hallpike maneuver to check for positional vertigo. Acute vestibular neuronitis and labyrinthitis are caused by viral infections. They are temporary causes of vertigo and are not dependent on positional changes. Central vertigo

is caused by an acoustic neuroma on the VII cranial nerve. Usually, this is associated with unilateral hearing loss. *(Labuguen, 2006, pp. 244-251, 254)*

46. **(E)** A peritonsillar abscess often presents with trismus, "hot potato" voice, painful swallowing, and fever. Examination of the oral cavity will demonstrate protrusion of the lateral pharynx and unilateral tonsil with deviation of the uvula away from the mass lesion. A computed tomography (CT) scan is sometimes used to differentiate between a phlegmon (inflamed tissue) and a coalesced abscess. Treatment consists of steroids, intravenous antibiotics, and surgical drainage. *(Lustig and Schindler, 2010, p. 205)*

47. **(B)** Posterior bleeding is much less common than anterior bleeding and usually is treated by an otolaryngologist. However, vigorous bleeding cannot wait for the specialist. While getting intravenous access, type, and cross, the provider can provide an effective posterior pack. Posterior packing may be accomplished by passing a catheter through one nostril (or both nostrils), through the nasopharynx, and out the mouth. If a specialized balloon device is not available, a Foley catheter (10 to 14 French) with a 30-mL balloon may be used. The catheter is inserted through the bleeding nostril and visualized in the oropharynx before inflation of the balloon. The balloon then is inflated with approximately 10 mL of saline, and the catheter is withdrawn gently through the nostril, pulling the balloon up and forward. The balloon should seat in the posterior nasal cavity and tamponade a posterior bleed. After the balloon is situated, a nasal tampon can be inserted along the medial portion of the anterior nasal vault and both secured with tape. There are commercial products (eg, Epistat) that include both a posterior and anterior ballon. *(Kucik and Clenney, 2005, pp. 305-311, 312)*

48. **(D)** Persistent and repetitive use of topical α-adrenergic decongestant sprays (such as oxymetazoline) for more than 5 to 7 consecutive days is associated with rebound nasal congestion after withdrawal. This phenomenon is termed *rhinitis medicamentosa*. Extensive use of these over-the-counter sprays can cause inflammatory mucosal hypertrophy and chronic congestion. The patient should discontinue using the topical decongestant, which will resolve the problem. This can be difficult for patients. Use of steroidal nasal sprays can be helpful. *(Quillen and Feller, 2006, 1583-1590)*

49. **(A)** The diagnosis of acute bacterial sinusitis (ABS) is based on clinical signs and symptoms and does not require radiographic assessment. Having a cold and then suddenly worsening is called *second sickening* and is associated with a viral infection complicated by a secondary, bacterial infection. Treatment is with topical decongestants, oral decongestants, mucolytics, and antibiotics. Usually amoxicillin or amoxicillin–clavulanic acid (Augmentin) is the initial antibiotic followed by cephalosporins or fluoroquinolone. Antibiotic therapy should be reserved for patients who have had symptoms for more than 7 days and meet clinical criteria. Four signs and symptoms that are the most helpful in predicting ABS include purulent nasal discharge, maxillary tooth or facial pain (especially unilateral), unilateral maxillary sinus tenderness, and a sudden worsening of symptoms after initial improvement. *(Scheid and Hamm, 2004, pp. 1685-1692)*

50. **(E)** Infectious mononucleosis caused by Epstein–Barr virus is often associated with pharyngitis. Tonsils are often covered with exudates, and there is prominent anterior and posterior cervical adenopathy. Generalized lymphadenopathy and splenomegaly are frequently seen. An evaluation for the presence of heterophile antibodies (eg, monospot test) will confirm the diagnosis. Patients should be cautioned against sports activities if they have mononucleosis since this can cause a life-threatening splenic rupture. Also, be aware that primary human immunodeficiency virus seroconversion illness can present with a similar fashion. A high index of suspicion is essential, because this diagnosis is often missed in clinical practice. *(Corrales-Medina and Shandera, 2010, pp. 1243-1244)*

REFERENCES

Beal MF, Hauser SL. Trigeminal neuralgia, Bell's palsy & other cranial nerve disorders. In: Fauci AS, Braumwald E, DL Kasper E, et al., eds. *Harrison's Principles of Internal Medicine*. 17th ed. New York, NY: McGraw-Hill; 2008.

Bhattacharya N. Approach to epistaxis. In: Goroll AH, Mulley AG, eds. *Primary Care Medicine*. Baltimore, MD: Lippincott Williams & Wilkins; 2009;1383-1385.

Bhattacharya N. Approach to the patient with otitis. In: Goroll AH, Mulley AG, eds. *Primary Care Medicine*. Baltimore, MD: Lippincott Williams & Wilkins; 2009; 1400-1402.

Bhattacharya N. Evaluation of hearing loss. In: Goroll AH, Mulley AG, eds. *Primary Care Medicine*. Baltimore, MD: Lippincott Williams & Wilkins; 2009;1377-1382.

Boahene DK, Driscoll CL. Otosclerosis. In: Lalwani AK, ed. *Current Diagnosis & Treatment in Otolaryngology—Head & Neck Surgery*. 2nd ed. New York, NY: McGraw-Hill; 2008.

Chang CYJ. Cholesteatoma. In: Lalwani AK, ed. *Current Diagnosis & Treatment in Otolaryngology—Head & Neck Surgery*. 2nd ed. New York, NY: McGraw-Hill; 2008.

Corrales-Medina VF, Shandera WX. Viral & rickettsial infections. In: McPhee SJ, Papadakis MA, eds. *Current Medical Diagnosis & Treatment*. 49th ed. New York, NY: McGraw-Hill; 2010.

Ehlers JP, Shah CP, Fenton GL, et al. *The Wills Eye Manual*. Baltimore, MD: Lippincott Williams & Wilkins; 2008.

Goddard G. Temporomandibular disorders. In: Lalwani AK, ed. *Current Diagnosis & Treatment in Otolaryngology—Head & Neck Surgery*. 2nd ed. New York, NY: McGraw-Hill; 2008.

Grunstein E, Santos F, Selesnick SH. Diseases of the external ear. In: Lalwani AK, ed. *Current Diagnosis & Treatment in Otolaryngology—Head & Neck Surgery*. 2nd ed. New York, NY: McGraw-Hill; 2008.

Hellman DB, Imboden JB. Musculoskeletal & immunologic disorders. In: McPhee SJ, Papadakis MA, eds. *Current Medical Diagnosis & Treatment*. 49th ed. New York, NY: McGraw-Hill; 2010.

Horton JC. Disorders of the eyes, ears, nose, and throat. In: Fauci AS, Braumwald E, Kasper DL, et al., eds. *Harrison's Principles of Internal Medicine*. 17th ed. New York, NY: McGraw-Hill; 2008.

Johnson J, Lalwani AK. Vestibular disorders. In: Lalwani AK, ed. *Current Diagnosis & Treatment in Otolaryngology—Head & Neck Surgery*. 2nd ed. New York, NY: McGraw-Hill; 2008.

Kelly PE, Friedman NR, Yoon PJ. Ear, nose & throat. In: Hay WW Jr, et al., eds. *Current Diagnosis& Treatment Pediatrics*. 19th ed. New York, NY: McGraw-Hill; 2008.

Kucik CJ, Clenney T. Management of epistaxis. *Am Fam Physician*. 2005;71:305-312.

Labuguen RH. Initial evaluation of vertigo. *Am Fam Physician*. 2006;73:244-251, 254.

Lustig LR, Niparko JK. Disorders of the facial nerve. In: Lalwani AK, ed. *Current Diagnosis & Treatment in Otolaryngology—Head & Neck Surgery*. 2nd ed. New York, NY: McGraw-Hill; 2008.

Lustig LR, Schindler JS. Ear, nose & throat disorders. In: McPhee SJ, Papadakis MA, eds. *Current Medical Diagnosis & Treatment*. 49th ed. New York, NY: McGraw-Hill; 2010.

Mandpe AH. Paranasal sinus neoplasms. In: Lalwani AK, ed. *Current Diagnosis & Treatment in Otolaryngology—Head & Neck Surgery*. 2nd ed. New York, NY: McGraw-Hill; 2008.

Oghalai JS. Neoplasms of the temporal bone & skull base. In: Lalwani AK, ed. *Current Diagnosis & Treatment in Otolaryngology—Head & Neck Surgery*. 2nd ed. New York, NY: McGraw-Hill; 2008.

Oliver LC. Approach to the patient with sleep apnea. In: Goroll AH, Mulley AG, eds. *Primary Care Medicine*. Baltimore, MD: Lippincott Williams & Wilkins; 2009; 372-376.

Oliver LC. Evaluation of the subacute and chronic cough. In: Goroll AH, Mulley AG, eds. *Primary Care Medicine*. Baltimore, MD: Lippincott Williams & Wilkins; 2009; 351-355.

Pokhrel PK, Loftus SA. Ocular emergencies. *Am Fam Physician*. 2007;76:829-836.

Quillen DM, Feller DB. Diagnosing rhinitis: allergic vs. nonallergic. *Am Fam Physician*. 2006;73:1583-1590.

Riordan-Eva P. Disorders of the eyes & eyelids. In: McPhee SJ, Papadakis MA, eds. *Current Medical Diagnosis & Treatment*. 49th ed. New York, NY: McGraw-Hill; 2010.

Rubin MA, Gonzales R, Sande MA. Pharyngitis, sinusitis, otitis, and other upper respiratory tract infections. In: Fauci AS, Braunwald E, Kasper DL, Hauser SL, Longo DL, Jameson JL, Loscalzo J, eds. *Harrison's Principles of Internal Medicine*. 17th ed. New York, NY: McGraw-Hill; 2008.

Scheid DC, Hamm RM. Acute bacterial rhinosinusitis in adults, I: evaluation. *Am Fam Physician*. 2004;70:1685-1692.

Seidel HM, Ball JM, Dains JE, et al. *Mosby's Guide to Physical Examination*. 6th ed. St Louis, MO: Mosby; 2006.

Shah AR, Salamone FN, Tami TA. Allergic and non-allergic rhinitis. In: Lalwani AK, ed. *Current Diagnosis & Treatment in Otolaryngology—Head & Neck Surgery*. 2nd ed. New York, NY: McGraw-Hill; 2008.

Shah AR, Ryzenman JM, Tami TA. Nasal manifestations of systemic disease. In: Lalwani AK, ed. *Current Diagnosis*

& Treatment in Otolaryngology—Head & Neck Surgery. 2nd ed. New York, NY: McGraw-Hill; 2008.

Shah SB, Emanuel IA. Nonallergic & allergic rhinitis. In: Lalwani AK, ed. *Current Diagnosis & Treatment in Otolaryngology—Head & Neck Surgery*. 2nd ed. New York, NY: McGraw-Hill; 2008.

Shnayder Y, Lee KC, Bernstein JM. Management of adenotonsillar disease. In: Lalwani AK, ed. *Current Diagnosis & Treatment in Otolaryngology—Head & Neck Surgery*. 2nd ed. New York, NY: McGraw-Hill; 2008.

Sullivan EM. Emergency medicine. In: Ballweg R, Sullivan EM, Brown D, Vetrosky D, eds. *Physician Assistant: Guide to Clinical Practice*. 4th ed. Philadelphia, PA: Saunders; 2008.

Tiemstra JD, Khatkhate N. Bell's palsy: diagnosis and management. *Am Fam Physician*. 2007;76:997-1002, 1004.

Wilson WR. A brief review of nasal anatomy and physiology. In: Wilson WR, Nadol JB Jr, Randolph GW, eds. *The Clinical Handbook of Ear, Nose and Throat Disorders*. New York. NY: Parthenon; 2004;113-119.

Wilson WR. Nasal and facial emergencies. In: Wilson WR, Nadol JB Jr, Randolph GW, eds. *The Clinical Handbook of Ear, Nose and Throat Disorders*. New York, NY: Parthenon; 2004;145-158.

Wilson WR. Nasal and sinus congestion and infection. In: Wilson WR, Nadol JB Jr, Randolph GW, eds. *The Clinical Handbook of Ear, Nose and Throat Disorders*. New York, NY: Parthenon; 2004;127-144.

CHAPTER 21

Urology

Raymond Eifel, MS, PA-C

DIRECTIONS: Each of the numbered items or incomplete statements is followed by answers or by completion of the statement. Select the ONE lettered answer or completion that is BEST in each case.

1. What is the most common composition of renal calculi?

   (A) cystine
   (B) calcium
   (C) struvite
   (D) uric acid

2. Which diagnostic finding is most indicative of acute pyelonephritis?

   (A) hematuria
   (B) pyuria
   (C) white blood cell casts
   (D) epithelial cells

3. What is the most likely pathogen associated with acute cystitis?

   (A) *Escherichia coli*
   (B) *Pseudomonas* species
   (C) *Staphylococcus epidermidis*
   (D) *Chlamydia trachomatis*

4. What is the chief symptom associated with bladder cancer?

   (A) pyuria
   (B) hematuria
   (C) dysuria
   (D) urinary frequency

5. Which condition is suggested by urethritis, arthritis, and conjunctivitis?

   (A) chlamydial infection
   (B) gonococcal infection
   (C) reactive arthritis
   (D) tertiary syphilis

6. Which of the following is a painless lesion of the penis?

   (A) chancre
   (B) chancroid
   (C) granuloma inguinale
   (D) Lymphogranuloma venereum

7. Inability to retract the foreskin from the glans penis due to inflammation or infection is often an indication for circumcision. Which condition does this describe?

   (A) phimosis
   (B) paraphimosis
   (C) balanitis
   (D) urethral meatal stricture

8. Which of the following would be of most concern if found while examining a 26-year-old healthy male patient?

   (A) tender epididymis
   (B) enlarged, fluid-filled scrotum
   (C) nontender mass on the testes
   (D) mass that feels like a "bag of worms"

9. The anatomical portion of the prostate that becomes hyperplastic with benign prostatic hyperplasia is the

   (A) anterior fibromuscular area
   (B) central zone
   (C) transition zone
   (D) peripheral zone

10. A 38-year-old man presents with an abrupt onset of myalgia and low back/perineal pain. The patient also reports urinary symptoms of frequency, urgency, and dysuria. A urinalysis reveals pyuria; urine culture reveals the presence of gram-negative bacteria. What is the initial therapeutic approach for this patient?

    (A) hospitalization with administration of intravenous antibiotics
    (B) trimethoprim–sulfamethoxazole (TMP/SMZ) or a fluoroquinolone for 4 weeks
    (C) a fluoroquinolone and α-blocker for 8 to 12 weeks
    (D) nonsteroidal anti-inflammatory drugs (NSAIDs) and hot sitz baths

11. A 20-year-old college football player presents with a chief complaint of a dull ache in his scrotum after prolonged standing on the sideline. It seems to get worse with vigorous activity and is relieved by lying down. Dilated veins in the left scrotum are observed on inspection, and both testicles are palpable and without masses. What is the most likely diagnosis?

    (A) varicocele
    (B) spermatocele
    (C) hydrocele
    (D) testicular mass

12. A 72-year-old man presents to the office with a chief complaint of a 3 month history of nocturia. He states that his urine stream is weak, has been increasingly slow to start during this time, and sometimes he finds himself straining to void. What is the most reasonable initial therapeutic approach for this patient?

    (A) watchful waiting
    (B) trial of tamsulosin
    (C) trial of finasteride
    (D) Transurethral resection of the prostate (TURP)

13. A 6-month-old boy is brought to the office by his mother for a follow-up check for a right undescended testicle that has been absent since birth. This examination is consistent with previous examinations, revealing an empty right hemiscrotum. Even with treatment, which of the following is most likely to occur to this patient in future years?

    (A) testicular torsion
    (B) epididymitis
    (C) orchitis
    (D) acute appendicitis

14. A 65-year-old woman presents with a complaint of blood in her urine, intermittently for the last month. The patient denies any fever, chills, flank pain, or dysuria. Social history is positive for tobacco use (45 pack years), but patient reports stopping her tobacco use last year. What is the most likely cause of her hematuria?

    (A) urinary tract infection (UTI)
    (B) bladder cancer
    (C) renal calculi
    (D) pyelonephritis

15. A 32-year-old man presents severely worried with a complaint of increased urinary frequency and bladder pain. He states that he has been feeling poorly for the past 4 days with intermittent fever, chills, and persistent malaise. He states never feeling this way before. Physical examination is significant for a temperature of 101°F. Genital examination is normal except a gentle rectal examination reveals an enlarged and tender prostate. What is the most likely diagnosis?

    (A) acute bacterial prostatitis
    (B) chronic bacterial prostatitis
    (C) prostatic abscess
    (D) benign prostatic hypertrophy (BPH)

16. A 66-year-old man with a 15 year history of hypertension and status postinferior myocardial infarction 4 months ago presents for a follow-up office appointment. He has been feeling well, without chest pain or shortness of breath, and has returned to his work as a salesman at a local insurance company. He reports being compliant with his prescription of isosorbide and denies any side effects. He says that he is nervous about resuming sexual activity with his wife since the heart attack because he wonders whether sexual relations can hurt his heart. He has tried a couple of times to have sexual relations with his wife but has been unable to achieve a full erection. What is the most reasonable initial therapeutic approach for this patient's erectile dysfunction?

    (A) tadalafil
    (B) vardenafil
    (C) sildenafil
    (D) alprostadil

17. A 16-year-old girl presents to the emergency department with a 1 day history of severe right flank pain with associated vomiting. She denies any fever, urgency, or dysuria. Her past medical history (PMH) is unremarkable. Physical examination reveals she has guarding, and rebound is present on the right, along with severe right costovertebral angle (CVA) tenderness. Which of the following radiographic studies is indicated for this patient?

    (A) KUB (kidneys, ureter, and bladder)
    (B) intravenous pyelogram (IVP)
    (C) noncontrast spiral computed tomography (CT)
    (D) flat plate

18. A 75-year-old woman, mother of four, presents to your office to establish care. Appearing healthy, she reports a past medical history positive for hypertension and denies any additional problems. However, when specifically asked she admits to having urinary incontinence for "a couple of years" and now describes symptoms that have recently worsened, with the patient experiencing the need to void almost hourly. These desires to urinate are so severe that she is now using four to five adult incontinence pads per day to manage the urine she leaks. What is the most likely diagnosis?

    (A) urge incontinence
    (B) stress incontinence
    (C) overflow incontinence
    (D) functional incontinence

19. A patient with a history of multiple episodes of renal calculi secondary to hypercalcemia also has repeatedly corresponding suppressed levels of parathyroid hormone (PTH). What is the most likely cause for the low level of PTH?

    (A) malignancy
    (B) primary hyperparathyroidism
    (C) vitamin D intoxication
    (D) hyperthyroidism

20. A 54-year-old woman presents with gross hematuria and flank pain. Physical examination is positive for a RUQ (right upper quadrant) palpable mass and negative for costovertebral angle tenderness. Gross blood is observed in the urine specimen. What is your most likely diagnosis?

    (A) renal abscess
    (B) renal cyst
    (C) angiomyolipoma
    (D) renal cell carcinoma

21. A 32-year-old man presents to the urgent care center with a concern of scrotal tenderness that began 3 days ago and has now worsened. Physical examination reveals a temperature of 100.7°F, positive tenderness in the posterolateral aspect of the right testis with swelling, negative spermatic cord tenderness with palpation, and no transillumination. What is this patient's most likely diagnosis?

    (A) epididymitis
    (B) orchitis
    (C) epididymo-orchitis
    (D) testicular torsion

22. A 21-year-old sexually active female student presents to the university clinic with recurrent pain with urination. Initially treated with trimethoprim–sulfamethoxazole, her follow-up urine culture was negative. What is the most likely organism causing her discomfort?

    (A) *Escherichia coli*
    (B) *Chlamydia trachomatis*
    (C) Candida species
    (D) Proteus species

23. A 43-year-old female patient presents with back pain and hematuria. The patient reports having this problem earlier this year and recalls her previous clinician telling her, "they're just cysts." Denying any history of urinary tract infections, the patient reports her mother was on dialysis before passing away. The patient is afebrile and her physical examination is positive for diffuse back tenderness and bilateral flank masses with palpation. Urine dipstick is positive for 3+ blood and is negative for leukocytes and nitrites. What is this patient's most likely diagnosis?

    (A) adult polycystic kidney disease
    (B) renal cyst
    (C) horseshoe kidney
    (D) renal cell carcinoma

24. A 37-year-old woman returns to your office a week after being treated for a urinary tract infection. She reports her symptoms have not gotten better and have even gotten worse with a fever and flank pain. A urine specimen is obtained and viewed under a microscope. Which type of casts would you expect to observe in this patient's urine sediment?

    (A) white blood cell
    (B) epithelial cell
    (C) red blood cell
    (D) hyaline

25. When treating a patient for benign prostatic hypertrophy (BPH), which of the following medical therapies affects the patient's prostate-specific antigen (PSA) level?

    (A) phytotherapy
    (B) α-adrenergic antagonists
    (C) 5α-reductase inhibitors
    (D) saw palmetto

26. A male patient with the bone scan shown in Figure 21-1 has metastatic bone cancer. Which of the following is the most likely source of the disease?

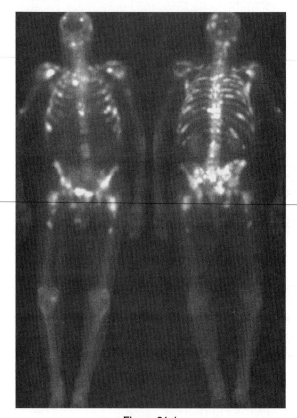

Figure 21-1
(*Reproduced, with permission, from Tanagho EA, McAninch JW, eds. Smith's General Urology. 17th ed. New York, NY: McGraw-Hill; 2008:359.*)

    (A) renal cell carcinoma
    (B) bladder cancer
    (C) prostate cancer
    (D) testis cancer

27. A 32-year-old female patient presents to a family practice office with claims of "another UTI." The patient's complaint is narrowed to dysuria and increased frequency for the last 2 days. The patient denies fever and none is assessed by the nurse. The chart review reveals that this is the patient's fourth visit to the clinic in the last 9 months. Which of the following should be done next?

    (A) Send the urine for culture and sensitivity test and treat for the most common organism.
    (B) Refer the patient to a urologist for an evaluation.
    (C) Give the patient a prescription for a 3 day course of a fluoroquinolone.
    (D) Treat the patient with nitrofurantoin (100 mg bid $\times$ 7 days) and refer to urology.

28. What is the most common cause for recurrent urinary tract infections in a 4-year-old girl?

    (A) bladder diverticulum
    (B) vesicoureteral reflux
    (C) renal calculus
    (D) resistant organism

29. A 27-year-old woman with recurrent urinary tract infections comes to the office concerned about another infection. In previous infections, the patient has always been treated with the correct antibiotic according to culture and sensitivity results. Also, a recent work-up for genitourinary anatomic abnormalities was negative. Which of the following disorders listed in her PMH is most commonly associated with these recurring infections?

    (A) systemic lupus erythematosus
    (B) partner associated
    (C) renal abscess
    (D) type 2 diabetes mellitus

30. A 33-year-old patient presents to the office with a complaint of a "bladder infection." She reports irritative symptoms of dysuria and increased frequency. Her physical examination is positive for suprapubic tenderness and she is afebrile. Her urine dipstick is positive and her urine is sent for culture and sensitivity test. Which of the following values is considered positive for an offending organism in a urine culture?

    (A) $<10^2$/mL colony forming units
    (B) $<10^4$/mL colony forming units
    (C) $>10^4$/mL colony forming units
    (D) $>10^5$/mL colony forming units

31. A 42-year-old woman, with a history of struvite renal calculus, calls the office with a complaint of a urinary tract infection. As part of the interview, she reports intermittent, mild right flank pain for 4 days. Her urine dipstick is positive for microscopic hematuria, and the urine pH is 7.5. The KUB film is positive with two visible stones in the right kidney. Which of the following organisms is most likely to be cultured from the urine specimen?

    (A) *Escherichia coli*
    (B) *Klebsiella*
    (C) *Proteus*
    (D) *Chlamydia trachomatis*

32. A 57-year-old female patient presents to the office with a complaint of increasing urinary urgency and pelvic pain. These symptoms have gradually progressed and worsened to the point the patient gets up at night to void. The pain improves after voiding. The patient is postmenopausal and denies any history of UTIs. There is no suprapubic pain with palpation. Which of the following is the most likely diagnosis?

    (A) urinary tract infection
    (B) endometriosis
    (C) bladder cancer
    (D) interstitial cystitis

33. Which of the following laboratory findings will be observed in a patient with noninflammatory nonbacterial prostatitis?

    (A) positive bacterial culture from postmassage urine (chronic)
    (B) positive bacterial culture with expressed prostatic secretions (chronic)
    (C) negative bacterial culture with elevated leukocytes
    (D) negative bacterial culture with normal leukocytes

34. Which of the following radiographic studies is indicated for the initial evaluation of a questionable palpable mass in the area of the kidney, with no other complaints by the patient?

    (A) renal ultrasound
    (B) intravenous pyelogram (IVP)
    (C) abdominal computed tomography
    (D) magnetic resonance imaging

Answers and Explanations

1. **(B)** Eighty to eighty-five percent of all kidney stones are composed of calcium. Another 5% of kidney stones consist of uric acid. Calcium and uric acid stones are more common in male population. One to two percent of kidney stones consist mainly of cystine. Less than 2% are made of struvite, a combination of magnesium, ammonium, and phosphate. Struvite stones frequently present as staghorn calculi, are associated with urinary tract infections, and are more common in women. Stones containing calcium are radiopaque; others are radiolucent. *(Stoller, 2008, pp. 249-254)*

2. **(C)** White blood cell casts, in the presence of the acute symptoms (fever, chills, flank pain, and dysuria), usually provide strong evidence of acute pyelonephritis. Although observed in many patients, the finding of pyuria is non-specific and a patient with pyuria may or may not have infection. Hematuria is rarely seen in acute pyelonephritis. The presence of hematuria usually suggests the presence of calculi or tumor. Epithelial cells are not associated with pyelonephritis. *(Stoller et al., 2009, p. 829)*

3. **(A)** Women experience urinary tract infections at a much higher rate than do their male counterparts. Cystitis most commonly is due to ascending colonization of the lower urinary tract. In women, the urethra is shorter and easily contaminated with fecal flora. Other factors that increase the risk of cystitis include extremes of age, sexual intercourse, diaphragm use, and pregnancy. *Escherichia coli* is the most common pathogen in uncomplicated cystitis. *Pseudomonas* is more likely in patients with recurrent urinary tract infections and in hospitalized patients. *Staphylococcus epidermidis* may indicate a contaminated specimen. *Chlamydia trachomatis* is more likely in sexually transmitted urethritis. *(Nguyen, 2008, p. 207)*

4. **(B)** The most common presenting symptom of bladder cancer is painless hematuria, which occurs in 85% to 90% of patients. Additional symptoms of bladder irritability, and urinary frequency, urgency, and dysuria are the second most common presentation and are usually associated with invasive bladder cancer. *(Rugo, 2009, p. 1461)*

5. **(C)** Both chlamydia and gonorrhea infections can result in urethritis. Gonococci can disseminate to the joints and cause septic arthritis. Chlamydia is typically asymptomatic but can cause chronic conjunctivitis in adolescents and young adults. Reactive arthritis (also known as Reiter syndrome) is a result of an untreated chlamydia infection, and although typically characterized, in texts, by the triad of urethritis, arthritis, and conjunctivitis, all of the symptoms may not be present or not identified at the time of presentation. Tertiary syphilis is characterized by neurologic and cardiovascular disease, gumma, auditory and ophthalmic involvement, and cutaneous lesions. *(Gravel et al., 2007, pp. 936-938)*

6. **(A)** Chancre is the painless lesion caused by *Treponema pallidum* (syphilis). It occurs approximately 3 weeks after exposure to the bacteria. It often goes unnoticed and resolves without treatment in 3 to 6 weeks. Chancroid is the painful lesion of *Haemophilus ducreyi*. It is a large sloughing ulcer with secondary infection and inflammation of the inguinal lymph nodes.

The lesion of granuloma inguinale produces a shallow painful ulcer with a bright red base from which Donovan bodies from *Calymmatobacterium granulomatis* can be found in tissue scrapings and secretions. Lymphogranuloma venereum may be associated with multiple shallow painless lesions caused by *Chlamydia trachomatis*, which heal quickly. A painful unilateral adenopathy may follow the healing of the ulcerations. *(Krieger, 2008, pp. 240-242)*

7. **(A)** Phimosis is the condition in which the foreskin (prepuce) cannot be retracted because of adherence or fibrosis with acute or chronic inflammation. Recurrent balanitis, inflammation of the glans penis, is common. Paraphimosis is the inability to return the retracted foreskin over the glans. This is often iatrogenic following instrumentation or Foley catheter insertion. Urethral meatal stricture occurs following inflammation of the urethra. *(McAninch, 2008, p. 633)*

8. **(C)** Although all of these findings might elicit some concern, the nontender testicular mass would be of most concern because that should be considered testicular cancer until proven otherwise. Testicular cancer affects predominantly young men in the age group ranging from 20 to 35 years. These tumors can metastasize early in their development and almost all will require chemotherapy to treat. A tender epididymis might indicate epididymitis. A fluid-filled scrotum is likely due to a hydrocele and can be surgically repaired. The "bag of worms" mass is characteristic for a varicocele, a condition that usually does not require treatment unless considered a causative factor for infertility. *(Carter et al., 2007, p. 1248)*

9. **(C)** Benign prostatic hyperplasia develops in the transition zone and involves, to varying degrees, both stromal and epithelial tissue. The hyperplastic process results in increased cell numbers. As enlargement progresses, mechanical obstruction results from intrusion of the transition zone into the urethral lumen. The peripheral zone is the primary site for prostate carcinoma—approximately 60% to 70% occurs there. The remainder typically is found in the central zone. *(Presti et al., 2008, pp. 348-349)*

10. **(B)** Trimethoprim–sulfamethoxazole and fluoroquinolones have high drug penetration into prostatic tissue and are recommended for 4 to 6 weeks for patients with acute bacterial prostatitis. Patients presenting as acutely ill and febrile and exhibiting symptoms of acute urinary retention would benefit from hospitalization with parenteral antibiotics. Patients with chronic bacterial prostatitis may benefit from a longer course of antibiotics combined with an α-blocker to reduce urinary symptoms. NSAIDs and sitz baths may also relieve the symptoms associated with chronic prostatitis. *(Nguyen, 2008, pp. 208-210)*

11. **(A)** A varicocele can be recognized by the presence of scrotal enlargement caused by dilation of the pampiniform venous plexus. Varicoceles present as a "bag of worms" in the spermatic cord and are more prominent when the patient stands. More than 80% of the time, varicoceles occur on the left side. Hydroceles and spermatoceles are caused by fluid collection and are usually asymptomatic. Testicular masses must always be included in the differential diagnosis of scrotal masses, as they generally present as painless. *(Carter et al., 2007, p. 1231)*

12. **(B)** Watchful waiting, although an option, is unlikely to resolve the patient's moderate symptoms. A trial of tamsulosin, a selective α-blocker, is most reasonable, as it will provide the patient with the quickest improvement in symptoms without the systemic side effects (i.e., orthostatic hypotension) of a nonselective α-blocker. Finasteride, a 5α-reductase inhibitor, requires 6 months of therapy before seeing symptomatic improvement. Transurethral resection of the prostate (TURP) has higher rates of morbidity and mortality and includes risks of retrograde ejaculation, impotence, and incontinence. *(Presti et al., 2008, pp. 352-354)*

13. **(A)** An undescended testis can be brought down into the scrotum with an orchiopexy surgery, which is usually performed on babies between the age of 9 and 15 months. Even with treatment, there are several consequences associated with cryptorchidism including infertility, malignancy, associated hernia, and torsion of

the undescended testis. The risk of malignancy with a unilateral undescended testis is approximately 1 in 80. The most common tumor developing in an undescended testis is a seminoma. Orchiopexy does not change the risk of developing cancer of the testis. Cryptorchidism does not increase the likelihood of epididymitis, orchitis, or appendicitis. *(Elder, 2007, p. 2260)*

14. **(B)** Hematuria in women older than 60 years is consistent with a bladder malignancy. Bladder cancer causes episodic, gross hematuria that is usually painless. Cigarette smoking is a risk factor that also increases the incidence of bladder cancer. Painful hematuria associated with suprapubic discomfort or dysuria (or both) is more indicative of cystitis or calculi. Pyelonephritis is associated with chills, fever, and flank pain. *(Carter et al., 2007, pp. 1244-1245)*

15. **(A)** Acute bacterial prostatitis is the most common diagnosis in men younger than 50 years old. Patient presentation includes the sudden onset of constitutional and urinary symptoms. Chronic bacterial prostatitis presents without fever, and the digital rectal examination is often normal. Prostatic abscesses are a result of inappropriate treatment for a prior episode of acute bacterial prostatitis. The incidence of benign prostatic hypertrophy is age related, with symptoms presenting in the fifth decade of life. *(Nguyen, 2008, pp. 208-209)*

16. **(D)** All phosphodiesterase type 5 (PDE5) inhibitors (tadalafil, vardenafil, and sildenafil) are contraindicated in men taking organic nitrates (i.e., isosorbide dinitrate or nitroglycerin). Several second-line therapies exist, including alprostadil, vacuum-constriction devices, and penile implants. Referral to a urologist is recommended when considering these therapeutic options. *(Kolodny, 2009, pp. 718-719)*

17. **(C)** The preferred study for an adolescent with suspected renal colic is the spiral CT. This study is performed quickly, delineates the number and location of calculi, and demonstrates whether there is hydronephrosis in the involved kidney. It can also identify stones too small to be picked up on other diagnostic studies. In the past, an intravenous pyelogram was generally performed. A KUB (kidneys, ureter, and bladder) film may not pick up radiolucent stones. A "flat plate" is an older out-of-date term for a KUB. *(Elder, 2007, p. 2268)*

18. **(A)** Urinary incontinence is defined as involuntary urine loss. Urge incontinence is the result of uninhibited urge sensations that are so strong that the patient experiences an involuntary urine loss. Women particularly experience this problem with the changes associated with aging (weakened pelvic muscles secondary to childbirth as well as estrogen depletion causing weakening of the detrusor muscle). The problem may be worsened by the use of diuretics to treat hypertension. Stress incontinence is associated with increases in intra-abdominal pressure (laughing, sneezing, coughing, etc.). Overflow incontinence is associated with leaking small amounts of urine from mechanical factors that affect an already distended bladder. Functional incontinence is associated with patients who exhibit cognitive impairment (severe dementia). *(Johnston et al., 2009, pp. 66-68)*

19. **(A)** Malignancy and primary hyperparathyroidism account for more than two-thirds of the cases of hypercalcemia. Primary hyperparathyroidism is associated with an elevated PTH. Malignancy, vitamin D intoxication, and hyperthyroidism are associated with suppressed levels of PTH. However, malignancy is the most common of the three. *(Sheeler et al., 2007, pp. 1031-1032)*

20. **(D)** The triad of gross hematuria, flank pain, and palpable mass are the common findings, although rarely seen together, associated with renal cell carcinoma. Of the three, a palpable mass is the least likely to be found, but when present is significant for advanced disease. Most renal masses are simple cysts, which require no additional workup. Angiomyolipoma contains large amounts of fat as shown on CT. A renal abscess is associated with a patient presentation that includes fever and flank pain. *(Konety and Williams, 2008, p. 332)*

21. **(A)** Pain and swelling are prominent features of epididymitis; fever and abdominal pain may also be present. Epididymitis is caused by an ascending infection that without treatment will continue to the testicles, causing a significant swelling that will make it difficult for the clinician to distinguish between the epididymis and the testicles (epididymo-orchitis). Orchitis alone is most commonly viral (mumps) and observed in prepubertal boys. In men younger than 30 years, epididymitis can be confused with torsion. *(Krieger, 2009, pp. 696-699)*

22. **(B)** *Chlamydia trachomatis* should be considered in recurrent episodes of dysuria when urine cultures are found to be negative and the patient has failed to respond to therapy. All of the other organisms are treatable with trimethoprim–sulfamethoxazole. *(Cunha, 2009, p. 682)*

23. **(A)** Adult polycystic kidney disease is a hereditary condition that almost always has a bilateral presentation (95% of the cases). It does not appear until after the age of 40, and dialysis or kidney transplantation is necessary for survival. Renal cysts and renal cell carcinoma generally present unilaterally. A horseshoe kidney (fusion of the renal tissue) may be palpated bilaterally; otherwise, the patient is asymptomatic. *(McAninch, 2008, pp. 507-512)*

24. **(A)** Pyelonephritis results from an ascending urinary tract infection from the bladder via the ureter to kidney. Although not pathognomonic, white blood cell casts are suggestive of pyelonephritis. Red blood cell casts are highly suggestive of glomerulonephritis. Epithelial cell casts are typical in acute tubular necrosis. Hyaline casts in small numbers are insignificant and are commonly seen in patients who regularly exercise. *(Kreder and Williams, 2008, p. 51)*

25. **(C)** 5α-Reductase inhibitors (finasteride) can lower a patient's PSA level by 50% and a baseline PSA should be taken before beginning therapy. Doxazosin and terazosin (α-Adrenergic antagonists) relax prostate and bladder neck smooth muscles and may cause dizziness and orthostatic hypotension but do not affect PSA levels. Phytotherapy refers to the use of plants or plant extracts for medicinal purposes; saw palmetto is a popular treatment for BPH. *(Badlani and Karlovsky, 2009, p. 714)*

26. **(C)** Prostate cancer is the most common primary source for metastatic bone disease in men. Although rare, men may present with lumbar pain as their presenting symptom for prostate cancer and should be considered in the clinician's differential diagnosis. Renal cell carcinoma commonly metastasizes to the lungs. Germ cell tumors (testes) metastasize to the lymph nodes located along the renal hilum. Bladder tumors commonly metastasize to lung. Bone metastasis also occurs from breast cancer. *(Konety and Williams, 2008, p. 333; Presti, 2008, p. 377; Presti et al., 2008, p. 359)*

27. **(D)** This patient will receive both an antibiotic and referral, as this is her fourth recurrence for the same problem within the period of a year. A recurrence rate of more than three infections per year should be evaluated by a urologist to rule out any anatomic abnormality. Although an uncomplicated cystitis can be treated with TMP/SMZ, the clinician should use either a fluoroquinolone or nitrofurantoin because of increasing resistance to TMP/SMZ. *(Stoller et al., 2009, p. 828)*

28. **(B)** Vesicoureteral reflux is the retrograde passage of urine from the bladder to the kidneys via the ureter because of an incompetent vesicoureteral sphincter. It occurs in children 25% to 40% of the time. Although it occurs in both boys and girls, it is more common in girls, with the ratio of female/male occurrence being approximately 4:1 after 1 year of age. Most damage to the kidney occurs before the age of 5 years, as scarring leads to progressive renal deterioration. *(Tanagho, 2008, p. 187; Watnick and Morisson, 2009, p. 822)*

29. **(D)** UTIs are more common in patients with diabetes mellitus, resulting in a two- to fivefold increased frequency of UTIs when compared with nondiabetic patients. It is believed that two separate defects are responsible for this difference. First, there is a change in urinary cytokine secretions; and second, there is an

increased adherence of microorganisms to the uroepithelial cells found throughout the urinary tract. These patients are also more likely to have recurrent fungal infections. *(Nguyen, 2008, pp. 213-214)*

30. **(D)** A urine culture is positive for an offending organism when the colony forming counts exceed 10^5/mL, although this criterion is not essential in making the diagnosis. A clinical diagnosis may be made on the basis of patient's symptoms and physical examination. A urine dipstick screen with a positive leukocyte esterase indicates pyuria, and a positive nitrite test suggests the presence of more than 100,000 organisms per milliliter. *(Kreder and Williams, 2008, p. 48; Stoller et al., 2009, p. 828)*

31. **(C)** This patient has struvite stones. They are frequently associated with recurrent urinary tract infections, visible stones, and high urine pH. These stones are formed by urease-producing organisms including *Proteus* and *Pseudomonas* while being caused less commonly by *Klebsiella*. Struvite stones are not typically caused by *E. coli* and *C. trachomatis*. *(Stoller et al., 2009, p. 836)*

32. **(D)** This patient has interstitial cystitis (IC). Pelvic pain increases the differential to include all of the responses, but pelvic/suprapubic pain that decreases with voiding is associated with interstitial cystitis. The physical examination is usually normal, and a urine specimen for this patient will most likely be negative.

Endometriosis will present with pelvic pain but will most likely also have adnexal tenderness. A UTI will have increased frequency and urgency and a positive urine specimen. Patients with bladder cancer can also have urinary symptoms of frequency, urgency, and suprapubic pain and will also have a urine specimen taken with hematuria. *(Tanagho, 2008, pp. 576-577)*

33. **(D)** Prostatitis includes a continuum of prostate characteristics ranging from acute episodes to prostatodynia, a noninflammatory disorder. Patients with acute bacterial prostatitis will have an exquisitely tender prostate gland, and prostatic massage is contraindicated in these patients. Chronic prostatitis patients may have no evidence of an acute infection but will have increased leukocytes. Nonbacterial prostatitis is broken into two subcategories with the noninflammatory classification having neither bacteria nor leukocytes. *(Nguyen, 2008, pp. 208-210; Stoller et al., 2009, pp. 830-832)*

34. **(A)** Renal masses are initially identified by ultrasound. Ultrasound will be able to distinguish between a solid mass and a cyst. It is not uncommon to find some texts state that an intravenous pyelogram is noted as the initial test. Intravenous pyelograms have limited value, especially in differentiating small tumors. Whether a mass or a cyst, these findings are usually referred to a urologist who will follow-up with their own IVP and CT. *(McAninch, 2008, p. 511)*

REFERENCES

Badlani GH, Karlovsky ME. Benign prostatic hypertrophy. In: Rakel RE, Bope ET, eds. *Conn's Current Therapy 2009*. Philadelphia, PA: Saunders; 2009:712-715.

Carter C, Stallworth J, Holleman R. Urinary tract disorders. In: Rakel RE, ed. *Textbook of Family Medicine*. 7th ed. Philadelphia, PA: Saunders; 2007:1217-1252.

Cunha BA. Urinary tract infections in women. In: Rakel RE, Bope ET, eds. *Conn's Current Therapy 2009*. Philadelphia, PA: Saunders; 2009:682-686.

Elder JS. Disorders and anomalies of the scrotal contents. In: Kliegman RM, Behrman RE, Jenson HB, Stanton BF, eds. *Nelson Textbook of Pediatrics*. 18th ed. Philadelphia, PA: Saunders; 2007:2260-2265.

Elder JS. Urinary lithiasis. In: Kliegman RM, Behrman RE, Jenson HB, Stanton BF, eds. *Nelson Textbook of Pediatrics*. 18th ed. Philadelphia, PA: Saunders; 2007:2267-2271.

Gravel J, Comeau D, Gordon A. Rheumatology and musculoskeletal problems. In: Rakel RE, ed. *Textbook of Family Medicine*. 7th ed. Philadelphia, PA: Saunders; 2007:915-953.

Johnston CB, Harper GM, Landefeld CS. Geriatric disorders. In: McPhee SJ, Papadakis MA, eds. *Current Medical Diagnosis and Treatment*. 48th ed. New York, NY: McGraw-Hill; 2009:56-71.

Kreder KJ, Williams RD. Urologic laboratory examination. In: Tanagho EA, McAninch JW, eds. *Smith's General Urology*. 17th ed. New York, NY: McGraw-Hill; 2008: 46-57.

Krieger JN. Epididymitis. In: Rakel RE, Bope ET, eds. *Conn's Current Therapy 2009*. Philadelphia, PA: Saunders; 2009:696-699.

Krieger JN. Sexually transmitted diseases. In: Tanagho EA, McAninch JW, eds. *Smith's General Urology*. 17th ed. New York, NY: McGraw-Hill; 2008:235-245.

Kolodny L. Erectile dysfunction. In: Rakel RE, Bope ET, eds. *Conn's Current Therapy 2009*. Philadelphia, PA: Saunders; 2009:715-721.

Konety BR, Williams RD. Renal parenchymal neoplasms. In: Tanagho EA, McAninch JW, eds. *Smith's General Urology*. 17th ed. New York, NY: McGraw-Hill; 2008:328-347.

McAninch JW. Disorders of the kidneys. In: Tanagho EA, McAninch JW, eds. *Smith's General Urology*. 17th ed. New York, NY: McGraw-Hill; 2008:506-520.

McAninch JW. Disorders of the penis and male urethra. In: Tanagho EA, McAninch JW, eds. *Smith's General Urology*. 17th ed. New York, NY: McGraw-Hill; 2008:625-637.

Nguyen HT. Bacterial infections of the genitourinary tract. In: Tanagho EA, McAninch JW, eds. *Smith's General Urology*. 17th ed. New York, NY: McGraw-Hill; 2008:193-218.

Presti JC. Genital tumors. In: Tanagho EA, McAninch JW, eds. *Smith's General Urology*. 17th ed. New York, NY: McGraw-Hill; 2008:375-387.

Presti JC, Kane CJ, Shinohara K, Carroll PR. Neoplasms of the prostate gland. In: Tanagho EA, McAninch JW, eds. *Smith's General Urology*. 17th ed. New York, NY: McGraw-Hill; 2008:348-374.

Rugo HS. Cancer. In: McPhee SJ, Papadakis MA, eds. *Current Medical Diagnosis and Treatment*. 48th ed. New York, NY: McGraw-Hill; 2009:1417-1492.

Sheeler RD, Wermers RA, Flinchbaugh RT, Haugo A, Ackerman JM, Shafer HIL. Endocrinology. In: Rakel RE, ed. *Textbook of Family Medicine*. 7th ed. Philadelphia, PA: Saunders; 2007:1021-1073.

Stoller ML. Urinary stone disease. In: Tanagho EA, McAninch JW, eds. *Smith's General Urology*. 17th ed. New York: McGraw-Hill; 2008:246-277.

Stoller ML, Kane CJ, Meng MV. Urologic disorders. In: McPhee SJ, Papadakis MA, eds. *Current Medical Diagnosis and Treatment*. 48th ed. New York, NY: McGraw-Hill; 2009:827-847.

Tanagho EA. Disorders of the bladder, prostate, and seminal vesicles. In: Tanagho EA, McAninch JW, eds. *Smith's General Urology*. 17th ed. New York, NY: McGraw-Hill; 2008:574-588.

Watnick S, Morisson G. Kidney disease. In: McPhee SJ, Papadakis MA, eds. *Current Medical Diagnosis and Treatment*. 48th ed. New York, NY: McGraw-Hill; 2009: 794-826.

Health Promotion & Disease Prevention

CHAPTER 22

Preventive Medicine

James F. Cawley, MPH, PA-C

DIRECTIONS: Each of the numbered items or incomplete statements in this section is followed by answers or by completion of the statement. Select the ONE-lettered answer or completion that is BEST in each case.

1. Which disease/health threat is the leading cause of disability-adjusted life years (DALYs) in the United States?

   (A) lung cancer
   (B) ischemic heart disease
   (C) unipolar depression
   (D) road traffic injuries
   (E) HIV/AIDS

2. Which of the following statements related to the identification of intimate partner violence (IPV) is TRUE?

   (A) women are at less risk for violence during pregnancy
   (B) most cases of domestic violence are sporadic and isolated
   (C) victims of intimate partner violence are more likely to delay seeking care
   (D) patients with family history of IPV are less at risk

3. If death rates per 1,000 licensed drivers are plotted by age, the distribution of the curve is

   (A) bell shaped
   (B) J shaped
   (C) U shaped
   (D) unimodal

4. A group of physicians conducted interviews of their patients regarding symptoms of gastritis following use of two different types of NSAIDs for a research study. They found no difference in amount or frequency of symptoms between the two agents. An external reviewer concluded that the study was flawed because of assessment bias. What would have prevented this flaw?

   (A) random assignment of the patients
   (B) better training of the interviewers
   (C) masking interviewers to the treatment
   (D) using a case-control method

5. Which of the following risk factors for coronary heart disease has the highest attributable risk (risk of disease due to a specific factor)?

   (A) smoking
   (B) elevated cholesterol
   (C) lack of physical exercise
   (D) high blood pressure

6. One of your patients is a 30-year-old man who tells you he is planning to travel to the Dominican Republic for a 3-week hiking trip. The most appropriate medication to use for malarial prophylaxis is

   (A) atovaquone
   (B) chloroquine
   (C) mefloquine
   (D) doxycycline

7. Researchers wish to study the association between consumption of saturated fat and myocardial infarction. They administer a food frequency questionnaire to all patients ($n = 15,000$) who come to a large Health Maintenance Organization (HMO) practice for annual checkups in 1980. The researchers use the food frequency data to calculate the usual amount of saturated fat consumed by each participant per week. Then, they follow these patients for 15 years and determine the number of myocardial infarctions that occur in this group. What type of study is the study described above?

(A) case-control study
(B) cohort study
(C) randomized controlled trial
(D) cross-sectional study

8. Which tick-borne public health threat, especially prevalent in the upper Midwest, New England, and some of the Mid-Atlantic States, is a cause of an infection of neutrophils?

(A) human granulocytic anaplasmosis
(B) Rocky Mountain spotted fever
(C) psittacosis
(D) cryptococcosis

9. The medical evaluation of a 32-year-old HIV-infected male patient reveals a tuberculin skin test reaction at 5 mm and indurated. His chest x-ray is normal. He is currently taking antiretroviral therapy that includes protease inhibitors. He has not previously received antituberculous therapy nor had any known contact with people with tuberculosis (TB). Which is the most appropriate intervention at this time?

(A) isoniazid (INH) for 9 months
(B) no preventive therapy for TB needed
(C) rifampin for 9 months
(D) streptomycin for 6 months

Questions 10 and 11

On a Friday afternoon, a 30-year-old registered nurse is brought to your office in employee health for evaluation following a needle stick injury that occurred in the HIV clinic. The source patient involved is known to be infected with HIV and has advanced AIDS.

10. Which of the following factors carries the greatest risk for the transmission of HIV to the nurse?

(A) depth of injury
(B) presence of visible blood on the needle
(C) prior immune status of the nurse
(D) stage of illness of the source patient

11. What is the most appropriate course of action for this health worker?

(A) reassure her of the low risk of infection
(B) offer two-drug antiretroviral therapy (lamivudine [Combivir])
(C) draw HIV antibody test and refer to an infectious disease specialist on Monday
(D) offer triple drug therapy to prevent seroconversion

12. The prevention of shingles is best accomplished by

(A) administration of herpes zoster (HZ) vaccine (zoster vaccine live [Zostavax]) in patients older than 50 years
(B) prophylactic use of acyclovir (Zovirax) in patients older than 50 years who present with a painful rash
(C) use of vitamins to boost immunity in adults
(D) administration of measles–mumps–rubella–varicella (MMRV) (ProQuad) vaccine in children ages 1 through 10 years

13. What is the most prevalent sexually transmitted infection (STI) in the United States and also accounts for many observed complications such as pelvic inflammatory disease (PID), infertility, ectopic pregnancy, and chronic pelvic pain?

(A) syphilis
(B) chlamydia
(C) herpes simplex
(D) gonorrhea

14. In the course of investigating a 24-year-old HIV-infected male, it was observed that the

HBsAg was positive. The patient is asymptomatic, his physical examination reveals normal result, and has CD4 count of 800. Which test is the most helpful in determining if he is in the acute phase of viral hepatitis?

(A) HBeAg

(B) HBsAg

(C) IgG anti-HBcAg

(D) IgM anti-HBcAg

15. The most important risk factor for heat-related illness is

(A) age older than 65 years

(B) age younger than 1 year

(C) history of previous heat stroke

(D) obesity

Questions 16 and 17

A new screening program was instituted in Maryland. The program used a screening test that is effective in detecting cancer C at an early stage. Assume that there is no effective treatment for this type of cancer and, therefore, that the program results in no change in the usual course of the disease. Assume also that the rates noted are calculated from all known cases of cancer C and that there were no changes in the quality of the death certification of this disease.

16. What would happen to the apparent incidence rate of cancer C in Maryland during the first year of the program?

(A) increase

(B) decrease

(C) remain constant

(D) insufficient information to answer the question

17. What will happen to the apparent prevalence rate of cancer C in Maryland during the first year of the program?

(A) increase

(B) decrease

(C) remain constant

(D) insufficient information to answer the question

18. What is the protozoal infection, source of which is usually animal-urine-contaminated water and which causes an acute severe febrile icteric hepatitis?

(A) relapsing fever

(B) typhoid fever

(C) *Vibrio vulnificus*

(D) leptospirosis

19. The leading cause of childhood (*ages 5 through 14*) death in the United States is

(A) poisoning

(B) malignant neoplasms

(C) unintentional injury

(D) birth defects

20. The most powerful and consistent risk factor for the development of substance use disorders (SUD) is

(A) poverty

(B) age

(C) depression

(D) family history

21. Which of the following is the best example of primary prevention?

(A) immunization against smallpox

(B) mammography to detect breast cancer

(C) testing to detect C-reactive protein (CRP) for the identification of coronary heart disease

(D) performing carotid endarterectomy for the prevention of stroke

22. Which is the pathogenic pathway in the development of colorectal cancer accounting for 15% of sporadic cases and nearly all cases of hereditary nonpolyposis colorectal cancer (HNPCC)?

(A) chromosomal instability

(B) Familial Adenomatous Polyposis (FAP) mutation

(C) microsatellite instability

(D) telomere cutoff

23. Of the following major sexually transmitted illnesses, which has a safe and effective vaccine?

    (A) syphilis
    (B) chlamydia
    (C) hepatitis B
    (D) herpes simplex II

24. What is the type of rate that is defined as the number of new cases of a disease occurring in a population per unit time?

    (A) epidemic
    (B) prevalence
    (C) incidence
    (D) virulence

25. Which factor is most closely associated with the spread of tuberculosis?

    (A) poverty
    (B) alcoholism
    (C) poor hygiene
    (D) crowding

26. The proportion of nondiseased individuals who are correctly identified as negative by a test describes the test's

    (A) validity
    (B) specificity
    (C) reliability
    (D) sensitivity

27. For which patient is pneumococcal vaccine (PPV 23) *not* beneficial?

    (A) a 15-month-old HIV-infected child
    (B) a 20-year-old patient about to undergo a splenectomy for thrombotic thrombocytopenic purpura (TTP)
    (C) a 5-year-old patient with sickle cell disease
    (D) a 10-year-old child with nephrotic syndrome

Questions 28 through 30

A drug company sponsors and executes a randomized controlled clinical trial to assess the efficacy of a new topical cream medication aimed at inducing new hair growth in men with male pattern baldness. The researchers determine that new hair growth must increase by at least 20% in the treatment group (as compared to placebo) to be considered marketable. They determine a sample size that will ensure 80% power for the purposes of statistical testing and carry this out at the 5% level of statistical significance.

28. The probability that this statistical test will fail to detect a clinically important difference in hair growth between the two groups, given that such a difference actually exists between populations from which the samples were drawn

    (A) increases as the specific effect size decreases
    (B) increases as the sample size increases
    (C) increases as alpha, the level of significance, increases
    (D) increases as the power of the test increases

29. The probability that this statistical test will detect the specific difference in new hair growth, given that such a difference does actually exist between the populations represented in the study samples, is

    (A) 0.95
    (B) 0.05
    (C) 0.20
    (D) 0.80

30. Which of the following statements best describes alpha, the level of significance?

    (A) The chance of detecting a statistically significant difference between the two study groups is 95%
    (B) If new hair growth does not differ between the study and placebo groups, the chance of detecting a statistically significant difference between the two samples is 5% or less.
    (C) If new hair growth differs between the two groups, the chance that the statistical test will detect a true difference between the samples is at least 95%

(D) A statistically significant result will be obtained 5% of the time that a true difference exists between the study populations

31. The incidence rate of lung cancer is 120/100,000 person-years for smokers and 10/100,000 person-year for nonsmokers. What is the risk of developing lung cancer for persons who smoke?

    (A) 5
    (B) 12
    (C) 50
    (D) 100

32. The most prevalent arboviral disease in the United States is

    (A) West Nile virus encephalitis
    (B) anaplasmosis
    (C) Lyme disease
    (D) eastern equine encephalitis

33. Eating undercooked chicken or food that has been contaminated by the drippings of raw chicken is most commonly associated with infection with

    (A) *Salmonella*
    (B) *Giardia lamblia*
    (C) *Campylobacter*
    (D) *Escherichia coli* 0157:H7

34. The leading cause of blindness among adults (persons ages 20–74 years):

    (A) senile macular degeneration
    (B) diabetes mellitus
    (C) retinal artery thrombosis
    (D) glaucoma

35. A 60-year-old white man presents with a palpable prostate mass and a prostate specific antigen (PSA) level of 6.2 ng/mL. There are no indicators of high risk (ie, marked PSA elevation, other suspicious symptoms, positive family history, African American race).

The recommended next step is

    (A) observation
    (B) measuring the free-to-total PSA ratio
    (C) rechecking the PSA in 6 months
    (D) prostate biopsy

36. Which statement best defines a meta-analysis?

    (A) A collection of research evidence that combines quantitative and qualitative methods
    (B) A long-term examination of a cohort studied longitudinally without a comparison group
    (C) An examination of research data already collected
    (D) An investigation that pools data gathered from multiple studies

37. An investigation is begun to identify the cause of lung cancer among ship workers. Workers with the disease were matched with controls by age, place of residence, and type of occupational category. The frequency of smoking and exposure to asbestos was then compared in the two groups. This is what type of study?

    (A) retrospective cohort
    (B) case-control
    (C) controlled clinical trial
    (D) observational

38. In the United States, the largest proportion of TB cases occur among

    (A) HIV-infected persons
    (B) foreign-born persons
    (C) IV drug abuses
    (D) the incarcerated

39. Which of the following is classified as a zoonotic disease?

    (A) *Clostridium difficile*
    (B) typhoid fever
    (C) plague
    (D) listeriosis

40. Level of resistance of a community/group of people to a particular infectious disease beyond that afforded by protection of an immunized individual defines

    (A) community protective effect
    (B) innate immunity
    (C) herd immunity
    (D) natural resistance

Answers and Explanations

1. **(B)** Burden of disease studies have been implemented in many countries using the disability-adjusted life year (DALY) to assess major health problems and estimate the leading causes of morbidity. The leading cause of morbidity is the United States for both males and females by a wide margin is ischemic heart disease. *(McKinna et al., 2005, pp. 415-423)*

2. **(C)** Domestic (or intimate partner violence) violence is prevalent among women; with up to 50% lifetime prevalence being reported. It is often misdiagnosed. Many studies have demonstrated that women are at a higher risk during pregnancy. Patients with a positive family history of violence are at an increased risk for violence even if not currently in an abusive relationship. *(Feldman, 2008, pp. 380-385)*

3. **(C)** Fatalities per 1,000 licensed drivers in the United States are highest among the youngest and oldest drivers, the graph plotting fatalities by age shows a U-shaped distribution. *(Messinger-Rapport and Baker, 2004, p. 267)*

4. **(C)** This study is flawed because the investigators making the assessments were aware of the treatments the patients were receiving. This is called assessment bias and can be minimized by masking (blinding) the assessment team to the treatment. Training the interviewers will help improve interrater reliability. *(Riegelman, 2005, pp. 25-29)*

5. **(A)** When assessing the impact of a risk factor on a group of individuals, the use of the concept of attributable risk is useful. Attributable risk is the percentage of the risk, among those with the risk factor, associated with exposure to the risk factor. If a cause-and-effect relationship exists, then attributable risk is the percentage of disease that can be potentially eliminated if the risk factor is completely eliminated. *(Riegelman, 2005, pp. 60-65)*

6. **(B)** Chloroquine is a standard prophylaxis for the prevention of malaria. The Dominican Republic is a country with a high risk for malaria; it is also a chloroquine-susceptible region as are most parts of Central America and Mexico. It is safe, efficacious, and has few major side effects. It is ideal for short visits to endemic regions. Mefloquine and doxycycline are medications generally used in chloroquine-resistant regions. *(White and Breman, 2008, pp. 192-193; http://www.cdc.gov/malaria/diagnosis_treatment/treatment.html)*

7. **(B)** Cohort studies typically observe study subjects and follow them forward in time. Case-control studies compare the experiences of cases of a disease and controls and measure exposures using past records. Cross-sectional studies observe or measure population characteristics at one point in time. *(Gordis, 2009, pp. 167-170)*

8. **(A)** Human granulocytic anaplasmosis (formerly known as "ehrlichiosis") is caused by a rickettsial bacterium and transmitted by the bite of various tick species that often overlap with those that transmit other diseases such as Lyme disease and babesiosis. Rocky Mountain spotted fever is also a tick-borne infection and is also rickettsial in origin and causes a systemic febrile syndrome and a rash. Psittacosis is associated with exposure to parrots and other

birds and is primarily pneumonia illness; cryptococcal disease typically causes fungal meningitis in immunosuppressed persons. *(Walker et al., 2008, pp. 1059-1061)*

9. **(A)** A positive tuberculin skin test of 5-mm induration or more is considered positive in a person who has HIV infection, has had contact with a person with TB, or who has a positive chest x-ray. HIV-infected persons are at an increased risk of TB and should be screened on a regular basis. Prophylaxis is warranted in this patient, and it is recommended that INH be used for 9 months. Rifampin is not recommended for use in patients taking protease inhibitors, as this reduces effective levels of the antiretroviral drug. *(Raviglione and O'Brian, 2008, pp. 1006-1009)*

10. **(A)** and **11 (D)** The risk of HIV transmission following a needle stick with the blood of an HIV-infected patient is about 1:300. Risks are higher with deep punctures, large inocula, and source patients with high viral loads. While treatment with zidovudine decreases seroconversion by 79%, some clinicians recommend triple combination therapy in high-risk situations as described in the case. *(Zolopa and Katz, 2010, pp. 1220-1221)*

12. **(A)** The use of the HZ vaccine is a useful option for the prevention of herpes zoster infection in older adults. The HZ vaccine was licensed in 2006 and has 14 times the antigenicity of the varicella-zoster virus (VZV) vaccine used in children. The MMRV vaccine or the VZV vaccine used in children would be inappropriate for use in an adult. Treating an older adult suspected on developing zoster with acyclovir may moderate the length and severity of the illness but would not prevent it. *(Wolfe, 2008, p. 410)*

13. **(B)** Chlamydia is by far the most prevalent STI in the United States, with over 900,000 cases reported to the Centers for Disease Control and Prevention (CDC) in 2004. By comparison, in the same year, there were 330,000 cases of gonorrhea reported. Approximately 70% of chlamydia and 50% of gonorrheal infections are asymptomatic. If not adequately treated, 20% to 40% of women with chlamydia and 10% to 40% of women with gonorrhea will develop PID. Syphilis is much less common and is not associated with the cited complications. *(Kodner, 2008, p. 297)*

14. **(D)** Antibodies to the hepatitis B core antigen appear early in the infection with the IgM fraction being the most prominent. The presence of the surface antigen and/or the e antigen does not provide sufficient information regarding the timing of the acquisition of the infection. *(Dienstag, 2008, pp. 1932-1935)*

15. **(A)** Older adults are the most susceptible to heat-related illness because of decreased response of the cardiovascular system during hot weather. *(Lang and Hensrud, 2004, p. 257)*

16. **(A)** and **17 (A)** In this example, given the stated assumptions, it is likely that the incidence (the number of newly diagnosed cases) would increase due to heightened awareness of the cancer brought about by the screening program. This sometimes is called overdiagnosis, and the rise in incidence represents an artifactual, not real, increase in the occurrence of the disease. If the duration of the disease was relatively long, for instance, more than a year, it is also likely that the prevalence of the disease would also rise (incidence = prevalence × duration). *(Riegelman, 2005, pp. 175-183)*

18. **(D)** Human leptospirosis typically presents as an acute illness with high fever, jaundice, abdominal pain, and myalgia and is caused by one of three spirochetal serovars. Leptospires are typically transmitted by the ingestion of food or drink contaminated by the urine of varies animals including cattle, dogs, swine, and rats. The most severe form is anicteric hepatitis (Weil syndrome), which carries a 5% to 40% mortality rate. Typhoid fever is caused by *Salmonella* and presents with acute then chronic severe diarrhea. Relapsing fever is caused by a tick-borne spirochete of the *borrelia* species and causes a systemic febrile illness. *Vibrio vulnificus* is caused by a cholera-related bacterial

species that causes a necrotizing cutaneous infection. *(Speelman and Hartskeerl, 2008, pp. 1048-1049)*

19. **(C)** Unintentional injuries comprise the leading cause of mortality in the childhood age group followed in rank order by malignant neoplasms, congenital malformations, homicide, and suicide. *(Woolf, 2008, p. 12)*

20. **(D)** While there are a wide array of factors including biologic factors, gender, age, employment status, education, and psychiatric history, the strongest association identified for substance use is a positive family history of either drug or alcohol abuse. *(Brown and Fleming, 2008, p. 266)*

21. **(A)** Primary prevention is the concept of preventing disease before it occurs. Immunization prevents infectious diseases such as smallpox. Because of immunization strategies, smallpox has been eradicated from the globe. Mammography and testing for CRP are forms of secondary prevention, as disease already exists in the patient, and the goal is identification of disease at the earliest stage; surgery for carotid artery stenosis is essentially a therapeutic procedure consistent with tertiary prevention. *(Aschengrau and Seage, 2003, pp. 405-406)*

22. **(C)** Microsatellite instability due to mismatch repair gene inactivation is present in approximately 15% of sporadic CRCs and is the major cause of hereditary nonpolyposis colorectal cancer (HNPCC). Other distinct pathways involving genetic alterations in the development of colon cancer include chromosomal instability which arises from an accumulation of allelic losses or mutation and accounts for a small number of cases of sporadically occurring colon cancer. Hypermethylation of promoter regions of genes contributes to some sporadic cases. *(Burke, 2004, p. 544)*

23. **(C)** Hepatitis B is commonly sexually transmitted, accounting for roughly 55% of all cases. Hepatitis B is more efficiently transmitted through sexual contact than HIV. The likelihood of sexual transmission of hepatitis B is reduced with condom use. The hepatitis B immunization is a safe and effective vaccination and has been shown to decrease rates of transmission. No vaccines are available for syphilis or chlamydial infections. An effective vaccine for herpes simplex II, a viral infection, is still under development. *(Kasten, 2004, p. 597)*

24. **(C)** Incidence rates reflect the occurrence of new cases of a disease in the population and are often used to assess the risk of a disease to the public's health. Virulence refers to the pathological properties of infecting microorganisms. Epidemic refers to outbreaks of disease above normal levels. Prevalence is the number of existing cases of a disease in a population per unit time. *(Gordis, 2009, pp. 38-52)*

25. **(D)** While poverty, alcoholism, and poor hygiene are all known risk factors for contracting tuberculosis, it is crowding that has the highest correlation with the transmission of the tubercle bacillus. Making crowding the primary factor stems from evidence that shows that it is coughing from individuals with active tuberculosis that aerosolizes tubercle bacilli that are then inhaled by a susceptible person. Thus, close contact among individuals substantially enhances the likelihood of this occurrence. *(Raviglione and O'Brian, 2008, pp. 1006-1009)*

26. **(B)** Specificity describes the test's ability to identify the absence of disease in nondiseased individuals. It is typically expressed as a percentage. Sensitivity is defined as the ability of the test to detect the presence of disease in those who have it. Reliability is the ability of a test to reproduce similar results in similar situations over time. Validity is a broad concept that describes the ability of a test to distinguish between those who have a disease and those who do not. Sensitivity and specificity are components of validity. *(Gordis, 2009, pp. 85-103)*

27. **(A)** Pneumococcal vaccine is not recommended for children younger than 2 years or less. This would include the 15-month-old child with HIV infection. The other three patients should receive the immunization. The spleen is important

in the immune defense of infections with polysaccharide antigens. Protection with pneumococcal vaccination is important in persons with various conditions conferring higher risk of pneumococcal infection such as those who are asplenic, have sickle cell disease, or who have chronic diseases such as renal failure (or the nephritic syndrome). *(Woolf, p. 392)*

28. **(A), 29 (D),** and **30 (B)** The probability that the statistical test will fail to detect a clinically important difference, given that this difference actually exists is the beta, shows the chance of a type II error. As the sample size or level of significance—the alpha—increases, the chance of a beta error decreases. Because it is the complement of power, beta decreases as power increases. The probability that the statistical test will detect a true difference is the power of the test, and in this question, is equal to 0.80. A statistical test carried out on these two samples will erroneously detect a difference between the two groups 5% of the time. The highly significant result of the statistical test indicates that the observed effect of the new medications unlikely to have occurred by chance (less than 0.05% of the time). *(Riegelman, 2005, pp. 18, 68-73)*

31. **(B)** The formula for the calculation of relative risk is I_e/I_{non-e}, where I represents the incidence of disease and e represents exposure. In this case, $120/100,000 \div 10/100,000 = 12$. This indicates that the risk of developing lung cancer among those exposed is 12 times that of the rate of those not exposed. *(Gordis, 2009, pp. 203-205)*

32. **(A)** West Nile virus has become the most common mosquito-borne (arthropod-borne or arboviral) infectious disease in the United States since the 2002 epidemic and is far more prevalent than eastern equine encephalitis. Between 2001 and 2004, it spread progressively annually across the United States and is now endemic in most parts of the United States. Anaplasmosis is a bacterial infection transmitted by ticks and infects white blood cells producing a systemic febrile illness. Lyme disease is caused by tick bites, usually produces a vivid

rash, and is endemic particularly in states on the Eastern seaboard. *(Barlem, 2009a, p. 595)*

33. **(C)** *Campylobacter* is a bacterial pathogen that causes fever, diarrhea, and abdominal cramps and is the most commonly identified bacterial cause of diarrheal illness in the world. They live in the intestines of healthy birds, and most raw poultry meat has *Campylobacter* on it. Eating undercooked chicken, or other food that has been contaminated with juices dripping from raw chicken, is the most frequent source of this infection; this accounts for 70% of cases. Salmonellosis typically includes fever, diarrhea, and abdominal cramps. *E. coli* O157:H7 has a reservoir in cattle and other similar animals. Illness typically follows consumption of food or water that has been contaminated with microscopic amounts of cow feces and consists of a severe and bloody diarrhea and painful abdominal cramps. Giardia is associated with contaminated water supplies and causes a chronic diarrheal disease. (CDC, 2008; *Barlem, 2009b, pp. 456-458*)

34. **(B)** Diabetes mellitus is a prevalent disease and is by far the leading responsible factor for blindness in adults aged 20 through 65 years. It is classified as either proliferative or nonproliferative. The latter form is characterized by dilation of veins, microaneurysms, retinal hemorrhages, retinal edema, and hard exudates. It is the most common cause of legal blindness in maturity-onset diabetes. *(Powers, 2008, pp. 2287-2288)*

35. **(B)** If the patient is considered at low risk, that is does not have the aforementioned risk factors, it seem most appropriate to measure the free-to-total PSA level. If it is normal, then recheck the PSA level within 3 to 6 months. A less-aggressive approach is supported by evidence that men with prostate cancer who defer treatment demonstrate no increase in mortality from prostate cancer for 8 to 15 years. This may also be appropriate management in patients with apprehension about unnecessary diagnostic or therapeutic procedures. *(Molella, 2008, p. 479)*

36. (D) A meta-analysis is a study that combines data obtained from multiple studies. By combining data from two or more studies, the power of the inquiry is increased, thus allowing for a more accurate estimate of the strength of an association. A collection of research evidence that combines quantitative and qualitative methods refers to a systematic review. A long-term examination of a cohort studied longitudinally without a comparison group describes a prospective cohort study. A study that is an examination of research data already collected is usually referred to as a secondary data analysis. *(Riegelman, 2005, pp. 99-102)*

37. (B) This is an example of a case-control study. Case-control studies begin by identifying those who have developed or failed to develop the disease being investigated. After identifying those with and without the disease, they look back in time to determine the characteristics of individuals (such as smoking or exposure to asbestos) before the onset of disease. Controls are individuals who are matched with cases in all respects except that they are free of disease. A retrospective cohort study, also called a historic cohort study, is one where the medical records of groups of individuals who are alike in many ways but differ by a certain characteristic (such as smoking) are compared for a particular outcome (such as lung cancer). The key distinction from a case-control study is the time of collection of outcomes and exposure

data. Observational studies are those in which the investigator does not have the capability to manipulate the studies' subject but instead simply observes the outcomes of various effects. *(Gordis, 2009, 177-198; Riegelman, 2005, pp. 11-13)*

38. (B) Foreign-born individuals comprise more than a third (36%) of new cases of reported TB in the United States. Individuals in the other categories have a high risk for the development of TB. *(Raviglione and O'Brian, 2008, pp. 1006-1009)*

39. (C) Zoonotic diseases are infectious diseases that can be transmitted or shared by animals and humans. Plague is a classic zoonosis caused by a bacterium transmitted by fleas that are carried by rats. The others are primarily infections of the gastrointestinal tract secondary to either antibiotic overgrowth or food-borne contamination. *(Dennis and Campbell, 2008, pp. 980-981)*

40. (C) Herd immunity is defined as the resistance of a group of individuals to a disease when there is a large proportion of the group being immune. This concept is important because it is nearly impossible to achieve 100% immunization rates. Therefore, when random mixing occurs, it is possible to halt the spread of a particular communicable disease because the infected person is likely to encounter fewer individuals who are susceptible. *(Gordis, 2009, pp. 24-25)*

REFERENCES

Aschengrau A, Seage GR. *Essentials of Epidemiology for Public Health*. Sudbury, MA: Jones and Bartlett; 2003.

Barlem TF. Insect-and-animal-borne viral infections. In: Fauci AS, Braunwald E, Kasper DL, et al., eds. *Harrison's Manual of Medicine*. 17th ed. New York, NY: McGraw-Hill; 2009a.

Barlem TF. Inflammatory diarrhea. In: Fauci AS, Braunwald E, Kasper DL, et al., eds. *Harrison's Manual of Medicine*. 17th ed. New York, NY: McGraw-Hill; 2009b.

Brown RT, Fleming MF. Substance abuse. In: Woolf SH, Jonas S, Kaplan-Liss E, eds. *Health Promotion and Disease Prevention*. 2nd ed. Philadelphia, PA; Lippincott Williams & Wilkins; 2008.

Dennis D, Campbell G. Plague and other Yersinia infections. In: Fauci A, Braunwald E, Kasper DL, et al., eds. *Harrison's Principles of Internal Medicine*. 17th ed. New York, NY: McGraw-Hill; 2008.

Dienstag J. Acute viral hepatitis. In: Fauci A, Braunwald E, Kasper DL, et al., eds. *Harrison's Principles of Internal Medicine*. 17th ed. New York, NY: McGraw-Hill; 2008.

Feldman MD. Intimate partner violence. In: Feldman MD, Christensen JF, eds. *Behavioral Medicine: A Guide for Clinical Practice*. 3rd ed. New York, NY: McGraw-Hill; 2008.

Gordis L. *Epidemiology*. 4th ed. Philadelphia, PA: Saunders Elsevier; 2009.

Kodner CM. Sexually transmitted infections. In: Woolf SH, Jonas S, Kaplan-Liss E, eds. *Health Promotion and Disease Prevention.* 2nd ed. Philadelphia, PA: Lippincott Williams & Wilkins; 2008.

Lang RS, Hensrud DD. *Clinical Preventive Medicine.* 2nd ed. Chicago, IL: AMA Press; 2004.

McKinna M, Michaud C, Murray CJL, et al. Assessing the burden of disease in the US using DALYs. *Am J Prev Med.* 2005;28:415-423.

Messinger-Rapport BJ, Baker PT. Safety in the home and automobile. In: Lang RS, Hensrud DD, eds. *Clinical Preventive Medicine.* 2nd ed. Chicago, IL: AMA Press; 2004.

Molella RG. Health and genetic risk assessment instruments. In: Woolf SH, Jonas S, Kaplan-Liss E, eds. *Health Promotion and Disease Prevention in Clinical Practice.* 2nd ed. Philadelphia, PA; Lippincott Williams & Wilkins; 2008.

Powers AC. Diabetes mellitus. In: Fauci A, Braunwald E, Kasper DL, et al., eds. *Harrison's Principles of Internal Medicine.* 17th ed. New York, NY: McGraw-Hill, 2008.

Raviglione MC, O'Brian R. Tuberculosis. In: Fauci A, Braunwald E, Kasper DL, et al., eds. *Harrison's Principles of Internal Medicine.* 17th ed. New York, NY: McGraw-Hill; 2008.

Riegelman RK. *Studying a Study and Testing a Test.* 5th ed. Philadelphia, PA: Lippincott Williams & Wilkins; 2005.

Speelman P, Hartskeerl K. Leptospirosis. In: Fauci A, Braunwald E, Kasper DL, Hauser SL, et al., eds.. *Harrison's Principles of Internal Medicine.* 17th ed. New York, NY: McGraw-Hill; 2008.

Walker DH, Dumler SJ, Marris T. Rickettsial disease. In: Fauci A, Braunwald E, Kasper DL, et al., eds. *Harrison's Principles of Internal Medicine.* 17th ed. New York, NY: McGraw-Hill; 2008.

Wallace RB, Doebbling BN, Last JM, et al. *Maxcy-Rosenau-Last Public Health and Preventive Medicine.* 14th ed. Stamford, CT: Appleton and Lange; 1998.

White NJ, Breman JG. Malaria. In: Fauci A, Braunwald E, Kasper DL, et al., eds. *Harrison's Principles of Internal Medicine.* 17th ed. New York, NY: McGraw-Hill; 2008.

Wolfe R. Immunizations. In: Woolf SH, Jonas S, Kaplan-Liss E, eds. *Health Promotion and Disease Prevention.* 2nd ed. Philadelphia, PA; Lippincott Williams & Wilkins; 2008.

Woolf SH. Principles of risk assessment. In: Woolf SH, Jonas S, Kaplan-Liss E, eds. *Health Promotion and Disease Prevention.* 2nd ed. Philadelphia, PA: Lippincott Williams & Wilkins; 2008.

Woolf SH, Jonas S, Kaplan-Liss E. *Health Promotion and Disease Prevention.* 2nd ed. Philadelphia, PA: Lippincott Williams & Wilkins; 2008.

Zolopa AR, Katz MH. HIV Infection and AIDS. In: McPhee SJ, Papadakis MA, eds. *Current Medical Diagnosis and Treatment.* 49th ed. New York, NY: McGraw-Hill; 2010.

CHAPTER 23

Basic Science

Raymond J. Pavlick Jr., PhD

DIRECTIONS: Each of the numbered items or incomplete statements in this section is followed by answers or by completion of the statement. Select the ONE-lettered answer or completion that is BEST in each case.

1. A 24-year-old woman with newly diagnosed schizophrenia has been treated with chlorpromazine for the past 4 weeks to control her symptoms. The patient has been experiencing a great deal of dry mouth, a common adverse effect of the drug, which has prompted her to drink copious amounts of water. As a result of this excessive water ingestion, what changes most likely occurred in the patient's plasma osmolality and level of antidiuretic hormone (ADH) secretion?

   (A) both plasma osmolality and ADH secretion decreased
   (B) both plasma osmolality and ADH secretion increased
   (C) plasma osmolality increased and ADH secretion decreased
   (D) plasma osmolality decreased and ADH secretion increased
   (E) plasma osmolality remained the same and ADH secretion increased

2. A 37-year-old man with a history of Paget disease presents with a deviation of the tongue to the right side upon sticking it out. The right side of the tongue is also observed to have slight atrophy. These symptoms most likely point to a lesion of which of the following cranial nerves?

   (A) left hypoglossal nerve
   (B) left vagus nerve
   (C) left glossopharyngeal nerve
   (D) right glossopharyngeal nerve
   (E) right hypoglossal nerve

3. Which of the following serves as the precursor for the synthesis of adrenocortical hormones such as cortisol and aldosterone?

   (A) amino acids
   (B) cholesterol
   (C) glucose
   (D) phospholipids
   (E) triglyceride

4. A 29-year-old woman presents to the clinic with a complaint of severe diarrhea occurring over the last 3 to 4 days. Upon examination, the patient displays poor skin turgor and has a temperature of 100.2°F. In the supine position, the patient's blood pressure is 88/64 mm Hg and her heart rate is 112 beats/min. Upon standing, her heart rate further increases to 126 beats/min. Which of the following accounts for the further increase in the patient's heart rate upon standing?

   (A) decreased systemic vascular resistance
   (B) decreased venous return
   (C) increased preload
   (D) increased myocardial contractility
   (E) increased peripheral vasodilation

5. A 54-year-old woman has suffered a stroke that has resulted in dramatic changes to her personality, left leg and foot weakness, loss of sensation in the left leg, and apathy. Which of the following arteries was most likely affected by the stroke?

   (A) left anterior cerebral
   (B) left middle cerebral
   (C) right anterior cerebral
   (D) right middle cerebral
   (E) right posterior cerebral

6. A 56-year-old man with a 17-year history of type 2 diabetes mellitus presents with bilateral swelling of his ankles and calves. A dipstick urinalysis reveals 3+ protein and glycosuria. Which of the following is most likely responsible for the patient's edema?

   (A) a decrease in capillary hydrostatic pressure
   (B) a decrease in capillary oncotic pressure
   (C) an increase in capillary hydrostatic pressure
   (D) an increase in capillary oncotic pressure
   (E) an increase in interstitial hydrostatic pressure

7. According to the Frank–Starling law of the heart:

   (A) the majority of ventricular filling occurs passively
   (B) the ventricles completely empty with every beat
   (C) the ventricles eject more blood with increases in end-diastolic volume
   (D) the ventricles eject more blood with sympathetic stimulation
   (E) venous return decreases with an elevated central venous pressure

8. A premature infant is born with the inability to produce adequate amounts of pulmonary surfactant. Which of the following is the primary function of pulmonary surfactant?

   (A) increase the solubility of carbon dioxide in the alveoli
   (B) increase the solubility of oxygen in the alveoli

   (C) prevent infectious organisms from infiltrating the alveoli
   (D) prevent the collapse of small lung alveoli
   (E) stimulate the unloading of carbon dioxide from hemoglobin

9. Which of the following is the major determinant of resistance to blood flow in the arterial circulation?

   (A) blood volume
   (B) length of blood vessels
   (C) plasma protein concentration
   (D) radius of blood vessels
   (E) viscosity of the blood

10. A 48-year-old man presents to the emergency department with acute right upper quadrant tenderness, fever, and mild jaundice. Which of the following is most likely to be elevated in the blood?

    (A) bilirubin
    (B) creatinine
    (C) glucose
    (D) ketones
    (E) uric acid

11. A 52-year-old woman presents with vaginal discharge that is white curd-like in appearance but is not malodorous. She has a 19-year history of obesity and poorly controlled type 2 diabetes mellitus. Microscopic examination of the discharge with 10% potassium hydroxide demonstrates filaments and spores. Which of the following is the most likely etiologic agent?

    (A) *Candida*
    (B) *Gardnerella*
    (C) *Lactobacillus*
    (D) *Staphylococcus epidermidis*
    (E) *Trichomonas vaginalis*

12. A 9-year-old girl with glycosuria is newly diagnosed with type 1 diabetes mellitus. The patient's glycosuria most likely occurred when the

    (A) adipocytes elevated their rate of lipolysis
    (B) kidneys decreased their filtered load of glucose

(C) liver enzymes that normally degrade glucose decreased their activity

(D) liver hepatocytes elevated their rates of glycogenesis

(E) transport maximum of glucose was reached in the kidneys

13. A 17-year-old girl starts her normal menstrual flow this month. Which of the following is the normal, physiological trigger for this event?

(A) a failure of corpus luteum functioning

(B) a rising progesterone level in the blood

(C) an increase in luteinizing hormone secretion

(D) increased frequency of myometrial contractions

(E) the formation of the Graafian or mature follicle

14. A 58-year-old man with a medical history of gouty arthritis presents with a red, swollen joint at the base of the great toe. His diet for the past 7 to 10 days consisted of large quantities of organ meats and fresh seafood. The increased metabolism of which of the following most likely contributed to the patient's symptoms?

(A) amino acids

(B) polysaccharides

(C) purines

(D) pyrimidines

(E) triglycerides

15. The sinoatrial (SA) node is the heart's normal pacemaker and controls the heart rate because it

(A) develops the fastest rate of depolarization

(B) is located in the right atrium of the heart

(C) is the only cardiac pacemaker that causes atrial depolarization

(D) is unaffected by hormonal regulation

(E) receives both sympathetic and parasympathetic innervation

16. A 42-year-old man is prescribed a drug classified as a "bile acid sequestrant." Which of the following will most likely be diminished as a result of administering this drug?

(A) activity of pancreatic amylase

(B) bile flow from the gall bladder to the duodenum

(C) emulsification of triglycerides

(D) secretion of gastric acid

(E) synthesis of plasma proteins

17. A 74-year-old man with end-stage renal failure is suffering from a number of bone abnormalities, including osteomalacia. Which of the following is most likely diminished in this patient?

(A) blood urea nitrogen (BUN)

(B) production of 1,25-dihydroxycholecalciferol

(C) secretion of parathyroid hormone (PTH)

(D) secretion of thyroid hormones

(E) serum concentration of creatinine

18. High-density lipoproteins (HDLs) are considered good cholesterol because they

(A) decrease lipoprotein lipase activity in adipocytes

(B) inhibit chylomicron synthesis in the small intestine

(C) inhibit endogenous cholesterol production by the body

(D) prevent cholesterol absorption from the intestines

(E) transport excess cholesterol to the liver for biliary excretion

19. Administration of a drug that inhibits acetylcholinesterase would most likely lead to which of the following?

(A) bronchodilation

(B) decreased lacrimation

(C) decreased salivation

(D) increased gastric juice secretion

(E) increased heart rate

20. A 48-year-old woman has been taking gentamicin for the last several weeks for a serious *Pseudomonas aeruginosa* infection. She presents today with a complaint of tinnitus. After further evaluation, it is determined that, in addition, she is also suffering from a bilateral high-frequency sensorineural hearing loss. The patient denies any dizziness or balance disturbances. Which of the following structures is most likely affected?

    (A) ear ossicles
    (B) organ of Corti
    (C) saccule
    (D) semicircular canals
    (E) tympanic membrane

21. A 58-year-old man presents with a recent onset of erectile dysfunction. He has a 20-year history of type 2 diabetes mellitus and was last seen in clinic 2 months ago when he was suffering from dizziness associated with postural hypotension. Physical examination reveals normal detection of sensation of both feet using monofilaments. A glycated hemoglobin test reports a current level of 10.8%. Which of the following set of spinal nerves is most likely affected?

    (A) T5–T8
    (B) T11–L2
    (C) L1–L4
    (D) L5–S2
    (E) S2–S4

22. Which of the following is the major method by which carbon dioxide is transported in the venous blood?

    (A) as bicarbonate ions
    (B) bound to albumin
    (C) bound to carbonic anhydrase
    (D) bound to hemoglobin
    (E) dissolved in the plasma

23. A 45-year-old woman with complaints of palpitations, heat intolerance, and nervousness is diagnosed with Graves disease. Which of the following set of serum laboratory values support this diagnosis?

    (A) elevated TSH; elevated free T4
    (B) elevated TSH; low free T4
    (C) low TSH; elevated free T4
    (D) low TSH; low free T4
    (E) low TSH; normal free T4

24. During a spirometry test, a patient is asked to forcibly expel as much air from the lungs as possible. Which of the following represents the amount of air that remains in the patient's lungs following this maximal forced expiration?

    (A) expiratory reserve volume
    (B) functional residual capacity
    (C) residual volume
    (D) tidal volume
    (E) vital capacity

25. A 38-year-old woman diagnosed with pancreatic cancer 2 months ago develops jaundice and steatorrhea. Which of the following is most likely to be diminished in the blood?

    (A) calcium
    (B) iron
    (C) vitamin B_{12}
    (D) vitamin C
    (E) vitamin K

Answers and Explanations

1. **(A)** Ingesting large volumes of water typically causes a decrease in plasma osmolality, as solutes such as sodium and chloride become more dilute in the blood. An increase in plasma osmolality (>295 mOsm/L) is the primary stimulus for ADH secretion from the posterior pituitary; hence, a decrease in plasma osmolality leads to reduced ADH secretion. In addition, volume expansion also reduces ADH secretion to allow for more water excretion via the urine. This patient would be expected to produce large volumes of urine in an attempt to maintain water homeostasis due to the excessive intake of water. *(Giebisch and Windhager, 2009, pp. 874-877)*

2. **(E)** One of the many clinical manifestations of Paget disease is narrowing of cranial foramina. The 12th cranial nerves (hypoglossal nerves) pass through the hypoglossal canals of the occipital bones. The hypoglossal nerves innervate many of the extrinsic muscles that move the tongue, including the genioglossus, hyoglossus, and styloglossus. Each hypoglossal nerve supplies the ipsilateral extrinsic muscles. Hence, the tongue deviates to the paralyzed side during protrusion because of the actions of the unaffected extrinsic muscles on the other side. *(Beal and Hauser, 2008, pp. 2586-2587; Favus and Vokes, 2008, p. 240; Nolte, 2010, pp. 88-89; Snell, 2010, p. 362)*

3. **(B)** Cortisol and aldosterone are examples of steroid hormones that, as a class, are all derived from cholesterol. The steroid hormones contain the basic four-ringed structure (A, B, C, and D rings) of cholesterol, with each individual hormone having different chemical modifications emanating from these rings. These various modifications confer different functions to each of the steroid hormones. *(Barrett, 2009, p. 1023; Costanzo, 2006, pp. 408-409)*

4. **(B)** The patient is displaying signs of hypovolemia likely because of her chronic diarrhea. Upon standing, most of her low blood volume pools in the veins of her lower extremities because of the effects of gravity. As a result, even less blood returns to the heart, which leads to a decrease in both stroke volume and cardiac output as well as orthostatic hypotension. This elicits the baroreceptor reflex, which attempts to increase and maintain arterial blood pressure by raising the heart rate. *(Costanzo, 2006, pp. 176-178)*

5. **(C)** The anterior cerebral arteries supply the frontal lobes as well as the medial aspects of the parietal and occipital lobes rostral to the parietooccipital sulcus. The prefrontal cortex of the frontal lobe is concerned with a person's personality, depth of feeling, and initiative. Hence, occlusion of an anterior cerebral artery can cause neuronal injury to this area, leading to feelings of apathy and personality changes. The paracentral lobule represents the medial aspects of the precentral gyrus (frontal lobe) and postcentral gyrus (parietal lobe), which are responsible for motor control and somatosensory perception, respectively, of the leg and foot. Hence, occlusion of an anterior cerebral artery can produce contralateral hemiparesis and hemisensory loss involving the leg and foot. With the 54-year-old patient, the symptoms were occurring on the left side, which points to a right anterior cerebral artery occlusion. *(Snell, 2010, pp. 475, 478, 483)*

6. **(B)** Capillary oncotic pressure (also known as "plasma colloid osmotic pressure") is a Starling force determined by the concentration of plasma proteins and causes fluid to move from interstitial spaces into capillaries. As the concentration of plasma protein decreases in this patient due to proteinuria, there is less absorption of fluid into the capillaries and more net filtration of fluid out of the capillaries. This excess volume of interstitial fluid exceeds the ability of the lymphatic system to return it to the circulation, resulting in the patient's edema. *(Boulpaep, 2009, p. 493; Costanzo, 2006, pp. 164-166)*

7. **(C)** The Frank–Starling law of the heart explains the relationship between end-diastolic volume and stroke volume. According to the relationship, the more the ventricles fill with blood during diastole (within physiological limits), the more forceful they will contract during systole. This is an intrinsic mechanism the heart uses to match cardiac output with venous return without any neural or hormonal influences. *(Costanzo, 2006, p. 143)*

8. **(D)** Because of their small size, many lung alveoli are prone to collapse. Pulmonary surfactant contains a high concentration of amphipathic phospholipid molecules, which lowers the surface tension of alveoli. According to the law of Laplace, a reduction of surface tension reduces the collapsing pressure on small alveoli and allows them to remain open. Pulmonary surfactant production does not typically begin until the 24th week of gestation; hence, an infant born before this time is at great risk for having collapsed alveoli. *(Costanzo, 2006, pp. 197-198)*

9. **(D)** The relationship between the major factors causing resistance to blood flow can be summarized with Poiseuille equation:

$$\text{Resistance} = \frac{8VL}{\pi r^4}$$

where V is the viscosity of blood; L the length of blood vessel; and r the radius of blood vessel.

When the radius of an arterial blood vessel decreases (as in vasoconstriction), the resistance increases tremendously because the radius is raised to the fourth power. This same effect, in terms of magnitude, would not be achieved with changes to blood viscosity or blood vessel length according to Poiseuille equation. *(Costanzo, 2006, pp. 116-118)*

10. **(A)** This patient's signs and symptoms correlate with a suspected case of cholecystitis. Jaundice is associated with hyperbilirubinemia, in which the excess bilirubin can deposit in tissues such as the skin, sclera, and nails, causing a yellowish discoloration. Bilirubin is the waste product generated from the metabolism of hemoglobin. *(Greenberger and Paumgartner, 2008, pp. 1995-1996; Pratt and Kaplan, 2008, p. 261)*

11. **(A)** This case has several clues pointing to a *Candida* infection, including the fact that diabetes mellitus can predispose patients to *Candida* infections and the presence of the white curd-like discharge that is not malodorous. In *Trichomonas vaginalis*, the discharge is malodorous and yellow–green in color. With *Gardnerella*, there is also a malodorous discharge. *Lactobacillus* is the predominant, normal microorganism of the vagina and keeps it slightly acidic to help reduce the growth of potentially harmful organisms. *Staphylococcus epidermidis* is also part of the natural flora of the vagina. *(MacKay, 2008, pp. 637-638)*

12. **(E)** The transport maximum (T_m) represents a point where a carrier-mediated transporter has reached saturation. In the kidney, glucose reabsorption occurs via the Na^+–glucose cotransporter (SGLT) located on cells lining the proximal convoluted tubules of nephrons. At normal plasma–glucose concentrations, all of the glucose filtered at the glomeruli is reabsorbed and none is excreted, in large part because of these cotransporters being able to function normally. In type 1 diabetes mellitus, the absence of insulin raises the plasma–glucose concentration. As a result, the filtered load of glucose increases and exceeds the reabsorptive capacity of the kidneys. This corresponds to the transport maximum for SGLT being reached and exceeded. Hence, glucose appears in the urine and is usually accompanied by an osmotic diuresis. *(Costanzo, 2006, pp. 6, 258-261)*

13. **(A)** If a woman does not become pregnant during her menstrual cycle, there is a lack of human chorionic gonadotropin (HCG) production, as the trophoblast never formed. HCG normally maintains functioning of the corpus luteum and is the signal for the corpus luteum to continue synthesizing progesterone and estradiol, which maintain the endometrial lining. Regression of the corpus luteum and the subsequent loss of progesterone and estradiol cause the endometrial lining to degenerate and menstrual bleeding to occur. (*Costanzo, 2006, pp. 456-458*)

14. **(C)** Purines are normally metabolized into uric acid by the liver and can be found in high amounts in several foods, including organ meats, seafood, beans, peas, and many others. Higher levels of meat and seafood consumption are associated with an increased risk of gout because of the hyperuricemia that can occur via purine metabolism. (*Hellman and Imboden, 2008, pp. 706-708*)

15. **(A)** The SA node functions as a pacemaker because it exhibits automaticity, which means that it can fire action potentials spontaneously without requiring neural or endocrine input. However, the cells comprising the SA node are not the only myocardial cells that demonstrate automaticity. The heart also has latent pacemakers such as the AV node, bundle of His, and Purkinje fibers. While these tissues can exhibit automaticity and function as a pacemaker, they generally do not because of a physiological concept known as "overdrive suppression." Fundamental to this concept is the fact that the cells that have the fastest rate of depolarization are the ones that control the heart rate. The cells of the SA node generate the fastest rate of depolarization and, as a result, the latent pacemakers' ability to spontaneously depolarize is suppressed. (*Costanzo, 2006, pp. 130-131*)

16. **(C)** Bile acids are constituents of the bile that are synthesized into bile salts by liver hepatocytes or by intestinal bacteria. One of the major roles of bile salts is to emulsify dietary lipids within the lumen of the small intestine. Emulsification is an important first step in lipid digestion, as it increases the surface area for lipases to function.

Bile salts also help to form micelles, which transport the products of lipid digestion from the lumen and into the cells (enterocytes) lining the small intestine. Without bile salts, digestion and absorption of dietary lipids is incomplete and therefore decreased. (*Costanzo, 2006, p. 358*)

17. **(B)** Osteomalacia represents a softening of the bone due to inadequate amounts of calcium. Hypocalcemia often develops in end-stage renal failure due to the inability of the kidneys to activate vitamin D into the form known as 1,25-dihydroxycalciferol. The kidneys possess an enzyme (1-alpha-hydroxylase) that performs this activation, but in end-stage renal failure, the activity of this enzyme declines. 1,25-Dihydroxycalciferol is essential for adequate calcium absorption in the small intestine. Without 1,25-dihydroxycholecalciferol, calcium is excreted in higher amounts in the feces. The secretion of PTH is likely to be elevated (and not diminished) in patients with end-stage renal failure, as the main stimulus for PTH secretion is hypocalcemia. Thyroid hormones do not play a role in calcium homeostasis. Both the BUN and the serum creatinine level would elevate in the patient with end-stage renal failure, as the glomerular filtration rate is diminished to the point where both urea and creatinine cannot be adequately filtered from the plasma. (*Costanzo, 2006, pp. 435-437*)

18. **(E)** High-density lipoproteins (HDLs) are considered "good" when elevated in the blood because of their ability to lower the risk of coronary heart disease. HDLs accomplish this through a series of biochemical reactions that enable them to target excess cholesterol present in the blood for biliary excretion. (*Baron, p. 1074; Suchy, 2009, p. 1005*)

19. **(D)** Acetylcholinesterase is the enzyme responsible for metabolizing acetylcholine, which is the major neurotransmitter released from postganglionic neurons of the parasympathetic nervous system. Inhibition of acetylcholinesterase increases the level of acetylcholine at target tissues and can thereby create parasympathomimetic effects. These would include bronchoconstriction, increased lacrimation, increased

salivation, bradycardia, and increased gastric juice secretion. *(Costanzo, 2006, pp. 51-54)*

20. **(B)** Gentamicin belongs to the class of antibiotics known as "aminoglycosides," which are capable of producing ototoxicity as an adverse effect. Ototoxic agents target the hair (receptor) cells of the inner ear. Hair cells are found in organs involved in hearing (eg, cochlea) and balance (eg, semicircular canals, utricle, and saccule). This patient complains only of tinnitus and has sensorineural hearing loss. She denies any symptoms associated with a balance disturbance. The structure within the cochlea that contains the hair cells is the organ of Corti. *(Costanzo, 2006, pp. 87-88; Schindler et al., 2008, p. 176)*

21. **(E)** A history of diabetes mellitus is associated with autonomic neuropathy, which can lead to postural hypotension, diarrhea, constipation, incomplete bladder emptying, and erectile dysfunction. The parasympathetic control of erection occurs by way of the pelvic nerve, pelvic plexus, and cavernous nerve to the penile corpora and vasculature. These nerves derive from the sacral division of the parasympathetic nervous system, which is represented by the S2–S4 sacral segments of the spinal cord. The parasympathetic activity originating from these sacral segments and their corresponding spinal nerves normally results in vasodilation of penile blood vessels to cause erection. Thoracic and lumbar spinal nerves do not contain parasympathetic fibers. *(Jones, 2009, pp. 1141-1143; Masharami, 2008, p. 1058)*

22. **(A)** Carbon dioxide is carried in three different forms within the blood: dissolved in plasma,

attached to proteins such as hemoglobin and albumin, and as bicarbonate ions. Carbon dioxide is converted into bicarbonate ions because of the activity of carbonic anhydrase, which is present in red blood cells. Approximately 70% of the total carbon dioxide in the blood is carried as bicarbonate ions. *(Costanzo, 2006, pp. 215-217)*

23. **(C)** Graves disease is an autoimmune disorder that leads to hyperthyroidism. In Graves disease, autoantibodies bind to thyroid stimulating hormone (TSH) receptors, causing the thyroid gland to synthesize and secrete abnormally high amounts of triiodothyronine (T3) and thyroxine (T4). The elevated levels of T3 and T4 feedback onto the anterior pituitary to decrease the secretion of thyroid stimulating hormone (TSH). *(Fitzgerald, 2008, pp. 965-967)*

24. **(C)** By definition, residual volume is the volume of air remaining in the lungs after a maximal forced expiration. The residual volume is important physiologically, as it prevents total collapse of the alveoli and minimizes the pressure and energy required to inflate the lungs during inspiration. *(Boulpaep, 2009, pp. 625-626; Costanzo, 2006, pp. 185-187)*

25. **(E)** Tumors in the pancreatic head region can often block the flow of bile from the gall bladder and liver to the duodenum, resulting in jaundice and steatorrhea. The bile salts are important for micelle formation within the lumen of the small intestine. Micelles provide a mechanism whereby the hydrophobic products of lipid digestion as well as fat-soluble vitamins (eg, A, D, E, and K) can be absorbed in the small intestine. *(Costanzo, 2006, pp. 368-369; Rugo, 2008, pp. 1420-1421)*

REFERENCES

Baron RB. Lipid abnormalities. In: McPhee SJ, Papadakis MA, eds. *Current Medical Diagnosis and Treatment.* New York, NY: McGraw-Hill Medical; 2008.

Barrett EJ. Organization of endocrine control. In: Boron WF, Boulpaep EL, eds. *Medical Physiology.* 2nd ed. Philadelphia, PA: Saunders Elsevier; 2009.

Beal MF, Hauser SL. Trigeminal neuralgia, Bell's palsy, and other cranial nerve disorders. In: Fauci AS, Braunwald E, Kasper DL, et al., eds. *Harrison's Principles of Internal Medicine.* 17th ed. New York, NY: McGraw-Hill Medical; 2008.

Boulpaep EL. The microcirculation. In: Boron WF, Boulpaep EL, eds. *Medical Physiology*. 2nd ed. Philadelphia, PA: Saunders Elsevier; 2009.

Costanzo LS. *Physiology*. 3rd ed. Philadelphia, PA: Saunders Elsevier; 2006.

Favus MJ, Vokes TJ. Paget disease and other dysplasias of bone. In: Fauci AS, Braunwald E, Kasper DL, et al., eds. *Harrison's Principles of Internal Medicine*. 17th ed. New York, NY: McGraw-Hill Medical; 2008.

Fitzgerald PA. Endocrine disorders. In: McPhee SJ, Papadakis MA, eds. *Current Medical Diagnosis and Treatment*. New York, NY: McGraw-Hill Medical; 2008.

Giebisch G, Windhager E. Integration of salt and water balance. In: Boron WF, Boulpaep EL, eds. *Medical Physiology*. 2nd ed. Philadelphia, PA: Saunders Elsevier; 2009.

Greenberger NJ, Paumgartner G. Diseases of the gallbladder and bile ducts. In: Fauci AS, Braunwald E, Kasper DL, et al., eds. *Harrison's Principles of Internal Medicine*. 17th ed. New York, NY: McGraw-Hill Medical; 2008.

Hellman DB, Imboden JB Jr. Arthritis and musculoskeletal disorders. In: McPhee SJ, Papadakis MA, eds. *Current Medical Diagnosis & Treatment*. New York, NY: McGraw-Hill Medical; 2008.

Jones EE. The male reproductive system. In: Boron WF, Boulpaep EL, eds. *Medical Physiology*. 2nd ed. Philadelphia, PA: Saunders Elsevier; 2009.

MacKay HT. Gynecology. In: McPhee SJ, Papadakis MA, eds. *Current Medical Diagnosis and Treatment*. New York, NY: McGraw-Hill Medical; 2008.

Masharmi U. Diabetes mellitus & hypoglycemia. In: McPhee SJ, Papadakis MA, eds. *Current Medical Diagnosis & Treatment*. New York, NY: McGraw-Hill Medical; 2008.

Nolte J. *Essentials of the Human Brain*. Philadelphia, PA: Saunders Elsevier; 2010.

Pratt DS, Kaplan MM. Jaundice. In: Fauci AS, Braunwald E, Kasper DL, et al. eds. *Harrison's Principles of Internal Medicine*. 17th ed. New York, NY: McGraw-Hill Medical; 2008.

Rugo HS. Cancer. In: McPhee SJ, Papadakis MA, eds. *Current Medical Diagnosis & Treatment*. New York, NY: McGraw-Hill Medical; 2008.

Schindler J, Lustig L, Jackler RK, Kaplan MJ. Ear, nose & throat. In: McPhee SJ, Papadakis MA, eds. *Current Medical Diagnosis & Treatment*. New York, NY: McGraw-Hill Medical; 2008.

Snell RS. *Clinical Neuroanatomy*. 7th ed. Philadelphia, PA: Wolters Kluwer Lippincoptt Williams & Wilkins; 2010.

Suchy FJ. Hepatobiliary Function. In: Boron WF, Boulpaep EL, eds. *Medical Physiology*. 2nd ed. Philadelphia, PA: Saunders Elsevier; 2009.

Index